NURSING RESEARCH

A Qualitative Perspective

FIFTH EDITION

PATRICIA L. MUNHALL, EdD, ARNP, PsyA, FAAN
President
International Institute for Human Understanding
Miami, Florida

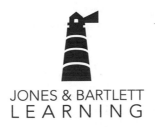

JONES & BARTLETT
LEARNING

World Headquarters

Jones & Bartlett Learning
40 Tall Pine Drive
Sudbury, MA 01776
978-443-5000
info@jblearning.com
www.jblearning.com

Jones & Bartlett Learning
Canada
6339 Ormindale Way
Mississauga, Ontario L5V 1J2
Canada

Jones & Bartlett Learning
International
Barb House, Barb Mews
London W6 7PA
United Kingdom

Jones & Bartlett Learning books and products are available through most bookstores and online booksellers. To contact Jones & Bartlett Learning directly, call 800-832-0034, fax 978-443-8000, or visit our website, www.jblearning.com.

Substantial discounts on bulk quantities of Jones & Bartlett Learning publications are available to corporations, professional associations, and other qualified organizations. For details and specific discount information, contact the special sales department at Jones & Bartlett Learning via the above contact information or send an email to specialsales@jblearning.com.

Production Credits

Publisher: Kevin Sullivan
Acquisitions Editor: Amy Sibley
Associate Editor: Patricia Donnelly
Editorial Assistant: Rachel Shuster
Production Editor: Amanda Clerkin
Associate Marketing Manager: Katie Hennessy
V.P., Manufacturing and Inventory Control:
   Therese Connell
Composition: Arlene Apone
Cover Design: Timothy Dziewit
Cover Image: © Excellent Backgrounds/
   ShutterStock, Inc.
Printing and Binding: Malloy, Inc.
Cover Printing: Malloy, Inc.

Library of Congress Cataloging-in-Publication Data
Nursing research : a qualitative perspective / [edited by] Patricia L. Munhall. — 5th ed.
   p. ; cm.
Includes bibliographical references and index.
ISBN 978-0-7637-8515-4 (pbk.)
1. Nursing—Research. I. Munhall, Patricia L.
[DNLM: 1. Nursing Research—methods. WY 20.5 N9735 2011]
RT81.5.N866 2011
610.73072—dc22
                          2010019181
6048
Printed in the United States of America
14 13 12 11 10   10 9 8 7 6 5 4 3 2 1

Contents

2   *Language and Nursing Research: The Evolution*   **33**
Patricia L. Munhall

3   *Epistemology in Nursing*   **69**
Patricia L. Munhall

4   *Postmodern Philosophy and Qualitative Research*   **95**
Joy Longo and Lynne M. Dunphy

10 *Ethnography: The Method* **285**
Zane Robinson Wolf

11 *Exemplar: War Stories: Frontline Reports of the Daily Experiences of Low-Income, Urban, Black Mothers* **339**
Roberta Cricco-Lizza

12 *Case Study: The Method* **359**
Patricia Hentz

PART III   INTERNAL AND EXTERNAL CONSIDERATIONS IN QUALITATIVE RESEARCH   489

20   Ethical Considerations in Qualitative Research   491

Patricia L. Munhall

21   Institutional Review of the Qualitative Research Proposals: A Task of No Small Consequence   503

Patricia L. Munhall

25 *Combining Qualitative and Quantitative Methods for Mixed-Method Designs*   **571**
Janice M. Morse and Linda Niehaus

Epilogue: In Coming to an Open Closing   **585**
Patricia L. Munhall

Index   **589**

Prologue

Welcome to a most meaningful prologue for me personally. The first edition of this book was published in 1986 and I never anticipated that in 25 years from that date I would be writing the prologue for a fifth edition! I feel overwhelmingly privileged to have had this opportunity to "meet" in this way a new generation of students and faculty. Beyond my own experience is the context of the history of qualitative research in nursing, which was greeted with puzzlement at first to the present recognition, respect, and appreciation of the importance of qualitative research to nursing science and to the art of nursing. If this book has played a small part in that recognition, it is because of the very many wonderful and excellent contributing authors who have generously shared their expertise and research to make all five editions possible. I indeed feel both grateful and humble. For sure, one never knows what is ahead in life!

This fifth edition, like the preceding ones, is written with an unwavering and overwhelming concern for the experience of individuals, groups, and cultures—concern about the attribution of meaning individuals and groups give to their experiences. This concern is grounded in human compassion and caring. It is further grounded in concern for social justice, quality of care for all individuals, and care that is based on individual choice. When we conduct qualitative research, we come to understand what is needed for human understanding, nursing care practice, healthcare policy, and social policy. Qualitative research studies have the critical potential to influence and change for the better the nurse–patient discourse as well as public health and social policy discourse.

And it does so without any preconceived notions, assumptions, or prejudices—it does so with an open-mindedness to all possibility. Qualitative researchers, no matter their level of intelligence, begin with a "beginner's mind," as in the Zen quote by Suzuki:

> *"In the beginner's mind there are many possibilities, but in the expert's mind there are very few."*

To image this, we can think of a beginner's mind actually having a lot of space to come to know and see phenomena afresh, where in the expert's mind, it is crowded with information. This information can actually prevent a person from considering new and foreign alternatives. Many times the expert has the answers, purely theoretical but not experiential. That is the *crux* of the qualitative perspective, to hold the beginner's mind, where the researcher listens with the third ear (defined in Chapters 1 and 5), one without any noise, to hear the experience of the one who has experienced some phenomenon, the one who happens to be the *real* expert!

I believe through the lens of the philosophical underpinnings of qualitative research that qualitative nurse researchers contribute in a very meaningful way to an incredibly humanistic form of nursing practice and healthcare policy. We use our different ways of seeing to uncover and discover meaning through understanding, which is the essential core, from my perspective, to authentic compassion and caring.

Qualitative researchers have a different worldview, paradigm, and research traditions than our quantitative colleagues. Given the proper encouragement, freedom, and resources to grow and develop in their methods, these researchers provide understanding, description interpretation, the ground work of new theory, and direction encompassing the intricacies and interconnectedness of being in this world—a world that is not one but many, made of multiple realities emerging from multiple perceptions. Qualitative researchers search for the differences not only *between* individuals and cultures but also *within* the same individual and cultures. In understanding this complexity, there is recognition of multiplicity (Chapter 1). In so doing, they challenge stereotypes, presuppositions, and assumptions, and they discover in-depth understanding that comes from the human source of experience—the individuals or culture are the knowers, the researchers are the unknowing ones.

Inherent, then, in qualitative methods is the potential for liberation and emancipation from the constraints of outdated beliefs, myths, and theories. The sands of nursing science must keep shifting to breathe new life into the ever-changing and evolving world around us, as well as the worlds of those we serve.

Qualitative researchers break new ground by revealing what had been concealed. They look beyond appearance. They provide the reconstruction that time demands of us as these sands shift and knowledge changes. In their quest for discovery, qualitative researchers legitimize the existence of others in their differences. Conformity and generalizability are not the aims of our research: we know that a universal concept of meaning in experience is not possible and doubt that it would even be desirable. I believe we are attuned to our place in the universe, and while we may appear similar from a distance, we must move beyond appearances to embrace and celebrate the nuances of existence, and to understand the subtle and not-so-subtle differences between you and me and all members of the human race.

Because qualitative research has the power to liberate us from biases and prejudices that oppress people, research studies can expose the dark side, where a need for change is illuminated and a call for action results. Part of the intrigue of our work is understanding a "newness," a very different negotiation of meaning. I sometimes think of our studies as "awakenings," and very significant ones. The newness of or about some thing or experience awakens and expands our consciousness of others and self. The results from qualitative research raise our consciousness to what was not known; the unbeknownst becomes understood, the concealed becomes seen, the silence given voice.

About This Edition

The first edition of this book was written in 1986, and as I write that date, I think writing and doing qualitative research has encompassed much of my professional life. If you ever see the first edition, you will not believe its size. First of all, it is in hardcover, reflecting the economics of the time, and it is composed of about 280 pages. The size, of course, reflects its stage of development in nursing. For those of you who might not have even been born, it may be hard to conceive of a nursing world without qualitative research, but it did exist. Actually, it was a struggle at first for our legitimacy. Qualitative research in nursing at that time was emerging as a "home" for many nurse researchers for reasons discussed in Part I of this volume. Looking at the authors in that edition, however, one sees accomplished qualitative researchers as the pioneers and leaders in what really was a "movement" in nursing research.

The second, third, and fourth editions followed the format of that text with additions to make the book as inclusive as possible. This aim continues in this edition. Every edition requires choices about what to include or leave out. Very important chapters often have to be removed to make room for new and current content. However, those chapters continue to be important, and if in this edition you do not find what you are looking for, there is a very good chance that it is in a previous edition.

New chapters build a library of this particular qualitative book. For instance, if you are interested in the grounded theory method, you could return to the other four editions and find different authors for the method chapter and four other grounded theory research exemplars, plus the one in this edition. If you wanted to find information on using the Internet for qualitative research, you can return to the fourth edition. One more example to demonstrate how rich this library is: If you wanted to find a chapter on analyzing data from interviews, you could return to a chapter in the third edition titled: "Types of Talk: Modes of Responses and Data-Led Analytic Strategies" (Morse, in Munhall, 2001). All these editions have very impressive authors whose work has always been and still is the best in qualitative research.

I am not always sure if students understand the concept of different editions of the same book. In the field of qualitative research, knowledge continuously expands and what is most critical to share cannot be added to a single edition. The book would soon be over 3,000 pages. Instead chapters are chosen to be replaced with content that was not widely known in an earlier edition. That brings this new edition up to date, but with this particular subject, the material in the other editions is not out of date. I encourage you to look at the Table of Contents for each edition so that you can widen your knowledge of qualitative research, additional topics, and also different ways of writing about methods and different exemplars of research methods.

As with previous editions, this edition is divided into three sections. Part I attempts to provide the essential foundational content and groundwork to understand the qualitative research perspective and qualitative research itself. I believe Part I is essential to understanding, because it presents the origin, the rationale, and the philosophical and epistemological underpinnings of qualitative research. In essence Part I demonstrates to you why we need qualitative research in nursing, why it is congruent in language and philosophy of nursing, and how it fits into today's postmodern world. The content of Chapter 1 "The Landscape of Qualitative Research" (Munhall) is different in this edition not so much because it has changed from the fourth edition, but because I wanted to add to the perspective of the landscape. If you were to return to the fourth edition you would find out more still about the landscape or the context of qualitative research. Chapters 2 and 3 (Munhall) have been updated but cannot be substantively changed because these two chapters are foundational to understanding qualitative research. You will see different language systems employed that are often diametrically opposed in Chapter 2. Following the same method of comparing and contrasting philosophical systems that are representative of different worldviews, the third chapter ends with the philosophical fit for qualitative research and nursing philosophy. The fourth chapter (Longo & Dunphy) of Part I, expands on Chapter 3 as a continuum of philosophical thinking, which brings us into the postmodern period, and the different components that comprise postmodernism. When reading about postmodernism as a contemporary philosophy it is interesting to note how much is congruent with nursing philosophy and qualitative research.

As an aside, postmodern philosophy provides a critical perspective to understanding the world in which we are now living. I hope you might be stimulated to read more on this perspective. It is so illuminating and aids us in understanding the complexities and interconnectedness of all humans and the world we inhabit. When I was a student, even in high school, I was very interested in the philosophy of existentialism and continued to be so in college. I now can see how that interest evolved into a profound interest in postmodernism and particularly in phenomenology. I begin this prologue with a common concept that no one knows where he or she will be 25 years from now. Perhaps you can keep that in mind as you read the chapters. This knowledge is not stagnant—it requires insight, interpretation, exploring meaning, asking questions, and then asking some more questions.

Part II presents the more prevalent qualitative research methods, and with each chapter an exemplar of the method follows. The exemplar might not precisely follow the method chapter, because interpretation of methods can be different. You will also see this in prior editions. However, each exemplar is an example of current research reflecting the underlying tenets and aims of the method. Chapter 5 (Munhall) is the phenomenological method chapter, and, as I have mentioned many times in this book, the philosophy of phenomenology underpins qualitative methods, though often they are not spelled out in each method. It is the best foundation to the open mind or the beginner's mind that is required for conducting qualitative research. Chapter 5 includes listening techniques, a discussion on the process of "unknowing," additional discussion on life worlds, contingencies, the situated context, and the importance of critiquing the meaning of qualitative research study to determine its significance. All of this content I believe is essential to the carrying out of each qualitative method that follows. The phenomenological method has two exemplars. Chapter 6 (Lauterbach & Frank) is an exemplar for linguistic transformation in phenomenology and longitudinal phenomenology. The second exemplar (Chapter 7; Harner, Heinz, & Evangelista) is an example of descriptive phenomenology and discusses the significance of this description.

Chapters 8 (Wuest) and 9 (Beck) represent grounded theory and the exemplar is another form of longitudinal work that demonstrates how a researcher develops a research program. Beck continues work on a study from the previous edition that has resulted in a second study, furthering development of new knowledge. This is how a researcher becomes an authority on a subject. If this interests you, visit the fourth edition and also the many articles by Beck in her reference section. Similarly, Wuest is also considered an expert on the grounded theory method. Chapters 10 (Wolf) and 11 (Cricco-Lizza) present ethnography and a moving exemplar of that method, which calls for policy change. Both chapters exemplify how critical the role of culture is in experience. Chapters 12 (Hentz) and 13 (Hentz) are about the case history method, and once again the exemplar is extremely moving and revealing, revealing of what is and what is concealed.

Chapters 14 (Lundy) and 15 (Rutherford) represent the historical method and demonstrate to us how critical history is to nursing practice. It is always important to be reminded of the place of history. In our hurried world we often repeat the same self-defeating actions because we are not aware of our history. Historical accounts as in the exemplar often read like a story, but one that was actually lived and can give us an appreciation for those that came before us in new and different ways. Narrative inquiry and the exemplar comprise Chapters 16 (Duffy) and 17 (Gallant). Narratives and narrative inquiry research are becoming increasingly important not only as a research method but as a teaching method used in nursing and medical schools in the endeavor to help students to understand the experiences of their patients and patients' families. Chapters 18 (Chenail, St. George, Wulff, & Cooper) and 19 (Valade) cover action research. They demonstrate to us that in qualitative research we can implement new practices and policies (based on the underpinnings of qualitative research) to understand and evaluate how people experience these actions. Action research is just what it says—it is actively done with participants (with strict ethical standards)!

Part III of the book explicates some critical considerations about qualitative research for all the methods studied thus far. Ethical considerations and how to implement them in qualitative research are a vital component of your study. The utmost of care must be taken and Chapter 20 (Munhall) presents the most important ethical considerations. Chapter 21 (Munhall) assists you in the ways to guide your research proposal through an Institutional Review Board and offers some practical suggestions. Evaluation of our research studies is where we hold our research to its highest standards, which we all must be committed to, and Chapter 22 (Mackey) provides different sets of criteria for doing just that.

Today's most current demand in health care is to provide evidence-based practice. Chapter 23 (Zuzelo) shows the valuable contributions that qualitative research can make toward that goal. The newest movement in qualitative research since the last edition is combining different qualitative methods in one research study, thus enriching it beyond measure. Chapter 24 (Morse) presents a model for accomplishing this. Another mixing of methods occurs when you combine a qualitative and quantitative method in one study—this is explicated for you in Chapter 25 (Morse & Niehuas). It is important to note that Chapter 24 is combining *qualitative* methods in the same study and Chapter 25 is about combining *qualitative and quantitative* methods in a study. This way Morse in Chapter 24 and Morse and Niehuas in Chapter 25 have covered the whole gamut!

The world has changed dramatically since 1986, and one of the largest influences is, the use of personal computers and helpful software packages. Around the third edition of this book, software packages specific to qualitative research were being developed. I remember a colleague who was one of the first to master the computer when many of us feared it and hoped it would go away who encouraged me to at least try to learn to use it. Can you imagine that? Now I cannot imagine living without a computer! I also imagine some of you do not remember a world without computers! In qualitative research, this phenomenon is called the situated context (I am always slipping material in!).

Thinking back, I was being resistant, and my contributions to that first edition were handwritten on my treasured yellow legal pads, which I placed on a chessboard I had given to my late father as a gift. I would write in these early morning hours, in the quiet which enabled reflection. I also remember in the predawn hours sitting in a chair near a window, surrounded by books on philosophy and ethics, drawn into a world of ideas. I use the Internet as much as the next person, but personally I recommend (and this believe it or not is for your own pleasure) that you lose yourself in these books. Some ideas just cannot be summarized. Also the idea of thinking or dwelling about your research during undisturbed times allows spontaneous interpretations and new ideas occur to you. Spending quiet time in contemplation is an important part of qualitative research, sometimes referred to as "dwelling with the data."

To paraphrase Husserl, remember, to the people themselves, to the experiences themselves. Stay close to your participants' stories, their language, descriptions, interpretations, and to their subjective perspective of their reality. Follow their emotions, their moods, and affect. If you are using software to categorize responses you are moving away from individual interpretations and subjective perspectives of reality toward a world that looks something like "word frequency": categories without context, which removes the experience from individual contingencies. It is like reading a summarization but not the whole book. I understand that it is tempting with efficiency, but I fear you will be losing the experience you are studying and at the same time miss something in your own experience of this phenomenal way of coming "to understand."

The essence of qualitative research is to embed yourself, your subjective self, into an intersubjective world with the subjective world of another. Also what is lost is intonation, body language, appearance, attitudes, moods, and humor. Maybe I am a dinosaur, but I did notice when reading the exemplars in this book (unless it was not mentioned) not one person was using the software (other dinosaurs?). Just to go on record, this is my personal and professional opinion.

I often think of qualitative research, because of our closeness with individuals, with reverence and awe. As researchers, we are given permission to enter the experience of others as they openly share with us their pain and joy. So, it is not the research per se that prompts my reverence and awe: It is the generosity and courage of our participants, who allow us to accompany them and who share with us, themselves. It is to these people to whom this book is dedicated and has always been dedicated, with much gratitude and appreciation.

Contributors

Editor and Contributing Author
Patricia L. Munhall, EdD, ARNP, PsyA, FAAN
President
International Institute for Human Understanding
Miami, Florida

Contributing Authors
Cheryl Tatano Beck, DNSc, CNM, FAAN
Board of Trustees
   Distinguished Professor
School of Nursing
University of Connecticut
Storrs, Connecticut

Ronald J. Chenail, PhD
Professor
Department of Family Therapy
Graduate School of Humanities
   and Social Sciences
Nova Southeastern University
Fort Lauderdale, Florida

Robin Cooper, PhD
Adjunct Professor
Department of Multidisciplinary
   Studies, Graduate School of
   Humanities and Social Sciences
Research Associate
Office of Institutional Effectiveness
Nova Southeastern University
Fort Lauderdale, Florida

Roberta Cricco-Lizza, PhD, RN, MPH
Adjunct Assistant Professor, Center
   for Health Equity Research
Associate Fellow, Center for Public
   Health Initiatives
School of Nursing
University of Pennsylvania
Philadelphia, Pennsylvania

Maureen Duffy, PhD
President, International Institute for
    Human Understanding
Miami, Florida
Professor, Postgraduate Certificate
    in Qualitative Research
Nova Southeastern University
Fort Lauderdale, Florida

**Lynne M. Dunphy, PhD,
    ARNP, FNP-BC**
Routhier Chair of Practice &
    Professor of Nursing
RWJ Executive Nurse Fellow
Center Director, Rhode Island Center
    for Nursing Excellence (RICNE)
College of Nursing
University of Rhode Island
Kingston, Rhode Island

Maria Carmela Evangelista
Faculty Nurse Practitioner &
    Clinical Instructor
Columbia University School
    of Nursing
New York, New York

**Deborah L. Frank, PhD,
    ARNP, MFT**
Professor
College of Nursing
Florida State University
Tallahassee, Florida

Paul Gallant, PhD
Associate Professor and
    Clinical Director
Master of Family Therapy Program
Department of Psychiatry and
    Behavioral Science
School of Medicine
Mercer University
Macon, Georgia

**Holly M. Harner, PhD, MPH,
    CRNP, WHCNP-BC**
Assistant Professor and Director,
    Master of Public Health
    (MPH) Program
School of Nursing and
    Health Sciences
La Salle University
Philadelphia, Pennsylvania

**Patricia Hentz, EdD,
    PMHCNS-BC, CRNP**
Practice Associate Professor,
    Program Director,
    Vice Chair of Curriculum
School of Nursing
University of Pennsylvania
Philadelphia, Pennsylvania

**Sarah Steen Lauterbach, EdD,
    RN, MN, MSPH, ARNP**
Professor
College of Nursing
Valdosta State University
Valdosta, Georgia

Joy Longo, DNS, RNC-NIC
Assistant Professor
Christine E. Lynn College of Nursing
Florida Atlantic University
Boca Raton, Florida

**Karen Saucier Lundy, PhD,
    RN, FAAN**
Professor
School of Nursing
University of Southern Mississippi
Hattiesburg, Mississippi

Marlene C. Mackey, PhD, RN, FAAN
Professor Emerita
College of Nursing
University of South Carolina
Columbia, South Carolina

Janice M. Morse, PhD (Anthro), PhD (Nurs), FAAN
Professor Emeritus
University of Alberta
Professor and Keith and Dotty
    Barnes Presidential Chair
College of Nursing
University of Utah
Salt Lake City, Utah

Linda Niehaus, PhD
Research Associate
University of Alberta
Edmonton, Alberta
Canada

Marcella M. Rutherford, PhD, MBA, MSN
Program Director RN to BSN and
    RN to MSN Programs
Health Professions Division, College
    of Allied Health and Nursing
Nova Southeastern University
Fort Lauderdale, Florida

Sally St. George, PhD
Associate Professor
Faculty of Social Work
University of Calgary
Calgary, Alberta
Canada

Rita M. Valade, RSM
Chair and Associate Professor
School of Social Work
Spalding University
Louisville, Kentucky

Zane Robinson Wolf, PhD, RN, FAAN
Dean and Professor
School of Nursing and
    Health Sciences
La Salle University
Philadelphia, Pennsylvania

Judith Wuest, PhD, RN
Professor
Faculty of Nursing
University of New Brunswick
Fredericton, New Brunswick
Canada

Dan Wulff, PhD
Associate Professor
Faculty of Social Work
University of Calgary
Calgary, Alberta
Canada

Patti Rager Zuzelo, EdD, RN, ACNS-BC, ANP-BC, CRNP
Professor, DNP Program Director
    and CNS Track Coordinator
School of Nursing and
    Health Sciences
La Salle University
Philadelphia, Pennsylvania
Associate Director of Nursing
    for Research
Albert Einstein Healthcare Network
Philadelphia, Pennsylvania

Acknowledgments

I have been extraordinarily blessed to come to the fifth edition of this book with individuals who are willing to share their concern for the human condition with compassion, caring, and the talent, creativity, and scholarship to put that concern into research and language. Through the writings of the contributors to this volume we once again show the ways to research and to write about the meaning of human experience so that we come to understand what it means to be human. Voice is given to those unheard, healthcare reform becomes possible through narratives, emancipation becomes possible through understanding the contexts of individual lives, and humanistic care for individuals and healthcare policy becomes achievable. The contributors to this book make this intricate and delicate task possible and understandable to you, the reader.

I am deeply grateful and appreciative to those contributors, who have been in past editions, for their loyalty and their continued research and scholarship. I thank Lynne Dunphy, Joy Longo, Sarah Steen Lauterbach, Patricia Hentz, Judith Wuest, Cheryl Tatano Beck, Zane Robinson Wolf, Roberta Cricco-Lizza, Maureen Duffy, Ronald Chenail, Sally St. George, Dan Wulff, Marlene Mackey, Patti Zuzelo, Janice Morse and Linda Niehaus for their continued presence in the past and present.

As with new editions, new contributing authors join us, enriching and enlarging our narrative. I welcome you and thank you for your wonderful contributions. Thank you to Deborah Frank, Holly Hunter, Maria Evangelista,

Kay Lundy, Marcie Rutherford, Paul Gallant, Robin Cooper, and Rita Valade. Also I would like to extend my deepest gratitude to Edward Freeman, a former contributor and close colleague for his assistance with the editorial process.

I want to extend my sincerest gratitude to all of you for contributing your time, expertise and scholarship to make this 25th anniversary edition perhaps the best! Also I want to acknowledge your patience for the writing process and my "oh no, it's her again!" emails so necessary to putting this volume together. Thank you from a very deep part of me.

"Putting together this volume" is no small task for the Jones & Bartlett Learning professionals who work as an outstanding group and who make this publication possible. I extend my sincerest appreciation to Amanda Clerkin, Production Editor, Rachel Shuster, Editorial Assistant, and thank Kevin Sullivan, Nursing Publisher for Jones & Bartlett Learning. Thanks Amanda and Rachel for all your patience and professionalism over this past year and thank you Kevin for your continued support of this work. I extend much appreciation to Wendy Swanson who must be the best copyeditor around and to talented Tim Dziewit who did the wonderful cover. These acknowledgments are in a way like film credits, the people behind the scenes that make producing a work such as this possible. I thank you all for the wonderful work you do.

As I wrote in the prologue of this book, qualitative research would not be possible without the willingness of our research participants to share their experiences, giving voice to their inner most thoughts, perhaps risking what comes along with reaching inside one's self to a deeper level and search for meaning. I more than acknowledge these people, who are often facing daunting challenges: I praise their courage, admire their generosity and give many thanks for their faith in us. To these individuals as always, and on behalf of all the people mentioned here, this book is dedicated to them.

Patricia L. Munhall

PART I

The Qualitative Perspective

In Part I of this edition of *Nursing Research: A Qualitative Perspective*, I invite you to contemplate the emergence of qualitative research in nursing, from the past to this most exciting time in our ever expanding history of qualitative research, where there seems to be a heightened search for meaning and understanding within the context of being. Today, more than ever, we see how individual meaning and understanding are fundamental to the caring and compassionate practice of nursing. In this section, the "why" of this will become explicit to you.

The chapters in this section provide you with the essential philosophical, epistemological, and contextual foundations critical to the doing of qualitative research. From the first chapter, which is a brush stroke of the landscape of qualitative research, to the last chapter of this section, which discusses contemporary postmodern philosophical thought, you should become grounded in the historical, the linguistic, the "how we come to know things" of epistemology and the philosophical underpinnings that comprise the qualitative research perspective. In the beginning of this section, you might encounter a newness of perception that might require you to reread different parts to gain a better understanding. The philosophical underpinnings of qualitative research does require a shift in perception from the positivist perspective. I think you will find it a most dynamic and humanistic shift!

I hope you will immerse yourself in these four chapters to the extent that you can actually feel what it means to be coming from a qualitative perspective. The paradigm shift in your thinking or worldview will be palpable! When you hear or perhaps you say, "I am coming from a qualitative perspective," you will understand the meanings underpinning this very profound way of seeing and understanding being and experience.

The Landscape of Qualitative Research in Nursing

Patricia L. Munhall

I want to welcome you, the student, as well as the faculty member who is guiding this study, to the landscape of qualitative research in nursing. Oftentimes when reading a text such as this the first question one might legitimately ask is, "What is qualitative research?" In this volume you will find many definitions, perhaps each differing in some ways, reflecting the many ways of defining or perceiving qualitative research. In fact each method included in this book will have a definition for the specific method. However, characteristics of qualitative research, or tenets, if you like, follow through all qualitative methods. I like this way of perceiving qualitative research because I have long supported the proposition that definitions limit possibilities. Definitions can box people into a formula, which is the antithesis of qualitative research.

What I hope to do as I describe the landscape of qualitative research as I perceive it to be lived today is to include in this discussion the various components, beliefs, values, and characteristics that comprise qualitative research. So, there will not be a one-sentence definition but instead an evolving sense of what qualitative research is, demonstrated throughout this chapter. When I write something that is not from a qualitative perspective, I will call your attention to it as distinct and probably belonging to the quantitative methods of research. Otherwise, this chapter is a reflection of the qualitative perspective, which shows itself through the content.

My intention in this chapter is to provide a holistic description and explanation—to the extent that one chapter can permit—of the qualitative research perspective in nursing and relate the discussion to your own world. I encourage you to begin thinking from a qualitative perspective as you read because this will help you understand the following chapters. Try to incorporate the concept being discussed into your thinking to other instances of a particular idea or activity.

For example, have you noticed that the first person "I" is being used? Qualitative research is known for giving voice to people, to hearing people's own personal narrative and using the *language of our participants* in research. Often, this is distinct from quantitative research, where, for example, a questionnaire might be derived from a theory developed by a researcher (for example, the Myers-Briggs Type Indicator). The outcome of this test, like other psychological measurement, results in the language of the researcher in the form of a category, stage, or type as a result of answers provided by participants. The voice of the person is for all practical purposes lost. So, in this class, if that is the case, or while reading this text, give yourself voice by using *I*: I see the world this way and I interpret the experience this way. Give your subjective experience voice. In this way you will also learn to give your research participants their voice, encouraging them to use their "I" and seeing through their eyes.

This chapter includes many cross-references to other chapters that explain specific concepts in greater depth. I want to reassure you that ideas discussed in Chapter 1 are further elaborated upon throughout the entire book. So, in reading this introductory chapter, please know that concepts that may seem puzzling now are covered in later chapters.

The Irreducible You

In this chapter and throughout the book, I hope you find the landscape you are traveling across interesting and stimulating, the methods challenging, and the exemplars revealing as well as quite meaningful. But let's begin with you, a place where thinking qualitatively is a natural place to start.

This might be your second or third course in nursing research, and you may have been introduced to qualitative research methods in your first course, which I assume was an overview. Here, I would like to emphasize one of the most important characteristics of qualitative research: Do not make assumptions! To demonstrate how assumptions made at the very beginning of a study could lead to erroneous findings, let's examine what might be wrong with this paragraph.

First, I do not know how many courses in research you have already had, if any! A second erroneous assumption I have made is that you may have had an overview of qualitative research. Preparing this chapter, I found many fundamentals of nursing research textbooks that did not address in any way qualitative research (which, of course, I find very distressful for many reasons, the most important of which is that it deprives you of the possibilities, pleasures, authenticity, and meaningfulness that come from qualitative research).

I suggest that not making assumptions is a very good idea for any endeavor in which you are involved. The practice of not making assumptions indicates that qualitative research is very close to real-life experiences, not ones that are assumed, which often means not based on anything but conjecture. Sometimes assumptions can reflect prejudice, biases, and stereotypes that, when acted upon, can be very unjust, unfair, and lead to all sorts of poor judgments. That is the downside of assumptions. Sometimes people make positive assumptions. Be wary of these, too!

Many introductory nursing research courses emphasize the scientific method, sometimes referred to as quantitative methods. You might remember discussions of independent variables and dependent variables, sampling techniques, statistical methods of analyzing data, and rules for reliability and validity, among other essentials of the scientific method.

Can you remember the difference between an independent variable and a dependent variable? For some reason, students find this distinction troublesome, perhaps because it does not actually follow real-life experiences. Experience is so multifaceted that breaking it down into parts, such as independent and dependent variables, does little to contribute to understanding the whole. David Bohm (1985), who calls this the implicate order of organisms, states: "The word implicate means to enfold, in Latin, to fold inward. In the implicate order, everything is folded into everything" (p. 12).

The Irreducible Whole

Another critical component of qualitative research is its emphasis on holism and what Bohm (1985) calls the constraining grip of objectivity as a myth. Not only is an individual a holistic system, but he or she is much more than that: The individual is engaged in the world of others, in interacting worlds of experience. We come to see that qualitative research does not practice reductionism, does not reduce human beings or experiences to parts that require separate investigation. That we leave to quantitative researchers, who do remember the difference between independent and dependent variables! Variables are parts that, in the strict scientific worldview, influence other parts and are reduced from the whole. An example might be when we ask, "Is there a relationship between exercise and obesity?" A simple quantitative research project would distinguish two variables. Objectivity would play an important part in choosing the sample population so it is homogeneous and results can be generalized, meaning they can be applied to other like individuals.

In contrast, a qualitative researcher might even call this project the experience of obesity and view obesity as a holistic phenomenon of not only embodiment, *the unity of body and mind*, but also the *unity of self with others and the environment*. What is very interesting and very distinctive is the focus of qualitative research on subjectivity and intersubjectivity. Stolorow and Atwood (2002) describe this as: "the subjective world of the individual as its central theoretical concept, envisioning the world as evolving organically from the person's encounter with critical experiences that constitute his unique life history . . . the perspective toward being" (p. 2). What does this mean? We know what it means because we subconsciously think this way and our lives unfold this way. We just may not have reflected on subjectivity and intersubjectivity before as concepts. As individuals we each have a perspective of ourselves and the world. This is the reason why we might agree or disagree with others, because others also have a perspective, or a subjective world, their own subjective perspective. Other words to describe this perspective might be a worldview or paradigm (discussed in Chapters 2, 3, and 5).

Our own subjective world evolves from all our previous experiences: our experiences as a child; our relationship with parents, siblings, and friends; the culture we grew up in or are currently a part of; the time in history we are situated in; the country, state, and town we are living in; our age; and the list goes on. The subjective perspective is the result of our experiences and forms the context of where we are at present. This is sometimes called the *situated context*, another critical consideration in qualitative research. Taking into consideration the situated context of participants in a study is imperative. Who they are is taken very seriously. More than just demographics, they are people who differ because of their subjective perspective, which evolved from their experiences. Considering the situated context demonstrates respect for these individuals by acknowledging their uniqueness and taking into consideration their personal narratives (an illustration of two subjective worlds can be found in Chapter 6).

The Situated Context

I would like to demonstrate a situated context that might apply to you and your colleagues. Let us begin with the personal and your probable context, the place you find yourself right now. Most likely, part of your context is that you are studying at the master's or doctoral level of nursing. I acknowledge here all the assumptions I am making, and this is not how I would conduct qualitative research, I would instead want to know the authentic situated context of the participants in my study. Actually, authors make all sorts of assumptions about readers (like I am doing); in fact, it is essential to ensuring that a book will be useful to its audience. Paradoxically, though, it does not always work out correctly because readers most often have had different experiences, even if they have been classmates for the past 3 years. Most important, students are different from one another, learn differently, and remember what they value most, which varies from individual to individual. I emphasize this more when we discuss right-sided and left-sided brain dominance; more and more brain research seems to bear out very different characteristics of each side of the brain.

In Chapter 5 on the phenomenological method, I argue that one needs to "be" phenomenological to conduct that kind of research. But as you can see, one might "be" qualitative in perspective when writing, speaking, and most importantly delivering nursing care, whether as faculty, administrator, or practitioner so actually "being" phenomenological has implications far beyond research. Thinking qualitatively is thinking of holistic beings that cannot be understood by reducing them to parts; each has a distinct situated context that will influence the individual's subjective world, perspective, and use of language. Perhaps this stance can be summed up by Bohm (1985) as he discusses enfoldment: "Language is implicit in feelings and thoughts . . . and words . . . move towards mutual enfoldment. Thoughts and feelings also enfold intentions" (p. 16).

For instance, it was not my "intention" to digress from considering your situated context, but obviously I kept writing words and using language that was in the moment reflecting thoughts and feelings that led to an intention to discuss "thinking qualitatively" which I thought was important. Now I return to your situated context!

Your Situated Context

When you first started your undergraduate education, I imagine you were not aware that nurses conduct research. I wonder how many of you went into nursing to do research! If you had a sister or friend, you may have had advance knowledge, but for the most part you did not enter the profession of nursing to become a researcher. And here you are, most likely in a class studying research and perhaps preparing now to do research.

Congratulations! Research is so exciting and rewarding when you contemplate the wondrous idea that something not known is going to be found out by you or by the group you are working with. You are actually going to be creating and contributing knowledge to the discipline of nursing. You have the opportunity to improve the quality of life for others, to prevent hardship, to liberate people, to further understanding of life's mysteries of experience . . . indeed these are tasks of no small consequence.

If you had entered a field such as physics or chemistry, you would have known at the outset that you were going to become a scientist, and indeed that would have been your dream. You would have already developed a propensity for logic and the rationality of the scientific method. You would have had visions of yourself in a white lab coat with microscopes and measuring tools around you. This would have been a focused choice for you: a vision of yourself more grounded in the expectations of your chosen field. Yes, you might also teach as a scientist, but you also knew you would be doing research. This is a field you could enter if you wanted or indeed were excited about doing research.

How different, then, for you and your colleagues in nursing. You enter the nursing profession with visions very different from our physics and chemistry friends. For the most part, you're not aware that nurses do research, and when you happen to hear that you are required to take nursing research courses, you could not imagine what nurses research. So, the initial socialization of nurses, from the perception of others (guidance counselors, peers, parents), is that nursing usually does not include research.

In your class ask how many of your colleagues, when they said, "I am going to be a nurse," heard, "Oh, that is wonderful—perhaps you will become a nurse researcher!" What most incoming nursing students envision is caring for people in need. It is not trite to say that the reason I went into nursing is that I wanted to help people. I think most students picture a more hands-on profession, perhaps encouraged by the media. I don't recall any episodes of hospital dramas showing nurses going off to do research, or nurses announcing that they are ready to start a research project. Way back when I was younger, there was a book series about a nurse, Cherry Ames . . . she was many things, but never *Cherry Ames: Nurse Researcher*!

At the undergraduate level, when you were introduced to the reality of research in nursing, the standard research textbooks, which are larger than this one, included perhaps 1 chapter out of 30 on qualitative research. A situated context had been created for you in which entering nursing students do not have awareness that research is a part of the nursing role. And then, when the research role is introduced, the scientific method of the natural sciences seems to be the method of choice for research. You have probably found that the most prevalent worldview, paradigm, or model for research in nursing is the scientific method.

A Fluke

Now another fluke that makes nursing students different in regard to research is that most will not make a career in research, unlike the aforementioned physics and chemistry students. Few will ever be solely nurse researchers, and those who do research will share their time between other responsibilities, such as being a faculty member. Because of these differences, your educational preparation does not include the inherent faculty–student expectation of research mentorship, where research is often the primary goal of education, as it is in the natural sciences. This is also part of your situated context.

Yet, research has become one of the many goals of your nursing education. Nurse educators expect you to read, critique, and utilize nursing research, and indeed the quality and effectiveness of your practice depend on keeping abreast of the new knowledge in the field.

However, is it realistic to think that graduates of undergraduate schools can understand and critique research? Especially if it is presented in an advanced mathematical format, which the student has had little preparation to understand? One course in research at the undergraduate level, not to mention statistics, usually conjures up confusing memories for most graduates. This I have observed many times, so it is not an assumption, so to speak! However, it does not apply to everyone (another point about assumptions, even if they appear well grounded).

You now find yourself in graduate school. You are finding research discussed and focused on in much greater depth. You are told that you are the future nurse researchers and are the ones who will make the changes necessary to address the critical problems that individuals at all developmental stages and throughout the healthcare delivery system present.

In this textbook, you will be introduced in much greater depth and detail to qualitative research, the philosophical underpinnings, methods, outcomes, and how critical this perspective of research is to our understanding of human experience. This book represents a continuing conversation on qualitative research, which started before 1987, the year in which the first edition of this book was published. The interest, growth, and recognition of the value of qualitative methods for nursing research are evident in the enlarging conversation, which has grown from an original 288 pages of the first edition to the 604 pages of this fifth edition. Today we have journals, conferences, and classes specifically focusing on qualitative research. The acceptance of qualitative research as legitimate in the discipline of nursing was not an easy task to accomplish, and even today some nurse researchers, journals, and granting agencies still place paramount importance on the scientific method and its worldview, even though I (and many others) have argued often that they are not congruent with our philosophy (see Chapters 2 and 3). However, I do believe that the Scientific Method, with capital letters, has its place in nursing research, as I do believe Qualitative Research Methods have. They lead us to different places, ask different kinds of questions, and together can provide a multifaceted view of human experience.

Broadening the Landscape

You might wonder what characteristics of qualitative research are different from the scientific method (from this point on, the capital letters are removed to indicate it is just one more method to be used, not *the* method). We have mentioned a few, such as not making assumptions, the concept of holism, the critical importance of the situated context, and the all-important worlds of subjectivity and intersubjectivity.

The qualitative research perspective recognizes the influences of a dynamic reality rather than a static one with the following five points, as articulated by Beneloiel (1984). These five points will help you differentiate between the scientific method approach and qualitative approach:

- Social life is the shared creativity of individuals and their perceptions.
- The character of the social world is dynamic and changing.
- There are multiple realities and frameworks for viewing the world: The world is not independent of humankind and objectively identifiable.
- Human beings are active agents who construct their own realities.
- No response sets are highly predictable. (p. 4)

Furthermore, in distinguishing between the two paradigms, it is important to understand that nursing is a human science. According to Dilthey (1926), the human sciences are to be distinguished from the natural sciences because of critical and fundamental differences in attitude toward their respective phenomena of research. Stated simply, *the natural sciences investigate objects from the outside to the inside, whereas the human sciences depend on a perspective from the inside to the outside.* The most important concern in the human sciences is that of meaning. Meaning exists within human subjectivity rather than in material nature. Thus, the aims of the two sciences are different. The natural sciences seek causal explanation, prediction, and control. The human sciences seek understanding, interpretation, and meaning.

Remember, this chapter is an introduction, and all these ideas are discussed in much greater detail as you go through the various chapters. In other words, if some of this sounds a bit foreign as far as research is concerned, it will be further clarified. However, for most of you, the preceding five characteristics will sound familiar because this is often how human beings are conceptualized in nursing philosophies and theories. You might wonder why it does not always follow into nursing research. It does, in qualitative nursing research, making much of nursing philosophy, theory, and research, philosophically and linguistically congruent.

So much difference goes unacknowledged as we try earnestly to create human laboratory systems untainted by the outside world. Then the human being must eventually return to the outside world, to the entire context and all the contingencies of his or her life. These are some of the important concerns of the qualitative researcher:

- Meanings within context for the individual person
- Interpretations by the individual person
- How a person narrates his or her own story
- How a self is socially constructed
- How truth is an interpretation

- The significance of meaning as an antecedent or precedent for change and understanding
- The critique to improve well-being through understanding
- The emancipation of those oppressed

Which leads to a different perspective of "truth". These two different world-views, the natural science perspective and the human science perspective, have not only different philosophical approaches underpinning their research methods but also a different interpretation of truth.

Seeking Truth

Truth arrived at by numbers is often held suspect by qualitative researchers because they worry about all the variables that were not factored into the equations. They also worry about how individual people interpret words differently and assign different values to numbers. Qualitative researchers have a different propensity and different worldview. Given the freedom to grow and develop in their methods, they can provide to the profession understanding, description, theory, interpretation, and direction concerned with the intricacy and inter-connectedness of being in this world that is not one but many in perception; a world that is not one but many in language. One language has many languages within that language, as does one culture. Qualitative researchers search for the differences not only between cultures but also within cultures. They challenge stereotypes, presuppositions, and assumptions.

Qualitative researchers break new ground by revealing what had been concealed because they look beyond appearance. They provide the reconstruction or deconstruction that time demands of us, as the sands shift and the known is no longer valid. In their quest for discovery, qualitative researchers legitimate the existence of others in their differences. Conformity is not the object; we know that a universal concept of meaning is not possible and doubt that it is desirable.

Since publication of the first edition of this book in 1987 nursing research has burgeoned. Doctoral programs for nursing, research journals, research conferences, and courses continue to expand. Research and the concomitant dissemination of results are required of faculty and are essential for promotion and tenure. You, as a graduate student, might write a research proposal; some of you will complete a master's thesis; and, of course, a dissertation must be completed for the doctoral degree. A profession that, 45 years ago, was once housed in 3-year diploma schools affiliated with hospitals is now ensconced in the university setting and has responsibly taken on the values of an academic profession.

One of the most important values in the academy is the search for truth. Broadly speaking, this search for truth is a search for new knowledge for the profession. One of the most remarkable changes since 1987 is what is sometimes called "the knowledge explosion," which is concurrent with the explosion of technology. Technology has enabled advances in the health sciences, changes in the healthcare system, and the rapid communication of knowledge moment to moment.

Today when we embark on a research project, we see a change more in how we believe something than in what we believe. There are shifts in belief about belief, questioning the idea of absolute truth and *acknowledging the possibility of many truths* (Anderson, 1995). Before the introduction of qualitative methods of research in nursing, the profession embraced the scientific method as the paradigm for nursing research. The reasons for this are discussed in Chapters 2 and 3 of this text. However, some nurse researchers had a bent, so to speak, to look for other ways of coming to know and other ways to search for truth or many truths.

Other Disciplines' Methods

Other disciplines, other than the natural sciences, had methods that interested nurse researchers*. For those pioneers of qualitative research in nursing, the rationale for their use was as strong and compelling as the use of a natural science method. As with most new ideas—and we need to remember that the pursuit of qualitative research was a new idea for nursing research—some conflict ensued. Professional legitimacy was seen as affiliation with the "hard" sciences. Linear progress, absolute truths, and rationality were all thought to be ideals for a science. Before nursing entered the academy, it was popular to say that nursing was an art and a science, but, once in the academy, the art component was subsumed and the science component was elevated for reasons that were socially constructed within the situated context. To follow this trajectory this science component became the stimulus for adopting the scientific method as validation for "nursing as a science." This social construction is explained in the beginning chapters of this book.

The Sands of Science

The sands of science itself are shifting as more and more scientists, including nurse scientists, realize that science cannot be a field of absolute and final truth but is an endeavor focused on *illuminating an ever-changing body of ideas*.

---

* Here I am not discussing the nurse researchers that received doctorates in other fields prior to nursing having their own doctoral programs, which is discussed in Chapter 2.

For many, though, this focus is still not accepted and is considered a grievous loss; others find the shifting sands exhilarating and liberating. In 1987, few dissertations and publications indicated an acceptance of qualitative methods of inquiry in nursing. Ironically and unfortunately, in the year 2010, qualitative nurse researchers and quantitative nurse researchers, who often call themselves nurse scientists, do not garner the same prizes. The National Institute of Nursing Research, a branch of the National Institutes of Health, mostly rewards quantitative/scientific research proposals, though some encouraging changes are occurring.

Colleges of nursing pride themselves on establishing centers for nursing science or the science of nursing. Of course, a Center for Nursing Research would be more embracing, at least in name, of various approaches to the pursuit of knowledge. As you will read in this text, the situated context in which we live influences what we want to be "like" and how we wish to "appear" in the academic or medical setting. Qualitative research methods *are* indeed scientific in that they have their own paradigmatic philosophical underpinnings consistent with the qualitative worldview and methods that stay true to these beliefs and values. The evaluation strategies for qualitative research are real-world oriented, rather than mathematically determined, and are as rigorous as any for the scientific method.

From this perspective, qualitative methods are as scientific as quantitative methods; however, the capital S seems to belong to the Scientific Method. Qualitative researchers are indeed doing scientific research as the word science is generally understood.

I have yet to meet a qualitative nurse researcher who believes his or her method of doing research is the "only" and the most legitimate way of coming to know and advancing knowledge. I suppose this belief itself is reflective of the philosophical underpinnings of qualitative research methods so that it should not come as a surprise that here we see the difference about "how" we believe. Following are more concepts that characterize qualitative research:

- Multiplicity of worldviews
- Simultaneity of different worldviews
- Perspectivity of phenomena
- Polyvocality of many voices
- Multiple realities held by individuals
- Individual and cultural social construction of reality leading to multiple realities

All lend themselves to a broader acceptance of the many and different ways of being in the world and, in this case, nursing research. We see the same entity differently, interpret it differently, talk about it with different language, have varying perceptions about the same person or event and our situated context and contingencies of our lives influence all these differences. Understanding this complexity actually makes understanding others possible!

The Multistoried World

It would certainly be unfair to portray all nursing scientists based in the natural science method as unreceptive to qualitative nurse researchers, but it would also be unfair to have you as a student of nursing research be unaware of the dichotomy that persists within the field. I am very encouraged that, in spite of what some may view as the superiority of the scientific method, more and more nurse researchers change their whole view of research once they become acquainted with this alternative paradigm. Some have said that they have found a home. They have found a home in this world of research.

Hence, the conversation enlarges and the possibility now includes you and your class. Perhaps this is true about the faculty member teaching this class.

Within the dialogue and within this text are many reasons to consider just how critical qualitative research methods are for a human science field, a profession dedicated to alleviating suffering and promoting well-being. The need for the scientific method is not in dispute here. In fact, it is celebrated for specific problems and questions. However, it is inappropriate for seeking answers and solutions to other problems and questions of equal if not greater significance to a human science.

Transitioning Within a Postmodern World

In today's world, we are acknowledging a multifaceted world embracing complexity, subjectivity, meaning heterogeneity, the myriad of perceptions, polyvocality, and the fact that we are overwhelmingly pluralistic and living multiple realities of experience, as mentioned earlier.

Science, with a capital S, fascinated us and was and still is an interesting story, but it is only one story to describe you and me and the world we inhabit. It is interesting to note that we discuss science in a somewhat dispassionate discourse, a statement of a discovery, a theory proved, a theory refuted, so to speak. And, though sometimes dispassionate, there are moments of passion when a cure for some terrible condition arrives and quality of life is improved. Ironically, many of these scientific discoveries are found by accident; while something else is being searched for, a serendipitous discovery is made. Thomas Kuhn (1970) in *The Structure of Scientific Revolutions* speaks of many discoveries as anomalies that lead to a new way of looking at a phenomenon. I think it is critical to read this work of Kuhn's, if you have not yet. You will really understand the nature of science as a process, a changing one, and a changing one that is not always rational!

As nurses, though, we have much to contribute to understanding the multistoried world, the diversity and the plurality of the people who we serve through other methods of science, through qualitative methods. I have seen the excitement of students when they come upon these methods. A body of students reflects this multistoried world within their individual situated contexts.

I would like to emphasize we are all blessedly pluralistic: students, faculty, patients, family, and the community. There is not one best answer and there is not one best way of doing research. For instance, because incoming nursing students are often not aware of the research component, when it is introduced students might separate into groups in which some seem mathematically inclined and the others seem linguistically inclined. It is imperative to sort that out, for ourselves and for our students.

Toward that end, our research endeavors become enlarged as we help to develop a multitalented group of students in their specific propensities. Because we have both the mathematically logic–minded student and the linguistically/philosophically interpretive–inclined student, our potential is magnified, as is our field of understanding. Those who are linguistically, interpretive, and philosophically inclined need our encouragement to develop their talents and propensities in their research endeavors. No one way is superior to another. Students and faculty alike might have noticed that many students develop a dislike for research. Perhaps this dislike is because only one language is spoken and those students need to hear and learn the other languages of discovery.

There is growing support for the idea that the left or right side of an individual's brain is dominant. We need both sides to function in this world, just like we need a science to indicate the hard sciences associated with strict adherence to the scientific method, and we need a science associated with qualitative methods, which are indeed scientific but more multidimensional.

The Problem with Generalizations

In our practice we are exposed to languages, semiotics, and beliefs of different cultures. We need to have nurses and nurse researchers who hear the differences and who question generalizations. These are additional characteristics of qualitative research. We need to have researchers who using qualitative research methods will assist people in interpreting the meaning of different realities and personal subjective realities, so that we can develop approaches for different individuals. We begin to understand the many meanings of experiences and the implications of these meanings. Such approaches then are based on respect and knowledge about individual perceptions and not based on preconceived protocols that provide a general way to proceed. Many if not most protocols are based on what is best for the average person. The average person is a mathematical concept. Then we wonder why there are so many complications in healthcare delivery!

Let us distinguish again between someone who thinks from a quantitative paradigm and one who thinks from a qualitative paradigm in relation to the idea of a protocol. A protocol for patients with a specific condition is a prescription for action and process. You may not know the patient, but you have the protocol with which to treat the person based on his or her diagnosis.

For most qualitative nurse researchers, the idea of a protocol without emphasis on individual differences characteristic of qualitative research can be daunting. That is because qualitative researchers do not claim to generalize their findings—how could they when there is such emphasis on individual interpretation and subjectivity? Simply stated: One size or explanation cannot fit all! So protocols attempt to be a one-size or one-way approach to very complex conditions.

Sometimes following a protocol works; often it does not. When it does not, instead of questioning the protocol, often we assume there is something different about the patient and the result then becomes a complication. Of course, there is something different; generalizations made, for example, for wound healing cannot possibly take into account all the different variables in process for a particular person. Often it is said we cannot afford individualized care, so there must be protocols and procedures. *I believe with the cost of complications that we cannot afford not to have individualized care.* It is from the philosophical underpinnings of qualitative research and subsequent research that we come to see there are many truths and limitless possibilities to meet the differences that occur among our patients. We respect the person, and we respect that there are many truths and limitless possibilities.

Today there is an emphasis on evidence-based practice. We must realize that approximately every 5 years, new phrases call for the same response, have the same purpose, and mean very much the same. We have lived through an emphasis on theory-based practice, and this may be a good question for you to address with your class. What is the difference between theory-based practice and evidence-based practice? With theory-based practice, there was also a focus on developing taxonomies, nursing diagnoses, and interventions based on diagnoses. The interventions came from accepted scientific practice or newly developed protocols based on the newest research. Whatever system you are using—today it is evidence-based practice—as an advanced practice nurse, faculty member, administrator, or researcher, you need to be particularly focused on meaning: meaning of what a person may be experiencing, how a person might behave, what meaning a person gives to health, and even "meaningless" information. If a person believes that your evidence-based practice is meaningless to him or her, that belief should become meaningful to you. It changes your approach to the person. A current example is what some believe to be occurring in the United States, and that is an obesity epidemic. We focus on all age groups but, for the sake of this example, consider: Do we have evidence-based practice means to reduce obesity specifically in adolescents? Without finding the meaning and motivation for why some adolescents may overeat, we may never understand this behavior and be able to design means to change it. Based on the philosophical underpinnings of qualitative research as well as postmodern thought we are very cognizant that we are not going to find *the* answer. We will find many answers congruent once again with a multi-storied world.

A critical component that differentiates quantitative, scientific method–driven research from qualitative (scientific) methods is the unequivocal focus on meaning. Without knowing the meaning of a patient's behavior, the evidence-based intervention that in some samples did change behaviors in certain circumstances will undoubtedly be meaningless for others.

This happens in hospitals and other healthcare settings. If the patient does not follow the practice or intervention, then the patient is labeled noncompliant, a negative judgment against the patient. Measures will be taken against such noncompliance, and they also will be doomed until a qualitative approach into the meaning of events or behavior of the patient is carried out. And this qualitative approach is done to acknowledge the plurality, the diversity, and the different ways of being that most nursing philosophies subscribe to in their descriptions of a human being.

Putting This "Thus Far" Together Qualitatively _____

> *"In the beginner's mind, there are many possibilities, but in the expert's mind there are few"*
>
> —(Suzuki, as quoted in Andersen, 2009, p. 68).

Zen master Shunryu Suzuki introduces us to the paradoxical nature of everything we have been taught. Knowledge is power; evidence-based nursing, protocols, and theories are other forms of knowledge. Quotations, to me are high in efficiency; they can succinctly express the wisest ideas to ponder. I also have great respect for people's narratives of their experiences in whatever context they may appear. Often these narratives lead to understanding new possibilities. Today's most popular literature is often first-person narratives of people's lives. Because they are "real," they grip us, hold us in awe or terror, and provide a path to understanding that I do not believe can be surpassed. The exemplars of the qualitative research methods reflect, the "realness" of people's lives. They grip us and hold us in awe. Some inspire great compassion. As you will read in Chapter 5, while narratives, stories, and culture are all part of our qualitative research, we are called upon as qualitative researchers to read through either description or interpretation to critique what was found in our studies and suggest recommendations for individuals, researchers, policy makers, and, of course, nurses.

A description of narrative or the narrative itself, even if interpreted in any of the methods in this book, must be followed by the meaning of the study, the answer to "so what?" In Part I you will find discussions and explanations of the language and philosophical underpinnings of qualitative research. Understanding these underpinnings is often a challenge to those of us brought up on the scientific method. However, they must be understood at a level where you automatically "think" in a most fundamentally new way. To understand others though, you need the beginner's mind, which is a fun place to be because all sorts of possibilities for understanding open up to you, things you might not have *possibly* imagined. The following quotation also illustrates the idea that if we think we know something we do not look for answers. This I call premature closure to understanding an experience to its fullest, in its richest depth.

"The greatest obstacle to discovery is not ignorance but the illusion of knowledge"
(Boorstin, as quoted in Andersen, 2009, p. 68)

There is a song by Tom Petty and the Heartbreakers titled, "You don't know how it feels to be me." Every time I have given a workshop on phenomenology I start with this song. The chorus of the song is repeated quite often and conveys in great clarity, what qualitative research as a perspective attempts to resolve. The individuals we encounter often feel as though we do not understand how they feel—this will be illustrated shortly in an example.

Sometimes we do not understand our own self. We might say to a friend, "I don't understand why I did that or said that," so to add to the idea of not understanding how another person feels, we also struggle to understand ourselves. Carter (2008), in her book about multiplicity, argues that most of us believe we have a single self and deems that to be an illusion. Think of the different personalities you adopt during a day as you go from perhaps home, to a professional setting, to a meeting with your staff, to a discussion with a patient, to being a faculty member or a student, to being someone's partner or spouse, and on and on we change during the day. You might say it is still me, and yes it is you but each one of those personalities in a specific context holds varying viewpoints, goals, values, and investment (Carter, 2008). If you have any doubts about this perspective, think of when you last said *"I wasn't myself today,"* well, then who were you?

Often we see personality changes in our patients and instead of accepting those changes as a reflection of the multiplicity of that person we note it as a symptom! When we speak of pursuing understanding of individuals and self as well, we can see the influence of the context that person was in or that we were in, we understand that contingencies change the self from day to day and within the day. Yes, we like to be stable but we are not robots. We respond to our environment and it shows itself in a different kind of self. All this is essential to understanding the complexity of human behavior and human "being" as well as to the work of the qualitative nurse researcher.

A Stirring Example

Here I provide a healthcare provider's own experience in thinking she understood herself and how this understanding of her self enabled her to predict understanding or what was best for her patients. Thinking she understood what was best for her patients while not understanding what her own *actual* reactions would be in a similar situation (another self in a different context), had what can be referenced as premature closure to other possibilities. Thus, she misunderstood many of her patients who in the end turned out to be much like her, the *her* she did not understand. Is this confusing? Let me make some qualitative philosophical points here about this convolution of misunderstanding. The healthcare provider was the knower as in Boorstin's quote and it prevented her from being enlightened by discovery—it closed off other possible knowledge.

She did not allow for the patient to be the knowledge holder, the knower. She did not understand what each person was about on an individual level. That was her personality at the time. She unfortunately experienced something (the actual details are coming next) that changed her personality (viewpoints, beliefs, values), and she became open to other ways of being and everything she had once believed was completely suspended as those beliefs did not apply to herself. This is an excellent example of our different selves responding to different contingencies.

The story appeared on the front page of *The New York Times,* with the headline: "Helping Patients Face Death, She Fought to Live" (Hartocollis, 2010). This physician was a leading expert in palliative care, counseling terminally ill patients regarding choices they made. She held a very strong belief that patients should confront their illness once deemed terminal, get their affairs in order, and spend their remaining time in comfort rather than unbearable pain or enduring interventions that would add to this pain with little or dubious promise. I think most of us are aware of the scenarios where patients are subjected or persuaded to undergo painful and questionable interventions with little hope of change. Their dying is prolonged, their last days spent in intractable pain and other horrendous conditions. We also know some of these patients are themselves ready to die and yet are encouraged to try one more procedure. Hospitals are not places patients come to die, so interventions continue to persist until the patient does die.

So here is this wonderful-meaning physician wanting to assist patients to achieve a peaceful, painless death. Then she herself unfortunately developed a terminal type of cancer, one that with treatment had only a 2% chance of survival. She was offered palliative care—her prescription for others. As we learn more about qualitative research we will learn to appreciate specific contexts and the nature of the lived body and temporality (do not fret if you do not know what that means right now). The temporality exemplified in this case is that she was 40 years old, so it was a powerful influence.

Her Discovery

The physician in our example refused palliative care and *with anger that this was suggested* to her despite the 2% survival rate with treatment that entailed a great deal of pain. Regardless, she wanted to fight the fight. While her work thus far had been helping patients accept death, this did not apply to her. She was a fighter. When her painful treatments failed she would find a doctor who would bombard her with more. No amount of pain and discomfort, no matter how excruciating would stop her pursuit. It came to a point where the interventions themselves were life threatening, but she insisted on them.

What This Has To Do with Qualitative Research

The "narrative" is replete with examples of what this has to do with qualitative research. Without qualitative research we do not know what the other person is thinking, we do not understand possible alternative interpretations by individuals; we do not let the patient be "the knower".

The most revealing part of the terminally ill physician being "the knowledge holder" and knowing what is best for the patient is that not only did it not apply to her, it did not apply to others she counseled for palliative care. Here is an illustrative quote:

> She remembered patients who complained to her *that she did not know them well enough* to recognize that they were stronger than she thought. Now she discovered that she felt the same way about her own doctors. "I think they underestimated me." (italics added, p. A1)

What is critical in this example is that we have a moral imperative to understand what it is our patients want even if we are fairly sure that there is little to gain in continuing treatment (cost considerations are excluded here) that some patients would rather fight to the very end. Dr. Desiree Pardi died on September 6, 2009 in what one healthcare provider described as, "unfortunately quite a painful scenario. Many people would not have chosen that route" (p. A2).

However, she was an autonomous being and we do not know the meaning of her choice, but most of us probably believe she had the right to make her own decisions. The question though still remains: Did she allow or give permission to others to pursue that same path—the ones who felt misunderstood and said, "that she did not know them well enough"?

This Is Why We Do Qualitative Research

Each person we encounter can help us discover what is best for him or her. The other person, not us, is truly the expert knower of himself or herself. We acknowledge the importance of the above, that we need to know our patients well enough before intervening. We often try in nursing and with patient care or community service to fit individuals or cultures into our theory when actually it is the individual and/or the culture that should provide direction for a particular individualizing of any theory. Once we understand the interior (subjective) world of the individual or culture, we have accomplished the first step of knowing the truth, the meaning, and the interpretation from the source. That source is not our textbooks or courses. That source of knowledge comes from the knower and the people who are the "knowers" provide the outcomes of qualitative research. This book is about gaining that understanding from first-person narratives, stories, and researching cultures. Qualitative researchers want to know what happened to the person, how it is for that individual person, what they feel like, how they experienced the event, and from the example given earlier, what it is they want. The latter is so critical. Healthcare providers, as well as any human service profession, must respect what the individual wants, their autonomy. Nurses profess to protect patient's autonomy. Yet, we often have definitive plans and protocols made and implemented before we "know" the patient.

The idea that professionals know what is best for a person comes from having knowledge. Individualizing patient care has been considered a critical value in nursing care. You will actually learn a new way of doing that when you come to understand the philosophical underpinnings of qualitative research.

Of course I hope you become inspired by reading about qualitative research, the methods and the actual exemplars, where experiences become so vivid and the need for change so apparent for qualitative research. As this chapter explains some of you might be (since you too are an individual!) more inclined to do quantitative research, especially if you are left-side brain dominant. Quantitative research is needed and in fact that is where many qualitative studies should lead as is described in Chapter 3 as the cyclical continuum. However, alluding to what is written in Chapter 5 about *becoming phenomenological,* this book can assist you and provide you a way of thinking about "knowing" and "unknowing." Learning the importance of the subjective world of individuals and the intersubjective world when we engage with one another, you might change profoundly in ways that will give your life and work new meaning. What I am hoping for you is that what you can learn in this book, whether you do qualitative research or not, will be of great influence to you in your life and in your practice.

Understanding the Other: The Third Ear

I would like to write about the idea of listening with the third ear because undergirding all qualitative research is the art of listening. Undergirding all effective communication is the art of listening. Understanding another in the deepest ways comes from the art of listening. This does not only mean listening attentively—that is only part of it! Yes, you need to do that, but there are other components that are essential to really hearing what the other person is saying and what they mean.

Have you ever noticed all the misunderstandings you experience just in one day? From home to the workplace to the classroom, these misunderstandings contribute to frustration, conflict, powerlessness, feeling like an object, inaccurate interpretation of others, feelings of isolation, prejudice, and oppression. On some critical occasions misunderstandings have had disastrous results, such as a violent outcome in the home, more frequently now in our schools, and of course in the world, a world where we take war as a given. Less dramatic perhaps but extremely damaging misunderstandings in the workplace or school can lead to labeling, gossiping, criticism, ostracism, and now I am right back to dramatic and tragic outcomes, suicide or homicide. When you hear or read the responses of individuals after a tragedy, there often were signs and things were said, but did anyone hear those hints with the third ear?

I am attempting to make a strong case in the promotion of listening with the aim of truly understanding the other, the foundation not only of qualitative research but apparently a safer, more humane world. So how do we listen with the third ear, which is different or more than listening attentively?

What is critical, in order to understand another *is to suspend our assumptions, presuppositions, even our book knowledge and listen with what has been called the "third ear," the ear that is completely open, the ear that is opened to discovery and possibilities.* Let's imagine this ear is always clear of noise, the noise of "knowing."

We place what we think or think we know on the shelf, in a box, someplace out of the way of influencing our listening. In the example with the physician, the way some patients described, it sounds as though she listened to her patients from the perspective that they will be best served with palliative care. This did not make her a bad person, she truly believed in the value of what she was promoting. However, some patients did not feel heard.

Listening with the third ear, she would have listened to them, the way she wanted to be listened to, the way she wanted to be heard in spite of all that was known about her condition. So the "known" is not a part of this type of listening, it is suspended as we come "to know" this individual. This does take practice and you can practice with a colleague or observe the frequency of phrases that are spoken indicating assumptions. We are speaking with what we know when we ask or say, "Don't you think?", "I understand, I was in the same situation," "There is a book out on that very topic," and perhaps you can identify other remarks that indicate the introduction of knowledge on the listener's part. Recall the quotation in this chapter about the *illusion of knowledge as the greatest obstacle to discovery*, or where in the *experts mind there are few possibilities* because they are filled with knowing. In qualitative research we adopt a perspective of unknowing and let our research subjects/participants be the knowers, the knowledge holders, the holders of meaning in their experience.

Listening and Interviewing

In qualitative research, interviews or conversations are often the way qualitative researchers collect material from research participants. There is much written on interviewing and new researchers take this step very seriously with interview schedules of questions that often contradict the very intention of listening with third ear and being "unknowing." The questions contain content, theory, and the researcher's hunches.

If you were to adopt the "unknowing" stance you would not write interview questions with content information. They would all reflect that you are the "unknower" almost unable to know what questions would be relevant. Questions without content include: "Could you tell me about _____?" "What is it like for you?" ("was" if in the past), "What meaning did this experience have for you?" OK, here is a quiz question for you. What is wrong with that last question? It assumes that the person attributed meaning to an experience. Often people do not always think of the meaning of experience in a conscious way. When asked they reflect and then often come upon the meaning. That question would be better asked: "Does this (or "did this") experience have meaning for you?" Open-ended questions without subtle guiding in a direction toward openness are critical to "hearing" authentic language.

I think the best interview or conversation for qualitative research studies are started with one question, "Could you tell me what this is like for you?" ("what it was like", if in the past) and from then on, prompting with, "Go on", some encouragement, "That sounds _____" to mirror what the individual seems to be conveying, and "Tell me more about that." I would like to emphasize the importance of mirroring the person you are interviewing, paying important attention to non-verbal cues, such as facial expressions and body language. Then you are able to comment in a question that includes empathy such as: "that sounds so difficult for you." This acknowledgment of your sensitivity to their feelings will gain you trust.

Since this is an introductory chapter you will be coming to many examples and more content about interviewing, especially from a stance of "unknowing."

Other Ideas You Will Be Reading About for Understanding

Throughout this book you will read how critical it is to take into account the contingencies of the lives of individuals we are attempting to understand. The contingencies and the context from which the individual or group is situated is another reason why a predetermined intervention or protocol might not be successful or result in a "complication." When we do qualitative research we are cognizant of what we call the life worlds of individuals, how they perceive time and the history they are living through, how their bodies give them access to experience, the relationships they have with others, and the world and the space in which they are located. This is amplified in Chapter 5. The qualitative researcher knows that understanding does not exist in a vacuum, like the individual, it is embedded in experience, the context and the world.

Now the Crux: Understanding Another

"Sit down before fact like a little child, and be prepared to give up every preconceived notion, following humbly wherever and to whatever abyss nature leads, or you shall learn nothing"

(Huxley, as quoted in Dossey, 1982, p. 225).

To understand another and even yourself, it is essential to acknowledge your preconceptions, beliefs, intuitions, motives, biases, knowledge base and to be open to a whole new perception of another or yourself. This is also a critical component of the phenomenological perspective. As I say in the introductory remarks to Part II, I believe that this perspective and phenomenological philosophy guides and forms the underpinnings of most qualitative research methods. To conduct a study from any of the many qualitative methods it is essential to have an understanding of this philosophy. Critiques of qualitative studies often point to this lack. I think, what a shame, because understanding phenomenological philosophy is so very interesting and compelling. I would suggest at the outset of your study of qualitative research to make a commitment to understanding the philosophical underpinnings of phenomenology so that they show in your research study. That the reasoning of your study flows phenomenologically and is evident. I do not pretend to be a philosopher. I can even imagine a philosopher having a field day with my presentation. However I have tried to take very complex thinking to a place where the intent is understandable to most of us who have not been educated in philosophy.

Phenomenology is a philosophy that can not only guide your research but your interactions with others, your understanding of yourself and others, and can guide your practice as well. So in this introductory chapter I am just going to give you a taste of what is to come, going along with the metaphor, hoping to whet your appetite!

Underpinning Qualitative Research

The Phenomenological Perspective: The Study of the Meaning of Experience

I consider myself privileged to have had the opportunity through different venues to present and explain phenomenology and help make the underpinnings assessable to nurses, many of whom actually came to embrace this perspective. They often embrace it for research but also as a perspective for living and working. My own bias is that this philosophy is the foundation not only of qualitative research but also humanistic nursing practice. When I say assessable I mean, taking it from the arguments that the many philosophers make using language that often obfuscates rather than illuminates the underpinnings that can be useful to qualitative researchers. Philosophers themselves have accused Heidegger, one of these philosophers who is referenced often in this book, of incomprehensive writing.

My attempt in this book is to introduce you to the philosophy at an introductory level that is understandable without losing the richness of its complicatedness. Actually, I do not believe it is complicated like a calculus problem, rather it reflects life, and that life, of course, is complicated.

Not everyone as previously mentioned is going to do qualitative research. Many nurses are attracted to fact seeking, correlative, experimental, quantitatively oriented studies. And they are needed so this is not a conversion-seeking discussion. This is a philosophy that has as its central aim, to understand the meaning of experiences of other people, to understand how individuals are experiencing what they have been confronted with, both positive and negative. You will hear/read this in this book, especially in the exemplar chapters the voices of individuals and groups in their own contexts and language give voice to their experience. This is so very different than viewing something and reporting what you saw and coming to your own conclusions. This is research originating from the "knowers" themselves.

As nurses and nurse researchers we are often with people/patients at very vulnerable times and sometimes individuals are in fragile condition. The exemplars in the book include so many of those times: the experience of nurses during Katrina, Chapter 6; understanding the world of incarcerated women, Chapter 7; the experience of post-partum depression, Chapter 9; the experiences of low-income, urban, black mothers, Chapter 11; how the body grieves,

Chapter 13; understanding the value of nursing service, Chapter 15; how students experience practica, Chapter 17; and understanding what some of life is like for people with disabilities, Chapter 19.

It is critical that we learn the interior of these people and others like them. What is it that they are experiencing? This is based on the unique experience of the individual or group. This is based on understanding the individual and his or her needs. There are no textbooks or protocols that can predict how an individual will interpret his experience or reality. This is where we listen with the third ear. Using phenomenological philosophy as the basis of qualitative research is essential to grasping the meaning of these experiences.

The Road to Understanding: The Intersubjectiveness of "We-ness"

I do hope that the argument for the importance of understanding the uniqueness of another and their perception of an experience has been "understood." Part of phenomenological philosophy is the emphasis on perception and intersubjectivity, where two or more perceptions interact. This is an important part of qualitative research when we are attempting to understand others and also interpret our research material.

Perception

Perception is largely how we view the world and all its parts, how we view and think about phenomena, experiences, and the components of the world. Throughout the course of our individual development we have appropriated various beliefs, values, intuitions, preconceptions, assumptions, book knowledge, inherited knowledge from others, biases, and anything else that might add up to how we view anything in life, from the content of this book to the color blue. Perceptions that are built on prejudices and biases (also addressed in this book) can be extremely harmful. However, we all have biases and prejudices and this is important to acknowledge. When we attempt to understand another individual, everything mentioned that contributes to our perceptions, but especially prejudices and biases, are all to be held in abeyance. That is, to the extent possible for us, we disregard and place aside anything that has contributed to a perception. This step is essential, and for further emphasis I repeat essential to obtaining a true understanding of another person.

In addition "what *we* would do" in that person's situation also must be placed aside (this was exemplified in the example given in this chapter with palliative care for late stage cancer). What might be good for us, could be a disaster or inappropriate for another person.

So in phenomenological understanding, the *knower* is the person whom we are trying to understand. We should not question the validity of the knower. Whether we agree or disagree with their perception, our aim is to understand how this individual is viewing the experience. Whether we agree or disagree we should not be thinking parallel to or comparing our own perceptions to the person talking with us.

Intersubjectivity

Each of us has a subjective world, our own subjective worldview, our own window to interpreting the world and once again all that it holds. Residing in our subjective world or the subjective part of our consciousness are our perceptions. The other part of our consciousness is sometimes referred to as an objective world. We might define objectivity as agreed upon facts. Once again philosophers have argued about objectivity or lack of it for eons. Objective facts are supposedly immutable so we don't have to argue about them like our subjective world. However, we do know how many objective facts have not held up through time so we must be cautious with "facts."

In our education we have been told to be objective or to give an objective opinion. From my perspective these two ideas are going to wind up being subjective, because in the end "objectivity is a subjective notion." Because some subjective being determines the objective stance, what it means to be objective is thus a subjective call.

Here though we are speaking about intersubjectivity. What this means is when two or more people come together there is a melding of the different subjectivities. So when we are conversing, each person speaks from their own subjective world with their respective perceptions.

Giving voice to another without your own overlap in an attempt to understand their experience means, you acknowledge your subjective consciousness and as with perceptions hold them in abeyance. Place your subjectivity on the shelf and listen without the noise of self and with your third ear. That is the phenomenological idea of the use of intersubjectivity in the pursuit of understanding the experience of another.

Listening to the interpretation by others of their experiences, spoken or through narratives, and responding with thoughtfulness, respect, kindness, compassion, generosity, caring, and authenticity is the path to individualized nursing practice and management and of course qualitative research. Using the phenomenological perspective to listen keeps the noise out, so that individual's voices are heard as they are spoken and interpreted by first the speaker.

A Cautionary Tale

Many activities we see in qualitative research studies actually evolve from the quest to appear scientific with the capital S. Usually, they can be quickly identified, such as lists of themes with frequencies and lists of words used with frequencies. The caution here is not that these activities are not part of the process, but they must be accompanied with the variation of meanings. For example, when I say I have experienced anxiety over an event and someone else says she has as well, there is no way for a researcher to know anything more than that two people used the same word in a description. A qualitative researcher must explore the meaning and manifestations of what the perception of anxiety is to a particular person. Sometimes, for the sake of efficiency in communicating results, tables accomplish that; I certainly use tables when writing space is limited. But qualitative researchers should be careful that their reports are not numerical (numbers can be part of the overall results) but are interpretive and written mostly as narrative.

Choosing a Qualitative or Quantitative Research Study

Qualitative research in nursing in the 1980s was relatively new and was sometimes viewed skeptically. However the acceptance of its value and the number of nurse researchers who embrace qualitative research has been astounding. Science, with the capital "S", always seemed to be the goal, and it has been a long road for most nurse scholars to recognize the importance of qualitative research, which *is also scientific* in that there are as many, if not more, qualifications and characteristics to ascertain in effective and well-done qualitative research.

When qualitative research was first introduced into the field of nursing, many students erroneously thought that doing qualitative research might be easier and more manageable, especially for those who were more right-sided brain dominant. And for them, it would be easier only because they had the capacities. However, those who wanted "to finish as soon as possible" and mistakenly decided to do a qualitative study would think quite differently in retrospect. It is definitely not a contest in difficulty but should be a choice of intellectual fit. The difficulty of one or the other research method has more to do with one's propensity for the different ways of being, and those ways need to be considered paramount to choice.

Some of those unfortunate students who wanted to finish as soon as possible found themselves in the world of uncertainty, multiple interpretations, and mountains of interview notes or transcripts. Today, reflecting on your own best talents is the way to choose your method, and I hope that more faculty will develop the curriculum you need.

We used to say, and perhaps still do, that your method should be determined by your question. From more than 24 years of working with students on dissertations, I can see how some students seem natural doing either quantitative or qualitative research. The latest brain research supports why this is so. Today I would advise you *to start your research project with reflection on where your talents lie and capacities are at their best.* Your research interests can be studied from many perspectives, so choose the one that flows from the "how" you think, your worldview, your propensities, that is, what you do best!

Those who know they are definitely going to be quantitative researchers need to understand this alternative worldview and how their qualitative colleagues will approach objectivity and subjectivity, for instance. It makes for rich conversations and understanding of one another's work because both worldviews are equally essential to nursing research.

Earlier I mentioned how the conversation on qualitative research expands in each new edition of this textbook. One critical question I want to discuss here (and in Chapter 5) is the question of the significance of qualitative research.

The Significance of Qualitative Research

Part of the intrigue of qualitative research is understanding a "newness," a very different negotiation of meaning. What I value about qualitative research is that I am constantly amazed about and awakened to new ways of being. I find that through the beginning stance of qualitative research, the "unknowing" stance, often what I "knew" cannot be substantiated, that preconceptions are often biased, that assumptions have been nothing but myth or prejudice upholding them, and that practice thought scientific is just ordinary tradition without evidence to support the practice. Qualitative research seeks new possibilities, frees us from the bonds of biases, allows us to understand what was a mystery beforehand and searches for the significance and the meaning of being.

Qualitative research methods have the potential to free us from these erroneous preconceptions, raise our consciousness, encourage emancipation, and even lift many from oppression (the exemplar chapters all have implications of oppression resulting from being misunderstood). How can I communicate how critical qualitative research is when it has all this potential? Here, my own language fails me. A paradigm that searches for meaning from the perspective of the individual or searches for what can give meaning to an experience sometimes defies description. *It is almost ethereal*, while maintaining the rigor of science.

Qualitative nurse researchers return the following through their research to practice, among many other things:

- Caring for the individual
- Legitimization
- Understanding of experience
- Acceptance
- Change
- Emancipation
- Compassion
- Understanding of meaning, whether experiential or spiritual
- Empathy

- Understanding the needs of individuals and groups
- Critical needs for policy and healthcare changes
- Meaning, description, and interpretation to generate hypotheses
- Generation of theory from the source, the individual or their culture

Qualitative nurse researchers want to provide the following to the knowledge base of nursing, among other things:

- Discovery
- Description
- Explanation
- Interpretation
- Critique
- Justice and Equality for Health and Social Policy
- Understanding
- Sensitization
- Emancipation
- The meaning of being within and among various cultures, genders, and religions
- Grounded theory
- Direction toward improving the quality of life for all people

The work of qualitative nurse researchers offers to us, through the interpretation of meaning and experience, as well as the critique of the researcher's own results, an expanding and wakeful consciousness of others and the self.

I would suggest to you, that after you read each exemplar chapter of a specific method in this text, as well as other qualitative research reports, you ask yourself, "What did this qualitative study result in?" Here, I do not mean for you to specify the specific results, but to decide whether there was an increase in understanding, a different way of perceiving an experience unknown to you prior to reading the study, a critique of an accepted practice, and/or an interpretation of experience otherwise not known to you. *We search for a significance*, different from statistical, that raises the consciousness to meaning. This meaning has the capacity to change the quality of life for all concerned. The significance of our research informs us how to make this world a better, more ethical, safe, equalitarian, and humane place for all of us.

Postscript

Remember what was written in the Prologue, and go back to other editions of this text for different interpretations of methods and different exemplars. Also recall, the beginner's mind as a place where endless creativity and openness to new and exciting possibilities can change the way you view understanding others and yourself, as well. Enjoy!

References

Andersen, K. (2009). The avenging amateur. *TIME, 8*(10), 68.

Anderson, W. (1995). *The truth about truth.* New York: Putnam.

Beneloiel, J. (1984, March). Advancing nursing science: Qualitative approaches. *Western Journal of Nursing Research in Nursing and Health, 7,* 1–8.

Bohm, D. (1985). *Unfolding meaning.* New York: Routledge.

Carter, R. (2008). *Multiplicity: The new science of personality, identity and the self.* New York: Little, Brown and Company.

Dilthey, W. (1926). *Meaning in history.* London: Allen and Unwin.

Dossey, L. (1982). *Space, time and medicine.* Boulder, CO: Shambhala.

Hartocollis, A. (2010). Helping patients face death, she fought to live. *The New York Times, 4*(4), A1.

Kuhn, T. S. (1970). *The structure of scientific revolutions.* Chicago: University of Chicago Press.

Paterson, J. A., & Zderad, L. J. (1976, reissued 1988). *Humanistic nursing.* New York: National League for Nursing.

Pink, D. (2005). *A whole new mind: Moving from the information age to the conceptual age.* New York: Riverhead Books.

Stolorow, R., & Atwood, G. (2002). *Contexts of being: The intersubjective foundations of psychological life.* Hillsdale, NJ: Analytic Press.

Additional Resources

Bohm, D. (1998). *On creativity.* New York: Routledge.

Heidegger, M. (1962). *Being and time.* San Francisco: Harper & Row. (Original work published 1927)

Morse, J. (2004). Editorial: Qualitative significance. *Qualitative Health Research, 14*(2), 151–152.

Morse, J. (2004). Editorial: Using the right tool for the job. *Qualitative Health Research, 14*(8), 1029–1031.

Munhall, P. (1994). *Revisioning Phenomenology: Nursing and Health Science Research.* Sudbury, MA: Jones and Bartlett.

Ricoeur, P. (1998). *Critique and conviction.* New York: Columbia University Press.

Smith, D. W., & Thomasson, A. L. (2005). *Phenomenology and philosophy of mind.* New York: Oxford University Press.

Stolorow, R., Atwood, G., & Orange, D. (2002). *Worlds of experience.* New York: Basic Books.

van Manen, M. (2002). *Writing in the dark: Phenomenological studies in interpretive inquiry.* Ontario, Canada: Althouse Press.

Watson, J. (1999). Postmodern Nursing and Beyond. New York: Churchill Livingstone.

2

Language and Nursing Research: The Evolution

Patricia L. Munhall

Discussing or talking is the way in which we articulate significantly the intelligibility of Being-in-the-world. The way in which discourse gets expressed is Language.
—M. Heidegger, Being and Time

So the main function of a language symbol is not to stand for or represent an object to which it corresponds. Rather, it initiates a total movement of memory, imagery, ideas, feelings, and reflexes, which serves to order attention to and direct action in a new mode that is not possible without the use of such symbols.
—D. Bohm, On Creativity

Being in the world holds many challenges for those nurse researchers who embark on the path of discovery through qualitative research designs or methods. One of these challenges has to do with the limits and power of language. Our world is narrated and organized through language. The use of language is one way in which we communicate meaning. We also experience moments when we cannot find the language to express a feeling, an emotion, or a response. So our language at once allows expression and also constrains expression. In the very way that we narrate with language, the particulars of our context, personal, social, and cultural agendas are set. So too in our research language: Values, beliefs, and aims are communicated from which varying meanings of being in the world will evolve.

For many years, nurse researchers and theorists have engaged in a lively and enlightening dialogue of various paradigms, the two most common being the logical positivist or empirical-analytic paradigm and the contrasting one, phenomenology. This dialogue was prompted by many nurse researchers who initiated what was to become an "interpretive turn" in nursing research (Munhall, 1989). These nurse theorists and researchers began to raise these questions:

- Was nursing a natural science, like that of chemistry and biology, and therefore based on similar linguistic assumptions?
- Was nursing a human science based on differing linguistic assumptions?
- Was nursing research ready for a poststructuralist perspective? (Dzurec, 1989)

The purpose of this chapter is to illustrate the words and perspectives that gave rise to these discussions and the evolution of nursing research. You will most likely see that much of the same language is relevant in today's historical context. Nursing language is both concealing and revealing of the stances and perspective that we pose to nursing as we interact with the phenomenon of concern. For some nurse researchers, this discussion will be historical because they have chosen one paradigm over another for various reasons. For other nurse researchers, it will also be historical because they see a postmodern perspective of multiple research paradigms as not only acceptable but essential.

At this point in time, many nurse researchers are encouraging moving beyond what they see as an unruly dualism between what in the early 1980s was structured as a debate. The debate was centered on two different research paradigms, the quantitative and the qualitative. These two research paradigms were often compared and contrasted, elucidating their different philosophical underpinnings. However, it remains extremely important to students studying qualitative research at the outset to become familiar with some of the fundamental and basic assumptions, beliefs, and outcomes of these two paradigms. Using the concreteness of placing paradigms in stark relief to one another should be of assistance to our beginning understanding of various worldviews.

In this chapter, we will see, in the form of contrasting systems of language, competing articulations in other fields as well as our own that are characteristic of various philosophical orientations. This particular focus on philosophical analysis is further elucidated in Chapters 3, 4, and 5.

Research in nursing is at the center of this linguistic exploration. Methods of doing research are still divided into two purportedly ideological (and thus far considered conflicting) schools of thought with two distinct language systems. These schools of thought have been categorized as the qualitative and quantitative approaches to research.

By quantitative methods of research we mean the traditional scientific methods as presented in most of the contemporary nursing research textbooks. These methods are characterized by deductive reasoning, objectivity, quasi-experiments, statistical techniques, and control. On the other hand, qualitative methods are characterized as employing inductive reasoning, subjectivity, discovery, description, and process orienting (Reichardt & Cook, 1979). The outcome, depending on the method, can be derived from description, interpretation, and analysis (Ashworth, 1997).

This chapter explores a qualitative-quantitative dichotomy and perhaps will appear culpable of unnecessary polarization. This is done for a pedagogical advantage of clearly revealing the possible differences between these two research traditions. I hope to resolve this polarization as the third chapter of this book begins. In that chapter a cyclical continuum is suggested that finds its origins in qualitative research and its validation in quantitative research. Advocating a cyclical continuum is congruent with calls to move beyond the debate, and thus enter post-positivism and reconciliation (Clark, 1998).

The present chapter begins with a discussion of the living aspect of language and then progresses to a contextual analysis of nursing research. The purpose is to ferret out the meanings of our linguistic expressions, their origins, and subsequent propulsions. This motion of transition from nursing's earliest identification with medicine represents a broad worldview transition or paradigmatic shift. Nursing research and the quest for nursing theory development are discussed from the perspective of language development and language usage as we seek out the pattern and process to articulate our meaning and experience.

Language and Lived Experience

Long before children speak actual words, they have learned effectively to express their physical, mental, and emotional states of being. Very early in our childhood we learn that laughing, crying, pouting, and looking quizzical stimulate a response from those who are "significant others." We are indeed beginning to learn the power of expressive language (Wells, 1985).

Eventually, we begin to develop a vocabulary and, interestingly, by the time we are 2 years of age or so, we have learned to treasure the word "no." Individuation, assertiveness, posturing, and a continuing desire for power in our environment render this one of the most important words in any language. People have written entire books on how, when, and where to say "no" effectively (Coventry & Garrod, 2005).

Nursing as a profession, concomitantly with women as a social force, is still very much involved in those processes of individuation, assertiveness, posturing, and claiming power in our environment. Like the significance of the word no, our language and the use of specific sets of words simultaneously reveal and conceal who we are, both to ourselves and to the world at large.

Thus, in our quest for individuation and, we might add, our autonomy (auto-**no**-my), we are in the process of developing a language system that defines our particular role with our clients. This focus on autonomy correlates well with the point of the revelatory and concealing power of language and the exemplary word no. Nursing has claimed the power to say no through the Greek word autonomous (*autos*–"self" and *nomos*–law or rule), meaning self-ruling. Whenever the Greek suffix *nomos* appears in an English word associated with a human quality, it addresses the rule of right or privilege that has been attributed to the prefix. Using autonomy as an example, "I have a right to be self-determined."

The living of autonomy expresses the position of a profession and, in nursing, has called attention to our transition from the physician's handmaiden (just look at that word!) to an independent self-ruling practitioner. This posturing of ourselves is consistently illustrated in our transition from the primary usage of medical language to our concerted efforts to develop a nursing language, taxonomy, nomenclature, and nursing diagnostic system.[1]

The moment-to-moment language that we choose defines the posture or stance that we assume in the space that we believe is ours in the healthcare _____ (fill in the blank from the choices below):

1. system
2. arena
3. delivery system
4. field

For example, in the preceding multiple-choice option, we find it most interesting to study such words in their starkness for their literal or metaphorical meaning. Is health care "delivered"? Is there a "system" of health care? The word *arena*, which is frequently used with health care, is a word that is often associated with a circus or sports. (The temptation is too great to resist pointing out how that word, with its noted association, may be the most apt description of the present so-called healthcare system.) The word *sports* is also associated with the word *field*, where many games are played, with winners and losers. So, of these words, which one or two or perhaps one not mentioned would characterize, for you, the reader, the state of health care today?

Each profession creates its own language, and nursing is no different. The language of nursing reveals how nurses view the phenomena of their experiences. The symbols that we choose as expressions expose our assertions, propositions, assumptions, beliefs, values, and priorities either implicitly or explicitly. The significance of such expressions manifests in our emergence:

Our expressions bring us into existence. The *noumenal*, or "thing in itself," depends on the phenomenal for its expression.

DeVries (1983) succinctly and humorously illustrated the noumenal emerging from felt obscurity into shared, understood experience in the following passage:

> In the beginning was the word. Once terms like identity doubts and midlife crisis become current, the reported cases of them increase by leaps and bounds, affecting people unaware there is anything wrong with them until they have got a load of the coinages. You too may have an acquaintance or even a relative with a block about paper hanging or dog grooming, a high flown form of stagnation trickled down from writers and artists. Once my poor dear mother confided to me in a hollow whisper, "I have an identity crisis." I say, "How do you mean?" and she says, "I no longer understand your father." Now we have burnout, and having heard tell of it on television or read about it in a magazine, your plumber doubts he can any longer hack it as a pipefitter, while a glossary adopted by his wife has turned him overnight into . . . a male chauvinist pig, something she would never have suspected before. (p. 4)

Satire in the preceding quotation is a useful adjunct to disclosing how concepts develop. Concepts such as "midlife crisis" have a sturdy sound to them. Such concepts seem to have existed like trusted monikers for more years than people can remember. However, midlife crisis was not coined until 1965 (Jaques, 1965). Long before 1965, Carl Jung and others had intimated a maturation crisis as occurring between ages 40 and 60, but Jaques gave it the name. Certainly the "thing itself" (the noumenon) existed before 1965. It was felt; yet we needed the description and language of shared experience to connect us within the world and provide a way of perceiving the phenomenon.

Writers of fiction provided glimpses of the noumenon called midlife crisis years prior to 1965. For example, Willa Cather (1873–1947), an American novelist, described the noumenon of midlife crisis on several occasions. In Book 1 ("The Family") of her novel, *The Professor's House*, Cather (2001) described an existential release from the claustrophobia of the family's home that creative writing provided the character of the professor. We see further examples below of how "something existed", an experience not yet named, has come into our common parlance by creating expressions of the experience through language.

1. Codependency (late 1970s, Beatty, 1989)
2. Deficit spending or "budgetary deficit" (Keynes, 1936)
3. Post-Traumatic Shock Syndrome (PTSS)

4. Premenstrual syndrome (serious study of PMS followed Brozan, 1982)
5. Attention Deficit Disorder (ADD)

Moreover, the proliferation of support groups for various conditions of life as well as the many 12-step programs speak to our need for shared language to connect us with one another within the world. The Internet has provided many ways of using language, ranging from informational purposes to allowing language to connect one human being to another once again. Blogs (Web logs) help form virtual communities. We now can find groups of people who believe and speak the same language, spending hours a day and "unqualitatively" most of the time substantiating their common beliefs.

An emerging field of graduate study today is Narrative Medicine, where people through their own personal experience gives voice to their experience through language that is made available to others. This assists those who identify with the experience so as not to feel alone or isolated in that experience or to assist others in understanding the trials and challenges of that experience. The qualitative method of Narrative Inquiry as illustrated in Chapters 16 and 17 demonstrates these purposes through research.

Language as Points of Contact

The various forms of language that we use, as with all disciplines, bring human experience into emergence. We need to recognize and articulate our points of contact in this pluralistic world, and we need referents to nursing phenomena in language to hold a recognized place in that world. Qualitative research is poised with its emphasis on language and meaning to assist us in understanding the meaning of our various places in experience.

For example, the word *undeveloped*, describing Third World countries, was judged to be a pejorative adjective and was discontinued. The word *emerging* was used instead to describe these countries and to express optimism. Our emergence, like that of children and emerging countries, will depend on our ability to express ourselves clearly within the context of this pluralistic world. Let us look at the lived experience of nursing through a contextual analysis of our language development.

The Context of Nursing Research

Stolorow and Atwood (2002) argue that there can be no meaning without context, and they question the myth of the isolated mind. Allen (1995) encourages us to recognize the social, political, and historical location in the role of nursing research. The historical context in which individuals live places them in a world specific to that time and place, of contingencies that must be recognized and acknowledged if research or discourse is to be meaningful (Rorty, 1991). So it appears appropriate, especially in a text on qualitative research that readily acknowledges and embodies its search within the context of "things," that we begin this exploration of language in nursing research by attending to the context in which it has occurred and is continuing to evolve.

Context is defined as "that which leads up to and follows and often specifies the meaning of a particular expression" and "the circumstances in which a particular event occurs" (*American Heritage Dictionary*, 1992). I believe that within this definition of context the following three antecedents and their evolutionary-concurrent factors should be acknowledged:

1. Research in nursing evolved predominantly when nursing education became a part of higher education and was seeking its own body of knowledge, different from that of medicine.
2. Nursing's first researchers were being prepared in fields other than nursing and have brought to nursing the various paradigms from those fields.
3. Derivation and/or deduction for nursing research was (is) being drawn from disciplines other than nursing. Each factor will be explored from the perspective of its contributions to our nursing research language.

Transition in Worldviews of Nursing

During the 1950s, as an outgrowth of the development and acceptance of new theoretical approaches to understanding physical and human phenomena emerging from other fields (approaches such as systems perspectives, quantum physics, adaptation, and ecological views), nurse scholars began questioning the prevalent acceptance and alignment of the medical model as the basis for nursing practice. Nursing was also entering the university setting at that time. These two historical events converged, and the need for our own distinct body of knowledge, a benchmark of a profession and the research imperative of the university, spurred a revolution in nursing.

These two factors, the acknowledgment of a major scientific revolution in other disciplines as well as our own, and the desire to attain a level of professionalism at which we would base practice on a distinct body of nursing knowledge, led to a perceptual shift in the way that we spoke about nursing phenomena and simultaneously led to the scientific investigation of nursing phenomena.[2] It seemed, though, that the way in which we spoke about nursing and the way in which we investigated nursing phenomena often reflected assumptions, propositions, beliefs, and priorities of two different worldviews, the first reflecting one worldview and the other reflecting a different worldview. We will see shortly that this is a characteristic of paradigmatic shift within a discipline.

The spoken language in nursing began to change, reflecting this perceptual shift from the medical, atomistic, causal model to a distinct nursing, holistic, interactive model. This represented a paradigmatic innovation for nursing. The way in which phenomena were viewed in nursing was changing in a way that was considered by some to be irrevocably conflictual in its basic premises and assumptions with the medical model.

This shift, which was well recognized in the discipline of physics, began to permeate the language of other fields as well as nursing. The change is representative of a transition from a mechanistic to an organismic perspective, from the reliance on objectivity to intersubjectivity, and from the received view to a nonreceived view (Watson, 1981). Today, Watson, Dossey, & Dossey (1999) urge us farther "away from the reaction worldview, past the reciprocal and into the transformative-simultaneous" and urge nurses to create nursing's own postmodern paradigm. Many of the qualitative methods of research, before the language of postmodernism became commonplace, have as underpinnings many of the values and beliefs of postmodernism.

Illumination of the differences between and among these worldviews and/or paradigms can be demonstrated in the scrutiny of the respective language systems. It seems appropriate, though, to be clear at this point as to what a worldview or paradigm is. Patton (1978), in terms consistent with those of Kuhn (1970), defines a paradigm as follows: "A worldview, a general perspective, a way of breaking down the complexity of the real world. As such, paradigms are deeply embedded in the socialization of adherents and practitioners: paradigms tell them what is important, legitimate and reasonable" (p. 203).

If we accept the premise that things come into being through language, the language paradigm of a discipline will tell the practitioner what is important, legitimate, and reasonable. Kuhn (1970) suggests that a paradigm is a discipline's specific method of solving a puzzle, of viewing human experience, and of structuring reality. It is a worldview, a way of viewing phenomena in the world.

Laudan (1977), in a similar vein, uses the phrase "research tradition" to communicate the same theme: "A research tradition . . . is a set of assumptions about the basic kinds of entities in the world, assumptions about how these entities interact, assumptions about the proper methods to use for constructing and testing theories about these entities" (p. 97). Morgan (1983) calls our attention to the significance of these assumptions. He states: "Assumptions make messes researchable, often at the cost of great simplification, and in a way that is highly problematic" (p. 377).

This reference about assumptions becomes more powerful when, as Morgan suggests, researchers choose their *own* assumptions on which to base their studies. One could then say that this latitude enables the means for achieving what the researcher values. In the paradigms introduced in this chapter are assumptions about the world, believed in some way to be true, though they are actually the "taken-for-granted" views of human scientists. In a fundamental sense, then, researchers choose the values, "truths," and perspectives on which they base their research endeavors.

Another way of expressing this shift was the idea that nursing was a human science. Nursing seems to be philosophically expressed through language to be compatible with the ideas and concepts of a human science. German philosopher–historian Wilhelm Dilthey (1926; as translated in Atwood & Stolorow, 1993) held these critical assumptions about a human science:

- "The supreme category of the human sciences is meaning" (p. 2).
- "The natural sciences investigate objects from the outside whereas the human sciences rely on a perspective from the inside" (p. 2).
- "The central emphasis in the natural sciences is upon causal explanation: The task of inquiry in the human sciences is interpretation and understanding" (p. 2).

Our transition in worldviews then seems to have moved from a narrowly defined type of science to a much broader connection of what constitutes science. However, in that broader view, there remain two very distinct sciences: natural science and human science. Some would even question the idea of a human science, if using the strict parochial rules of science. However, as the human sciences have evolved, there is little doubt that they have legitimated their place as a science, one with a different philosophy from the philosophy of natural science.

The Language of Worldviews

What follows are expressions belonging to different ways of viewing phenomena (worldviews). The language reveals different assumptions, beliefs, and values concerning human and physical reality. In essence, the paradigm or research tradition is a philosophy: It conceptualizes fundamental beliefs. For this reason, the research paradigm as a puzzle-solving method should be congruent with the discipline's larger paradigm, that is, the paradigm of nursing or nursing's philosophy.

Although this idea of congruency is not held as essential by all researchers, the most sophisticated or reasonable response to any either-or discussion would be to choose a dialectic approach (Moccia, 1988; Morgan, 1983). This approach, as Morgan (1983) states, "also accepts the diversity of assumption and knowledge claims as an inevitable future of research and attempts to use the competing perspectives as a means of constructing new modes of understanding" (p. 379). A postmodern perspective would transcend the either-or stalemate as an unnecessary obstacle to understanding and would beg the question with an emphasis on plurality of perspectives, which would be context dependent.

To assist students in understanding the different language systems of various fields, the tables included in this chapter present language in stark relief. They are purposely presented to demonstrate the different meaning systems and are more for explicitness than for the subtleties that, of course, also can be discussed. Each of the five tables (Tables 2–1 through Table 2–5) of paradigmatic-type language presents two contrasting belief systems. The language of the systems in the left-hand columns is often the same language or, if not literally the same, it is at least consistent in syntax and meaning, reflecting the underlying continuity of beliefs, values, and assumptions. The same continuity in language will be observed in the systems presented in the right-hand columns of the tables. The observations are important when we take into account that the paradigm preserves and perpetuates the disciplinary matrix of a field (Kuhn, 1970).

A major premise that this text suggests is that the language expressed in the left-hand columns and found within the paradigms of the mechanistic, the realists, the received view, behaviorism, and the medical model is consistent with the scientific method or quantitative research. In contrast, the language expressed in the right-hand columns reflects the paradigms of the organismic, the idealists, the nonreceived view, humanism, and many nursing models and is consistent with qualitative research methods.

We know well that there are more cultures than the two described by Snow (1959, 1993) in *The Two Cultures and the Scientific Revolution*. Today, there are hundreds, and there are disciplines and subdisciplines of those disciplines. Often, the subdisciplines of a discipline speak in foreign tongues to one another. For this reason, it is important to understand the overall fundamental differences so that we may intelligently see what Kirby (1983) calls "the points of contact in a plural world." Illustrating the plurality of worldviews, he optimistically states that "there could be an underlying unity . . . and thus a single earth-centered perspective from which all problems may be viewed" (p. 25). Three decades later, which is just a blip on the time screen, we have yet to come to this perspective. The following tables and the language should illustrate the fundamental differences. Perhaps the reader can surmise possible points of contact and propose an alliance where all sorts of evidence will contribute to the richness of our comprehension and our ability to make sense of the world around us.

Paradigms in Psychology

It has been said that all contemporary psychological systems are derivative of either the mechanistic or the organismic paradigms (Looft, 1973; see **Table 2-1**). Many philosophers and psychologists argue that the assumptions of each are unbridgeable. Either humans are reactive organisms, as Skinner (1953) would have them, or individuals are active and thinking organisms, as Piaget (1970) would predicate. One lays before us a thesis; the other, an antithesis.

The reader is asked to contemplate the differences in meaning as expressed in the descriptive language of the mechanistic and the organismic paradigms of psychology (see Table 2-1).

Are the perspectives unbridgeable? With these paradigms, as well as the ones that follow, discussion about the bridgeability of these perspectives should prove lively and fruitful.

Paradigms in Philosophy

Filstead (1979, p. 34) states that at the core of the distinction between the quantitative and qualitative methods of research lies the classical argument in philosophy between the schools of realism and idealism and their subsequent derivatives (**Table 2-2**). The Baconian reality of "seeing is believing" led to believing in the "real" as the only reality about which one could be positive. Hence, those who ascribed to that belief system were called "positivist." When reality could be held static, observations made, and experiments performed, science was done and the truth revealed. Those philosophers who questioned this positivist logic and method of science when it was applied to the understanding of human beings became known as "idealists" (Kneller, 1964). Today, the same questions asked by the idealists have been amplified by postmodernists. Science is no longer absolute or the final truth. Science is

TABLE 2-1 Paradigms in Psychology

Mechanistic	Organismic
Human being reacts and responds to the environment	Human being acts on and creates the meaning of an experience
Predictable response sets from human beings can be determined	Understanding comes from individual human perspective—variable responses
Empirical reality	Social construction of reality
One reality—same rules	Dynamic reality—different responses
Human beings can be controlled	Human beings are self-determined
Behavior—should be prescribed	Behavior—many possibilities acceptable and desirable

TABLE 2–2   Paradigms in Philosophy

Realism	Idealism
Static conception of world	Evolving conception of world
Seeing is believing	Truth as interpretation
Logical positivism	Dynamic, chaotic world
Social world as given	Social world as created
Independent physical reality	Reality is mentally perceived—sense perception
"At face value"	Approximate representational fit
Semantic truth-condition	Semantic relativism
Judgment-independent	Contingencies matter

an ever-changing body of ideas, and we have daily shifts about beliefs. The whole concept of universality and generalizability is put into question. We have come to see that "being in the world" may be more aptly stated as "beings-in-the-worlds." There are multiple worlds, multiple realities, and multiple perspectives (Anderson, 1995).

Although the idealists acknowledged the existence of a physical reality, they argued that the mind was the creator and source of knowledge. In addition to the language expressed in Table 2-2 from the idealist school, the following short Zen parable is indicative of idealists' ideas and the place of human perception (*Zen Buddhism*, 1959):

> One windy day two monks were arguing about the flapping banner. The first said, "I say the banner is moving, not the wind." The second said, "I say the wind is moving, not the banner." A third monk passed by and said, "The wind is not moving. The banner is not moving. Your minds are moving." (p. 52)

Although briefly presented, inherent here is the great debate between the objective and subjective means of knowing. We are about to see now how research methods as worldviews are an inherent outgrowth of a philosophical worldview that precedes it and establishes its epistemological ways of coming to know about the world.

Subsequent Paradigms in Epistemology

Flowing from the paradigms of philosophy should be congruent paradigms or research traditions for the way in which each school of thought establishes how it comes to know about its particular account of the world. Epistemology is the branch of philosophy that concerns itself with the nature of knowledge. Each school of philosophy will have an epistemology. In other words, each belief system will have a congruent belief system about coming to know about the world and the nature of knowledge.

For our purposes, the realist philosophy is connected with the epistemological paradigm of the received view, and the idealist is connected with the nonreceived view (**Table 2–3**). I must acknowledge at this point or perhaps call attention to this very simplified version of what is most complex to philosophers. We are examining the gist of language differences, yet I strongly recommend further study in this area for those who are interested in greater in-depth knowledge. (Chapters 3 and 4 provide a further base to this aspect of the discussion.)

The expressions of the received view are those of the positivists and/or realists (Suppe, 1977; Watson, 1981). They are consistent with the scientific method[3] and are representative of expressions found most often in our present nursing research texts. The nonreceived view of coming to know about nursing phenomena is emerging, and those expressions are found in the language of qualitative epistemology as well as most nursing philosophies.

Paradigms in Education

The mechanistic and organismic paradigms are reflected in the field of education as behaviorism and humanism (**Table 2–4**). Learning theories emerging from these two paradigms are distinctively different because they are reflective of differing beliefs, values, and assumptions about the world and the nature of human beings. You may find it interesting here to reflect on which paradigm is more prevalent in nursing education and discuss the relative merits of each and, again, the bridgeability or points of contact (Munhall, 1992).

TABLE 2–3   Paradigms in Epistemology

Received View	Nonreceived View
Logical positivism	Uncertainty
Materialism	Mental perception
Reductionism	Holism
Laws—quantification	Patterns—qualification
Predictions	Interpretations
Objectivity	Subjectivity
Neutrality	Human values
Operationalization	Context integration
Knowing something	Understanding meaning
Determinism, immutable	Variability, interpretations most possible

TABLE 2–4   Paradigms in Education

Behaviorism	Humanism
Homogeneous group	Heterogeneous group
Human reactiveness	Human activeness
Human malleability	Self-determination
Human passiveness	Unique interpretation of reality
Objectivity	Subjectivity
Shaping concrete behavior	Changes in consciousness
Measurable outcomes	Hoped-for outcomes—variable and many non-measurable
Preparation for specific roles	
Behavior must disclose state(s) of mind	Preparation for world at large
Can be conditioned to react	Behaviors and state(s) of mind may vary
Experience reduced to measurement	Reactions chosen by individuals
	Experience resists uniform measurement

Paradigms in the Health Professions

Table 2–5 seems to reflect nursing's congruity with the preceding paradigms of the organismic, the idealists, the nonreceived view, and humanism. In contrast, the language of medicine seems to be congruent with the mechanistic, the realists, the received view, and behaviorism. It seems important to note, then, that our language system is congruent with some paradigms and not logically consistent with other paradigms. This is particularly relevant when we acknowledge that each paradigm should have a compatible research paradigm or method. The relevance is demonstrated in the philosophical paradigms of the realistic and idealistic and in the concomitant epistemological paradigms of the received view and nonreceived view, respectively. The languages of the medical model and most nursing models are readily distinguishable as to their perspectives, worldviews, tradition, or paradigms.

It is important to return here to our first consideration: "Research in nursing evolved predominantly when nursing was in transition between broad philosophic worldviews." The language presented in Table 2–5 as the language of medicine was for a long time that of nursing. When the worldview for nursing began changing, as reflected in proposed nursing models, the activity of nursing research concomitantly was under way. Ironically, the research activities that occurred in a parallel fashion often were not congruent with the premises of the nursing model. However, this incongruity is quite understandable when we review the second consideration in our language development: Researchers in nursing were being prepared in fields other than nursing.

TABLE 2–5   Paradigms in Health Professions

Medicine	Nursing
Reductionism—treating the part; treating the symptom	Holism—care for the whole person, whether "sick" or well, person as integrated whole: more than sum of parts
Reactive human being—reacts as prescribed	Active human being—transformative and chooses action
Physical symptomatology	Integrated human being
Linear causality—cause and effect	Multiple interaction—self, others, environment, cosmos
Closed system	Open system
Steady state	Dynamic
Objective	Subjective
Manipulation	Self-determination
Control	Choice
Paternalism	Advocacy
Standardized protocols	Divergent trajectories

Early Preparation of Nurse Researchers

It is so commonplace today that our nurse scholars and researchers have doctorate degrees in nursing that we need to reflect on the influence of the earlier doctoral preparation of nurses. Before the opening of specific nursing doctoral programs in the United States, nurse faculty and others sought this degree in other disciplines that seemed to relate to nursing. On completing these degrees, many of those doctorally prepared nurses began to think of developing nursing's own degree, a doctoral degree in nursing. Because our doctoral education evolved in this way, we will proceed to examine its influence rather than discuss the merits and limitations of such evolution.

The outcome was the development of a community of nurse researchers who were educated in the better-established disciplines and who subsequently developed a commitment to that discipline's research method (Chinn, 1983; Corbin, 1999). Although this development offered nursing a wide array of methods from which to choose, it soon appeared evident that the scientific method, with its own language, was adopted to such an extent that, Watson (1981) reported, "The scientific method is considered the one and only process for scientific discovery, experimental quantitative research methodology and design" (p. 414). Swanson and Chenitz (1982) state: "While nursing exists almost exclusively in the empirical social world, the profession uses the laboratory method of the basic sciences in its research design" (p. 241).

Norris (1982) attributes this supremacy of the scientific method in part to nursing's "desperate attempt" to become a legitimate science by embracing the experimental research model as the way to proceed. Indeed, science and scientific cannot be considered neutral words (if there are such words). In today's world, they are extensively value laden as expressing truth, goodness, worthwhileness, and legitimacy. Kaplan (1964) emphasizes this legitimacy point: "There are behavioral scientists who in their desperate search for scientific status give the impression that they don't much care what they do if only they do it right: substance gives way to form" (p. 406).

However, as Norris (1982) points out in a discussion of nursing's leap to experimental research, many nurse researchers are hampered by the lack of concept clarification, theory development, and descriptive methods of research, all of which are linked to qualitative research methods. Norris (1982) observes that, during the period from 1958 to 1975, nursing scholars made a concerted effort to develop a body of nursing knowledge without the necessary training in the methods of concept clarification, which are prerequisite to experimental research. This "scientific" influence continues to exercise its exclusivity, as is evidenced in the following scenario (Tinkle & Beaton, 1983):

> It was her first dissertation committee meeting. The topic of discussion was the proposed research methodology. Two of the committee members (well-known for their "hard" research) began to dialogue about the "softness" of the approach in the proposal before them—the lack of control, the lack of quantitative measurement, and the lack of manipulation of variables. Before long, the committee was in accord about the relatively low scientific merit of this type of research methodology as opposed to an experimental approach. The student found herself agreeing to shift her methodology to one involving experimental manipulation. (p. 27)

What makes this anecdote relevant almost 3 decades later is that, in some colleges of nursing, this belief system has become even more prominent. The status and sometimes the requirement to attain National Institute of Nursing Research (NINR) or National Institutes of Health funding to advance, obtain a position, and even earn tenure demonstrate how fundamental to the research enterprise this commitment to "hard" science is.

Downs (1982) observed in response to a similar theme: "This distorted value system rode in on the coattails of the idea that scientific method was equivalent to experimental research" (p. 4). Bronowski (1965), with a broader conception of science, surpasses this narrow view of the scientific method and enlarges the aperture. Science, he says, is: "Nothing else than the search to discover unity in the world variety of nature or . . . in the variety of our experiences. Poetry, painting, the arts are the same search" (p. vi).

In a cogent argument for a poststructural perspective, Dzurec (1989) comments on the tenacity of logical positivist methodology in nursing:

> The period beginning in the 1960s and stretching to today is perhaps the first in which the power relations in nursing and in human sciences in general have allowed the recognition of logical positivism as a single philosophy of science rather than as science itself. (p. 74)

However, we do know that our worldview has opened to allow for other methods of research. Coming to know and coming to discover rather than verify have become acknowledged as essential to the base of nursing knowledge.

Watson (1981) attributes this increased acknowledgment to the same processes of scientific development that have taken place in other sciences. She states that our commonality with other fields lies in the process of first adopting the received-view idea and then undergoing processes of rejection of that particular paradigm. We would not advocate the abandonment of all the characteristics of the received view or the scientific method, but two important points need to be made about the early preparation of nurse researchers (and, to a large extent, the present preparation of nurse researchers). These points are still discussed today and will lead us into the next contextual consideration (Ashworth, 1997; Clark, 1998; Watson, Dossey, & Dossey, 1999). They are as follows:

1. Nurse researchers predominantly use the scientific method of inquiry and that language system.
2. The scientific method is used in nursing research prior to the description and understanding of the phenomenon within the nurse–patient context. In other words, we take leaps to a step without the necessary conditions for that step. Often we take those leaps within the context of deduction and derivation from theories from other disciplines and from nursing theories representing a totality paradigm (whose assumptions are congruent with those of natural science research).

A third possible point here is that some of nursing research is research done by nurses but is not research in nursing. An example of this is nurses participating in medical research studies.

Deduction and Derivation from Theories: From Then to Now

In this section I attempt to provide for you our origins in nursing research and theory development. Some educated in nursing research say they were spoon-fed these first pioneers. It is always critical to know the origins and history of your field, lest someone bring up old information as a new discovery!

Walker and Avant (2004/1983) define theory derivation as "the process of using analogy to obtain explanations or predictions in another field" (p. 163). These authors distinguish between theory derivation and borrowing theory (p. 163), but, for our purpose here, we are speaking about a process in which the description and explanation of phenomena for the development of nursing theory evolved from a discipline or field of knowledge other than nursing. Therefore, the language originates from a world other than the nurse–patient world. Nursing researchers identifying similarities from other fields believe a specific theory to be appropriate to a nursing or patient situation and proceed to generate deductions and/or hypotheses from that theory. This theory derivation is asserted to be useful when there are no available data or when the phenomenon is poorly understood (Walker & Avant, 2004/1983). Thus, we had almost 25 years of nursing research based on theoretical frameworks that did not originate within a nursing or patient context.

One point that should be considered is that many borrowed and derived theories in nursing are based first on the natural and behavioral sciences and, with that, a mechanistic paradigm. Subsequently, the hypothesis deduced from such theories originated from how physical matter behaves, how people respond to forced-choice questions, and, probably all too often, how college students respond to questionnaires and various experiments.

It is amazing to realize with a simple perusal of psychology texts that one experiment after another, leading to the development of theory, has been performed on college students. In these many instances, theories evolved from a very specific age sample and then were generalized to the population at large. The very specific sample has been for researchers of human behavior a real convenience sample, that is, their 19-year-old sophomore students.

Another potential problem with theory derivation and language development from other fields is the male bias inherent in many of our developmental theories (Belenky, Clinchy, Goldberg, & Taub, 1997/1986; Chinn, 1985; Gilligan, 1978). Pinch (1981) proposes that we should critically examine theories of development generated by Freud, Piaget, Erickson, and Kohlberg to recognize how we have accepted worldviews as developed and evolved from a male perspective. When we apply a hypothesis derived from such theory to individuals who may be ill—whether the derivation is from a male perspective, a college student's perspective, a well person's perspective, and so on—we will always have problems of authenticity, validity, and, most important, contextual meaning.

In our history of knowledge development, Dickoff and James (1968) propose a schema of four levels of theory: factor-isolating theories, factor-relating theories, situation-relating theories, and situation-producing theories. This schema dominated the development of nursing theory. We now need to evaluate how well we have proceeded with each of the four levels of theory. Often, when borrowing or deriving from theories from other fields, we proceed directly to situation-producing theories, sacrificing meaning and true significance to expedience. As far back as 1968, Dickoff and James cited this lack of attention to the beginning levels of theory development as being detrimental to the development of nursing theory. Wald and Leonard (1964) suggest that nurses develop their own concepts for nursing theory from inductive analysis of nursing experience rather than from deductive analysis from others' experiences. Perusal of many of the nursing research articles published today still indicates dependence on deducting hypotheses from unrelated contexts or unrelated populations.

Diers (1979), in a context correlative to the work of Dickoff and James, provides us with another classification of levels of theory (**Table 2–6**).

TABLE 2–6 Levels of Inquiry and Study Design

Level of Inquiry	Kind of Question	Study Design	Kind of Answer (Theory)	Study Design
1	What is this?	Factor-searching	Factor-isolating (naming)	Exploratory Formulative Descriptive Situational
2	What's happening here?	Relation-searching	Factor-relating (situation-depicting, situation-describing)	Exploratory Descriptive
3	What will happen if . . .?	Association-searching	Situation-relating (predictive)	Correlational Survey design Nonexperimental Natural experiment Experimental Explanatory Predictive
4	How can I make . . . happen?	Prescription-testing	Situation-producing (prescriptive)	

Source: From *Research in Nursing Practice* (p. 54), by D. Diers, 1979, Philadelphia: Lippincott.

Indeed, all the qualitative methods of research presented herein seem essential to the beginning steps of theory development. In the first and second levels of inquiry, the questions "What is this?" and "What's happening here?" are answered within our own nurse–patient context. With qualitative research methods, theory is not derived, borrowed, or modified from other fields but rather springs from observation of and participation in an actual phenomenon. Norris (1982) believes that the phenomena with which nurses have the social prerogative and mandate to manage concern human health, illness, and comfort. Newman (1983, 1999) identifies additional patient–nursing phenomena, such as reciprocities, patterns, configurations, rhythms, and composition, and emphasizes context dependency, recognizing the simultaneity of our human-environmental processes.

The Social Policy Statement of the American Nurses Association (1995) specifies that the phenomena of concern to nurses are human responses to actual or potential health problems. All are phenomena researchable through qualitative methods and in the end may well stimulate the development of knowledge grounded in the experience of the patient, in complex interactions, and situated in an individual life-world. In the last edition, I had voiced hope that these discussions and debates of a socially constructed dichotomy would be a historical curiosity. Although some literature speaks to moving beyond this debate (Clark, 1998), Watson, Dossey, and Dossey (1999) offers a strikingly contemporary worldview for nursing in which the old traditions largely dominate. What might influence the dominance of one paradigm over another or one theory over another is the importance placed today on interdisciplinary, multidisciplinary, or intradisciplinary theory and development. With the example of intradisciplinary theory, especially in nursing, we can actually come to see the benefit of combining or bringing together various theories, where there are philosophical consistencies or where one theory may be applicable to a particular experience and another theory better able to explain another area of experience.

Here is a place for human understanding in that nurse theorists who have devoted their life careers to development of their own theories are reluctant to let any part go or combine with another theorist. This is often unspoken, but for the sake of knowing, we need to be aware of this dynamic.

Intradisciplinary and interdisciplinary theory development and research could also come about with the six or so different specialty areas of nursing working together, which is so very complementary to the concepts of holism and the situated context.

Multidisciplinary theory development and research are also compatible with the ideas and tenets of qualitative research. Working with other human science disciplines enriches our understanding and broadens the possibilities by incorporating the many facets of being human. A suggestion, though, if you are to embark on multidisciplinary work, is to think of the following two considerations. First, is your project multidisciplinary because a granting agency is calling for that? If so, are you committed to a multidisciplinary approach beyond that requirement? Second, it is very helpful to work with an established or experienced researcher who has done multidisciplinary research previously. This can also be said for mixed-method research, which is discussed in Chapter 24 and Chapter 25.

A Transition: Nursing Worldviews, Nursing Researchers, and Theory Development

One of the purposes of this chapter is to explore nursing's coinages (language), its situatedness in this world, and how we choose to express ourselves. The foregoing discussion is an attempt to place in context our present posture in nursing research and to suggest the origin and evolution of how we have come to express ourselves and the language that we use to bring nursing phenomena into being. I suggest that this and other texts on qualitative research methods are a natural outgrowth of this context. It is contemporary, evolutionary, and congruent with changing worldviews. Expanding research horizons, acquiring new languages, and bringing phenomena into view constitute a reconstructing process.

Transitions in worldviews or paradigms are a gradual process wherein beliefs, values, and practices of the old and the new overlap (Kuhn, 1970). This continues to be a time when there is often conflict, incongruity, and confusion. However, these times are good times for self-reflection, self-consciousness, and clarification. Thesis, antithesis, and paradigmatic shifting are all parts of scientific revolutions or, in Laudan's (1977) terminology, the evolution of research traditions. They are the history and essence of science.

Returning now to the three identified factors that seem to influence the context of nursing research most, let us consider them from the perspective of Kuhn's language in an application to nursing research. Kuhn (1970) observes:

> During the transition period [of worldviews] there will be a large but never complete overlap between the problems that can be solved by the old and by the new paradigm. But there will also be a decisive difference in the modes of solution. When the transition is complete, the profession will have changed its view of the field, its methods and goals. (p. 84)

Perhaps for very good reasons we have not reached this stage, with the two main paradigms still being taught simultaneously: the totality paradigm and the simultaneity paradigm. Each of these paradigms indicates a method of research. The former yields best to the scientific method and the latter to qualitative methods of research. Today in our schools or colleges of nursing the research curricula often reflect the supremacy of the totality or scientific method, or the supremacy of the simultaneity or qualitative methods (very rare) or a combination of the two paradigms with a subtle or not so subtle preference for the scientific method. As in Chapter 1, I mention this so that you as a student understand the context of where qualitative research is placed in our present time. However, you are studying in a time when qualitative research is scientifically accepted, respected and sought after by journals and research conferences. The recognition of what qualitative research has to offer is being recognized more and more in all our scholarly venues. Once again though and as stated in Chapter 1, we must be rigorous in the use of our methods, grounding them congruently with the philosophical underpinnings of the methods and emphasizing significance.

Returning to Chapter 1 and before Chapter 3, teaching both paradigms is from my perspective a valid one. What is not valid is to ask a research question and then attempt to answer it prematurely with the wrong method or just to answer any research question or aim with the wrong method. As we discussed in Chapter 1, some research question and aims require a qualitative approach, while others a quantitative approach. In the scheme of things most knowledge in nursing would best be obtained with a preliminary understanding of the phenomenon or phenomena under study with a qualitative research study and then if necessary followed by a quantitative study. When this is not done we have the results as discussed above with borrowed theory. We find quantitative research derived from theories that do not originate in the patient/nursing world and the fit can be disastrously poor. On the other hand qualitative research does not require theory, such research is atheoretical and can be the origin of theories based in patient/nursing experience.

While Chapter 3 entertains epistemology in nursing and qualitative and quantitative methods of knowing, the task before us next in this chapter is a discussion of the linguistic transition in nursing away from language of the medical model. So whether the method we choose is qualitative or quantitative we still must concern ourselves with the development of our own language. As this chapter opened, we must concern ourselves with bringing nursing and our patient's authentic experience into existence, into being, into theory through language and this you will find within the exemplar chapters of this book and all the previous editions. This is important to understand, we are in the business of bringing the unknown, without language to describe it, into our everyday practice through newly discovered language and phrases. The earlier illustrations in this chapter demonstrate how phenomenon enters our nomenclature and we all have a way of understanding something we had not prior. This is very critical. *If* an entity is not given a name, a "something" to direct our attention to we will simply not even look for it! How significant is that?

Nursing Worldviews

Nursing has attempted to abandon the language of the medical model and, concomitantly, to reject the mechanistic paradigm expressed by that language. To a lesser extent, medicine itself appears to be in transition from its own medical model to one that seems more aligned with some of the beliefs that we have most recently been espousing. There is within that field an emerging language that focuses on holism, psychosomatic phenomena, and the influence of environmental factors.

Even though nursing has attempted to develop nursing language, it often continues to retain the philosophical foundations of the medical model for research and to express its significance and importance in the symbols and practices that traditionally belong to medicine. Perhaps readers will consider some of these nonverbal symbolic forms of language that nursing continues to use and even seeks to acquire from the perspective of paradigmatic transition (Roberts, 1973).

In view of Kuhn's (1970) suggestion that when "the transition is complete, the profession will have changed . . . its methods" (p. 84), let me repeat a question I asked a while back (Munhall, 1982): "Could it be that when nursing abandoned the medical model and the language of that discipline, it retained the research paradigm that perpetuated what nursing was seeking to dissociate from?" (p. 68). Today I would ask the question, not so much regarding an abandonment of the medical model but the hard scientific research model, vis-à-vis logical positivism/scientific method. Is that what we are invested in because of the academic scientific community giving primacy to the natural sciences and not to the human sciences or arts? Is it even more ingrained because research grant money has become a way to attain faculty positions and tenure and research grant money still favors the scientific method?

Because transitions are gradual and because of the aforementioned contextual variables, I am inclined to view this question as characteristic of a trajectory of transition in worldviews. Things do not change at once; Kuhn's (1970) words were: "When the transition is complete, the profession will have changed . . . its methods" (p. 84). Our transition is far from complete. However, many nurse researchers and scholars are catalyzing the progress and process of this transition. Many of them are in every edition of this book!

Nurse Researchers and Scholars

Many of our nurse researchers and scholars, many of whom were socialized in the scientific method, are emerging strongly from that orientation (often meaning experimental research) and are contributing now to the logical shift in research paradigms that would be congruent with the shift in the larger philosophical worldview and new perspective of viewing phenomena. What seems to have occurred is that questions and problems of the profession with its new and unique nursing perspective, that is, holism versus reductionism and/or simultaneity versus totality, cannot be answered or solved by the old methods, at least not at first.

Laudan (1977) reassures us with the following observation: "But there are times when two or more research traditions, far from mutually undermining one another, can be amalgamated, producing a synthesis which is progressive with respect to both the former research traditions" (p. 103).

We seem to have divided ourselves into two different schools of how to think about what we study. Certainly we have moved from what Norris (1982) identifies as "the occasional nurse who used the podium or the literature to support a descriptive route to knowledge [as] a 'voice crying in the wilderness'" (p. 6). Our progress now includes regular publication of the merits of qualitative research, the need for qualitative methods, research programs highlighting qualitative research, and general recognition of the advantages of a broadened repertoire of research methods.

When we first debated the various methods, it was as though we were seeking a place for each method for a specific purpose. As previously noted today, we see conferences, journals, and particular programs specializing in either quantitative or qualitative methods. It is an interesting evolution, and we need to be cognizant of the need to hear one another's voices, regardless of the orientation.

Hardly hidden in the agendas of various schools or organizations is a strong bias toward one orientation as previously alluded to, and unfortunately there may even appear to be suspicion toward or disrespect for the other. Such suspicion or disrespect is counterproductive, and just as tolerance for individual differences is part of our nursing philosophy and ethos, the same must extend to differences in research orientations. These differences need to enrich us and assist us in ultimately meeting the needs of our patients.

At this point it might be helpful to analyze not only the syntactical parallelism but also the contextual congruence of our larger philosophical paradigm with our most prevalent research method. The language that we use to express the philosophical paradigm and the research method demonstrates the emergence of a new worldview and the residue of the old.

The expressions in **Table 2–7** are provided to demonstrate the transitional nature of our worldviews and research paradigms. Table 2–7 illustrates the expressions of competing paradigms and Kuhn's overlap as we examine the contextual parallelism for logical syntax. This contrast has stimulated for many nurse researchers the proliferation of competing views, debates about methods, and discontent over the effect of nursing research on practice. Kuhn (1970) believes such debates are symptomatic of a "transition from normal to extraordinary research," but, as just mentioned, we should beware of splintering. The

TABLE 2–7   Expressions in Nursing Philosophy and Research Paradigms, and Contextual Parallelism

Expressions of Contemporary Nursing Philosophy

Humanism	Uniqueness
Individualism	Relativism
Self-determination	Autonomy
Active organism	Advocacy
Open system	Organismic
Holism	Situated context
Life-worlds	Simultaneity
Multiple realities	Multiplicity
Self-interpretive	

Expressions of the Scientific Method

Reductionism	Theory for the average
Objectivity–positivism	Categorization
Delimited problems	Prediction
Reality reduced to the measurable	Control
Human and environmental passivity	Mechanistic
Manipulation	Totality

Conceptual Parallelism

Nursing Philosophy	Nursing Research Based on the Scientific Method
Individualism	Commonalities
Uniqueness	Generalizations
Relativism	Categorization
Open system	Closed system
Holism	Reductionism
Individual interpretations	Statistical analysis
Active organism	Reactive organism
Organismic	Mechanistic
Self-determination	Control
Simultaneous interaction	Totality
Situated context	Acontextual
Multiple realities	Objective reality
Subjective perceptions	Objectivity

wholeness and the interaction that we propose in nursing models should be reflected in our own community of nurse researchers.

For the sake of conceptual clarity, the various paradigms have been presented in a dichotomized way. However, the practice is used more for its illustrative purposes. The goal here is to build bridges rather than erect walls. The bridge may well represent a transcendence of the two competing worldviews with the emergence of a research paradigm that either utilizes the two views or goes beyond them.

Theory Development

The transition from one paradigm to another paradigm or to the inclusion of another paradigm will be reflected, as has been suggested, in our language and expressions. We previously mentioned the borrowed theoretical frameworks that are used so prevalently in nursing research. We borrow freely from physics, biology, physiology, psychology, and sociology. We seem, as was mentioned, to also have two different nursing paradigms: the totality and the simultaneity. These practices often lead to fuzzy language. For example, in doing interdisciplinary research it is important that the situated context be similar to each discipline. The situated context of our patients' worlds is, in some instances, so very dramatic. The individuals are very vulnerable and there are family threats among contingencies that we must be extremely cautious in choosing what disciplines we do research with in these kinds of matters. On the other hand, if we are researching how to assist people to have a better quality of life then doing research with colleagues from public health, psychology, nutrition, among other fields makes perfect sense. The advantage of interdisciplinary research is that we do not have to reinvent the wheel, so to speak!

Paterson (1978) compiled a list of nursing phenomena (**Table 2–8**) selected by practicing nurses as being essential to nursing. I ask you to compare these expressions with the expressions found in many of our contemporary research titles. It bears repeating that we must recognize just how pioneering Paterson (1978) and Zderad (Paterson & Zderad, 1976) were. To pay tribute to them, their jointly written book, *Humanistic Nursing*, was reissued in 1988 as being contemporary and relevant for the present after its first publication in 1976. Read, think about, and respond to these words in Table 2–8 as perhaps the quintessence of nursing. Could any of us argue that they do not constitute nursing phenomena?[4] Would we not want them to? Are these not the words that express caring in experience? To those who wonder why there is not adequate description of such experiences in nursing literature, I believe the answer lies in the arguments for qualitative research. Qualitative researchers eagerly await the extraordinary research that Kuhn promises as the outcome of scientific revolutions. I believe the quality of patient care and outcomes depend on it.

TABLE 2–8   The Quintessence of Nursing

Acceptance	Give and Take
Authenticity	Laughing–crying
Awareness	Loneliness
Becoming	Openness
Caring	Patience
Charge	Readiness
Choice	Response
Commitment	Responsibility
Confirmation	Self-recognition
Confrontation	Sustaining
Dedication	Touching
Dying and death	Trust
Meaning	Understanding
Freedom	Waiting
Frustration	

Source: Reprinted with permission from "The Tortuous Way Toward Nursing Theory," in *Theory Development: What, Why and How?* (p. 65), by J. Paterson, New York: National League for Nursing, 1978, 1988.

Language and Comprehensibility

The existential-ontological foundation of languages is discourse or talk.
(Heidegger, 1962, p. 203)

Discourse is existentially language, because that entity whose disclosedness it articulates according to significations, has, as its kind of being, being-the-world and being which has been thrown and submitted to the world.
(Heidegger, 1962, p. 204)

For in conversation, as in research, we meet ourselves. Both are forms of social interaction in which our choice of words and actions return to confront us in terms of the kind of discourse or knowledge we help to generate.
(Morgan, 1983, p. 406)

And where does a nurse researcher thrown into and submitted to the world learn to speak? In the pedagogical world of research, a new language is learned. We noted earlier that this language is sometimes chosen freely, sometimes encouraged in one or another direction, and sometimes "raised" to such high levels of abstraction that it becomes incomprehensible. From a qualitative perspective, language and the ability to express oneself to others is the only way in which we can bring experience into a form that creates in discourse a conversational relation (van Manen, 1990, 1997).

Before this chapter ends, it seems essential to mention an obvious inherent component of language: listening. Discourse and conversing include keeping silent and hearing. The openness that is required for new ideas to penetrate into a belief system requires silence and hearing. Additionally, when considering language, many people silence themselves, they do not give voice to their experience, and what may be meaningful in the "said" may even be more meaningful in the "unsaid."

The language of human science or phenomenology may at first sound strange to people who are steeped in a natural-science language (see **Table 2–9**). Paterson and Zderad's (1976) first attempts to introduce this language into nursing were often met with firm preconceptions and assumptions about being in the world that were dramatically different.

TABLE 2–9   Expressions* of Qualitative Research Methods

Subjective experience	Closeness to the data
Intuition	Process orientation
Variability	Dynamic reality
Communication	Open system
Individual perceptions	Time and space considerations
Shared language	Patterns
Interrelatedness	Polyvocality
Situated context	Configurations
Lived experience	Context dependence
Holism	Complementarity
Naturalism	Human development
Nonmanipulated observation	Life-worlds
Self-interpretation	Contingencies
Multiple perspectives	Multiple realities
Intersubjectivity	Narratives/stories
Existential meaning	Emergence/Convergence

* All these terms will be explained within the text.

As I suggest in Chapter 1, one key idea is to lay groundwork in many curricula to assist students in the language of understanding the meaning of both being human in our different perspectives and understanding those differences in nursing and nursing research. The symbols, signs, and words that we use have inherent meaning. They are signifiers of who we are, what we are, and what is meaningful to us.

Summary

The intent of this chapter can be summarized by borrowing Paterson's (1978) words: "For responsible, effective existence the professional requires language to relate authentically the purposes, beliefs, concerns, and events experienced continually to the nursing world" (p. 51). A mystery exists in those phenomena listed by practicing nurses, but each seems to be a "thing in itself," something waiting for description to bring it into our everyday awareness and to give it significance. It is as though we need to assert these events as belonging to nursing, to articulate our authentic experience with patients, and to claim what we and our patients believe to be essential to health and to our quality of existence. We then assign language to what is uniquely the abstract and the concrete, the enduring and the relevant meanings of shared human experience between patient and nurse. It is indeed a privilege and a calling to assist a patient in finding meaning in experience.

Qualitative research methods have much to offer as a research paradigm that is congruent with nursing's larger worldview, paradigm, or model. These methods offer ways to approach individuals in experiences, to encourage them to give voice to their experiencing, and to care enough to search for meaning within the experience. I refer again to Table 2–9 as an illustration of the language of the qualitative research methods and leave you to draw your own conclusions.

References

Allen, D. (1995). Hermeneutics: Philosophy, traditions, and nursing practice research. *Nursing Science Quarterly, 8*(4), 175–181.

The American Heritage Dictionary of the English Language, Third Edition. (1992). New York: Houghton Mifflin.

American Nurses Association. (1995). *Nursing: A social policy statement.* Washington, DC: Author.

Anderson, W. T. (1995). *The truth about the truth.* New York: Putnam.

Ashworth, P. D. (1997). The variety of qualitative research (Part 2: Non-positivist approaches). *Nurse Education Today, 17*(3), 219–224.

Atwood, G., & Stolorow, R. (1993). *Structures of subjectivity: Explorations in psychoanalytic phenomenology*. New York: Routledge.

Beatty, M. (1989). *Beyond codependency*. San Francisco: Harper & Row.

Belenky, M., Clinchy, B., Goldberg, N., & Taub, J. (1986). *Women's ways of knowing: The development of self, voice and mind*. New York: Basic Books [(1997, *10th Anniversary Edition*). New York: Basic Books.]

Bohm, D. (2004). *On creativity* (2nd ed.). New York: Routledge.

Bronowski, J. (1965). *Science and human values* (Rev. ed.). New York: Harper & Row [Re-released (2008). London: Faber Finds.]

Brozan, N. (1982). "Premenstrual syndrome: A complex issue." *The New York Times*, July 12, 1982 edition.

Cather, W. (2006). *Death comes for the Archbishop*. London, U.K.: Virago, U.K.

Cather, W., Woodress, J. (history essay & explanatory notes), Ronning, K. (explanatory notes), Link, F. (Ed.) (2001). *The professor's house*. Lincoln, NE.: University of Nebraska Press.

Chinn, P. (1983). Editorial. *Advances in Nursing Science, 5*(2), ix.

Chinn, P. (1985). Debunking myths in nursing theory and research. *Image: The Journal of Nursing Scholarship, 17*(2), 45–49.

Clark, A. M. (1998). The qualitative-quantitative debate: Moving from positivism and confrontation to post-positivism and reconciliation. *Journal of Advanced Nursing, 27*, 1242–1249.

Corbin, V. (1999). Misusing phenomenology in nursing research: Identifying the basic issues. *Nurse Researcher, 6*(3), 52–65.

Coventry, K. R., & Garrod, S. C. (2005). *Saying, seeing, and acting: The psychological semantics of spatial prepositions*. Hove, U.K.: Psychology Press.

DeVries, P. (1983). *Slouching towards Kalamazoo*. Boston: Little, Brown.

Dickoff, J., & James, P. (1968). A theory of theories: A position paper. *Nursing Research, 17*, 197–203.

Diers, D. (1979). *Research in nursing practice*. Philadelphia: Lippincott.

Dossey, L. (1982). *Space, time and medicine*. Boulder, CO: Shambhala.

Downs, F. (1982). It's a great idea but it won't work. *Nursing Research, 31*(1), 4.

Dzurec, L. (1989). The necessity for and evolution of multiple paradigms for nursing research: A poststructuralist perspective. *Advances in Nursing Science, 11*(4), 69–77.

Filstead, W. (1979). Qualitative methods: A needed perspective in evaluation research. In C. Reichardt & T. Cook (Eds.), *Qualitative and quantitative methods to evaluation research*. Beverly Hills, CA: Sage.

Gilligan, C. (1978). In a different voice: Women's conception of self and of morality. *Harvard Education Review, 47,* 481–517.

Heidegger, M. (1962). *Being and time* (J. Macprairie & E. Robinson, Trans.). New York: Harper & Row.

Kaplan, A. (1964). *The conduct of inquiry*. Scranton, PA: Chandler.

Kaplan, A., & Wolf, C. (1998). *The conduct of inquiry: Methodology for behavioral science*. Piscataway, NJ. Transaction Publishers.

Keynes, J. M. (1936). *The general theory of employment, interest and money*. New York: Harcourt, Brace and Company.

Kirby, D. (1983). Seeing the points of contact in a plural world. *Chronicle of Higher Education, 26*(7), 25.

Kneller, G. (1964). *Introduction to the philosophy of education.* New York: Wiley.

Kuhn, T. S. (Ed.). (1970). *The structure of scientific revolutions.* Chicago: University of Chicago Press.

Laudan, L. (1977). *Progress and its problems: Toward a theory of scientific growth.* Berkeley, CA: University of California Press.

Looft, W. (1973). Socialization and personality throughout the life span: An examination of contemporary psychological approaches. In P. Baltes & K. Schaie (Eds.), *Life-span developmental psychology* (pp. 210–227). New York: Academic Press.

Matson, F. (1964). *The broken image: Man, science and society.* New York: George Brazillier.

Moccia, P. (1988). A critique of compromise: Beyond the methods debate. *Advances in Nursing Science, 10*(4), 1–9.

Morgan, G. (1983). *Beyond method: Strategies for social research.* Newbury Park, CA: Sage.

Munhall, P. (1982). Ethical juxtaposition in nursing research. *Topics in Clinical Nursing, 4*(1), 66–73.

Munhall, P. (1989). Philosophical pondering on qualitative research methods in nursing. *Nursing Science Quarterly, 2,* 20–28.

Munhall, P. (1992). A new ageism: Beyond a toxic apple. *Nursing and Health Care, 13*(7), 370–375.

Newman, M. A. (1983). Editorial. *Advances in Nursing Science, 5*(2), x–xi.

Newman, M. A. (1999). The rhythm of relating in a paradigm of wholeness. *Image: Journal of Nursing Scholarship, 31*(3), 227–230.

Norris, C. (1982). *Concept clarification in nursing.* Rockville, MD: Aspen.

Norwood, R. (1990). *Women who love too much.* New York: Pocket Books.

Page, A. (Ed.) (2004). Nurses caring for patients: Who they are, where they work, and what they do. In *Keeping patients safe. Transforming the work environments of nurses* (pp. 65–107). Washington, DC: The National Academies Press.

Paterson, J. (1978). *The tortuous way toward nursing theory. In theory development: What, why and how?* New York: National League for Nursing.

Paterson, J. A., & Zderad, L. J. (1976, reissued 1988). *Humanistic nursing.* New York: National League for Nursing.

Patton, M. Q. (1978). *Utilization focused evaluation.* Beverly Hills, CA: Sage. [(1996 – 3rd ed.). The New Century Text, Sage.]

Piaget, J. (1970). *Structuralism.* New York: Basic Books.

Pinch, W. (1981). Feminine attributes in a masculine world. *Nursing Outlook, 12,* 29–36.

Reichardt, C., & Cook, T. (Eds.). (1979). *Qualitative and quantitative methods in evaluation research.* Beverly Hills, CA: Sage.

Roberts, S. (1973). Oppressed group behavior: Implications for nursing. *Advances in Nursing Science, 5*(4), 21–30.

Rorty, R. (1991). *Essays on Heidegger and others.* New York: Cambridge University Press.

Skinner, B. (1953). *Science and human behavior.* New York: Appleton-Century-Crofts.

Snow, C. P. (1959). *The two cultures and the scientific revolution.* Cambridge, U.K.: Cambridge University Press. [Re-issued: (1993). Cambridge edition: The two cultures (Canto). Cambridge, U.K.: Cambridge University Press.]

Stolorow, R., & Atwood, G. (2002). *Contexts of being: The intersubjective foundations of psychological life.* Hillsdale, NJ: Analytic Press.

Suppe, F. (Ed.). (1977). *The structure of scientific theories* (2nd ed.). Champaign, IL: University of Illinois Press.

Swanson, J., & Chenitz, C. (1982). Why qualitative research in nursing? *Nursing Outlook, 30*(4), 241–245.

Tinkle, M., & Beaton, J. (1983). Toward a new view of science: Implications for nursing research. *Advances in Nursing Science, 5*(2), 27–36.

van Manen, M. (1990). *Research lived experience: Human science for an action sensitive pedagogy.* New York: SUNY Press. [(1997—2nd ed.), London, ON.: The Althouse Press, University of Western Ontario.]

Wald, F., & Leonard, R. (1964). Towards development of nursing practice theory. *Nursing Research, 13,* 4–9.

Walker, L., & Avant, K. (1983). *Strategies for theory construction in nursing.* Norwalk, CT: Appleton-Century-Crofts. [(2004—4th ed.). Upper Saddle River, N.J.: Prentice Hall.]

Watson, J. (1981). Nursing's scientific quest. *Nursing Outlook, 29*(7), 413–416.

Watson, J., Dossey, B., & Dossey, L. (1999). *Post modern nursing and beyond.* New York: Churchill Livingstone.

Wells, G. (1985). Language and learning: An international perspective. In G. Wells & J. Nicholls, *Language and learning: An international perspective* (pp. 21–40). Philadelphia: The Falmer Press.

Woolf, V. (2005). *A room of one's own: Annotated* (Eds., Hussey, M. & Gubar, S.). New York: Mariner Books.

Zen Buddhism. (1959). Mount Vernon, NY: Peter Pauper Press.

Additional Resources

Allen, D., Benner, P., & Diekelmann, N. (1985). Three paradigms for nursing research: Methodological implications. In P. Chinn (Ed.), *Nursing research methodology issues and implementation.* Rockville, MD: Aspen.

Asp, M., & Fagerberg, I. (2005). Developing concepts in caring science based on a lifeworld perspective. *International Journal of Qualitative Methods, 4*(2), article 5. Retrieved December 14, 2005, from http://www.ualberta.ca/~ijqm/backissues/4_2/html/asp.htm

Baer, E. (1979). Philosophy provides the rationale for nursing's multiple research directions. *Image, 2*(3), 72–74.

Barbour, R. S. (2000). The role of qualitative research in broadening the "evidence base" for clinical practice. *Journal of Evaluation in Clinical Practice, 6*(2), 155–163.

Benner, P. (Ed.). (1994). *Interpretive phenomenology: Embodiment, caring, and ethics in health and illness.* Thousand Oaks, CA: Sage.

Benner, P., Sutphen, M., Leonard, V., Day, L., & Schulman, L. S. (2009). *Educating nurses: A call for radical transformation.* Edison, NJ: Jossey-Bass.

Benoliel, J. (1984). Advancing nursing science: Qualitative approaches. *Western Journal of Nursing Research, 6*(3), 1–8.

Byrne, M. M. (2001). Linking philosophy, methodology and methods in qualitative research. *AORN, 73*(1), 207–210.

Cheek, J. (2002). Advancing what? Qualitative research, scholarship and the research imperative. *Qualitative Health Research, 12*(8), 1130–1140.

Chenitz, W. C., & Swanson, J. M. (1986). *From practice to grounded theory: Qualitative research in nursing.* Menlo Park, CA: Addison-Wesley.

Clark, C. L., & Wilcockson, J. (2002). Seeing need and developing care: Exploring knowledge for and from practice. *International Journal of Nursing Studies, 39*(4), 397–406.

Creswell, J. (2008). *Research design: Qualitative, quantitative and mixed methods approaches* (3rd ed.). Thousand Oaks, CA: Sage.

Davies, D., & Dodd, J. (2002). Qualitative research and the question of rigor. *Qualitative Health Research, 12*(2), 279–289.

Fawcett, J. (1983). Hallmarks of success in nursing theory development. In P. Chinn (Ed.), *Advances in nursing theory development* (pp. 3–17). Rockville, MD: Aspen.

Field, P., & Morse, J. (1985). *Nursing research: The application of qualitative approaches.* Rockville, MD: Aspen. [cf. new ed. (2003), Morse, J. & Field, P., below]

Foucault, M. (1977). *Language, counter memory, practice: Selected essays and interviews.* Ithaca, NY: Cornell University Press.

Foucault, M., & Bouchard, D. F. (Ed.). (1980). *Language, counter memory, practice: Selected essays and interviews.* Ithaca, NY: Cornell University Press.

Gaita, R. (2002). *A common humanity: Thinking about love and truth and justice.* London: Routledge.

Gorenberg, B. (1983). The research tradition of nursing: An emerging issue. *Nursing Research, 32,* 347–349.

Harden, J. (2000). Language, discourse and the chronotope: Applying literary theory to the narratives in health care. *Journal of Advanced Nursing, 31,* 506–512.

Jacobs-Kramer, M. K., & Chinn, P. L. (1988). Perspectives on knowing: A model of nursing knowledge. *Scholarly Inquiry for Nursing Practice: An International Journal, 2*(2), 129–139.

Johnson, J. (1991). Nursing science: Basic applied or practical implications for the art of nursing. *Nursing Research, 14,* 7–15.

Leininger, M. (1985). *Qualitative research methods in nursing.* New York: Grune & Stratton.

Light, R., & Pillemer, D. (1982). Numbers and narrative: Combining their strengths in research reviews. *Harvard Education Review, 51*(1), 1–23.

Lock, L. F., Silverman, S. J., & Spirduso, W. W. (2009). *Reading and understanding research* (3rd ed.). Thousand Oaks, CA: Sage.

Ludemann, R. (1979). The paradoxical nature of nursing research. *Image, 2,* 2–8.

MacPherson, K. I. (1983). Feminists methods: A new paradigm for nursing research. *Advances in Nursing Science, 5,* 17–25.

Maggs-Rapport, F. (2001). "Best research practice": In pursuit of methodological rigour. *Journal of Advanced Nursing, 35*(3), 373–383.

Meleis, A. (2006). *Theoretical nursing: Development and progress* (4th ed.). Philadelphia: Lippincott, Williams & Wilkins.

Meshier, E. (1979). Meaning in context: Is there any other kind? *Harvard Education Review, 49*(1), 1–19.

Moccia, P. (Ed.). (1986). *New approaches in theory development.* New York: National League for Nursing.

Morse, J. M. (1999). Qualitative methods: The state of the art. *Qualitative Health Research, 9,* 393–406.

Morse, J. M. (2002). Enhancing the usefulness of qualitative inquiry: Gaps, direction, and responsibilities. *Qualitative Health Research, 12*(10), 1419–1426.

Morse, J. M. (2003). Toward holism: The significance of methodological Pluralism. *International Journal of Qualitative Methods, 2*(3), Article 2.

Morse, J., & Field, P. (2003). *Nursing research: The application of qualitative approaches.* Rockville, MD: Aspen.

Morse, J. M. (2004). Constructing qualitatively derived theory: Concept construction and concept typologies. *Qualitative Health Research, 14*(10), 1387–1395.

Munhall, P. (1982b). Nursing philosophy and nursing research: In apposition or opposition? *Nursing Research, 31*(3), 176–177, 181.

Munhall, P. (1986). Methodological issues in nursing: Beyond a wax apple. *Advances in Nursing Science, 8*(3), 1–5.

Munhall, P. (1992). Holding the Mississippi River in place and other implications for qualitative research. *Nursing Outlook, 10*(6), 257–262.

Munhall, P. (1993). Toward a fifth pattern of knowing: Unknowing. *Nursing Outlook, 41,* 125–128.

Munhall, P. (1994). *Qualitative research: Proposals and reports.* New York: National League for Nursing.

Munhall, P. (1997). De ja vu, parroting, buy-ins, and opening. In J. Fawcett & I. King (Eds.), *The language of nursing theory and metatheory.* Indianapolis, IN: Sigma Theta Tau International.

Newman, M. A. (1979). *Theory development in nursing.* Philadelphia: Davis.

Newman, M. A. (1992). *Health as expanding consciousness* (2nd ed.). Thousand Oaks, CA.: Sage.

Oiler, C. (1982). The phenomenological approach in nursing research. *Nursing Research, 31*(3), 178–181.

Oiler, C. (1986). Qualitative methods: Phenomenology. In P. Moccia (Ed.), *New approaches to theory development.* New York: National League for Nursing.

Omery, A. (1983). Phenomenology: A method for nursing research. *Advances in Nursing Science, 5*(2), 49–64.

Patterson, D., & Brogden, L. M. (2004). Living spaces for talk with/in the academy. *International Journal of Qualitative Methods, 3*(3), Article 2.

Reeder, J. (1987). The phenomenological movement. *Image, 19,* 150–152.

Sandelowski, M. (2004). Using qualitative research. *Qualitative Health Research, 14*(10), 1366–1386.

Sandelowski, M., & Barosso, J. (2002). Reading qualitative studies. *International Journal of Qualitative Methods, 1*(1), Article 2.

Sarter, B. (1988). Philosophical sources of nursing theory. *Nursing Science Quarterly, 1,* 52–59.

Silva, M. C. (1977). Philosophy, science, theory: Interrelationships and implications for nursing research. *Image, 9*(5), 59–63.

Stolorow, R., & Atwood, G. (2002). *Contexts of being: The intersubjective foundations of psychological life.* Hillsdale, NJ: Analytic Press.

Thorne, S., Joachim, G., Paterson, B., & Canam, C. (2002). Influence of the research frame on qualitatively derived health science knowledge. *International Journal of Qualitative Methods, 1*(1), Article 1.

Walters, A. J. (1996). Nursing research methodology: Transcending Cartesianism. *Nursing Inquiry, 3*(2), 91–100.

Watson, J. (2008). *Nursing: The philosophy and science of caring.* Boulder, CO: University Press of Colorado.

Watson, J. (1985). *Nursing: Human science and human care and theory of nursing.* Norwalk, CT: Appleton-Century-Crofts.

West, M. (1983). *The world is made of glass.* New York: Morrow.

Wolf, S. (2010). *Meaning in life and why it matters.* Princeton, NJ: Princeton University Press.

Endnotes

[1] There is considerable ambivalence within the profession about the usage of the term nursing diagnosis and developing taxonomies. Many view these systems as reductionistic, acontextual, and a continued imitation of medicine. In addition, a long history of debate over whether to identify the recipient of nursing care as "patient" or "client" follows a similar vein.

[2] For a more detailed explanation of the scientific revolution that eclipsed determinism and objectivism, the reader is referred to works on quantum physics, Heisenberg's principle of uncertainty, and Bohr's principle of complementarity. In Floyd Matson's *The Broken Image* (1964), a most readable discourse can be found, and Larry Dossey's *Space, Time and Medicine* (1982) is wonderfully explicit and enjoyable reading on this topic.

[3] As defined in the traditional sense. All the methods presented in this text are considered scientific methods of research.

[4] Additional phenomena are discussed in Chapter 3.

3

Epistemology in Nursing

Patricia L. Munhall

Since we have come to the understanding that science is not a description of "reality" but a metaphorical ordering of experiences, the new science does not impugn the old. It is not a question of which view is "true" in some ultimate sense. Rather, it is a matter of which picture is more useful in guiding human affairs.
—Willis Harman, Symposium and Consciousness

I noted in Chapter 2 that I intended to resolve an unnecessary polarization of worldviews. To that end, I hope you will understand that any indulgence in polarizing worldviews provides conceptual clarity for pedagogical purposes, and little else. Furthermore, I could not agree more with Gould (1984) when he observed,

> Dichotomy is the usual pathway to vulgarization. We take a complex web of arguments and divide it into two polarized positions—them against us. We then portray "them" as a foolish caricature of extremes in order to put "us" in a better light. (p. 7)

However complex they may be, webs become differentiated when placed against contrasting systems. The differences between the systems assume greater focus. Our goal in observation, then, is not to see one system as the truth, but to see each as different. As Harman (1977) states, "It is not a question of which view is true [but which] is more useful in guiding human affairs." Usefulness in guiding human affairs serves as an axis of a shared connectedness, rather than dichotomous worldviews.

In this chapter, I propose an epistemology for nursing research that, as a whole, incorporates the qualitative and quantitative methods of research. This does not represent a conciliatory effort at compromise, but rather a belief in a cyclical continuum that begins with discovery and moves toward verification. These activities represent, respectively, the first- and second-order activities of science.

I believe that specific research methods are better suited to answering certain questions. Failing to match questions and research methods results in faulty conclusions because a method might have been used prematurely or a-contextually to answer a question or solve a problem. As long as there are times when two research traditions are amalgamated to produce a synthesis that is progressive to both traditions (Laudan, 1977), risk of inadequate alignment of research questions and methods diminishes. As the fire of debates over opposing methods dies, there are now opportunities for methodological synthesis along with wider acknowledgment of a need for multiple ways to study being and knowledge in the human sciences. The philosophy of postmodernism has served as common ground in which partisans of years gone by no longer need to raise swords in conflict. Postmodernism "is an intellectual movement (and as such) challenges the ideas of a single correct approach to knowledge development, of a single truth, and a single meaning of reality, rejecting the ideal that there is one true story about reality" (Uris, 1993, p. 95). A more explicit discussion of postmodernism follows in Chapter 4.

In this chapter, there will be an overview discussion of paths to knowledge, the purpose of science, research paradigms, and research traditions. I will attempt to answer the questions "Knowing about what?" and "How do we get to know?" as well as "Toward what end?" and will then propose a qualitative-quantitative cyclical continuum for knowing. Emphasis throughout is on qualitative research methods as beginning points. Too often we engage in experimental research before the variables significant to that research have been determined, or we conduct quantitative studies based on our own knowledge of the world and not the knowledge of "experiencers" of phenomena. Currently, because of the situated context of the necessity of grant funding, we are witnessing once again the dominance of the scientific method for funding purposes. Following is from an email I received, not one word changed:

> I am putting together my tenure portfolio and feel great trepidation. There is such an emphasis on grants and, as you know, qualitative research does not receive much funding of note. Someone told me that without an NIH grant I am not going to get tenured. In the criteria for tenure, it does mention "evidence of external funding," and I did get a small grant from Sigma Theta Tau, but supposedly that does not count or measure up. I have actually received awards for my research but the secret message seems to be that the gold standard is the NIH grant. It's

as though a wall is closing in on me, and I worry if I don't comply with doing quantitative research, which is the paradigm rewarded, I am not going to make it. Perhaps I should ask for an extension and quickly send in a grant proposal for a quantitative study, though it compromises who I am as a researcher. No. I believe in my work.

—*Sandy*

Sandy, a qualitative researcher in nursing, recognizes what she wants to do, which should be promoted in her scholarly unit to assure academic freedom. However, what she spent years in formal education and research apprenticeship to master is being corrupted by outside influences. A principal corrupting influence is a return of quantitative research or the scientific method as not only dominant, but also exclusive in an academic economy of restrictive rewards and negligible incentives. Some nurse researchers have argued that a pure-experimental design with methods and measurement instruments for interval-level data are essential to build an evidence-based practice. (This chapter as well as Chapters 1, 2, and 23 discusses how essential qualitative research is to evidence-based practice.)

Yet many questions cannot be answered in a true experimental design. These questions are no less substantive or important to nursing, and skilled researchers such as Sandy must risk animus or indifference from tenure and promotion committees that do not share her core values of caring and compassion. The same values envelop Sandy's approach both to caring for others and to sensitive application of research methods that are congruent with her questions. From the preceding testimony, we can ascertain the writer's concern for what she believes to be the central values in nursing: caring and compassion. Indeed, even if you did not think that caring and compassion were central, most of us would agree that caring and compassion are high on the list of our aspirations.

Ironically, for any research enterprise to be authentic, we must begin with qualitative inquiry as a foundation from which we can identify variables, understand the context of experiences, and develop instrumentation. That is exactly the kind of research the preceding nurse researcher wants to do, and from my perspective we need to encourage and support this work if we are actually going to have research that is applicable. In this chapter, a theme as articulated by Morgan (1983) will guide us: "To steer clear of the delusion that it is possible to know in an absolute sense of 'being right' and devote our energies to the more constructive process of dealing with the implication of our different ways of knowing" (p. 18). I also envision a postmodern perspective where the necessity for and evolution of multiple paradigms for nursing research will create new possibilities of coming to understand and develop the knowledge that is necessary to nursing practice par excellence. This is the study of nursing epistemology, that branch of philosophy that deals with knowledge and how we come to know about the world as we experience it. P.S. Sandy received tenure AND special recognition for her research! Not only that, a year later she received a NIH grant to continue her qualitative research project. "Times, they are a-changing."

Paths to Knowledge

From where does knowledge *for* nursing, *about* nursing and *in* nursing come? In Chapter 2, I mentioned knowledge (theory) borrowed from related disciplines. Other disciplines are indeed sources of knowledge, perhaps more accurately called "shared knowledge" (Stevens, 1979, p. 85): because disciplines have indistinct boundaries, there are areas "where the inquiries and answers of one field overlay those of another." At the turn of the 21st century, we have almost abandoned the term borrowed theory, recognizing the interconnectedness of various disciplines, and so today interdisciplinary research is encouraged by nurse researchers and sometimes is a requirement for funding. Wilson (1998) states this so clearly:

> Most of the issues that vex humanity daily, ethnic conflict, arms escalation, overpopulation, abortion, environment, endemic poverty to cite several most persistently before us cannot be solved without integrating knowledge from the natural sciences with that of the social sciences and humanities. (p. 13)

However, caution must be used when integrating similarities from other disciplines and then utilizing those respective theoretical frameworks to derive hypotheses for nursing. We need to understand that if the first- and second-order activities are not from the same world or discipline, there is a risk that the inquiry will not be logically consistent or experientially valid. For example, if the first-order activities of coming to know, discovering, and understanding come from another discipline and from that discipline's perspective and the second-order activities of validation and verification are then performed within the nursing discipline and apply nursing's particular perspective, you can see the risk. Before we go further, however, let us in a foundational manner consider where knowledge generally comes from and some of the structures of knowing. In a pedantic fashion, philosophers who study the way that we come to know (epistemologists) have identified specific sources of knowledge, generally acceptable as structures of knowing. Among them are the following (Kneller, 1971):

1. Revealed knowledge—knowledge that God has disclosed. Revelations of truth are found in the Bible, the Koran, and the Bhagavad-Gita. In the past decade, we have seen a growth of research on spirituality—for example, religion as a source of comfort and inspiration; belief as having curative power; and so on. We do know that from revealed knowledge comes the imperative to care for and about one another.

2. Intuitive knowledge—knowledge within a person, in the form of insight that becomes present in consciousness; an idea or thought produced by a long process of unconscious work. This process of discovery is nurtured through experience with the world.
3. Rational knowledge—knowledge from the exercise of reason. This knowledge takes the form of abstract reasoning and is exemplified in the principles of formal logic and mathematics.
4. Empirical knowledge—knowledge formed in accordance with observed or sensed facts and associated with scientific hypotheses that are tested by observation or experiments.
5. Authoritative knowledge—knowledge accepted on faith because it is vouched for by authorities in the field.

In the foregoing brief description of the sources of knowledge, the one least attended to, but the one holding much potential for nursing, is intuitive knowledge, which for the purpose of this text will be experiential knowledge. The repudiation of intuition as a source of knowledge was one of the major themes when nursing moved toward establishing itself as a science. Intuition was unscientific; it was associated with women, who themselves were thought to be unscientific. More confident today, women of science—including nurses—recognize the vitalness of intuition and have come to trust and value this important source of knowledge.

Belenky, Clinchy, Goldberg, and Taub (1986), in describing the different ways in which women come to know, have legitimized to a great extent the place of intuition, personal meanings, and the connection to ideas as means of knowing. Rather than focusing on proof, these women scientists seek understanding. The work of Gilligan (1982), Belenky et al. (1986), and Freire (1971) challenges us all to rethink our concepts about epistemology—underlying assumptions and the critical consequences. Critical theory (discussed in Chapter 4) is one way to analyze the underlying structural and power relations inherent in the sanctioned ways of knowing (Allen, 1991). Allen (1995) expands the importance of critique in his discussion of critical hermeneutics with great emphasis on the subjective reality that research can socially construct.

Carper's (1978) framework of four fundamental patterns of knowing, based on the work of Philip Phoenix, continues to this day to be a way in which nursing identifies its epistemological interests. These patterns of knowing are described as follows:

1. Empirics—the science of nursing; emphasis is on the generation of theory and of research that is systematic and controllable by factual evidence. Within this pattern of knowing, there is a need for emphasis on knowledge about the empirical world, knowledge that will be organized

into general laws and theories for the purpose of describing, explaining, and predicting phenomena of concern to nursing.

2. Esthetics—the art of nursing; emphasis is on expressiveness, subjective acquaintance, individual perceptions, and empathy. Rather than uniformity and general laws, there is recognition of alternative modes of perceiving reality, which then clearly asks for a "many different ways" approach to designing and participating in nursing care.

3. Personal knowledge—the focus is on the importance of the interpersonal process and the "therapeutic use of self"; on knowing the self, knowing the other as a subject, and striving toward authentic personal relations.

4. Ethics—the focus is on matters of obligation or what ought to be done. Knowledge within this domain requires an understanding of ethical theories, conditions of society, conflicts between different value systems, and ethical principles.

All of the foregoing patterns are rich and essential sources of nursing knowledge that can be studied from various perspectives of science.

I have suggested a fifth pattern of knowing, while at the same time questioning the categorization of knowledge in this way (Munhall, 1993). The fifth pattern is one of "unknowing." "Knowing," in contrast with "unknowing," leads to a form of confidence that has the potential of a state of closure to alternatives and differences. Unknowing, from an epistemological perspective, is a condition of openness and seems essential to the understanding of intersubjectivity and perspectivity (discussed further in Chapter 5). Kurtz (1989) states: "Knowledge screens the sound the third ear hears, so we hear only what we know" (p. 6). *We can become limited by our own belief systems.* Often, once we believe something or think we know something, we cease further exploration or explanation. Many practitioners in all fields will continue to hold the body of knowledge that they attained in their formal education. The impracticability and danger of continuing to do so in an unsurpassed age of knowledge explosion are apparent.

Only by unlearning comes wisdom.
—James Russell Lowell

Although the patterns of knowledge are presented for historical and pedantic reasons, they are organized as categories; I think we can see them as mutually interdependent, not mutually exclusive. Intuiting in the empirical world while using one's personal knowledge embedded in an ethical context or founded on a philosophical perspective is a holistic approach to theory development.

We move now from general structures of knowing to the purpose of exploring those structures. Because nursing has identified itself as a science, let us review the purpose of science or science in general. How does nursing conceptualize itself as a science?

Purpose of Science

Laudan (1977), a philosopher, simply states that the purpose of science is to solve problems, and theory tells us how to do so. He further proposes that the rationality and progressiveness of a theory are not linked with its confirmation or its falsification but instead with its problem-solving effectiveness. This conception of science opens the windows and doors in the hallowed halls of science to include important nonempirical and even nonscientific knowing in the traditional sense. This provides a broader perspective that Laudan suggests is necessary to the rational development of science. Insight, spontaneity, accidental findings, mutability, vicissitude, and fortune all play a role in science.

On the basis of this conception of science and theory, it seems that all sources of knowledge and patterns of knowing are essential sources for problem solving. Nursing research, in its earliest years, began its quest to become a legitimate science with an almost unilateral pattern of knowing that can be categorized as empirics, logical empiricism, logical positivism, or, as described in most nursing research textbooks, the scientific method.

Laudan (1977) sets forth—in contrast or in explanation—a philosophy of science of historicism that incorporates the human elements of science; the study of scientific knowledge is often fostered by illogical and nonrational decision making. The following two quotations may illuminate this point:

> *That no major scientist ever has proceeded in his work along either Baconian or Cartesian lines has not prevented the consecration of method by these two powerful minds from exacting a dismal toll.* (Nesbitt, 1976, p. 14, italics added)

> *Insight announces itself in mental images. Newton's conception of gravity and Einstein's notion of the constant speed of light came to them as perceptions, as images, not a hypothesis or conclusions drawn from logical deduction. Formal logic is secondary to insight via images, and is never the source of new knowledge.* (Bohm, cited in Smith, 1981, p. 444, italics added)

van Manen (1990), in contrast with Laudan's emphasis on problem solving, summarizes what a phenomenological human science cannot do: "Phenomenology does not problem solve" (p. 23). van Manen believed, from a research perspective, that phenomenological questions are meaning questions. However, as addressed in Chapters 1 and 5, if we understand the meaning of specific phenomena, might we not have the basis for problem solving or other types of interventions? In fact, do we not have a responsibility to attempt to problem solve as Crotty (1996) maintained? Furthermore, might we also have understanding that could significantly contribute to the promotion of health and well-being? This does not mean we change the meaning an experience has for a person, perhaps it means based on that meaning we create a unique response. Although, van Manen does not include problem solving, instead understanding of how humans experience being is what is paramount when he states:

> Natural science studies objects of nature, "things," "natural events" and the way that objects behave. Human science, in contrast, studies "persons" or beings that have "consciousness" and that act purposefully in and on the world by creating objects of "meaning" and that are expressions of how human beings exist in the world. (p. 4)

However, this compliments Laudan's science of historicism, of not only incorporating the vicissitudes of the scientist, and so forth, but also to enlarge; what is necessary to knowing something is the essential nature of also knowing what is going on in the contingencies of history and life-worlds when that knowing something occurs (see Chapter 5 for further discussion). We return to the postmodern idea that truth is not immutable and is indeed an ever-changing body of ideas and meaning contingent on multiple factors.

These ideas are not necessarily contradictory; rather, they seem to be woven together as a whole. In addition, discussions about sciences and methods of sciences often seem to lead us away from concrete, lived experiences unless that lived experience is the discussion of sciences. Researchers, I believe, need to be well grounded in the pedantic and philosophical underpinnings of the research enterprise but not for conformity, which can sacrifice creativity. I suggest to students that it is far more scientific to find a phenomenon that interests them, piques their curiosity, and perhaps even fills them with passion than it is to become befuddled by method.[1] Substance should lead the way to form. Interest in some thing or experience should light many sparks of imagination and light the path to method.

However, it is essential to understand the influence and power of research paradigms and traditions in interweaving the ways of knowing and shaping them into a body of knowledge. They can be restricting or liberating, depending on their own ontology and supporting constituencies. Qualitative research methods seek to be of the liberating, illuminating, and emancipatory kind. The critical nature embedded in research paradigms and traditions is found in the circumstance that they are rarely questioned in the study of a discipline. It is a rare undergraduate or graduate student in any field who questions the research methods prevalent in that field. If most of us find guidelines helpful and a research tradition provides us with those guidelines—and if success within the field will be determined by how well one follows those guidelines—the importance of those guidelines can hardly be overstated! The next section describes the nature of research paradigms and traditions connected with our discussion of paths to knowledge and the purpose of science. It is paradoxical to hear the purpose of education to be one of liberation and then to hear students cite the common wisdom of "just do what they tell you to do," subsuming to the unfair power structure that we often encounter in our educational settings.

Paradigms and Research Traditions ⸻

Kuhn (1970) believes that a paradigm structures the questions to be asked within a discipline and systematically eliminates those kinds of questions that cannot be stated within the concepts and tools supplied by the paradigm. This function then is enormously powerful. A paradigm can actually prevent questions from being answered! Laudan (1977), elaborating on his definition of a research tradition, writes: "A research tradition is a set of general assumptions about the entities and processes in a domain of study, and about the appropriate methods to be used for investigating the problems and constructing the theories in that domain" (p. 81). In both these ways, as suggested by Kuhn and by Laudan, the research paradigm and tradition will specify the domain of study, the legitimate modes, and the methods of inquiry open to a researcher within a discipline. This directedness is seldom questioned; in fact, complicity is usually required as well as rewarded.

Why one proceeds in this fashion is explained by Laudan's idea that we need to explore the scientists' work and their reasoning processes. Laudan suggests that scientific knowledge is often developed by illogical and nonrational decision making. Let us now tie together that idea with nursing's historical acceptance of the logical empiricist's worldview or, as stated, the large reliance on logic and empirics as our primary paths to theory development.[2]

The preparation of many nurse researchers in fields in which the research tradition was one of logical empiricism was considered in Chapter 2. Let us look for evidence that supports the further use of this tradition and that may exemplify the nonrational or illogical side of science. This evidence is not always negative, but let us reflect on nursing research and on the subtle and not so subtle ways in which this paradigm or tradition has been perpetuated and still prevails today.

The answers to the following questions, which were asked in the first edition of this book (1987), demonstrate how the values of scientists and their practices influence the general account of human nature. I believe it is quite significant that the same questions are relevant 24 years later. I attempted to explain the reason for their relevance in a discussion of life-world fittingness (Munhall, 1992):

- If you were to request a research grant from the Division of Nursing of the Department of Health and Human Services or the National Institute of Nursing Research (NINR)–National Institutes of Health (NIH), which research method do you believe would be viewed most favorably?

- If you wanted guidelines for doing research and consulted the most prevalent nursing research textbooks, which research method would seemingly be the only one available? What is the research method most taught in research classes?
- If you wish to submit an abstract of research for a general research conference, which research method is represented in the format for the abstract?
- If you wanted to critique a research study, which method is most represented under criteria for evaluation?

Now in the fifth edition of this book, I might ask you to consider additional questions:

- If you are enrolled in a PhD program, which method do your required courses support and prepare you for? (There are exceptions!) We looked at this problem in Chapter 1.
- If you are seeking a faculty position, how will you get the evidence of extramural funding that is required to be demonstrated?
- Peruse the list of recent NINR grants and ask: Which paradigm is most rewarded?
- Here is progress: Many NINR grants today require a qualitative research section. Yay!

For those nurse researchers who have been questioning the general acceptance of the answers to these questions, I suggest we enlarge our lens, broaden our scope, and widen our perspective. Furthermore, the answers to these questions demonstrate the subjectivity of the entire research enterprise. Human beings determine which paths to explore. We need to explore all the paths to knowledge and all the patterns of knowing because we would then be researching the whole of the human condition, both the subjective and objective worlds of our research endeavors.

Capra (1982) stated our need almost 3 decades ago:

> What we need, then, is a new vision of reality—a fundamental change in our thoughts, perceptions and values. The beginnings of this change, of the shift from the mechanistic to the holistic conception of reality, are already visible in all fields and are likely to dominate the entire decade. (p. ix)

My endeavor here, built upon the works of many nursing scholars, among them the contributors to this book, is to encourage this vision, to incorporate the qualitative and quantitative methods of research as representative of an epistemology of wholeness, and to respect and reward all patterns of knowing. Despite the answers to the preceding questions, the processes and rewards of doing qualitative research certainly have continued to grow, and we have become more sophisticated and savvy. As stated above, many NINR grants today require a qualitative section. That is progress. Yet, it still seems we qualitative researchers have to defend our work to a much greater extent. So many scholars are calling for this consilience, we need to heed their wisdom. Reread Wilson's quote in the section titled "Paths to Knowledge" and the preceding quote by Capra.

It has been said that your research question should determine your research method. Today I am not sure that is the best way to think about choosing a research method. Over many years, I have seen that students have specific leanings toward one or another way of thinking, as was discussed in Chapter 1. I believe these leanings reflect a natural attitude toward the world at large, and students—just as we acknowledge students have different ways of learning material—have different philosophical orientations toward questioning and how one answers those questions. I believe most of my colleagues respect these innate tendencies. Actually recognizing individuals as being more left-sided brain dominant and others as more right-sided brain dominant should make the whole research enterprise holistic, more consistent with the times in which we live, and contribute to a much greater depth and breadth of knowing and understanding. Our differences enrich us and inspire us to see the new.

Let us move now to a consideration of two epistemological questions: What is it that we want to know about? and What is it that we wish to understand?

Epistemological Interests of Nursing

As stated earlier, one of the purposes of science is to solve problems, and the subsequent theory development involves the solution of problems (Laudan, 1977). Qualitative researchers can qualify that purpose with the caveat that, before you can solve a problem, you need to understand the many facets of a problem. In this section, we explore schemata that have been developed by nurses in an effort to focus nursing research on nursing phenomena.

Six nursing perspectives are summarized in an effort to identify our epistemological interests. They are presented chronologically and may demonstrate consistency, overlap, complementarity, and/or much variation. Also they are presented here as a demonstration of our historical evolution. I begin with Paterson and Zderad, out of great respect for their major groundbreaking work of 1976, in which they were the first nurses to actually use the language and the method of phenomenology. It is important to understand these different perspectives so that one can debate the merits or lack of merit of the various perspectives. Each provides varying answers to the question, "What do nurses study?" We will also reexamine the ideas of Donaldson and Crowley (1978), the American Nurses Association's Social Policy Statement (1995), Fawcett's (1984) metaparadigm for nursing, and the emphasis on care (Newman, Sime, & Corcoran-Perry, 1991; Watson, 1985). We conclude with Watson's (1999) ideas of what nurses should be studying at the beginning of this new century.

This summary does not do justice to the field of theory development, nor does it intend to; the intent of this section is to consider exemplars and a historical perspective. Undoubtedly, if you are reading this book, you probably are very knowledgeable about theory and can ask, "What does a particular theorist think we should 'know' and 'how' should we research particular phenomena?" These questions could provide a good seminar discussion.

Paterson and Zderad (1976), to the question "What do nurses study?" (or "What should nurses study?"), might reply in this manner. Because the act of nursing is "the intersubjective transactional relation, a dialogue experience, lived in concert between persons where comfort and nurturance produce mutual human unfolding" (Paterson, 1978, p. 51), nurses would do well to study the following situations:

- Comfort—persons being all that they can be in particular life situations
- Nurturance—promoting growth through relating
- Clinical—presence in the health situation, reflected and acted upon
- Empathy—imaginative moving toward oneness with another, sharing his or her being in a situation, resulting in an insightful knowledge of another's perspective

From these situations, the phenomenon of concern to nurses is the need for quality nursing descriptions of those experiences inherent in the preceding situations and suggested in Table 2–7 in Chapter 2. Paterson and Zderad (1976) call our attention to existential, humanistic, phenomenological phenomena that should be our epistemological interests. This they did in 1976, and you can see how future oriented they were. I urge students of current theory to read through their pioneering book, which was reissued in 1988.

Widely cited and more traditional, yet showing promises of a new worldview, were Donaldson and Crowley (1978), who identified three major themes of nursing:

1. Concern with the principles and laws that govern the life processes, well-being, and optimal functioning of human beings, sick or well.
2. Concern with the patterning of human behavior in interaction with the environment in critical life situations.
3. Concern with the processes by which positive changes in health status are affected.

Concepts within the nurse–client world that relate to the preceding themes need to be discovered, and the methods of the first order of scientific activity, the qualitative methods of science, are essential to this process. Within this book, an effort is made to demonstrate this basic activity of discovering what is there, naming it, understanding it, and explaining it. We can then give examples of what is meant and what is the potential within the scope of these themes.

Our own professional organization, the American Nurses Association, has consistently revised its definition of nursing according to society's needs and has focused nurse researchers' perspectives on human responses within the following context: "Nursing is the diagnosis and treatment of human responses to actual or potential health problems" (American Nurses Association, 1995). Possible phenomena that bear investigation from this perspective of nursing are further suggested, including the following:

- Self-care limitations
- Impaired functioning—physiological needs
- Pain and discomfort
- Emotional problems, such as anxiety, loss, loneliness, and grief
- Distortion of symbolic functions   *roles &*
- Deficiencies in decision making   *transitions*
- Self-image changes
- Dysfunctional perceptual orientations
- Strains related to life processes
- Problematic affiliative relations

Readers familiar with the works of Rogers (1970), Roy (1976), Johnson (1980), Orem (1980), King (1981), Watson (1985), and other nursing theorists can readily see the influence of these theorists on the various phenomena that would constitute human responses.

Fawcett (1984) identifies in her earlier works a metaparadigm for nursing in pursuit of establishing boundaries within which the purview of nursing can be delineated. She proposes that the metaparadigm comprises the central concepts and themes that represent the phenomena of interest to the discipline. Paradigms, then, are the conceptual models that provide "distinctive contexts for the metaparadigm concepts and themes" (p. 2).

The metaparadigm of nursing that has evolved, according to Fawcett (1984, p. 2), consists of four major concepts: person, environment, health, and nursing. These central concepts are defined as follows:

1. Person—the recipient of care
2. Environment—significant others and the surroundings of the recipient of care; the setting in which nursing care takes place
3. Health—the wellness or illness state of the recipient at the time when nursing occurs
4. Nursing—actions taken by nurses on behalf of or in conjunction with the recipient of care

Fawcett (1984) adds the themes explicated by Donaldson and Crowley, presented earlier, to the metaparadigm of nursing by indicating the central concepts and the themes that should represent the phenomena of interest to nurse investigators. She then suggests that the four patterns of knowledge, as discussed by Carper (1978), link the concepts and themes. With these varying perspectives have come articles that call for a focus of the discipline of nursing. Newman et al. (1991) point out that nursing's domain of inquiry distinguishes it as a discipline. As is readily apparent in the foregoing paragraph, nursing has a rather large domain of inquiry. Newman et al. (1991) suggest that nursing should have a focus statement. They point out that, from the time of Florence Nightingale to the present era of Leininger (1984), Watson (1988), and Benner and Wrubel (1989), health and caring have been linked. Incorporating Pender's (1987) use of the term health experience, Newman's focus statement at the time was this: "Nursing is the study of caring in the human health experience" (p. 3).

Nursing's domain of inquiry was then stated as "caring in the human health experience" (p. 3). Present-day perspectives in nursing research and theory seem to have evolved from this eclecticism of thought. This eclecticism is philosophically congruent with the world at large. Today the prefixes 'multi' and 'poly' are frequently used to reflect the shift from foundationalism to hermeneutics, or interpretation of phenomena. Newman (1986) and Watson (1999) are among the many nursing scholars who have expanded the worldview of nursing and the domains for nursing inquiry. Postmodern in their perspectives, they recognize that whatever is studied must be viewed within the context and possibility of multiple realities. The idea that individuals, families, cultures, and societies construct their own realities is readily evident in a world that all of a sudden has found itself so interconnected—that what we hear is polyvocality, what we see is individually perspectival, and what we read is contextually interpreted. Multiple realities are recognized as being based on subjective experience; so multiplicity and multimind emerge. Qualitative researchers are most synchronous with these conditions of uncertainty, flux, discontinuity, and indeterminacy. Qualitative researchers have long recognized the social construction of reality, contingencies, and the situated context as critical parts of their research efforts. This topic will be further considered in the next section, but, for our purposes here, whatever domains or phenomena nurses want to research, it is most important for them to take into account the situatedness of a person in a multiworld of endless variations.

We should enjoy the complexity of our profession because it affords us an opportunity to study and research an almost infinite variety of human and environmental phenomena. Some could say we are "all over the place;" and, in actuality, nurses themselves are all over the place, in every developmental phase of an individual's life, in health and in crisis, in private practice, in schools, in hospitals, in foreign countries, and in the homes of patients. They are practitioners, educators, administrators, writers, researchers, and politicians. With all this complexity, it is quite understandable why nurses would need a variety of research methods or approaches from which to choose.

Epistemological Commitments to Qualitative Research _____

In the preceding discussion, I present different perspectives on what nurses might investigate. The broad scope reflects the expansiveness of the profession of nursing. Discussions among theorists and researchers often revolve around narrowing this scope, perhaps by adopting one model or accepting, for equally good reasons, a multiple-perspective approach. I do not think we have any choice but to be representative of the world, and, being in the world, that demands a multiperspectival epistemological commitment. In Chapter 2, I defined quantitative methods of research as "the traditional scientific methods as presented in most of the contemporary nursing research textbooks. These methods are characterized by deductive reasoning, objectivity, quasi-experiments, statistical techniques, and control." In contrast, I defined the qualitative methods, many of which are described in this text, as "characterized by inductive reasoning, contingency, subjectivity, discovery, description, and process orienting." Benoliel (1984) enhances that description in this observation: "Qualitative approaches in science are distinct modes of inquiry oriented toward understanding the unique nature of human thoughts, behaviors, negotiations and institutions under different sets of historical and environmental circumstances" (p. 7).

We should view these two approaches from a historical perspective. During the 17th century, empiricism, as the scientific method, reigned supreme. That form of empiricism proceeds through sense knowledge, and that which connects with our senses is matter. This often is the origin of conceived objectivity, in which the physical world can be seen, touched, or measured. The hold that matter (materialism) has on us is connected with the simple fact that we think we can get hold of matter and control it. Thus, we have the controlled experiment with validation, significance, and the premises of confidence and prediction. As has been suggested, nursing research has, to a large extent, aligned itself with this positivistic and materialistic view of science. In the preceeding editions of this book, I discussed the postpositivistic perspective articulated by Polkinghorne (1983), who cited recognition and acceptance of the following factors as enlarging the scope of science:

- Different language systems reflect different perceptions of the same reality (as was illustrated in Chapter 2).
- The essential study of complex wholes is through system theory, and human beings are complex wholes.
- The ideas of purposive and intentional activity explain human action.
- All knowledge, instead of being truth, is an expression of interpretation.

Such beliefs and assumptions have contributed to the acceptance of the worthiness and credibility of methods of knowing other than the positivistic worldview. Additionally, there has been growing acceptance and recognition of the differences between the material and the experiential nature of human behavior and relationships. Benoliel (1984, p. 4) cites some of these differences as follows:

- Social life is the shared creativity of individuals and their perceptions.
- The character of the social world is dynamic and changing.
- There are multiple realities and frameworks for viewing the world: the world is not independent of humankind and objectively identifiable.
- Human beings are active agents who construct their own realities.
- There are not any response sets that are highly predictable.

Since earlier editions, one can easily see how these ideas have come to expression in most contemporary philosophies of nursing. Because the emergent nursing philosophies reflect, whether stated or not, poststructuralist or postmodern perspectives, the stated beliefs and values about the individual are congruent with the research methods presented in this text. We are involved in an emergent shift from the modern characteristics of science to a postmodern perspective of science. This shift is not a negation of science but recognition of a "more." Science expands its boundaries from strict materialism and recognizes the need for accommodating a dynamic reality and describing individual situatedness to be essential to good research.

The shifts that are most prevalent in the qualitative domain are the focus on meaning of experience; understanding what it means to be in this world, or that world; listening to others to provide us with this material; and interpretation by both the research participant and the researcher. Contrary to the traditional scientific method, where the problem is stated at the outset of the research project by the researcher, the qualitative researcher usually begins with a phenomenon or an experience. Going to the people who are involved in the phenomenon or experience, the qualitative researcher engages with the participant and the environment and lets both speak to her or him. The narratives, semiotics, and interaction allow for the development of coming to understand some "thing." Problems may emerge as part of the wholeness of the experience, but the identification of a problem comes from the source, the individual in experience.

This involvement calls for the nurse researcher to have many characteristics. It is important for qualitative researchers to grasp the complexity of experience, of its wholeness. Rather than compartmentalizing experience into two or three different variables, which may be necessary in experimental research, experience needs to be met with openness by the researcher. In addition to being open, the researcher needs to be the one who is unknowing. The participant is the expert who is imparting to the researcher existential material that should be co-interpreted and then interpreted for its implications for nursing practice.

Before specific questions for research are formulated, overarching questions and commitments should guide researchers in choosing a research method. What is it that interests you? Do you think of yourself as more concrete and more comfortable with structure? Do you like discovering relations, correlations, and possible solutions to problems? Do you find beauty in a perfect scientific design with complex statistical analysis? If you have these propensities, then what we are calling quantitative designs are probably what you will enjoy doing and be successful at, as well as contributing to nursing's body of knowledge.

Those considering qualitative research methods need to be more comfortable with uncertainty and unpredictability. The primary focus is on meaning (and the implications of the meaning), and the aims of inquiry are found in understanding and interpretation. A critical commitment is to faithfully, without your own presuppositions or judgments, represent another's experience, meaning, and interpretation. There needs to be an authentic caring about how another person perceives his or her world, and there needs to be authentic respect for many differences, as was discussed in Chapter 1.

These considerations do not in any way imply that a nurse researcher cannot combine these commitments. Indeed many hold all these commitments toward research. Yet, in the years of my own experience, students and researchers seem to show different ways of being in the world, and one should reflect on and recognize one's leanings before embarking on learning a specific method, which is its own commitment.

And that brings us to considering the last commitment in this section. This text is an overview, as are many textbooks. If you are interested and excited about a specific method, this is your first step: read the particular chapter on that method and the following exemplar. The real commitment is to further in-depth study of the particular method; its philosophical, ontological, theoretical, and conceptual underpinnings; and the human requirements, abilities, and characteristics needed to implement the method well. With more and more reading and practice, you will evolve, change, have your own insights, and truly understand what you are doing in a way that becomes a part of you. The first meaning, understanding, and interpretation are those of the experience itself, those of grasping the wholeness and complexity of the method.

An Epistemological Circle: Circle and Re-Circle _____

Questions are often asked about the relatedness of quantitative and qualitative methods, if there is a relation at all. Chapter 25 addresses this question. A mental representation of an epistemological circle could be one perspective. This conceptualization is one of process and demonstrates how theory evolves, is revised by a nuance, and is first discovered through qualitative inquiry and can be validated in some way by quantitative inquiry. We can visualize a qualitative-quantitative cyclical continuum where qualitative inquiry could lead to a hypothesis and a quantitative study. Quantitative inquiry in a human science, I believe, should always have its origins in qualitative inquiry. Otherwise, the researcher is the knower of the experience and the phenomenon, and therefore, whatever instrument is developed or intervention tested, it is grounded in the life-world of the researcher rather than in the life-world of those experiencing knowers who can inform, through their sharing with us, the descriptions and interpretations necessary for congruency grounded in specific contexts.

What I Did Not Know

My own dissertation was an example of not following this sequence. It is an example of a quantitative study as will be described without the necessary qualitative research. Furthermore it is an example of what was required at the time of my doing a dissertation. From the critique that follows my own impetus to the importance of qualitative research was born. All sorts of realizations took place based on recognizing the lack of logic and understanding.

Using an instrument, which was derived and tested on an all-male population, Kohlberg (1976) derived a theory of moral development. Not knowing its origin, which unfortunately is the case with many instruments used in quantitative research, I used this instrument on women, an instrument based on his theory, and the women participants performed much "lower" in scores than the norms. The norms, I did not realize, were based on only males, and only males were utilized to develop and evaluate the instrument. The males like so many studies where theory has been developed were from a university class of men about 20 years of age or so. After Carol Gilligan's (1982) groundbreaking work, *In a Different Voice*, I came to realize why my own sample of nurses did not seem to fare so well in the test scores. This too provides another example or question: are all things measurable? Context and contingency were also absent for the responders, they were to use logical thinking without experience.

Calling Generalizations Into Question

I wrote an article critiquing my own study and illustrating that using a theory and instrument derived from another population and applied to a different population is a serious epistemological error. The article was rejected by a very prominent nursing research journal on the grounds *"that the last thing we need in nursing research is to start criticizing ourselves."* The manuscript did find a home (Munhall, 1982), and I do hope it called attention to the need for a self-reflective epistemological circle and the thorough thinking through of any method, as well as the critical need for self-critique of one's research.

In a nonlinear schema, qualitative descriptions, interpretations, and understandings lead to quantitative analysis (when that is appropriate), and from that analysis, nuances, or what Kuhn (1970) terms *anomalies*, become sources of further qualitative inquiry. For example, many studies statistically support the proposition that preoperative teaching reduces anxiety for the majority of preoperative patients. However, the same teaching can increase anxiety in some patients. This is a nuance and calls us back to a qualitative study: "What about those patients?" We need to discriminate further within our populations. We need to call into question generalizations. Theories always need reevaluating, and the nuances or the exceptions often alert us to alternative or evolving ways of viewing phenomena. Thus, thinking about research as a qualitative-quantitative cyclical continuum represents the dynamic and changing life-worlds. Circularity does not have to be the outcome of all qualitative research, where quantitative research follows. The findings of qualitative research can stand on their own merit with implications for nursing practice found in the descriptions, interpretations, and narratives by the researcher. However, for congruency in arriving at a hypothesis, a qualitative base line from the same situated context—that is, people, place, time, culture, sex, and other characteristics—should be the origin of good quantitative research. Perhaps Campbell (1975) summarizes this point best when he says:

> *After all, man in his ordinary way is a very competent knower, and qualitative common sense is not replaced by quantitative knowing. Rather quantitative knowing has to trust and build on the qualitative, including ordinary perception. We methodologists must achieve an applied epistemology which integrates both.* (italics added) (p. 191)

Summary

I hope that you hold with me a belief in the rich potential that qualitative methods of research have to offer to our practice and our understanding of ourselves, our patients, the multi-worlds in which we live, and what it means to be human at this time in history. I think we have come to understand the importance of the subjective experience of the one who experiences to the development of nursing theory. In Chapters 2 and 3, I have attempted to provide the background necessary for you to understand the differences in language, the philosophical perspectives, and the contexts in which nursing research first developed and continues to grow and evolve. Additionally, an effort has been made to explicate patterns of knowing, the purpose of science, what it is we want to know about, how we go about knowing, and what commitments are needed to engage in qualitative research.

References

Allen, D. (1991). Applying critical social theory to nursing education. In N. Greenleaf (Ed.), *Curriculum revolution: Redefining the student–teacher relationship.* New York: National League for Nursing.

Allen, D. (1995). Hermeneutics: Philosophy, traditions, and nursing practice research. *Nursing Science Quarterly, 8*(4), 175–181.

American Nurses Association. (1995). *Nursing: A social policy statement.* Kansas City, MO: Author.

Belenky, M., Clinchy, B., Goldberg, N., & Taub, J. (1986). *Women's ways of knowing.* New York: Basic Books [(1997—10th Anniversary Edition). New York: Basic Books].

Benner, P., & Wrubel, J. (1989). *The primacy of caring.* Menlo Park, CA: Addison-Wesley.

Benoliel, J. (1984, March). Advancing nursing science: Qualitative approaches. *Western Journal of Nursing Research in Nursing and Health, 7,* 1–8.

Campbell, D. J. (1975). Degrees of freedom and the case study. *Comparative Political Studies, 8,* 178–193.

Capra, Z. (1982). Foreword. In L. Dossey (Ed.), *Space, time and medicine* (p. ix). Boulder, CO: Shambhala.

Carper, B. A. (1978, October). Fundamental patterns of knowing in nursing. *Advances in Nursing Science, 1,* 13–23.

Crotty, M. (1996). *Phenomenology and nursing research.* South Melbourne, Australia: Churchill Livingston.

Donaldson, S. K., & Crowley, D. M. (1978). The discipline of nursing. *Nursing Outlook, 26,* 113–120.

Dzurec, L. (1989). The necessity for and evolution of multiple paradigms for nursing research: A poststructural perspective. *Advances in Nursing Science, 11*(4), 69–77.

Fawcett, J. (1984, October). Hallmarks of success in nursing research. *Advances in Nursing Science, 7,* 1.

Freire, P. (1971). *Pedagogy of the oppressed.* New York: Seaver.

Gadamer, G. H., Sheed & Ward, Ltd. (1975). *Truth and method.* New York: Crossroad.

Gilligan, C. (1982). *In a different voice: Psychological theory and women's development.* Cambridge, MA: Harvard University Press.

Gould, S. J. (1984, August 12). Review of the book Science and gender. *New York Times Book Review.*

Harman, W. (1977). *Symposium and consciousness.* New York: Penguin.

Johnson, D. E. (1980). The behavioral system model for nursing. In J. P. Riehl & C. Roy (Eds.), *Conceptual models for nursing practice* (2nd ed.). Norwalk, CT: Appleton-Century-Crofts.

King, I. M. (1981). *A theory for nursing: Systems, concepts, process.* New York: Wiley.

Kneller, G. (1971). *Introduction to the philosophy of education.* New York: Wiley.

Kohlberg, L. (1976). Moral stages and moralization. In T. Lickona (Ed.), *Moral development and behavior.* New York: Holt, Rinehart and Winston.

Kuhn, T. S. (Ed.). (1970). *The structure of scientific revolutions.* Chicago: University of Chicago Press.

Kurtz, S. (1989). *The art of unknowing.* Northvale, NJ: Aronson.

Laudan, L. (1977). *Progress and its problems: Toward a theory of scientific growth.* Berkeley, CA: University of California Press.

Leininger, M. (Ed.). (1984). *Care: The essence of nursing and health.* Thorofare, NJ: Slack.

Morgan, G. (1983). *Beyond method.* Newbury Park, CA: Sage.

Munhall, P. (1982). Methodic fallacies: A critical self appraisal. *Advances in Nursing Science, 5*(4), 41–47.

Munhall, P. (1992). Holding the Mississippi River in place and other implications for qualitative research. *Nursing Outlook, 10*(6), 257–262.

Munhall, P. (1993). Toward a fifth pattern of knowing: Unknowing. *Nursing Outlook, 41,* 125–128.

Nesbitt, R. (1976). *Sociology as an art form.* New York: Oxford University Press.

Newman, M. (1983, January). Editorial. *Advances in Nursing Science, 5*(2), x–xi.

Newman, M. (1986). *Health as expanding consciousness.* St. Louis, MO: Mosby.

Newman, M., Sime, A., & Corcoran-Perry, S. (1991). The focus of the discipline of nursing. *Advances in Nursing Science, 14,* 1–5.

Orem, D. E. (1980). *Nursing: Concepts of practice* (2nd ed.). New York: McGraw-Hill.

Paterson, J. (1978). *The tortuous way toward nursing theory. In Theory development: What, why and how?* New York: National League for Nursing.

Paterson, J., & Zderad, L. (1976). *Humanistic nursing.* New York: Wiley.

Pender, N. J. (1987). *Health promotion in nursing practice.* Norwalk, CT: Appleton-Lange.

Polkinghorne, D. (1983). *Methodology for the human sciences.* Albany, NY: SUNY Press.

Rogers, M. E. (1970). *An introduction to the theoretical basis of nursing.* Philadelphia: Davis.

Roy, C., Sr. (1976). *Introduction to nursing: An adaptation model.* Englewood Cliffs, NJ: Prentice Hall.

Silva, M., & Rothbart, D. (1984, January). An analysis of changing trends in philosophies of science on nursing theory development and testing. *Advances in Nursing Science, 6*(2), 1–12.

Smith, H. (1981). Beyond the modern Western mind set. *Teachers College Record (Columbia University), 82*(3), 444.

Stevens, B. J. (1979). *Nursing theory: Analysis, application, evaluation.* Boston: Little, Brown.

Uris, P. (1993). Postmodern feminist emancipatory research. Unpublished doctoral dissertation, University of Colorado, Denver.

van Manen, M. (1990). *Research on lived experience: Human science for action-sensitive pedagogy.* New York: SUNY Press.

Watson, J. (1985). *Nursing: The philosophy and science of caring.* Boulder, CO: Colorado Associated University Press.

Watson, J. (1988). New dimensions of human caring theory. *Nursing Science, 1*(4), 175–181.

Watson, J. (1999). *Post modern nursing and beyond.* New York: Churchill Livingstone.

Wilson, E. (1998). *Consilience.* New York: Knopf.

Additional Resources

Anderson, W. (1995). *The truth about truth.* New York: Putnam.

Appleton, J. V., & King, L. (1997). Constructivism: A naturalistic methodology for nursing inquiry. *Advances in Nursing Science, 20*(2), 13–22.

Arslanian, C. (1998). Taking the mystery out of research: Qualitative nursing research. *Orthopaedic Nursing, 17,* 31.

Ashworth, P. D. (1997). The variety of qualitative research (Part 2): Non-positivist approaches. *Nurse Education Today, 17,* 219–224.

Atkinson, P., Coffey, A., & Delamont, S. (2003). *Key themes in qualitative research: Continuities and changes.* New York: Rowman & Littlefield.

Bohm, D. (1998). *On creativity.* New York: Routledge.

Bolster, A. (1983). Toward a more effective model of research on teaching. *Harvard Education Review, 53*(3), 294–308.

Boulton, M., & Fitzpatrick, R. (1994). Quality in qualitative research. *Critical Public Health, 5*(3), 19–26.

Benner, P. (Ed.). (1994). *Interpretive phenomenology: Embodiment, caring, and ethics in health and illness.* Thousand Oaks, CA: Sage.

Bunkers, S. S., Petardi, L. A., Pilkington, F. B., & Walls, P. A. (1996). Challenging the myths surrounding qualitative research in nursing. *Nursing Science Quarterly, 9,* 33–37.

Byrne, M. M. (2001). Evaluating the findings of qualitative research. *AORN Journal, 73*(3), 703–706.

Carey, M. A., & Swanson, J. (2003). Funding for qualitative research. *Qualitative Health Research, 13*(6), 852–856.

Carnevale, F. A. (2002). Authentic qualitative research and the quest for methodological rigour. *Canadian Journal of Nursing Research, 34*(2), 121–128.

Chan, G., Benner, P., Brykczinski, K., & Malone, R. (2010). *Interpretive phenomenology in health care research: Studying social practice, lifeworlds, and embodiment.* Indianapolis, IN: Sigma Theta Tau International.

Charmaz, K. (2004). Premises, principles and practices in qualitative research: Revisiting the foundations. *Qualitative Health Research, 14*(7), 976–993.

Clark, A. M. (1998). The qualitative-quantitative debate: Moving from positivism and confrontation to post-positivism and reconciliation. *Journal of Advanced Nursing, 27,* 1242–1249.

Cook, S. D. N., & Brown, J. S. (1999). Bridging epistemologies: The generative dance between organizational knowledge and organizational knowing. *Organization Science, 10*(4), 381–400.

Coyle, J., & Williams, B. (2000). An exploration of the epistemological intricacies of using qualitative data to develop a quantitative measure of user views of health care. *Journal of Advanced Nursing, 31,* 1235–1243.

Cutliffe, J. R., & Mckenna, H. P. (2002). When do we know that we know? Considering the truth of research findings and the craft of qualitative research. *International Journal of Nursing Studies, 39*(6), 611–619.

Dahlberg, K., & Drew, N. (1997). A lifeworld paradigm for nursing research. *Journal of Holistic Nursing, 15,* 303–317.

Davenport, J., & Rudd, A. (2001). *Kierkegaard after MacIntyre: Essays on freedom, narrative and virtue.* Chicago: Open Court.

Dews, P. (Ed.). (1999). *Habermas: A critical reader.* Malden, MA.: Blackwell.

Diers, D. (1979). *Research in nursing practice.* Philadelphia: Lippincott.

DiGiacomo, S. M. (1992). Metaphor as illness: Postmodern dilemmas in the representation of body, mind and disorder. *Medical Anthropology, 14,* 109–137.

Drew, N., & Dahlberg, K. (1995). Challenging a reductionistic paradigm as a foundation for nursing. *Journal of Holistic Nursing, 13,* 332–345.

Efinger, J., Maldonado, N., & McArdle, G. (2004). PhD students' perceptions of the relationship between philosophy and research: A qualitative investigation. *Qualitative Report, 9*(4), 732–759.

Estabrooks, C., Rutakumwa, W., O'Leary, K., Profetto-McGrath, J., Milner, M., Levers, M., & Scott-Findlay, S. (2005). Sources of practice knowledge among nurses. *Qualitative Health Research, 15*(4), 460–476.

Farrel, G. A., & Gritching, W. L. (1997). Social science at the crossroads: What direction mental health nurses? *Australian New Zealand Journal of Mental Health Nursing, 6,* 19–29.

Findlay, S. (2005). Sources of practice knowledge among nurses. *Qualitative Health Research, 15*(4), 460–476.

Forbes, D. A., King, K. M., Kushner, K. E., Letourneau, N. L., Myrick, A. F., & Profetto-McGrath, J. (1999). Warrantable evidence in nursing science. *Journal of Advanced Nursing, 29,* 373–379.

Frank, A. W. (2004). After methods, the story: From incongruity to truth in qualitative research. *Qualitative Health Research, 14*(3), 430–440.

French, P. (2002). What is the evidence on evidence-based nursing? An epistemological concern. *Journal of Advanced Nursing, 29*(1), 72–78.

Greene, G., & Freed, S. (2005). Research as improvisation: Dancing among perspectives. *Qualitative Report, 10*(2), 276–288.

Habermas, J., Nicholsen, S., & Stark, J. A. (Trans.). (1996). *On the logic of the social sciences.* Cambridge, MA: The MIT Press.

Hall, E. O. C. (1996). Husserlian phenomenology and nursing in a unitary-transformative paradigm. *Vard-I-Norden Nursing Science and Research in the Nordic Countries, 16*(3), 4–8.

Holliday, A. (2001). *Doing and writing qualitative research.* London: Sage.

Hones, M. L. (2004). Application of systematic review methods to qualitative research: Practical issues. *Journal of Advanced Nursing, 48*(3), 271–278.

Irving, J., & Klenke, K. (2004). Telos, Chronos, and Hermeneia: The role of metanarrative in leadership effectiveness through the production of meaning. *International Journal of Qualitative Methods, 3*(3), Article 3.

Johnson, D. E. (1978). *State of the art of theory development. In Theory development: What, why, how?* New York: National League for Nursing.

Kearney, M. H. (2001). *Levels and application of qualitative research evidence. Research in Nursing and Health, 24*(2), 145–153.

Letourneau, N., & Allen, M. (1999). Post-positivistic critical multiplism: A beginning dialogue. *Journal of Advanced Nursing, 30,* 623–630.

Light, R., & Pillemer, D. (1982). Numbers and narrative: Combining their strengths in research reviews. *Harvard Education Review, 52,* 1–23.

Lincoln, Y., & Guba, E. (1985). *Naturalistic inquiry.* Newbury Park, CA: Sage.

Lutz, K. F., Jones, K. D., & Kendall, J. (1997). Expanding the praxis debate: Contributions to clinical inquiry. *Advances in Nursing Science, 20*(2), 23–31.

MacIntyre, A. (1988). *Whose justice? Which rationality?* South Bend, IN: University of Notre Dame Press.

MacIntyre, R. (1999). *Mortal men: Living with asymptomatic HIV.* Piscataway, NJ: Rutgers University Press.

Madjar, I., Taylor, B., & Lawler, J. (2002). The role of qualitative research in evidence based practice. *Collegian, 9*(4), 7–9.

Madjar, I., & Walton, J. A. (1999). *Nursing and the experience of illness: Phenomenology in practice.* New York: Routledge.

Mantzoukas, S. (2004). Issues of representation within qualitative inquiry. *Qualitative Health Research, 14*(7), 994–1007.

Marks, M. D. (1999). Network. Reconstructing nursing: Evidence, artistry and the curriculum . . . including commentary by L. Nyatanga & M. Johnson. *Nurse Education Today, 19,* 3–11.

McAllister, M., & Rowe, J. (2003). Blackbirds singing in the dead of night? Advancing the craft of teaching qualitative research. *Journal of Nursing Education, 42*(7), 296–303.

Monti, E. J., & Tingen, M. S. (1999). Multiple paradigms of nursing science. *Advances in Nursing Science, 21*(4), 64–80.

Morse, J. (2005). Decontextualized care. *Qualitative Health Research, 15*(2), 143–144.

Morse, J., & Chung, S. (2003). Toward holism: The significance of methodological pluralism. *International Journal of Qualitative Methods, 2*(3), Article 2.

Morse, J. M. (1999). Qualitative methods: The state of art. *Qualitative Health Research, 9,* 393–406.

Munhall, P. (1982a). Nursing philosophy and nursing research: In apposition or opposition? *Nursing Research, 31*(3), 176–177, 181.

Munhall, P. (1982b, April). Ethical juxtapositions in nursing research. *Topics in Clinical Nursing, 4,* 66–73.

Munhall, P. (1986). Methodological issues in nursing: Beyond a wax apple. *Advances in Nursing Science, 8*(3), 1–5.

Munhall, P. (1989). Philosophical pondering on qualitative research methods in nursing. *Nursing Science Quarterly, 2,* 20–28.

Munhall, P. (1992). A new ageism: Beyond a toxic apple. *Nursing and Health Care, 13,* 370–376.

Munhall, P. (1994a). *Qualitative research: Proposals and reports.* New York: National League for Nursing.

Munhall, P. (1994b). *Revisioning phenomenology: Nursing and health science research.* Sudbury, MA: Jones and Bartlett.

Munhall, P. (1997). Déjà vu, parroting, buy-ins, and opening. In J. Fawcett & I. King (Eds.), *The language of nursing theory and metatheory.* Indianapolis, IN: Sigma Theta Tau International.

Munhall, P. (1998). Qualitative designs. In P. Brink & M. Wood (Eds.), *Advanced designs in nursing research* (2nd ed.). Newbury Park, CA: Sage.

Munhall, P. (2000a). *Qualitative research reports and proposals: A guide.* Sudbury, MA: Jones and Bartlett.

Munhall, P. (2000b). Unknowing. In W. Kelly & V. Fitzsimons (Eds.), *Understanding cultural diversity.* Sudbury, MA: Jones and Bartlett.

Munhall, P., & Oiler, C. (1986). *Nursing research: A qualitative perspective.* Norwalk, CT: Appleton-Century-Crofts.

Munhall, P., & Oiler, C. (1993). *Nursing research: A qualitative perspective* (2nd ed.). Sudbury, MA: Jones and Bartlett.

National Institutes of Health. (2001). *Qualitative methods in health research: Opportunities and consideration in application and review* (NIH Publication No. 02-5046). Washington, DC: Author.

Newton-Smith, W. H. (1981). *The rationality of science.* New York: Routledge & Kegan Paul.

Norris, C. (1982). *Concept clarification in nursing.* Rockville, MD: Aspen.

Oakey, A. (2004). Qualitative research and scientific inquiry. *Australian and New Zealand Journal of Public Health, 28*(part 2), 106–108.

Plack, M. (2005). Human nature and research paradigms: Theory meets physical therapy practice. *Qualitative Report, 10*(2), 223–245.

Reichardt, C., & Cook, T. (Eds.). (1979). *Qualitative and quantitative methods in evaluation research* (pp. 33–48). Beverly Hills, CA: Sage.

Rorty, R. (1991). *Essays on Heidegger and others.* New York: Cambridge University Press.

Sandelowski, M. (1995). On the aesthetics of qualitative research. *Image: Journal of Nursing Scholarship, 27*(3), 205–209.

Sandelowski, M. (2002). Reembodying qualitative inquiry. *Qualitative Health Research, 12*(1), 104–115.

Sandelowski, M. (2004). Using qualitative research. *Qualitative Health Research, 14*(10), 1366–1386.

Sandelowski, M., & Barroso, J. (2002). Finding the findings in qualitative studies. *Journal of Nursing Scholarship, 34*(3), 213–219.

Schultz, P. R., & Meleis, A. I. (1988). Nursing epistemology: Traditions, insights, questions. *Image: Journal of Nursing Scholarship, 20*(4), 217–221.

Silva, M. C. (1997). Classic image. Philosophy, science, theory: Interrelationships and implications for nursing research. *Image: Journal of Nursing Scholarship, 29*(3), 210–215.

Thomas, S. P., & Pollio, H. R. (2004). *Listening to patients: A phenomenological approach to nursing research and practice.* New York: Springer.

Thorne, S. E., Kirkham, S. R., & Henderson, A. (1999). Ideological implications of paradigm discourse. *Nursing Inquiry, 6*(2), 123–131.

Thorne, S., Jensen, L., Kearney, M., Noblit, G., & Sandelowski, M. (2004). Qualitative metasynthesis: Reflections on methodological orientation and ideological agenda. *Qualitative Health Research, 14*(10), 1342–1365.

Tobin, G. A., & Begley, C. M. (2004). Methodological rigour within a qualitative framework. *Journal of Advanced Nursing, 48*(4), 388–396.

Turner, D. S. (2003). Horizons revealed: From methodology to method. *International Journal of Qualitative Methods, 2*(1), Article 1.

Wainwright, S. P. (1997). A new paradigm for nursing: The potential realism. *Journal of Advanced Nursing, 26*, 1262–1271.

Waterman, H. (1998). Embracing ambiguities and valuing ourselves: Issues of validity in action research. *Journal of Advanced Nursing, 28*(1), 101–105.

Watson, J. (1995). Postmodernism and knowledge development in nursing. *Nursing Science Quarterly, 8*(2), 60–64.

Wilson, L., & Fitzpatrick, J. (1984, January). Dialectic thinking as a means of understanding systems in development: Relevance to Rogers' principles. *Advances in Nursing Science, 6*(2), 41.

Endnotes

[1] van Manen's (1990) interpretation of why Gadamer's (1975) book *Truth and Method* became popular in North America is relevant and recommended to readers.

[2] Silva and Rothbart (1984) have written a most readable and highly recommended work synthesizing this material. Dzurec (1989), presenting a poststructural perspective, should also be considered.

4

Postmodern Philosophy and Qualitative Research

Joy Longo and Lynne M. Dunphy

In the realm of science, authority is given to the empirical-analytic paradigm. In research, knowledge produced within this paradigm is regarded as real science, and randomized controlled trials are considered the gold standard. Nursing occurs not in a laboratory but within the nurse–patient interaction which is laden in social context; therefore, knowledge that is generated within a positivistic framework fails to fully embrace the perspectives of the real world. Critical science is a critique of social conditions for the purpose of creating social and political change (Chinn & Kramer, 2004). For nurses the interest lies in the ability to achieve social justice, which Kagan, Smith, Cowling, and Chinn (2009) describe as: "objectives and strategies that are explicitly directed toward changing practices and social structures that sustain advantage for some and disadvantage for many in health care" (p. 74) with the purpose of overcoming healthcare disparities that exist due to social structures.

Critical scientists look for truth in the real world and not in laboratories (Ritzer & Goodman, 2004). Maxwell (1997) states:

> Knowledge development in nursing is traditionally constructed from the perspective of modern thought, which is embedded in a social order that perpetuates dominant interests. Focus on the individual, a tendency toward realism and universalism, has produced knowledge that serves the dominant interests by expressing ideologically frozen relationships of dependence and by silencing the oppressed. (p. 215)

The application of a philosophical framework of postmodernism, critical social theory, and feminist theory in research allows for critique of social factors, such as class, and values imposed by dominant groups leading to emancipation. This ideology fits well into a qualitative research realm as it allows for subjectivity and context to enter into the development of knowledge. The subjectivity may not be a single point of view but rather a collective picture of a group or community. Nurses have embraced a global responsibility to health while identifying the disparities that often exist among those of various races, cultures, and economic groups or between the genders. A description of context and critique of factors within that context can contribute to an understanding of their impact on health and health care and the implementation of actions to overcome barriers.

Postmodernism

The very term *postmodernism* implies that one is "beyond" the modern; that one has grasped the limitations of positivistic modes of knowledge acquisition and dissemination; that one recognizes multiple voices, multiple views, and multiple methods when analyzing any aspect of reality, and that one challenges the assumptions of modernist thought and reality. Disowning ideas of universal truths, postmodernism, as Cheek (2000) notes, "challenges the notion of a rationale and unified subject that is so central to modernist thought" (p. 6). Defined by what it comes after, postmodernism is a self-consciously transitional moment, "the boundary between the 'not yet' and the 'no longer'" (Lather, 1991, p. 87). The exhaustions of the paradigms of modernity create an affective space where we feel we cannot continue as we are. The modernist endeavor of control through knowledge has imploded. Lather (1991) describes the postmodern project as a "turning away from the enormous pretensions of positivism . . . to the development of a human science much more varied and reflexive about its limitations" (p. 102). Postmodern thought has infiltrated any number of disciplinary fields, most commonly since WW II. Initially influencing art and architecture, it spread rapidly to philosophy and literary studies in the 1950s and 1960s and since then, it has influenced all fields, including health care, nursing, and feminism (Cheek, 2000; Fraser & Nicholson, 1990).

Method

According to Bauman (1992) postmodernism is an unstable concept, difficult to define. It does not represent a unified position or coherent school of thought; indeed, it is notable for its incoherence. Likewise, there is no one postmodern "method." According to Foucault (1980), postmodern and post-structural approaches become "instruments of analyses" (p. 62) rather than rigid set of rules. If one links positivism to prediction, post-positivist inquiry, encompassing postmodern and poststructural approaches, may be said to aim to understand, emancipate, and/or deconstruct. According to Lather (1991) each of these three post-positivist "paradigms" offers a different approach to generating and legitimating knowledge (p. 7). See **Table 4–1**.

Postmodern thought argues that "knowledge is contextualized by its historical and cultural nature" (Agger, 1991, p. 117). Thus, researchers must expose rather than conceal (for instance behind methodological frames) "their own investment in a particular view of the world" (Agger, 1991, p. 117). Personal values manifest themselves in the very research questions posed as well as the methods used to seek answers to those questions. It is a short leap from postmodern thought to critical social theory, and further to feminist approaches. They spring from similar soil and intermingle in ways that enrich the growth of each.

Critical Social Theory

Existing sociopolitical restraints limit individual freedoms. These limitations often remain hidden within the dominant societal structure allowing for a continuous oppressive presence. Critical examination of a situation brings recognition to these constrictions and provides a path to emancipation. The purpose of critical social theory (CST) is to provide a framework for examining and critiquing these socially constructed borders that are placed on human freedom (Kendall, 1992). For nurses, critical social theory is a pathway to come to understand how dominant societal values impact the profession and the health and welfare of patients. Critical reflection that raises awareness of the social constraints becomes an emancipatory action known as praxis (Freire, 1970/2003). An important focus of critical social theory is dialectics,

TABLE 4–1	Post-positivist Inquiry		
Predict	**Understand**	**Emancipate**	**Deconstruct**
Positivism	Interpretive	Naturalistic	Poststructural
	Naturalistic	Neo-Marxist	Postmodern
	Constructivist	Feminist	Post-Paradigmatic
	Phenomenological	Praxis-Oriented	Diaspora
	Hermeneutic	Educative	
		Freirian Participatory	
		Action Research	

Source: Lather (1991), p. 7.

which can be defined as the need to look at broad context and not focus on a specific aspect of social life but to look for inconsistencies between ideology and social reality (Browne, 2000; Ritzer & Goodman, 2004). Knowledge is contextual so standards of truth require interpretation in a social, historical, economic, and cultural perspective (Allen, 1986). Browne (2000) states:

> Praxis refers to the dialectical relationship among knowledge, theory, and practice that can precipitate emancipator changes in relation to clients, nursing and health care. At the very least, praxis from a CST perspective necessitates a critique of the ideological assumption that drive nursing research, theory and practice. (p. 44)

Critical social theory originated as a German intellectual movement in the 1920s in response to the growing appeal of logical positivism in intellectual thought in Europe and its influence on working class oppression (Campbell & Bunting, 1991). Critical social theory began at the Institute for Social Research in Frankfurt, Germany, and is often referred to as the Frankfurt School. The underlying conviction of CST is that history and structure need to be known to understand social phenomena (Fulton, 1997). The principles originated from critical Marxist principles and Hegelian dialectics stressing contradiction, change, and movement (Stevens, 1984; Kuokkanen & Leino-Kilpi, 2000). In the beginning The Institute followed traditional Marxist belief, but around 1930 shifted focus from the economy to the cultural system (Ritzer & Goodman, 2004). In acknowledgment of its Marxist roots, the epistemology of critical social theory has been to dictate that knowledge should be used for emancipatory political aims with the goal to free one's perceptions from ideological constraints, which often are produced by the ruling elite, to allow for evaluation of the true situation (Campbell & Bunting, 1991; Ritzer & Goodman, 2004).

According to Weber (2005) the first generation of the Frankfurt School was characterized by the conceptual framework of deconstruction and "salvage operation" of Marxism/Hegelianism, but the second generation of the Frankfurt School signaled a shift to a focus on epistemological problems. This directed critical social theory away from the concentration on method and ontology, which dominated the first generation and returned it to an understanding of intersubjectivity of social life. The second generation of critical social theory was introduced in the 1960s by German theorist Jürgen Habermas. Habermas wanted to base knowledge in the social sciences as intended by Marx while looking at power structures that oppress within social systems with the goal of self-reflection about ideas clouded by values imposed by society, allowing for disempowered groups to reflect and find sources of oppression (Seidman, 1989; Welch, 1999).

Habermas focused his concerns on communication believing it was foundational for sociocultural life and human sciences (Ritzer & Goodman, 2004).

He believed communication can help to maintain power relations and internalize ideologies (Wilson-Thomas, 1995). Communicative action is assumed to achieve emancipation through a process of mutual understanding (Welch, 1999). The task set forth by Habermas was to understand how people communicate and develop symbolic meanings. An understanding of this process would uncover the constraints which impede equal, free, and uncoerced participation in society (Stevens, 1984). Through this recognition, rationality became a central issue in Habermas's work. Ritzer and Goodman (2004) define rationality as: "removal of the barriers that distort communication, but more generally it means a communication system in which ideas are openly presented and defended against criticism; unconstrained agreement develops during argumentation" (p. 146). In regard to Habermas, Bernstein (1983) states:

> Habermas, who discovered that hermeneutics not only helps to highlight the limitations of positivist modes of thought but that there is also an essential hermeneutic dimension in all social knowledge, has been primarily concerned with the question of the foundation of a critical theory of society. From his perspective, neither the critique of ideology, as developed by Marx, nor the critical theory of the older Frankfurt thinkers is sufficient to provide a satisfactory answer to this foundational question. Habermas gradually came to realize more and more clearly the need to elaborate a comprehensive theory of rationality. (pp. 180-181)

Allen, Benner, and Diekelmann (1986) assert that rationality and lack of coercion are imperative for knowledge development and evidence. Two key values of rationality are autonomy, which is being free from conscious or unconscious restraints, and responsibility, which is the creation of an environment for others to freely speak (Allen, Benner, & Diekelmann, 1986). Rationality occurs when conscious and unconscious restraints are removed and a critique of ideological assumptions about knowledge, theory, and practice occur leading to emancipatory changes for clients, nursing, and health care (Allen et al.; Browne, 2000).

Critical Social Theory and Nursing Science

Habermas attempted to establish knowledge that leads to autonomy and responsibility by examining lived experiences while reflecting on concealed domination (Welch, 1999). Habermas identified three categories of knowledge that are based on the interest they serve: 1) empirical/analytical, which serves an interest of technical control through the use of empirical hypothesis or theses thus contributing to oppression; 2) historical/hermeneutical knowledge, which serves as an interest in understanding subjective experiences and is neither oppressive nor liberating, and 3) critical social theory, which aims to free persons from unacknowledged domination and transforming conditions (Ray, 1992; Ritzer & Goodman, 2004; Stevens, 1984). Knowledge that is gained through empirical means soon adheres to consensual means when actually its acceptance constrains or limits autonomy and responsibility within societal groups (Allen, 1986). Traditional notions of evidence such as that gathered through empirical inquiry do not account for the complexity of everyday lives (Kirkham, Baumbusch, Schultz, & Anderson, 2007). A driving force in health care today is the use of evidence-based practice (EBP) in order to deliver the most economic and scientifically grounded care. The emphasis that is placed on EBP and standardized care demonstrates the power of science (Sumner & Danielson, 2007). Kirkham et al. (2007) caution that: "For care to be efficient, it has to be effective, and for care to be effective, it means that it has to be appropriate to the context" (p. 28). Health care practiced within an evidence-based framework can support economic restrictions and decentralization of governance, and standardized care can lead to external controls (Kirkham et al.). The CST framework and inclusion of qualitative research methods can provide a way to establish evidence without the implications of dominance.

Browne (2000) suggests that critical social theory and the emancipatory advancement of nursing science needs to occur on two levels: 1) to generate emancipator knowledge in relation to client groups particularly disadvantaged groups, and 2) to require nurses to critique the ideology of nursing science. Without this critique, the status quo may be maintained and continue the oppressive patterns established by individuals and institutions. In addition to providing nurses a framework for examining issues of social injustice in regard to health, critical social theory provides a means for critical examination of the role of nursing in health care through the examination of social constructs placed on nursing. Allen (1986) asserts that though constraints on knowledge development can be created by dominant social values, it is the responsibility of nurses to examine the power issues that exist within their own profession. Emancipation from these constructs lead to empowerment and the ability to engage in autonomous practice and knowledge development. It has been theorized that nurses are an oppressed group as a result of their position in the medical hierarchy and the majority of nurses being female (McCall, 1996; Roberts, 1983; Skillings, 1992). The domination of this hierarchy suppresses the recognition of nurses and what nursing can bring to health care. Freire (1970/2003) states:

> As long as the oppressed remain unaware of the causes of their condition, they fatalistically "accept" their exploitation. Further, they are apt to react in a passive and alienated manner when confronted with the necessity to struggle for their freedom and self-affirmation. Little

by little, however, they tend to try out forms of rebellious action. In working towards liberation, one must neither lose sight of this passivity nor overlook the moment of awakening. (p. 64)

By reflecting on the oppression that is present and taking actions against such boundaries, nursing can move beyond oppressive ideologies to development of nursing science. Frameworks for emancipation such as critical theory fit well with research concerning nurses' workplaces (Rose & Glass, 2008). It is through an emancipatory framework that nurses can recognize dominant ideologies that exist in their work environments impeding their ability to deliver nursing care. For nurses it is not just the sociopolitical and economic contexts that must be appreciated but also the underlying gender issues that exist. Gender implications of oppression will be discussed in the next section of this chapter. This paradigm shift can begin during the educational process. In nursing education, critical social theory represents a shift from one of teaching-directed learning to one where there is an equal partnership between student and teacher. A critical view based on reflection, insight, and consciousness raising allows one to see socially dominant forces that exist and influence an individual's growth. This helps in making power relations and modes of domination visible to the nurse (Thompson, 1987). A traditional nursing education deemphasizes the subjective needs of the students. The ideal is to create an autonomous and socially responsible nurse which requires the provision of an unconstrained learning environment that seeks to uncover hidden meanings and nurture critique (Duchscher, 2000). It is imperative that students also learn to critique the environment in order to analyze the sources of their own interrelations, to question and to resist predefined meaning that educators encourage them to adopt and to develop tools to negotiate the world of nursing (Allen, Benner, & Diekelmann, 1986).

Nursing must look at its own self-limiting measures in terms of theory and practice. Ideally, theory should be applicable to the practice situation in which nurses engage and reflect on the lived experience of the nurse. According to Wuest (1994), nursing theories evolved from an "elite group" of nurse educator/academicians are often far removed from the reality of the practice world thereby endorsing a patriarchal structure. Critical social theory suggests that there must be a relationship between theory and practice, yet a disconnect occurs because practice is often delegated to a less powerful group (Ritzer & Goodman, 2004). Thus, nursing theory is often developed in the halls of academic institutions while the practice of nursing occurs during the nurse–patient interaction. The goal is to join theory and practice by developing partnerships between nurse scientists and those who are in practice and empowering each to overcome social constraints to work together for the betterment of their patients.

Feminist Approaches as Part of the Postmodern Enterprise ___

Feminist inquiry, as it relates to nursing, can be viewed from several perspectives. It can shed light on issues of gender that enable us to provide better care to our female patients, as well as their families and loved ones; and it can, like critical social theory, shed insight on sources of our own oppression/experiences as nurses and/or as women. The aims of feminist inquiry are clearly *emancipatory*, as are the aims of critical social theory. In a wonderful, and not very widely available (in this country) chapter, "Women and the politics of career development: The case of nursing," Ellen Baer, nurse historian, relates a quote from Ethel Manson Fenwick, the organizer of the British Nurses Association and editor of the *Nursing Record,* later to become the *British Journal of Nursing.* Fenwick was a strong antagonist of her contemporary Florence Nightingale regarding the state registration of nurses. According to Baer, Fenwick aptly summed up the situation when she said in 1887: "The Nurse question is the Women question, pure and simple. We have to run the gauntlet of those historic rotten eggs" (Fenwick, quoted in Baer, 1997, pp. 256–257).

In the words of Lather (1991), to do feminist research is "to put the social construction of gender at the center of one's inquiry" (p. 71). Feminists see gender as a basic organizing principle which profoundly shapes, and mediates, the concrete conditions of our lives. Gender is seen as central in the shaping of our ideas of the world, the skills we acquire, the institutions in which we reside and work, as well as the distribution of power and privilege. According to Callaway (1981), this entails the substantive task of making gender a fundamental category for our understanding of the social order, "to see the world from women's place in it" (p. 460). An overt ideological goal of feminist research in the human sciences, according to Lather (1991), is "to correct both the *invisibility* and *distortion* of female experience in ways relevant to ending women's unequal social position" (p. 71). The focus on gender as a social constraint goes beyond the social, political, and economic ideologies explored in critical social theory to provide a more complete picture of the experience of women.

The relatively short history of feminism is often described in "waves," the first wave being the 19th- and early 20th-century Women's Rights movement that ultimately led to voting rights for women in Great Britain and the United States . The second wave commonly refers to the 1960s and early 1970s when Women's "Lib" (Women's Liberation) as it came to be called, burst across the nation's consciousness along with the anti-war protests of the same era. Then came the birth control pill and the legalization of abortion (*Roe vs. Wade,* 1973). The genie was out of the bottle; Pandora was out of the box. Women's Studies formally entered the academy.

As a consequence of the methodological legacies which early feminist scholars inadvertently took from their teachers, feminist theory from the late 1960s to the mid-1980s tended to exhibit the problematic universalizing tendencies of academic scholarship in general. Additionally, its analyses tended to reflect the viewpoint of the largely privileged, white, middle-class women of North America and Western Europe who composed this group of early scholars, and these women tended to reflect "liberal" feminist thought. This perspective views women's oppression as stemming from a lack of equal civil rights and educational opportunities, thus channeling women into "traditional" roles.

This may account for some of the differences that existed between the early feminist movement of the 1970s and 1980s and nursing. This was a point that Baer (1997) was to make, taking mainstream feminism to task. Arguing that the "women as equal" perspective seemed to have greater resonance with feminists than "women as different," she notes that this perspective has had the

> effect of seeming not to comprehend or support the values and ideas of people who *choose* society's care-taking roles. In fact, such feminists seem to refuse to believe that women who engage in "women's work" chose it, thoughtfully and happily, with full consideration of other possibilities, and were not merely following their biological destiny. (Baer, 1997, pp. 245–246)

This continuing disdain for "women's work," she pointed out, threatens the entire healthcare system which relies heavily on nursing expertise, as well as recipients of care and their families.

Even more strikingly, according to Fraser and Nicholson (1990), these early scholars tended to repeat the specific types of universalizing found in the particular schools of thought to which their work was most closely allied. They use the examples of Marxist-feminist scholarship suffering from the same faulty universalizations found in non-feminist Marxist scholarship, as well as feminist developmental scholarship, mimicking, early on, the same mistakes present in developmental psychology: "The irony was that one of the most powerful arguments that feminist scholars were making was the limitation of scholarship which falsely universalized on the basis of limited perspectives" (Fraser & Nicholson, 1990, p. 1). Feminist scholars were becoming increasingly aware that the problem with much existing scholarship was that the voices of many other social groups were not represented. Clearly, new methods were necessary. The time was ripe for a fusion of postmodern perspectives and feminist approaches, each able to enrich the other.

An Emancipatory Agenda for Healthcare Delivery _____

In addition to providing a lens for self-reflection, critical social theory and feminist theory provide a means for nurses to critically evaluate the social context of health in hopes of improving health and healthcare delivery. Social structures are often at the root of human problems. Nursing has attempted to change these structures to improve health and quality of life for patients (Kagan, Smith, Cowling, & Chinn, 2009). Emancipatory nursing actions are those actions that allow the oppressed and disenfranchised to come to understand social reality and recognize the people or situations that are oppressing them and help them gain freedom (Kendall, 1992). Within the current healthcare system, disparities and injustices exist based on gender, race, and social situations. Critical theory offers a way to examine and critique inequalities by critiquing the historical, cultural, and social context of the patient (Browne, 2000). In order to improve health outcomes, power shifts must occur that contribute to equal power and lack of domination of one group (Boutain, 2005). Kirkham, Baumbusch, Schultz, and Anderson (2007), propose that rather than focusing on the implications of cultural beliefs or practices based on individuals that the focus shifts to population-based studies that look at the root causes of disparities. Emphasis should be placed on social inequalities to address problems related to population and socioenvironmental views of health (Maxwell, 1997).

Applying Postmodern Philosophies to Research

The application of critical social theory to research is the use of a conceptual framework in a manner that is consistent with the philosophy and beliefs of the approach. It is not a mechanistic application of a methodology for emancipatory insight. The purpose of the analysis of the issues is the emphasis on the context and historicity in order to increase the emancipation of individuals and groups. Critical theory is a use of narrative analysis that illustrates how social practices that are housed in political or educational institutions allow for unjust practices that benefit the dominant group (Chinn & Kramer, 2004). To fully understand phenomena of life, there must be an understanding of the historical and contextual whole, that is, the social structure conceived as a global entity (Hedin, 1986). The process itself is *praxis,* or critical reflection, on the ends and means of activity for the purpose of transformation, and it is a means of consciousness raising where theory and action become one. Research and analysis within a critical social theory framework promote a consciousness among persons who are impeded by oppressive constraints. This framework brings about conditions in which oppressive elements are brought forth to initiate a dialogue about action so change occurs. This can only aid in the anticipation of strategic action but not compel action. If it were to compel this action, those doing the research and theorizing would be placed above those who are experiencing the phenomenon addressed by the theory, which itself creates a state of domination (Stevens, 1984).

Habermas contends that certain conditions have to be met to make research *critical.* These include: a) analysis and unveiling of hidden power sources, b) commitment of the study to fill and equal participation of the researcher and the observed, and c) commitment to a mutually agreed upon plan for change (Welch, 1999). There is not one method to be used in conducting research using a critical social theory framework. The methods can include qualitative methods in the historical/hermeneutic tradition and quantitative methods in the empirical/analytic tradition (Stevens, 1984).

Feminists, like postmodernists and critical social theorists, have sought to develop new paradigms of social criticism that do not rely on traditional philosophical underpinnings. Both schools of thought have criticized modern epistemologies and universal and ahistorical "truths." There has been a "growing interest among feminists in modes of theorizing which are attentive to differences and to cultural and historical specificity" (Fraser & Nicholson, 1990, p. 33).

Women comprise more than half of our population. Research approaches to issues of gender, whether conducted by women or men, may vary. Feminist empirical work, as nursing research, is multi-paradigmatic (Dzurec, 1989; Lather, 1991). Westcott (1977) situates the feminist scholarship of the 1970s and 1980s as operating largely within the conventional positivist frame, whereas for many current feminist researchers, the methodological task has become generating and refining more contextualized, interactive methods in the search for pattern and meaning rather than prediction and control (Lather, 1991).

> When we began theorizing our experience during the second women's movement a mere decade and a half ago, we knew our task would be a difficult though exciting one. But I doubt that in our wildest dreams we ever imagined we would have to reinvent both science and theorizing in order to make sense of women's social experience. (Harding & O'Barr, 1987, p. 251)

One could extrapolate the words "we [i.e., nursing] would have to reinvent in medicine and therapeutics in order to make sense of the human experience of health care." This is the main point of Jean Watson's 1999 book *Postmodern Nursing;* she writes:

> Nursing is presented as a paradigm case for women and the caring-healing dimensions of women's work, work that has been expunged from the traditional western world cosmology, and particularly the modern masculine archetype of traditional science and medicine—the latent and not so latent, archetype under which nursing has located itself within this modern era of the 20th century. (p. 6)

Kroker and Cook (1986) state that "Feminism is the quantum physics of postmodernism" (p. 22) while others postulate a "post-feminism," enveloping issues beyond gender. According to Flax (1990), feminist theories, like other forms of postmodernism, including critical social theory, should encourage us to tolerate and interpret ambivalence, ambiguity, and multiplicity as well as to expose the roots of our needs for imposing order and structure. Flax concludes, "If we do our work well, reality will appear even more unstable, complex, and disorderly than it does now. In this sense perhaps Freud was right when he declared that women are the enemies of civilization" (p. 57).

None of the approaches discussed earlier are axiomatic. This is not a time for a new orthodoxy. Uncertainty and dissonance will persist. Lather (1991) states that her goal is to move research in many different and occasionally contradictory directions in the hope that "more interesting and useful ways of knowing will emerge" (p. 69). She supports experimentation, collaboration, and sharing, enterprises supported by feminist approaches. And she quotes Polkinghorne (1983):

> What is needed most is for practitioners to experiment with new designs and to submit their attempt and results to examination by other participants in the debate. The new historians of science have made it clear that methodological questions are decided in the practice of research by those committed to developing the best possible answers to their questions, not armchair philosophers of research (p. xi).

As nurses, and knowledgeable consumers of health care, there is very little chance of our becoming "armchair philosophers of research." There is too much important work to be done.

To further this train of thought, we would quote Salas (2005), "Toward a North-South Dialogue: Revisiting Nursing Theory (From the South)." Noting that nursing theories have "universalizing and generalizing" tendencies that do not address "the diversities of nursing phenomena . . . and thus offer little understanding of people's experiences" (Meleis, quoted in Salas, 2005, p. 19), the author claims, "the need to have an organizing framework to order the phenomena of interest for the discipline does not reflect an understanding of the way that nursing is lived in practice" (p. 22). This author suggests revisiting nursing theory in a "global world." What this means has relevance for us all, as nurses: attention to the marginalized and often exteriorized (Hall & Steven, 1991). A "path of solidarity" with the exteriorized is postulated as a way of coming to "a deeper understanding and appreciation of the interdependent character of the global community" (Smith, quoted in Salas, 2005, p. 23). Human interdependency demonstrates the need of the weak for the strong, and conversely, at the same time, the strong for the weak. This echoes the important theme of "cyclical continuum," identified by Munhall (2001)—the idea of "an absolution" to the eternal quantitative-quantitative polarization. Put another way, it suggests "moving to postpositivism and reconciliation" (Stevens, quoted in Munhall, 2001, p. 5). The global world is the postmodern. We are there. There is no going back. Take the plunge. The water is fine.

References

Agger, B. (1991). Critical social theory, post structuralism, post modernism: Their sociological relevance. *Annual Review of Sociology, 17,* 105–131.

Allen, D. G. (1986). Using philosophical and historical methodologies to understand the concept of health. In P. L. Chinn (Ed.), *Nursing research methodology: Issues and Implementation* (pp. 157–168). Rockville, MD: Aspen.

Allen, D., Benner, P., & Diekelmann, N. L. (1986). Three paradigms for nursing research: Methodological implications. In P. L. Chinn (Ed.), *Nursing research methodology: Issues and Implementation* (pp. 23–38). Rockville, MD: Aspen.

Baer, E. (1997). Women and the politics of career development: The case of nursing. In A. M. Rafferty, J. Robinson, & G. Elkan (Eds.), *Nursing history and the politics of welfare* (pp. 242–258). London: Routledge.

Bauman, Z. (1992). *Intimations of postmodernity.* London: Routledge.

Bernstein, R. J. (1983). *Beyond objectivism and relativism: Science, hermeneutics and praxis.* Philadelphia: University of Pennsylvania Press.

Boutain, D. M. (2005). Social justice as a framework for professional nursing. *Journal of Nursing Education, 44*(9), 404–408.

Browne, A. J. (2000). The potential contributions of critical social theory to nursing science. *Canadian Journal of Nursing Research, 32*(2), 35–55.

Callaway, H. (1981). Women's perspectives: Research as re-vision. In P. Reason & J. Rowan (Eds.), *Human inquiry* (pp. 457–472). New York: Wiley.

Campbell, J. C., & Bunting, S. (1991). Voices and paradigms: Perspectives on critical and feminist theory in nursing. *Advances in Nursing Science, 13*(2), 1–15.

Cheek, J. (2000). *Postmodern and poststructural approaches to nursing research.* Thousand Oaks, CA: Sage.

Chinn, P. L., & Kramer, M. K. (2004). *Integrated knowledge development in nursing* (6th ed.). St. Louis, MO: Mosby.

Duchscher, J. E. B. (2000). Bending a habit: Critical social theory as a framework for humanistic nursing education. *Nurse Education Today, 20,* 453–462.

Dzurec, L. (1989). The necessity for and evolution of multiple paradigms for nursing research: A poststructuralist perspective. *Advances in Nursing Science, 11*(4), 69–77.

Flax, J. (1990). Postmodernism and gender relations. In L. Nicholson (Ed.), *Feminism/ Postmodernism* (pp. 39–62). New York: Routledge.

Foucault, M. (1980). *Power/knowledge: Selected interviews and other writings 1972–1977.* New York: Pantheon Books.

Fraser, N., & Nicholson, L. (1990). Social criticism without philosophy: An encounter between feminism and postmodernism. In L. Nicholson, (Ed.), *Feminism/Postmodernism* (pp. 19–38). New York. Routledge.

Freire, P. (1970/2003). *Pedagogy of the oppressed.* New York: Continuum.

Fulton, Y. (1997). Nurses views on empowerment: A critical social theory perspective. *Journal of Advanced Nursing, 25,* 529–536.

Hall, J. M., & Steven, P. E. (1991). Rigor in feminist research. *Advances in Nursing Science, 13*(3), 16–29.

Harding, S., & O'Barr, J. F. (Eds.) (1987). *Sex and Scientific Inquiry.* Chicago: The University of Chicago Press.

Hedin, B. H. (1986). Nursing, education, and emancipation: Applying the critical theoretical approach to nursing research. In P. L. Chinn (Ed.), *Nursing research methodology: Issues and Implementation* (pp. 133–146). Rockville, MD: Aspen.

Kagan, P. N., Smith, M. C., Cowling, W. R., & Chinn, P. L. (2009). A nursing manifesto: An emancipator call for knowledge development, conscience, and praxis. *Nursing Philosophy, 11*, 67–84.

Kendall, J. (1992). Fighting back: Promoting emancipatory nursing actions. *Advances in Nursing Science, 15*, 1–15.

Kirkham, S. R., Baumbusch, J. L., Schultz, A. S. H., & Anderson, J. M. (2007). Knowledge development and evidence-based practice: Insights and opportunities from a postcolonial feminist perspective for transformative nursing practice. *Advances in Nursing Science, 30*(1), 26–40.

Kroker, A., & Cook, D. (1986). *The postmodern scene: Excremental culture and hyper-aesthetics.* New York: St. Martin's Press.

Kuokkanen, L., & Leino-Kilpi, H. (2000). Power and empowerment in nursing: Three theoretical perspectives. *Journal of Advanced Nursing, 31*, 235–241.

Lather, P. (1991). *Getting smart: Feminist research and pedagogy with/in the postmodern.* New York: Routledge.

Maxwell, L. E. (1997). Foundational thought in the development of knowledge for social change. In S. E. Thorne & V. E. Hayes (Eds.), *Nursing Praxis: Knowledge and Action* (pp. 203–219). Thousand Oaks, CA: Sage.

McCall, E. (1996). Horizontal violence in nursing: The continuing silence. *The Lamp*, April, 28–31.

Munhall, P. (2001). Language and nursing research. In P. Munhall (Ed.). *Nursing research: A qualitative perspective* (pp. 3–36). Sudbury, MA: Jones & Bartlett.

Polkinghorne, D. (1983). *Methodology for the human sciences: systems of inquiry.* Albany, NY: State University of New York Press.

Ray, M. A. (1992). Critical theory as a framework to enhance nursing science. *Nursing Science Quarterly, 5*(1), 98–101.

Ritzer, G., & Goodman, D. J. (2004). *Modern sociological theory* (6th ed.). Boston: McGraw Hill.

Roberts, S. J. (1983) Oppressed group behavior: Implications for nursing. *Advances in Nursing Science, 5*, 21–30.

Rose, J., & Glass, N. (2008). The importance of emancipatory research to contemporary nursing practice. *Contemporary Nurse, 29*, 8–22.

Salas, A. S. (2005). Toward a North-South dialogue. Revisiting nursing theory (from the South). *Advances in Nursing Science, 20*(23), 17–24.

Seidman, S. (Ed.). (1989). *Jürgen Habermas on society and politics: A reader.* Boston: Beacon Press.

Skillings, L. N. (1992). Perceptions and feelings of nurses about horizontal violence as an expression of oppressed group behavior. In J. L. Thompson, D. G. Allen, & Rodrigues-Fisher (Eds.), *Critique, Resistance, and Action: Working Papers in the Politics of Nursing* (pp. 167–185). New York: National League for Nursing Press.

Stevens, P. E. (1984). A critical social reconceptualization of environment in nursing: Implications for methodology. In P. Chinn (Ed.), *Exemplars in criticism: Challenge and controversy, Advances in Nursing Science Series* (pp. 127–139). Gaithersburg, MD: Aspen.

Sumner, J., & Danielson, E. (2007). Critical social theory as a means of analysis for caring in nursing. *International Journal for Human Caring, 11*(1), 30–37.

Thompson, J. L. (1987). Critical scholarship: The critique of domination in nursing. *Advances in Nursing Science, 10,* 27–38.

Watson, J. (1999). *Postmodern nursing and beyond.* London: Churchill Livingstone.

Weber, M. (2005). The critical social theory of the Frankfurt School and the 'social turn' in IR. *Review of International Studies, 31,* 195–209.

Welch, M. (1999). Critical theory and feminist critique. In E. C. Polifroni & M. Welch (Eds.), *Perspectives on philosophy of science in nursing* (pp. 355–359). Philadelphia: Lippincott.

Westcott, M. (1977). Conservative method. *Philosophy of Social Sciences, 7,* 67–76.

Wilson-Thomas, L. (1995). Applying critical social theory in nursing education to bridge the gap between theory, research, and practice. *Journal of Advanced Nursing, 21,* 568–575.

Wuest, J. (1994). Professionalism and the evolution of nursing as a discipline: A feminist perspective. *Journal of Professional Nursing, 10,* 357–367.

PART II

Qualitative Methods and Exemplars

Part II of this text invites you to contemplate and explore different qualitative methods with a "how to" chapter followed by a "here is an example" chapter. You will become aware of the similarities among the qualitative methods as well as variations, which most often depend on the aim of the study. The first method chapter is on phenomenology, followed by two exemplar studies. There are two to illustrate—Chapter 6 highlights linguistic transformation and longitudinal phenomenology while Chapter 7 covers descriptive phenomenology. Other methods and exemplars include grounded theory, ethnography, case study, historical, narrative inquiry, and action research. With the exponential growth of qualitative methods there are many variations of these methods to be explored in other venues. These were chosen to represent the most popular and the most foundational methods. I think you will find the exemplars to be most revealing of the power of qualitative research. It is difficult not to be moved by people's stories and the way they find meaning in their experiences.

All the methods in this section are founded on the perspectives described in Part I of this text. Many methods philosophical underpinnings are similar to the phenomenological perspective and take into consideration the same concepts and activities described in Chapter 5.

You might notice that some of the exemplar chapters may not follow literally the method chapter because variations in methods exist. There are different ways of doing a specific qualitative research method, and as long as the researcher adheres to the philosophical, and in some cases theoretical, underpinnings of the method, it is acceptable and perhaps characteristic of the respect qualitative researchers have for variations in interpretation. I have encouraged you, especially if you have chosen a particular method to pursue, to return to the first four editions of this book and read the different interpretations or ways of "doing" a method and also additional examples of that method.

Studies can also vary from the method because a researcher is not aware at the start of a study where the participants may lead the researcher. However, evaluation criteria are available to ensure credibility, trustworthiness, and resonance so we can evaluate our research from the highest standards of research science.

I hope you will be intellectually stimulated as you read these chapters and gain appreciation for what qualitative research offers us as human beings, nurses, healthcare providers, and students of the human sciences. *We are always in experience* as our patients are always in experience, so it is incumbent upon us to understand and appreciate their life worlds, as well as our own, with all the variations and complexities.

To me it is this complicatedness—sometimes called the messiness of our human lives—the interconnectedness of phenomena, and the appreciation of intersubjectivity that give qualitative research the authenticity and existential humanness that has the potential to enrich our lives with the knowledge and insight essential for compassion, care, liberation, and finding meaning in everyday experience.

5

A Phenomenological Method

Patricia L. Munhall

To Think Phenomenologically

The chapters of Part I lay the foundation for our initial foray into the wonderful philosophical world of phenomenology. I hope you are beginning to feel well grounded in the history, language, and epistemology of the qualitative perspective. You will find that what we discuss in this chapter will also apply to the other qualitative methods discussed in this book because most interpretations of qualitative methods are rooted in phenomenological philosophy. However, some qualitative methods also have a theoretical component, such as grounded theory, whereas phenomenology is atheoretical. Phenomenology is a philosophical approach, based on philosophical propositions, rather than theoretical concepts.

As discussed in Chapter 2, a prerequisite to acceptance as a discipline in the academy or university is to have bona fide research or a "science" for research. To accomplish a respectable status in research, it seems one must use a method and use it correctly for the research to be valid. This we have inherited from the positivistic world—the scientific method as iconic and the necessity of method. We create knowledge from knowledge already accepted as truth, cumulatively, we test theories and either validate them or not, but from a phenomenological perspective we are asked to suspend this knowledge and these theories, to become a beginner in whatever we are approaching in research. The following Zen quote introduces us to the paradoxical nature of all we have been taught: *In the beginner's mind, there are many possibilities, but in the expert's mind, there are few"* (Anderson, 2009).

The cultivation of an empty mind receptive to new perceptions is discussed in this chapter. I suggest that as you read this chapter to actually think and become phenomenologic as if you are to embark on phenomenological research. This receptive perspective will guide your thoughts and your ways of seeing phenomena and understanding experience. This actually is not an unusual direction in that if you were to do scientific laboratory research, you would be encouraged "to think like a scientist." Here is the same helpful suggestion, "to think phenomenologically," and in this chapter it is my aim to help you understand what that means.

Thinking and Being Phenomenological

You will find in qualitative research a flexibility that is essential to the inductive approach as discussed in Chapter 3. Although we have formalized methods with suggested steps to follow and we most certainly have rules for rigor, we also understand that we are studying in order to understand a phenomenon not fully understood at present. If we start a research project for which not much is known about the subject, often as we explore, we come to "know" something that might make the planned next step of our proposal irrelevant or inappropriate. Whether using phenomenology or another qualitative method, flexibility to change your proposal is essential. This can have dramatic results, as when your initial study of an experience reveals a factor hidden in the experience that must be studied before you will be able to understand your first chosen study.

For example, one of my first phenomenological studies was going to be researching the experience of social isolation. When I began to realize that the real phenomenon undergirding this seemed to be the experience of anger, I changed my perspective to seeing when anger appeared, the various faces of anger, and concealed or repressed expressions of this emotion.

Thinking phenomenologically and being phenomenological often entail that in this process of discovery we discover the unexpected causing our whole focus to change. We might think we have a good hunch but having an open mind can allow the perception of something quite different to be revealed. For example, my one "detour" resulted in a long research program concerning and coming to understand the meaning of anger. What if I were to suggest that there really is no phenomenological method for research? That it is truly a way of thinking and of understanding experience without preconceived perceptions. If you are planning to do a phenomenological study, perhaps you would become dismayed. Now what are you to do? There must be a "way," a "group of steps," a path to follow.

As is mentioned later in this chapter, it is the latter that researchers seek, which is very understandable. We might intuitively know how to get to our destination, but it feels so much safer and secure if we have a map.

So we seek maps that include various roads to get to our destination, always remembering that the map is not the actual territory. Like language, it is a representation. So are research methods. However, before we use the map, we need to know how to interpret it, and also how to drive a car. Too simplistic? Often in the simplest statements are very important, though obvious, truths. I believe far more important than a "method" or maybe intrinsic to a "method" is to learn to think and to be phenomenological.

Before we embark on "doing" a phenomenological research study, we must know how to interpret the philosophical underpinnings of phenomenology. We must understand them, and more important, we must know how to "be" phenomenologic in our own being. This was quite a challenge to me, being brought up in one of the most scientific times in our history. Science was (and still is, to some) an icon, a single version of truth. The way the word has come to be used symbolizes a process and product of the material world, seen from an objective stance. As a nursing student, I can remember having the statement "be objective" drilled into my head from the very first day. Today it is easy for me to understand that objectivity is itself a subjective concept. But at 17 years of age, well, you can just imagine! But objectivity has to be subjective. Who defines it? Who gives a study that kind of status? A subjective opinion. Often those subjective opinions differ. If you have sat through presentations of research, you will recall the many different opinions of various people, which originated from their own perceptions concerning the many different parts of that research project. Granted, the more subjective opinions one can obtain that are similar, the more objective a phenomenon or truth will seem.

However, in my own journey from nursing student to doctoral student, being objective seemed to be the defining characteristic of what was good and scientific. The Heisenberg Principle of Uncertainty withstanding, a problem emerged: Often, objectivity is a sterile state, devoid of humanistic characteristics, and it ignores the situated context where the phenomenon is located. When directed to "be objective," what does that actually mean? Don't think about what? Oneself, the other person in context, what you would do since you are not the other person? To me it is a most puzzling directive, and I know I cannot be objective in the way the concept of objectivity is presently thought of and that is decontextualized. I want to understand the different reference points, the situated context, and the individual person.

An Overheard Encounter as Exemplar

"Becoming phenomenologic" toward the world is an entirely different view. Here is an example: A student said to a friend, "Why can't you answer me? Must everything be a secret? I was just asking you what you were doing."

For most of us, that kind of dialogue or a variant is not uncommon in communications with a friend or loved one. The scientist hearing the preceding questions might assume objectively that the person not answering seems, objectively speaking, simply does not want to reveal what he or she is doing. Actually, the questions would not have much interest at all to a scientist! However, for a student who is asking the questions, we have another story. The question could become more complex with an accusation such as: "You are deliberately hiding something from me, you do not like me, you want to be away from me," or more elaborately, "You have been ignoring me for weeks, you don't speak to me, you don't tell me anything, and I am only trying to be reasonable. Why can't you be reasonable as well?" The person asking the question assumes a rational stance to the question, expecting a rational response.

The response might be, "Don't you get it? I don't want to tell you," which is actually pretty rational. But then again it might be more elaborate, with a response, "Stop annoying me and asking me questions. If I wanted to tell you, I would tell you, and yes everything is a secret if I don't feel like telling you. Who do you think you are, my mother?"

Looking at this potential conflict from a phenomenological perspective, although it is a simple interaction at first glance, it becomes a very significant interaction of which we cannot determine knowledge about anything. Nothing from the questioner, nothing from the responder, until we elaborate and ask about or express concerns and feelings. This is context, the situation around the question. Return to this dialogue when you read about intersubjectivity on page 139. Knowing how to think phenomenologically has enormous potential not only to make you a great researcher *but a very understanding person*. Understanding the dynamics of intersubjectivity can help you avoid many of the conflicts and misunderstandings inherent in human relationships. Thus, becoming phenomenologic is a way of being in the world.

In the preceding interaction, the phenomenological researcher knows there is a situated context and it is embedded in time, space, embodiment, and relationships, all of which will be explained in this chapter. We also know that two perceptions are operating here—not an objective truth—two subjectivities, interacting and forming an intersubjective space. Two people are seeing the world through two different social constructions of reality and are even using language differently, though there might be an assumption that they are using the words in similar ways. The two people have two different experiences during this encounter. Perhaps the most important phenomenological realization is that the two different perceptions are going to result in two different interpretations of what seemingly looks like one reality. When doing phenomenological research, thoughts like this should come naturally to you, which is an understanding of communication unlike what might be necessary in doing quantitative research, for example.

This is just a brief synopsis of what it might mean to "think" and "be" phenomenologic. Nothing is taken for granted. Everything is held up for questioning. Of course, this would be exhausting if you did this with all communication; however, the more practiced you become with this view of the world, the more automatic this type of thinking becomes for you and the better your understanding and communication become. Here is another possible answer to the overheard dialogue: "You know, I had no idea that I was being secretive. I am just preoccupied with something. I would not keep secrets from you. I am going over to the cafeteria." What do you think a phenomenological-type person would think of that answer? It could be a true statement of innocence, but phenomenologically it would never be assumed to be true. By now you probably can think of all the variations that this simple answer might actually be concealing. "Being" phenomenologic is not only hearing language and believing something is being revealed that might be valid, but it is hearing and also contemplating what might be concealed in responses.

Researching a Phenomenologic Method

In 1994, in my book *Revisioning Phenomenology: Nursing and Health Science Research* (Munhall, 1994a), I did not articulate a method in a formalized structured manner. I refer you to that work to supplement this chapter, and my aim here is to present a very flexible method that attempts to embrace the possibilities of thinking and being phenomenologic from one's perspective toward living and being. This method has evolved from the work of innumerable doctoral students who used van Manen's method and often utilized work from the "revisioning" book but still raised questions and asked for clarification (van Manen, 1990). In *Revisioning*, I purposely attempted to guide students through the process of inquiry from a phenomenological perspective. I referred the reader to van Manen's approach on the basis of a subjective appraisal that his method was the most consistent with phenomenology as philosophy. Still, I received requests to articulate a method because in my teaching I was apparently guiding students with what they perceived as a method not yet written. Also, some students, as well as myself, in contrast to van Manen, did think phenomenologic research could be problem solving and illuminate needed changes in many areas, whether policy or practice. I had begun to respond to Crotty's (1996) emphasis on critique where he states: "The goal of phenomenological inquiry goes beyond identifying, appreciating, and explaining current and shared meanings. It seeks to critique these meanings" (p. 5). You will see, then, in this proposed method a "step" not ordinarily found in phenomenological studies, but one that could be added to other phenomenological methods or to any study: "Write a narrative about the meaning of your study." This answers the "so what?" question that has been asked after many research studies have been completed. Here, too, you will find an emphasis on critiquing the interpretations with implications and recommendations for political, social, cultural, health care, nursing, family, and other social systems, as well as the individual.

Methods and Themes and Meaning Units

What motivated me to move forward the third edition of this text (2001) were some criticisms that were leveled at many of our phenomenological studies. I hoped that, perhaps by integrating those criticisms into the development of this method, our phenomenological research would become more meaningful to practice and policy. I wanted to do this then and now because I do not want phenomenology to be misperceived or have its potential go unrecognized and unrespected, which unfortunately has happened in some instances.

After 24 years of assisting colleagues and students with master's theses and doctoral dissertations, I had become acquainted with common questions and frustrations and with sincere attempts to combine philosophy with method. If we were to accept the proposition that phenomenology as inquiry is aimed at understanding lived experience, as is sometimes written, or that the central purpose of phenomenology is to understand the meaning of being human, then the guiding phrase, I think, would be *a phenomenological approach*. We would approach the project, the study, and be guided by the emergent material. The experiences themselves would show the way to understanding meaning. However, approach does not do well in dissertation proposals or grant applications. The relevant section is simply not labeled "approach" but "method." For now, we must conform and hope the day will come when flexibility in proposal writing will be realized as an essential characteristic of phenomenological study.

"What is the meaning of being human?" is a phenomenal question. I believe the question is asked to come to a phenomenological answer: understanding the meaning of being human. For the most part, this question, *the meaning of being*,[1] is answered from different perspectives and much of the meaning remains a mystery. All the phenomenology in the world is not going to solve the mystery altogether, and I am not sure that we would want all mystery removed. Yet, in many human experiences, the desire for human understanding cannot and should not be ignored. What individuals have done with the foregoing question and its purpose has varied in responses and very different methods, even within the same philosophy of phenomenology. This chapter, though, is not to critique the various ways in which different schools of thought have developed methods to answer this question, but to give examples of how phenomenology has been done using the various humanistic psychological phenomenological methods. Studies following these "psychological" early methods, while well intended and deserving of our gratitude for opening the doors to phenomenologic research, unfortunately have sometimes left us open to a well-founded criticism that these methods reflect a form of reductionism and step-like studies that appear much like those based on logical positivism. Of course, using the same outlines for proposals and criteria for evaluation as those of the scientific method has not helped at all.

Many of these methods came about to gain acceptance within the academy. Many nurse researchers, when reviewing phenomenological research, come away wondering what it all means: lists of themes, lists of essences, structural definitions, categories of abstractions, meaning units, and other reductionist descriptions of experience. However, these methods eased qualitative research and, in this instance, phenomenology, into the world of nursing research with rules to give these methods as much credence and respectability as the icon of the scientific method.

The Unknown: Where Being Reveals Itself

To be true to the philosophy of phenomenology we must follow the thing itself wherever and whenever it appears, while being attentive, conscious, and alert to its appearance or concealment. Know that with appearance there is concealment as well. Explore that and all its possibilities. Liberate yourself from prescribed steps. Methods can place you in a formula where you cannot wander outside, and that critical limitation, while a safeguard in the laboratory, is what will handcuff you and keep you from the spontaneous recognition of the appearance and the crucial exploration of the unforeseen. A method unfortunately can provide a set of blinders and an ear plug for the "third ear," as discussed in Chapter 1. For years, I have urged my wonderful colleagues to liberate students and let them follow the phenomenological process so that they can be free to journey where "being" reveals itself. My main argument was that where "being" and "understanding" reveal themselves is largely unknown at the outset of a phenomenological inquiry.

In my own phenomenological studies and writing I reveal to the reader the situated context of my life experience that brings me to that very instant of interest. I have come to understand in the past 24 years that my own subjectivity, which is often the same as my interpretive belief about phenomenological inquiry as process and not as method, can be substantiated philosophically. I have, though, also come to understand that nurse researchers and other human science researchers do not have the freedom to go about any inquiry without a method.

More Concerns About Method

In the last edition of this text, I reflected on having a choice to be a purist or, because of my experiential phenomenological understanding of students' experiences, to act on the meaning of their experiences. Will that mean that I am compromising my beliefs? The answer is no. I still believe the phenomenological inquiry is a process of the unknown that gives direction to the study and cannot possibly be known at the outset. How could we possibly come to understand the meaning of being human in experience if we were to follow linear, prescribed steps that create boundaries to exploration?

Each step taken would close that door prematurely; or worse, if it opened another door, we could not go there because it would not be part of the "steps" of the "method." I also believed, at the same time, that such a liberated perspective was not going to be accepted in the academy, unless perhaps (and even this is debatable) one was in a philosophy program. I have also taken note of the phenomenological "methods" and, with the exception of van Manen's, have become sufficiently concerned about the problems inherent in them, such as naming "reactions" to an experience instead of the meaning or even an understanding of the reactions. Most methods, when carried out according to prescribed steps, often start data collection with a plan of 6 to 10 "transcribed interviews."

Proceeding in this linear way, one then "extracts" essences or themes and provides a list or, worse, a definition of the lived experience! It is here that we are being critiqued as not understanding phenomenology (Crotty, 1996). I am providing this background as an example of how I have come to use phenomenological understanding to justify presenting a more pliable method. I am troubled by so many studies that present themselves as phenomenological studies, when the researchers have followed a linear method and ironically can come out with, despite the experience under study, often the same list of what I have come to understand as "reactions," usually called themes, to experiences. For example, without naming the experience, studies often have the same essences or themes as findings: fear of the unknown, loneliness, anxiety, anger, depression, helplessness, powerlessness and isolation. Actually, one at this point could hypothesize what the experience might be that would produce those reactions and be correct. I imagine that there could be over one hundred common experiences that prompt those reactions. If this is the case then it seems to me we are only on the very surface of understanding.

Listing themes or essences has left us open to the criticism that we are categorizing human experience, much like reductionism, found in quantitative studies. If we recall that the major focus of phenomenological inquiry is understanding meaning of some "thing," some experience, something that is human so that we can better understand the meaning of being human, perhaps the fact that the responses to experiences are often similar may not be surprising. I would venture further and say that we have a fairly good sense of what kind of reactions (themes) people are going to have in a specific experience. However, meaningful studies demonstrate that our preconceived notions of reality can be very wrong.

Where many studies leave off—because, I would suggest, there is no "step" in the method the researcher may be following—is not to inquire into the meaning of these essences/responses for the particular individual. A researcher being phenomenologic however, demonstrates, with her participants, the meaning of isolation in that person's particular experience. She demonstrates the going back and forth, seeking further explanation, pondering the responses, bringing them to bear on the experience in a unique manner, unique in that experience for that particular person. Always keep in mind that we are not interested in generalizations but in the particular.

Isolation, for example, has a different meaning in different experiences. The researcher has to be able to narrate for the reader the understanding that enlightens the meaning of isolation in the experience of, for instance, losing a newborn, losing a parent, or having had a sense of losing oneself. Reasons are uncovered in the narrative of the participants that surprise us and give new direction to practice and, most important, to an understanding of human beings in experience and over time.

Search for Significance

All this needs to be said because it provides the "situated context" that inspired me to move toward a form of pragmatism and a search for significance for phenomenological research. Rochberg-Halthon claims that pragmatism "speaks to the contemporary hunger for significance" (Crotty, 1996, p. 6). So it was from the perspective of two powerful beliefs of mine: that our phenomenological research is significant and that we can demonstrate its significance not by numbers, but by stating the implications for change that emerges from the interpretation we glean from our participants on the meaning of various experiences. Results from a phenomenological study can be used for policy development, change in practice, increasing our capacity for care and compassion, emancipation from oppression, and raising our consciousness of what was not known or otherwise erroneous.

On the very practical side of pragmatism, students and researchers are required to present a proposal, which must include a method that is clearly spelled out, that will lead to some kind of findings, and that must also pass the institutional review board. Ten years ago I came to a place where I realized that arguing that phenomenology was not a "method" but a process,[2] a way of being toward meaning and experience, was not pragmatic. And so I developed from a very holistic perspective the "suggestions" with which I have guided students and listened to their feedback and now have called a "method."

This flexible method is holistic in the sense that students and colleagues participated in a "going back and forth" with me and have been a greater part of this work than I have been. Because of their work, they have demonstrated the method. I have come to understand this experience, mostly from them, and unbeknownst to them and me, we were all participants! **Table 5–1**, which represents the broad outline of this method, and **Table 5–2**, which presents the method in greater detail, reflect this shared collaboration among former students, colleagues, and me.

Phenomenological Research Immersion

Immersion is an essential and critical beginning of a phenomenological study. Phenomenological inquiry just cannot be done well or have any meaning if the researcher has not learned the language and come to understand the philosophical underpinnings of phenomenology. This is the place where students often discover that qualitative research can be more difficult than quantitative research is. There may be many reasons for this, but surely one reason, as discussed in Chapter 1, is that students are not prepared for qualitative research in the same way they are prepared for quantitative research, as far as course requirements. Students must master quantitative methods through courses and learn qualitative methods on their own. Thankfully, some changes in this curriculum area are taking place, as was discussed in Chapter 1.

All philosophies are based on assumptions about the world and contain abstractions and concepts to explain, describe, conceptualize, and analyze the nature of being, the universe, truth, meanings, knowledge, ethics, and the many pursuits of philosophy. Criticisms have been directed toward some researchers for simplifying the complexity and text of phenomenology. In fact, this chapter is one of simplification because it is an introduction.

It is absolutely critical that, if you use a method, you read, read, read about it. Perhaps you can take a course at your university, or you could request a course or workshop. Online courses are also available. Of course, there is nothing like time and experience to really "get it," and even then there will be people who

---

TABLE 5–1   Method for Phenomenological Inquiry Broad Outline

I.	Immersion
II.	Coming to the phenomenological aim of the inquiry
III.	Existential inquiry, expressions
IV.	Phenomenological contextual and processing*
V.	Analysis of interpretive interaction
VI.	Writing the phenomenological narrative
VII.	Writing a narrative on the meaning of your study

*Concurrent processes.

TABLE 5–2   Method for Phenomenological Inquiry

I.   Immersion

   A.   Describe and interpret the philosophical assumptions and underpinnings of a particular phenomenological perspective.

   B.   Exemplify the meaning of phenomenological concepts.

   C.   Elucidate the worldview of phenomenology as an approach to answering questions. (If you know the experience in which you are interested, use it as an example.)

II. Coming to the phenomenological aim of the inquiry

   A.   Articulate the aim of your study.

   B.   Distinguish the experience that is part of your study.

      1.   Describe, if circumscribed experience, or delimit context, if broad experience.

      2.   Articulate the situated context that is available to you in the moment.

   C.   Decenter yourself and come to "unknow."

      1.   Reflect on your own beliefs, preconceptions, intuitions, motives, and biases so as to decenter.

      2.   Adopt a perspective of "unknowing."

   D.   Articulate the aim of the study in the form of a phenomenological question.

	III. Existential inquiry, expressions, and processing*	IV. Phenomenological contextual processing*
III. Existential inquiry, expressions, and processing* IV. Phenomenological contextual processing*	A. Listen to self and others; develop heightened attentiveness to self and others. B. Reflect on personal experiences and expressions. C. Provide experiential descriptive expressions: "the experiencer." D. Provide experiential descriptive expressions: "others engaged in the experience." E. Provide experiential descriptive expressions: the arts and literature review.	A. Analyze emergent situated contexts. B. Analyze day-to-day contingencies. C. Assess life worlds.

(continues)

TABLE 5–2   Method for Phenomenological Inquiry *(continued)*

F. Provide anecdotal descriptive expressions: as experience appears.

G. Record ongoing reflection in your personal journal.

V. Analysis of interpretive interaction
   A. Integrate existential investigation with phenomenological contextual processing.
   B. Describe expressions of meaning (thoughts, emotions, feelings, statements, motives, metaphors, examples, behaviors, appearances and concealments, voiced and nonvoiced language).
   C. Interpret expressions of meaning as appearing from integration.

VI. Writing the phenomenological narrative
   A. Choose a style of writing that will communicate an understanding of the meaning of this particular experience.
   B. Write inclusively of all meanings, not just the "general" but the "particular."
   C. Write inclusively of language and expressions of meaning with the interpretive interaction of the situated context.
   D. Interpret with participants the meaning of the interaction of the experience with contextual processing.
   E. Narrate a story that at once gives voice to actual language and simultaneously interprets meaning from expressions used to describe the experience.

VII. Writing a narrative on the meaning of your study
   A. Summarize the answer to your phenomenological question with breadth and depth.
   B. Indicate how this understanding obtained from those who have lived the experience calls for self-reflection and/or system reflection.
   C. Interpret meanings of these reflections to small and large systems within specific context.
   D. Critique this interpretation with implications and recommendations for political, social, cultural, health care, family, and other social systems.

*Concurrent processes.

have really "gotten it" and still do not come to the same interpretation of phenomenology, and that is fine. If we believe all our voices express a polyvocality, then we respect varying interpretations of method. Almost all methods have their own controversies, as mentioned in Judith Wuest's chapter on the grounded theory method (Chapter 8).

In this chapter, I reference material presented in my own text titled *Revisioning Phenomenology: Nursing and Health Science Research* (Munhall, 1994a) and am very open with the reader that reading that book does not in any way suffice as the process step of immersion. However, I have been very gratified that readers have thanked me for simplifying what might be more obtuse in other writings on understanding phenomenology. With modesty, I would say that it is a good first book to read. It is conversational and friendly. However, demonstrating the temporal nature of our situated context, it was written before I had read and taken to heart Crotty's (1996) critique and other critiques of phenomenological studies that were being done. If I was to write that book today it would contain many more additions and I hope important insights. When we continue to study we witness our own writings being outdated, or at least not up to our present understanding. I urge you always to continue to evolve in your knowledge, whatever path you choose to take.

Reading van Manen (1990) or Benner (1994) also do not fulfill the requirement for immersion, however they provide essential thoughts and insights for you to ponder and incorporate into your thinking. For example, to demonstrate how important immersion is to good phenomenological research, the philosophers described in the following paragraphs are essential to your knowledge base. Because this is not a text on phenomenology, I have compressed some of the most prevalent names and schools to impress upon you what you would read during your immersion process. You need to become familiar with these philosophers, methods, and the different interpretations of phenomenology.

This way, you will have a solid foundation on which to make your own choice of method or focus. This is incredibly important and vital. For some of you, this may seem daunting, but if you find your "home" here, you will enjoy the challenge, thoughtfulness, and ideas that reflect the search for meaning and understanding. However, not all philosophers are easy to read. Philosophers trained in the discipline find reading Heidegger exasperating at times. I am aware of the emphasis I have placed on reading the original works of these philosophers, but at the same time I encourage you to read authors who have interpreted the philosophers' works in an understandable format.

In the process of immersion, the following two paragraphs would be easily understood and you would be conversant with the material. For example, as part of your immersion you would read Merleau-Ponty, who is considered more of an existential phenomenologist. His focus is on the importance of perception and the individual's situatedness in the world through experience. Husserl, absolutely essential reading, is thought of as a transcendental phenomenologist for whom consciousness is not empirical but "pure" consciousness.

Hermeneutical phenomenology is most often associated with Heidegger, where the focus is on understanding "being," and you can see that his philosophical influence is prevalent in this chapter. Within Heidegger's phenomenology, one views all phenomenological description as interpretation. As you travel in the immersion process, you will come to ask, "What about analytical phenomenology as contrasted to interpretative? Are they the same?" The answer to those questions would vary, depending on the philosopher. Different answers to the same questions are, in my experience, part of the complexity of phenomenology. Yet, one could continue to categorize these different schools and arrive at one answer to the preceding questions and say that analytical phenomenology has more to do with the semiotic meaning structures of cultural practices, or that gender phenomenology is most concerned with context sensitivity and is truth tentative (M. van Manen, workshop, 1998).

The state of the art of phenomenology reflects the postmodern world that we inhabit in that there are multiple interpretations and multiple realities, as Lynne Dunphy and Joy Longo discussed in Chapter 4. Phenomenology is like a mirror in that it celebrates reflection, where differences and the "particular" are unveiled.

Nursing Research and Phenomenology

My own observations of phenomenological inquiry by nurses include references to one of the French or German phenomenologists, say, the first generation, and then these nurse researchers move to a phenomenologist who has proposed a "method" for inquiry. Among them (for the sake of simplicity, I choose four and refer to them as second-generation phenomenologists) are Georggi, Colaizzi, van Kaam, and van Manen. The first three are from the United States; they became the most influential methodologists for nurse researchers in the 1970s and 1980s. Faced with the requirement of finding a method to conduct a phenomenological study and lacking formal training themselves in this area, nurse researchers understandably chose one of these three phenomenological methods. Many problems seemed to have arisen from this attempt at articulation. Although the researchers became well versed in phenomenological thought by reading the first generation of phenomenologists, the transition to these other methods was often limiting and incongruent with the philosophy.

Historically, this outcome is understandable if we remember the pedestal that "method" was put upon; perhaps more influential and costlier, the closer a method could look like a "scientific method" or "the scientific method," the more acceptable it was in the academy. The last phenomenologist mentioned, Max van Manen (1984, 1990), changed this situation dramatically with a human science approach, where his views were often consistent with many of the first-generation phenomenological philosophers. The reason that he is an outstanding phenomenologist for those in the human sciences to follow is that he views phenomenology as a philosophy of being as well as a practice. From this perspective, any methodic location can give a view of experiential understanding by questioning lived experience through reflective writing.

Here, and in this way, meaning can be understood and we can become practitioners of the ever-fragile exercise of phenomenological wisdom (van Manen, 1998). Nurse researchers have elaborated on these various methods, including fine works by Paterson and Zderad (1976, 1988), Benner (1994), Parse (1987), Ray (1990), Watson (1985), Newman (1986), and many others. To reiterate, this chapter cannot prepare you entirely to do a phenomenological study. It is an overview, and the whole text is an introduction to many different qualitative methods. In this overview, I would like to place some basic phenomenologic concepts as they appear in Revisioning Phenomenology (1994a). To really understand these concepts is to dedicate yourself to following up on reading more and more, and then some more.

The Phenomenological Paradigm

As an alternative and a historical reaction to the then prevailing hegemony of the positivist perspective, phenomenology construed itself as a philosophy, a perspective, and an approach to practice and research. Philosophically, phenomenology seems to undergird many of the qualitative research approaches (although some argue this point). Because of its importance as a philosophy, some key concepts are presented here. Recognition needs to be given to Husserl, who introduced the idea of phenomenology in response to or in reaction to the context-free generalizations of the positivist approach of the natural sciences. Husserl attempted to restore the "reality" of humans in their "life worlds," to capture the "meaning" of this, and to revive philosophy with new humanism. Spiegelberg (1976), Cohen (1987), and Reeder (1987) provide excellent discussions of the history of the phenomenological movement. These concepts then, as outlined, reflect an acknowledgment of the inevitability of subjectivity in any exploration or description of reality. This inevitability is not stated with resignation but with the idea that subjectivity expands and enriches the authenticity of perceptions and understandings of phenomenology. It is this perspective that is both essential and desirable.

Key Concepts of Phenomenology as Philosophy

As defined by Merleau-Ponty (1962), consciousness is sensory awareness of and response to the environment. Consciousness is life: it is not an interior or inner existence, it is existence in the world through the body. The unity of mind and body becomes a means of experiencing, thus eliminating the idea of a subjective and objective world. A person cannot step out of consciousness and be sure of anything. The world is knowable only through the subjectivity of being in the world. Objectivity as a quest for reliability and validity depends on the recognition of this relationship between mind and body, subject and object, and the knowledge that this or any knowing comes about through consciousness.

Embodiment explains that through consciousness we are aware of being-in-the-world, and it is through the body that we gain access to this world. We feel, think, taste, touch, hear, and are conscious through the opportunities the body offers. There is talk sometimes about expanding the mind or expanding waistlines. The expansion is within the body, within consciousness. At any point in time and for each individual, a particular perspective or consciousness exists based on the individual's history, knowledge of the world, and perhaps openness to the world. Human science's focus on the individual and on the meaning events may have for an individual reflects the recognition that experience is individually interpreted.

The natural attitude (Schutz & Wagner, 1970) is a mode of consciousness that espouses interpreted experiences. The world as experienced and interpreted by preceding generations is handed down, teaching a great deal about reality in the process. These teachings become assumptions, unquestioned meanings about phenomena, that are a part of a person's "natural attitude" toward the world. To hear or see something contrary to the natural attitude can be disconcerting. This attitude of being in the world is deeply ingrained and usually unquestioned. Understanding the concept of natural attitude can help in understanding, at the individual level, responses to change. Both the perspectival and the physiological alterations associated with a life change are often the result of a disruption of the natural attitude.

Experience and perception are our original modes of consciousness. Perception, which takes place through the body, is an individual's access to experience in the world. Perception of varying objects depends also on the context in which they are experienced for interpretation and meaning. A person who says the aim of phenomenology is to describe lived experience may be describing his or her own or another's perceptions of that lived experience.

Perception of experience is what matters, not what in reality may appear to be contrary or more "truthful." If a person perceives danger when "in fact" there may be none, in the reality of that person's lived experience, there is danger. Perhaps that is why saying "this won't hurt" or "this will only hurt for a little while" is often ineffective in allaying a person's fear. The perception of the lived experience may not even be of pain; the perception may be of a danger far worse than being hurt or feeling pain. Interpretation of the experience from the individual's unique perception of an event is critical. What is important from this worldview, therefore, is not what is happening, but what is perceived as happening. That is the reality to be concerned with—the experience as the individual is perceiving it.

As a philosophy, phenomenology demonstrates these major concepts in the many interpretations that exist concerning its meaning. A phenomenological question here might be asked: "What is it like to try to understand phenomenology?" or, "What makes someone think and talk about phenomenology?"

The answers are found in the themes of consciousness, embodiment, the natural attitude, perception, and experience. Again, these two questions would be good grist for the phenomenological perspective as a qualitative approach to research.

Phenomenology as Philosophy: More Key Concepts

The relational view of the person posited by Heidegger (1962) further elaborates on the philosophical theme of phenomenology. Because an individual participates in cultural, social, and historical contexts of the world, to be human is to "be-in-the-world." Language, cultural, and social practices are handed down to individuals who embody the meanings and interpretations of these practices. In Heideggerian phenomenology, the interpretation and self-understanding handed down through language and culture are called the "background" (Allen, Benner, & Diekelmann, 1986). The idea of the background (like the natural attitude) is critical because it provides conditions for human actions and perceptions. It is where the individual is, a history to the present moment, and a view of "what can be." Other Heideggerian ideas include the following:

- Meaning is found in the transaction between an individual and a situation so that the individual both constitutes and is constituted by the situation.
- Human purposes and concerns "prestructure" the human world so that what is considered significant about an event or object is a function of or embodies that concern (Dreyfus, 1972). The perception of meaning follows from this understanding.
- This understanding is predicated on the belief that immediate experience is embodied with organization and meaning, with linguistic, social, and cultural patterning, and with characteristics intrinsic to the experience.
- A critical assumption of this phenomenological perspective is its emphasis on language, which imbues and informs experience. Language does not exist apart from thought or perception, for language generates and constrains the human life world.

Key Concepts of Phenomenology as Research

Max van Manen (1984) offers the following observations about phenomenological research:

- Phenomenology is the study of the individual's life world, as experienced rather than as conceptualized, categorized, or theorized. Phenomenology aims for a deeper understanding of the nature or meaning of everyday experiences.
- Phenomenological research is the study of essences of experience. In phenomenology, the researcher does not ask, "How do nursing students

learn to nurse?" but asks instead, "What is the nature of the experience of becoming a nurse?" The aim is to understand the experience. The opportunities for plausible insights bring the investigator in more direct contact with the world.

- Phenomenological research is the attentive practice of thoughtfulness— a minding, a heeding, a caring attunement, a wondering about the project of living. When the language of a lived experience awakens a person to the meaning of the experience, he or she gains a fuller understanding of what it means to be human.

- Phenomenological research is a quest for what it means to be human. The more deeply a person understands human experience, the more fully and uniquely he or she becomes human. Such individuals learn to notice and to make sense of the various aspects of human existence. Of course, the more often a person engages in such attentiveness, the more he or she should be able to understand the details as well as the more global dimensions of life. The corollary is that such previously unreflected upon phenomena, the "taken for granted," assume richer meaningfulness.

- Phenomenology has been called "the science of examples." Phenomenological descriptions are often composed of examples that permit readers "to see" the deeper significance or structure of the lived experience being described.

As emphasized earlier in this book, our colleagues who are preparing to do quantitative studies do so with many methods and statistics courses, and we cannot expect less when we embark on qualitative research. We do ourselves a disservice from the beginning if this formal study of qualitative research is not part of immersion. Reading unfamiliar language leaves the interpretation up to the reader, and it is in this particular activity where caution, in particular in the beginning of learning, needs to be taken. Speaking and hearing others speak of the philosophical ideas, concepts, and assumptions must be part of immersion. This is the area where I have found the most breakdown in phenomenological studies.

I want to again emphasize that the preceding didactic material on phenomenology, concepts, and origins is an abbreviated description, much too little content to really understand the concepts. Unfortunately, some students move directly from reading about a method and how to carry out the method to doing the study. Please don't miss the experience of delving deeper into understanding these concepts. Studying these concepts will eliminate frustration or confusion, and you will be confident in knowing that phenomenology is more than the study of lived experience. If you should do a dissertation using phenomenology, you will be comfortable in the knowledge and understanding you have acquired. Am I lecturing? Probably, but it is in your best interest. It is also from my own perspective and experience. For the student who does immersion, all else falls naturally into place. That student has become phenomenologic in being and continues, like Sarah discusses in the next chapter, to continue to become more so and to be in a very good place in this world.

The Aim of Immersion

The goal of immersion, then, is not unlike the goal of phenomenology: understanding. If you are going to embark on phenomenological inquiry, I urge you to find courses specific to phenomenology. They are becoming more widespread, and you may even find them online. In addition, participating in workshops provides an interaction that enlarges the processes in phenomenological research.* Immersion also requires reading phenomenological studies, which can be a curious sort of immersion. Some of these studies can teach you that some studies are not good ones, such as when you wonder what the point was.

Other studies resonate with you and, after reading such a study, you come to realize that you understand the meaning of being in some experience or another much better than you ever had before, or that you understand a human experience in a way that conflicts with what you once thought, as happens when people read, for example, Sarah's studies; this is good phenomenology. Immersion also means learning what may be called good phenomenology perhaps by reading articles from journals that discuss this topic, provide constructive criticism, and remind researchers what must be of importance. The references in the chapters in Part I and this chapter contain important readings and I urge you to read with wonder!

The process of immersion is ongoing. I have found in my own life that the interest in the literature and the pursuit of greater understanding has become a part of who I am as a person. It is as though phenomenology becomes part of who you are, and you become phenomenologically present to and in the world.

Immersion enables you to understand what becoming phenomenologically present to the world means. This is the part that really is a process and cannot be reduced to a method. Over time, one who comes from this perspective will begin to interact differently with others, whether in research or practice. One begins to become less assuming, often abandoning assumptions about another or another's experience, and adopts a stance of "unknowing" (Munhall, 1993, 1994a). In this place, a person can be phenomenologically present to another person. Toward what end? To understand the other. To be open, nonjudgmental, and compassionate.

How can one act toward another in a caring, compassionate way if one has not suspended assumptions or judgments? How can one understand what kind of meaning an experience has for a person unless one suspends one's own preconceptions? In giving of ourselves in nursing and in our personal lives, how do we know what to do, what to say, and when it is better not to say any-thing if we do not understand the meaning of "something" for the other? This is why immersion is so critical. Becoming phenomenologically oriented re-quires a new and different way of perceiving reality. Part of immersion is to practice being phenomenological, which is a challenge, but one that is essen-tial to the interviewing step in phenomenological methods. To interview in phenomenological inquiry is to be able to "decenter" and to be fully present to another (this topic is discussed further in this chapter).

If you are philosophically inclined toward understanding, once again I say immersion will be one of the most intellectually stimulating and affectively moving experiences of your educational experience. Without this step, phe-nomenological inquiry is not possible. Without this step, you will be doing storytelling, journalism, and impressionistic writing. Worse, you will be doing logical positivistic quasi-qualitative research! None of those activities on their own are negative; but they are not phenomenology.

How to Accomplish the Step of Immersion in an Actual Study

Remember, this method as discussed in this context is for new researchers and for those who might be doing a study for a dissertation or a master's thesis. Once this step is in process and has become a part of one's ongoing research program, the step itself does not have to be on every proposal or study. How-ever, it has been my experience that I continually enlarge my understanding with new literature as well as by returning to the classical literature. This step as presented here is for those embarking for the first or second time who have not done this step before.

Immersion is your research preparation for phenomenology (it is also preparation for any other method of inquiry; ironically, it is spelled out more clearly for quantitative studies but is never called immersion). Immersion as a step, then, is almost pedantic with the aim of achieving a dynamic deep un-derstanding; with practice it can be concretely reported as the first step for be-ginning researchers in the following ways. What we are about to do now is to articulate each step with an explanation of the step as well as the special con-siderations inherent in the process of the step of this method as illustrated in Tables 5–1 and 5–2.

I. Immersion

A. Describe and interpret the philosophical assumptions and underpinnings of a particular phenomenological perspective.
This section should include the evolution of phenomenology, the philoso-phers, the different schools of phenomenology, and how they differ from one

another. The assurance that section A is done well is that you, your colleagues, and your professor come away from reading this section and agree that you do have a good understanding of phenomenology. If this is not the case, more immersion is needed.

B. Exemplify the meaning of phenomenological concepts.

In the process of writing section A, you most likely did not discuss the meaning of the various concepts. In this section, explain what they mean. For instance, give the meaning of the following:

- Situated context
- Intersubjectivity
- Perception
- Decentering
- Unknowing
- Appearance–concealment
- Being-in-the-world
- Consciousness
- Life worlds: temporality, spatiality, corporeality, relationality
- Contingency
- Intentionality
- Preconceptions
- Shared perceptual fields

These and other phenomenological concepts are described in this chapter as well as in Revisioning Phenomenology (Munhall, 1994a) and other references. The assurance that section B is done well is that, with each concept, you demonstrate the meaning of the concept with a real-world example. Again, if colleagues and your professor understand you, you can be assured that you understand the meaning of specific concepts.

C. Elucidate the worldview of phenomenology as an approach to answering questions. (If you know the experience in which you are interested, use it as an example.)

This process prepares you for phenomenological dialogue/interviews/conversations. After studying decentering as an unknowing process and also understanding intersubjectivity, you practice conversations with others. The best person to practice with is someone who can critique your listening skills. That notwithstanding, after a conversation in which you practice decentered dialogue, write a description of the dialogue with an interpretation. Give this description to the person with whom you conversed to ascertain how and what you heard and whether you overlaid the description or interpretation of the dialogue with your own assumptions or preconceptions. This excellent exercise should be repeated. The assurance that section C is done well is that your description and interpretation of what the "other" was saying is validated by that person. This first step is critical. A lack of immersion is comparable to doing quantitative research without having taken research courses in the scientific method, statistics, and measurement. This step enables you to be the "instrument" for your study. Your role in the study requires high-level skills and learned sophistication in communication.

Existential Interaction. Remember, in phenomenological inquiry you are going to be in constant interaction in the existential processing of phenomenological material. You will also be in transaction with persons in interviews and conversations and need to develop the consciousness of one who does not know. The researcher is in search of the meaning of a phenomenon, the meaning of being human in experience (phenomenon). Whether the researcher has or has not experienced the phenomenon, he or she needs to come to the phenomenological question as free as possible from assumptions, preconceptions, and forethought about the phenomenon or experience. When you first begin phenomenological inquiry, it is important to be cognizant that you do not and should not have a hypothesis. To this, one may say, "Of course!" However, often we are not aware of some hidden belief we may have and then try to find ways to document that belief. That is why decentering yourself from your own world of knowledge and hunches is so important.

As you go on with these steps, it is important to understand that, as mentioned, they are not linear. There is a going back and forth, an examining and reexamining, a thought and then a change in thought, and there are many middle-of-the-night "ahas!"

A major component of phenomenological inquiry is a phenomenon that I call, for lack of a better description, "becoming your study." You become a repository for appearances of the experience or you become an example of the experience, and your attentiveness almost becomes unconscious. You are not actually looking for existential material for your study, but without notice, you will awaken to its presence. Some of us have marveled at the experience "of seeing it everywhere" or of realizing that "it was always there and I did not see it, hear it, understand it." Another way to describe this is to say that the subject of your study, the phenomenon, the experience, takes up residence within you. This will not occur if your inquiry is an academic exercise (although I have heard that, even then, it sometimes happens). The taking up of residence, to me, requires an intense longing to understand meaning—the meaning of something. It becomes a passion, and then the process is so much easier because you have become engaged with the philosophy of phenomenology. Philosophers are thinkers and questioners of a different sort than scientists. One very important distinction is this very lack of linearity.

Heidegger (1962) stated that language generates and constrains the human life world. As I was writing down a process as a method, I thought it was a wonderful example. I am constrained by language because it is expressed on paper in a linear way—line by line—when this method is, as mentioned, a back-and-forth and circular and sometimes even linear process.

II. Coming to the Phenomenological Aim of the Inquiry

The following four activities will assist you in focusing on the aim of your study. Your aim is to be understandable to others who are taking part in and who are interested in your work.

A. *Articulate the aim of your study.*

Be very clear about what you want to accomplish in conducting this inquiry. So often, the aim of a study is listed as studying the "lived experience" of some experience, but that is not an aim. It is a means toward an end. You think about what you are attempting to accomplish and for what purpose. Crotty's (1996) main concern about the way in which North American nurse researchers were conducting phenomenological studies is that phenomenology should offer a philosophical critique. Crotty asks for significance from phenomenological studies—that they go beyond describing and interpreting and suggest possibilities that may enhance or correct some experiences. Others who disagree say that their work is just to describe and interpret and that it is the work of other researchers to point out the problems inherent in the descriptions and to suggest actions leading to change.

My own concern is that, if we do not include critiques or suggestions to alleviate problems, question theoretical incongruencies, or pointedly demonstrate how our understanding illuminates a problem, the critical importance of our studies will go unfulfilled. A critique of the experience may offer infinite possibilities for needed change. At first I was defensive, like many other nurse researchers, in response to Crotty's criticism and leaned toward a purist perspective. But, after much reflection, I came to believe that the addition of critique would certainly have the benefit of increasing the significance of phenomenological work and, in a pragmatic way, provide direction to practice or to theory. Additionally, I was beginning to find it difficult to argue with a suggestion that would ultimately *enlarge our purpose* and assist individuals in attaining meaning and improve sensitivity, understanding, and change in conditions and approaches that were not enhancing the quality of their lives. In other words, we could use our understanding to improve the quality of life for people.

So, as a researcher, you need to enlarge your aim and be clear about which experience you are going to name, understand, and find the meaning of, as well as critique your findings for larger implications.

You can be assured that this section is complete when you can demonstrate to others the significance of your aim, and they agree that the way you have stated the aim lends itself to phenomenological inquiry.

B. Distinguish the experience that is your study.

1. Describe, if circumscribed experience, or delimit context, if broad experience. Describing the experience: Here is where researchers seem to go two different ways, and some methodologists may have rules here. From my perspective, either direction is fine. You might choose an actual experience in the form of an activity or procedure or, as in Sarah's study, a life event. Or you might choose an emotion, or feeling state, such as restlessness, comfort, pain, or anxiety. With emotions, or feelings, you must be clear in distinguishing the range of the study. For example: studying pain is an extremely broad experience. Think about what this inquiry is for and for what purpose. Then distinguish in some way the kind of pain or the pain associated with a specific kind of experience that you will focus on.

There is experience within experience, and this is not a problem. Actually, it is part of any experience. No experience occurs in isolation. With this in mind, you might decide to study the meaning of pain experienced in association with a specific condition. If you felt confident and grounded in phenomenology, you could study the meaning of pain to persons who have experienced pain and not actually distinguish a category or condition. That kind of study would be a grand study. All variations of experiences might be associated with pain and, in this type of study, you would distinguish the experience associated with the pain, but it would fall into the background and the meaning of pain would always be in the foreground. One advantage of doing a grand study is that it could become your research program, an area you continuously explore in ongoing studies. Certainly, this type of study requires more time, is a subject for a larger and continuing study, and would find its major understandings narrated in at least one volume.

The assurance that you have distinguished your phenomenon is when your colleagues or professor know that it is "this" that you are studying, not "that" or any other fringe phenomenon along with it. You are able to answer questions, clearly delineating what it is and what it is not that you are searching to find meaning in.

2. Articulate the situated context that is available to you in the moment. Experience is embedded in life worlds and various contingencies. In this part of the study, you need to describe the context in which you and the study will be taking place. Life worlds are described later in this chapter.

C. Decenter yourself and come to "unknow."

1. Reflect on your own beliefs, preconceptions, intuitions, motives, and biases so as to decenter. It has been said that phenomenology can liberate one from preconceptions. However, ironically, often without their knowing, researchers design their studies or "hear" in a way that substantiates their preconceptions. That is why this decentering process is so critical. The researcher in a phenomenological study is, to use a metaphor, the "research tool" or the "research instrument." To be truly authentic and effective, the researcher is asked to do something that is impossible to do, but to do it to the greatest extent that is possible.

Researchers are asked to clear their vision and thinking from their assumptions, from their prior knowledge, and from their belief systems. In this step, for that to happen, you need to adopt a perspective of "unknowing" in which you listen with "the third ear" free, to the extent possible, of any prejudice or bias. In your journal, record your beliefs, assumptions, preconceptions, what you expect your findings to be, and any other noise that might prevent you from hearing clearly, uninterrupted when you are listening to others by "noise" about the meaning of the experience. This is also an important step in seeing the experience in whatever forms it shows itself. Often, we see something and automatically overlay that sight with our own interpretation. We assumed we knew something about what we were seeing, only to find out that we had misperceived.

Two films come to mind to assist you in this step. The film *As Good as It Gets* is a wonderful portrayal of preconceptions, biases, and prejudices, and *The Tail Wagging the Dog* demonstrates to us that we are on thin ice, believing what we see! Many phenomenological concepts can be understood better by viewing these films from these two different perspectives. It is a wonderful learning experience.

The assurance that you have accomplished decentering is obtained through practice listening/interview/conversation sessions. As in section C of step I, immersion, you can practice decentering with a colleague or friend. Write in your journal what you are decentering from, listen to your friend describe an experience, write a description of what you heard and what meaning your friend ascribed to the experience. Let your friend evaluate how accurately you grasped the essence of what was said.

During this practice, do not use a tape recorder and do not repeat verbatim what was said. Listen to grasp the meaning. Listen to get inside the person's perceptions. This often takes practice with many different people and their experiences. It is quite a revelation to realize how different our perceptions of the same event are and how we take for granted that we both "saw" the same thing. My favorite example of differing perceptions of the same phenomenon are the following two descriptions.

The following passage, written by Jane Smiley (1989), describes the memory of a very young child:

> As I sit on this hard bench I suddenly yearn for one last long look and not only of the phenomenon of little Joe and little Michael, but of the others too; Ellen, four, and Annie, seven months, sharing a peach. . . . As I watch them now as adults the fact that I will never see their toddler selves again is tormenting. (p. 120)

Ann Beattie (1989) writes about the same kind of memory:

> When you are thirty, the child is two. At forty, you realize that the child in the house, the child you live with, is still, when you close your eyes, or the moment he has walked from the room, two years old. When you are sixty and the child is gone, the child will also be two, but then you will be more certain. Wet sheets, wet kisses. A flood of tears. As you remember him the child is always two. (p. 53)

2. Adopt a perspective of "unknowing." Decentering attempts to achieve the essential state of mind of unknowing as a condition of openness. In contrast, knowing leads to a form of confidence that has inherent in it a state of closure. The "art" of unknowing is discussed as a decentering process from the individual's own organizing principles of the world (Atwood & Stolorow, 1984). Unknowing is not simple but is essential to the understanding of subjectivity and perspectivity.

Unknowing paradoxically is another form of knowing. Knowing that you do not know something, that you do not understand someone who stands before you and who perhaps does not fit into some preexisting paradigm or theory, is critical to the evolution of understanding meaning for others.

To engage in an authentic encounter is to stand in your own socially constructed world and to unearth the other's world, saying: "I do not know you. I do not know your subjective world." A person who engages another human being to form impressions, formulate a perception, and theorize from a place called knowing has confidence in prior knowledge. Such confidence, however, has an inherent state of closure in it. To be authentically present to a person is to situate knowingly in your own life and interact with full unknowingness about the other's life. In this way, unknowing equals openness (**Figure 5–1**).

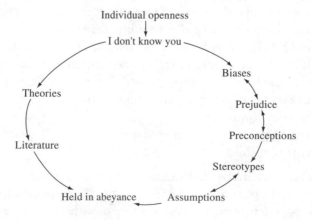

FIGURE 5–1   Unknowing Openness.

Unknowing. The state of being decentered and unknowing is challenging to achieve. Unknowing is an art and calls for a great amount of introspection. Unknowing is essential to the understanding of intersubjectivity and perspectivity. In other words, it is essential to understand ourselves and each participant in our study as two distinctive beings, one of whom the researcher does not know. Each of us has a unique perspective of our situated context and a unique perspective of who we are as individuals in the world. This is our perspectivity, our worldview, and our reality. When the researcher and the participant meet, two perspectives of a situation need to be recognized. Thus, the process of intersubjectivity begins to create a perceptual space (**Figure 5–2**).

Intersubjectivity. Intersubjectivity is not difficult to understand, though many writings seem intent on making the concept seem complex. What is complex is practicing it in a wide-awake manner. Intersubjectivity is the verbal and nonverbal interplay between the organized subjective worlds of two people in which one person's subjectivity intersects with another's subjectivity. The subjective world of any person represents the organization of feelings, thoughts, ideas, principles, theories, illusions, distortions, and whatever else helps or hinders that person. The real point here is that people do not know about anyone else's subjective world unless they are told about it. And even then, they cannot be sure. Figure 5-2 illustrates the concepts of intersubjectivity.

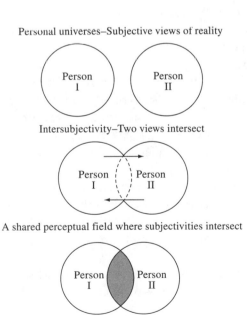

Personal universes–Subjective views of reality

Person I   Person II

Intersubjectivity–Two views intersect

Person I   Person II

A shared perceptual field where subjectivities intersect

Person I   Person II

FIGURE 5–2   Shared Perceptual Space of Intersubjectivity.*

*Visually the more interaction, the larger the shared perceptual space.

A film that illustrates how two subjectivities can be extremely different because of the situated context of various life contingencies for individuals is *Whose Life Is It Anyway?* In the perceptual space in which the characters engage in dialogue, there are good examples of how decentering and unknowing by the healthcare providers in the film would have contributed to an understanding of the patient. The patient is misunderstood, to the point of despair. Watch and listen to a person being heard in a phenomenological manner as the film comes to its conclusion.

D. Articulate the aim of the study in the form of a phenomenological question.

When you know the aim of your study, which is to understand the meaning of an experience, which you have clearly distinguished from other experiences, you are now able to begin to articulate questions. You have decentered yourself so as to be open and receptive to phenomenological material wherever and whenever it appears. These processes of phenomenological inquiry enable you to proceed to the question.

In Chapters 6 and 7 we can see the authors articulate the aim of their studies. Both chapters exemplify the freedom and opportunity to find meaning in experience and to understand what these experiences mean to individuals. This brings us to the critical aims of phenomenology: understanding the meaning of being human (Heidegger, 1962) and, as van Manen (1990) says, becoming more human. We can become more human only through understanding self and others in individual life worlds, situated contexts, and contingencies and caring about it all.

By internalizing the philosophy of phenomenology, distinguishing the phenomenon, and decentering from our own worldviews, we come now to the process of phenomenological questioning about the meaning of experience for individuals. We can have many questions and will have more as material evolves. However, it is often helpful to have one overarching question. This question can then guide other questions. We must use caution here and not plan more than a few questions. When the existential material "speaks" to us and begs our attention, it will be the material from the study itself that will guide you with questions and provide direction to the study as a whole. The overarching question, the question, should reflect the underlying aim, that of understanding the meaning of being human and focusing on the experience that you have chosen to study.

You can articulate the question in different ways, which often has to do with a particular philosopher or school of phenomenology in which you may be most interested. My own experience has led me to find personal meaning in the perspectives of Heidegger, Merleau-Ponty, and van Manen, among other philosophers including the postmodernists. For example, I find Heidegger's curiosity about the question on "being" very compelling. "What does it mean, this idea we call being? What is the nature of being? What is the meaning of being?" To wander down this path, one accepts that "beings" are always in experience. Therefore, we go to the experience in which the human being is to attempt to answer the question of meaning for that human being. The experience may not necessarily be concrete; it may be abstract, such as spirituality or even philosophizing. Beings are always being, even "being" asleep. It is in what beings are being that enables us to find meaning in being! The being is in experience.

The standard answer to the question "what is phenomenology?" evolved from there: It is the study of lived experience. That definition, I believe, has led many to miss the most critical "whatness" of phenomenology, as researchers focus more on the experience than on understanding human meaning in experience. Like "being," "experience" should never be simplified. Merlau-Ponty (1962) believed that experiences are layered with meanings, and he contributes to our understanding by emphasizing how these meanings create the ways in which we perceive experience. This is where the life worlds, contingency, and the situated context need to be addressed to assist us in understanding the many-layered multiplicity of considerations in any one person's perception of experience. I mentioned in Chapter 1 this multiplicity that resides within each of us—our multiple "beings" changing from day to day as different facets of who we are in that moment take precedence. We notice we feel different at different time periods. Time changes meaning. That is why Selen Lauterbach's study in the last edition of this text (2007) focusing on longitudinal phenomenology brings us even closer to understanding meaning. We need to understand that meaning is not permanent—it is fluid. Experience has meaning and continues to grow in meaning in different ways. For example, meaning can change, meaning can become more profound and/or meaning can be negotiated.

Articulating the research question calls on us to be very clear about what we are studying. The overall question, from a Heideggerian perspective, would be: "What is the meaning of being human in this experience (entity)?" Many studies begin with the question, "What is it like to be in this experience or to have had this experience?" After many years of reading studies that use the latter question, I have come to believe that if we keep *meaning* in the forefront of our study, we will have a richer study, one in which meaning is usually found in the participants' own words, as they form expressions of meaning. Keep in mind that you will have many questions that can be asked of participants in your study and, "What's it like?" could actually be the first question. Often this will lead to a description of the experience. I think we need to go further. Asking "How were you feeling? Thinking?" and other variations can lead to the meaning of the experience, which will then bring into play the life worlds, the situated context, and contingency.

Now, all this said, usually the academic world demands the question be clearly articulated. But too-strict guidelines might prevent you from following where the participant wants to go. Use common sense when trying to keep yourself and the participant focused. If the participant wanders from the experience, you must make a decision about the relatedness or, better yet, ask the participant how he or she sees what he or she is saying to be connected. A participant's wandering to areas whose relevance is not obvious to you can be extremely important to the participant. Refocusing participants needs to be done minimally. This wandering is part of the phenomenological study and, as such, has meaning that will be discussed in detail later in this chapter.

In one of my own studies, the question that was overarching was: What is the meaning of anger as it is experienced by women who are in therapy? The aim of that study was to begin to understand the meaning of anger of women who happened to be in therapy at the time (Munhall, 1994a).

You can see the difference in asking questions and stating aims, which are different from what we have become accustomed to reading. Remember the most frequent definition of phenomenology as the study of lived experience does not capture the essence of phenomenology. The "meaning as it is experienced" is a personal preference. I also believe that keeping meaning in the forefront of your study will produce a more phenomenological study. You will not be led astray to structures and categories. Phenomenological researchers do not want to know simply what it is like, but what the meaning of it is. They seek an understanding of the meaning of "things" to individuals. Within the method presented here, that is the ultimate aim and is reflected in the question.

III. Existential Inquiry, Expressions, and Processing

Steps III and IV are two process steps that are conducted simultaneously. Existential inquiry by nature requires our "being-in-the-world" and takes place in the life worlds of the researcher and the participant. When we engage in dialogue with our participants, in addition to hearing the linguistic expressions they use to describe and interpret their experience, we also need to hear the situated context of their being-in-the-world. This has been called the horizon, or the background, of the experience. Expressions of meaning cannot be acontextual. The thoughts, feelings, emotions, and questions are deeply embedded in the context of the participant's life, or life world. While we are doing the existential inquiry, we are also doing contextual processing. They are separated out for pedantic purposes here and for ease of understanding. This concurrent process can be imagined by overlaying **Figure 5–3** with **Figure 5–4**.

We begin with step III, the existential inquiry, expressions, and processing. Existential inquiry, expressions, and processing constitute the step in which you gather the existential material. This step requires specific processes, such as attentiveness, intuitiveness, constant reflection on decentering, active listening, interviews or conversations clarifying, synthesizing, writing, taking

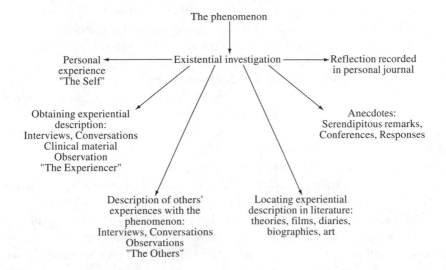

FIGURE 5–3   The Phenomenon—Existential Investigation.

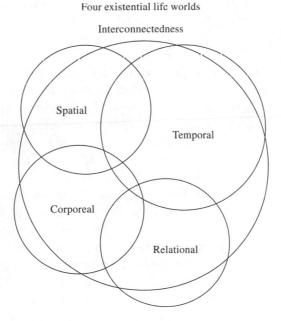

FIGURE 5–4   Four Existential Life Worlds.

photographs, creating verse, and almost anything that will reflect your participant's and your consciousness and awareness of the experience.

Most phenomenological studies at present use some technique to collapse the material into groupings. This is part of the confounding nature of phenomenological research. Originally, phenomenology was a method used to interpret texts. For example, "What is the meaning of this book?" However, since social and healthcare scientists started using the method to attempt to learn more about their clients' and patients' experiences, the problem of what to do with all the material has been approached in different ways.

Some methods call for collapsing or condensing the material into themes, essences, meaning units, and (probably the least phenomenological) structural definitions. In many phenomenological studies, we see the prevalence of these approaches in the discussion of themes, essential elements, labeling, clusters, categories—all attempts to provide a description of an experience in a clear, logical listing of some type. Sometimes whichever method the researcher used to organize the material is then placed into a narrative. If there were 10 participants, the researcher searched for similar themes among the 10 with perhaps a note or two about differences, but then wrote the narrative in a way that reflected the merging of 10 participants. Doing this is a profound disservice to the individual and to individual differences. Additionally it collapses language into universal meaning. We all use words or describe emotions with some of the same language but that does not mean we are using the language the same way to express the authentic experience.

In a field such as nursing, where we are strongly socialized in a world of signs and symptoms, lists of diagnoses, and other kinds of classifications, we tend to value this "shorthand" for its efficiency in communication. However, a major problem with this approach, especially in a phenomenological study, is that words and signs do not have the same meaning for everyone. Both the healthcare provider and the patient interpret words differently. These words and signs further lose meaning if they are acontextual. The signs and symptoms manifested by a patient have meaning only when placed in a historical, social, cultural, and individual context. So we have a dilemma. We cannot deliver a study of entire transcribed interviews. What are some alternatives? "Dwelling with the data" used to be a popular phrase, but not so much today. But it is here that I think we need to return. The researcher has either a transcribed interview of one person or notes taken over a series of interview dialogues. Within these texts are expressions of meaning. The expressions convey in words a manifestation of meaning. Throughout the material, the researcher can highlight such expressions. They come as participants express themselves with emotions, thoughts, desires, questions, wishes, hopes, and complaints. It is to this that we need to turn our attention. People do not talk in themes; we impose themes on their "language." It seems more authentic to stay close to the participant's language and search through the material for the expressions of meaning.

Dwelling. I believe it is essential to dwell. There are no shortcuts here. Those who invest the time and make the commitment to authenticity will serve well themselves and their participants. Once again the researcher is called on to be the "instrument." Each individual participant needs our reverence for his or her individuality and way of expressing meaning. You read the text of one participant, highlighting in your head the expressions of meaning, and then you actually do "dwell." Contemplation is another word that could be used to describe this part of the study. The researcher needs to be alone to contemplate over a period of time the meaning that this participant was attempting to convey. After a certain amount of time has passed—time not measured in hours—insights, intuitions, and understanding emerge. The researcher begins to write. The researcher returns to the material and uses the language of the participant to illustrate the particular meaning. The researcher also returns to the participant and, depending on the participant's evaluation, will either have successfully captured that individual's meaning or will return after clarification to writing once again. This is a departure from collapsing or categorizing interview materials in that there is no deliberate step of searching for similarities or differences. Each participant stands alone. The ending narrative does not homogenize 10 interviews but tells many different stories of meaning. Of course, the researcher will become aware of similarities and differences and write about them as well, while still holding the individual as the focus for meaning.

When I review some of my own work, I certainly see how I organized some material into categories, and I suppose for others and myself that there are times when this may be the most efficient way of organizing material. However, there is a chapter (Munhall, 1995) where I narrate Beverly's story, Lynn's story, Lisa's story, Victoria's story, and Carol's story. Each story is different, has different meanings, and challenges different normative commitments and unquestioned myths. Perhaps the experience that I was studying (women's secrets) allowed for the individualistic interpretations, but there is something about the heterogeneity that, for me, has a feeling of "the experiences themselves" and of phenomenology.

So in this part of the study, where the researcher is gathering material that is spoken before it is read, dwelling and contemplation of "the said" needs to take place. This is a thinking through and at the same time a freeing of the mind so that insights spontaneously arise. Every phenomenologist must carry a small notebook in which to write down insights for those spontaneous moments. It is like taking a picture: there is an opportunity, and if you don't capture it, you might lose it. This process will happen to you, I promise you.

This is also the step in which you may, in a proposal, use specific areas to indicate where there will be "human subjects"; in essence this is somewhat analogous to data collection. The difference in phenomenological inquiry is one of perception of the wholeness of the study. Once again, because the process is not linear, you are free to do the various processes of the existential process and phenomenological contemplation in a circular way. In actuality, all the steps should represent a circle. Toward the end of your study, you return to the earlier steps of immersion, coming to the phenomenological aim, and so on. From a language perspective, because phenomenological inquiry has at once a subjective, objective, and intersubjective quality to it, we call the individuals who participate in our study "participants" and we call data "material."

Researcher as participant and instrument. Not only is the researcher the most important "instrument," but he or she is a participant as well, as all functions come together to attempt to understand meaning in experience through this existential investigation. In this part of the study, you need to attend to the experience by amassing material and thought processes. Again, because this is not a textbook on phenomenology, I cannot possibly do justice to all that needs to be known. Hopefully, you understand the general framework of the inquiry and the processes that are critical to phenomenology. What follows are the process steps of the existential inquiry.

A. Listen to self and others; develop heightened attentiveness to self and others.
Listening and seeing in a phenomenological way need further description. Part of what is required is discussed earlier in the section on the decentering process. Oftentimes in phenomenological studies, as was mentioned, what we have seen consists of 10 or so transcribed interviews, with themes extracted, and then perhaps a discussion of those themes. As I said in *Revisioning Phenomenology* (Munhall, 1994a), if you feel you need to transcribe interviews in the beginning, you should go ahead and do that. As you progress with this method, taping interviews and writing transcriptions become less necessary because you are able to grasp meaning in what might become a conversation rather than an interview.

When you choose your participants, you do not need to follow the sampling rules of quantitative research. Instead, you need to find individuals who are willing to speak to you about the experience that you are interested in understanding. Another qualification is that the participants want to tell "their stories." Although many other sources assist you in attaining understanding, the language with all its intonation and inflection is the most revealing. Facial expressions and body language are also forms of languaging meaning. Needless to say, then, you want a willing and if possible enthusiastic participant.

Additionally, when you are listening, you must be cognizant that your participants are most likely telling you some things but not all things. As in any self-report, participants may think there is a "correct" way to respond to you. At the outset, this needs to be clarified, and the participants must be reassured that these stories are their own, that you are interested in their own meaning and their own personal experience. The participant is the repository of meaning through narrative. Reminding your participants of their generosity in sharing sometimes painful experiences demonstrates your sincerity. Clarify that there are no "right" answers or better answers and that what you value most is "their" exploring with you, in their own language, the meaning of the experience for them. If a participant asks you, "Is this what you want?" (which is often the case), you need to reassure the participant that it is "what" they want to share with you that you are interested in hearing.

At a dissertation hearing this past year, I heard a student say, "I had to keep bringing her back to the experience." This outcome is frequent; it merits a response and is somewhat like the participant looking for the right answer. Instead, here the researcher apparently had in mind the range of focus that she wanted her participant to stay within. Given that this is not psychotherapy but phenomenology, we do not have the luxury of free association. However, as mentioned earlier, we need to hear what the participant is moving away from and where the participant is going. This in itself can be material from which meaning may be gleaned, and sometimes that meaning is the participant's wish to avoid further discussion. If you ascertain that the participant's comfort level is being disrupted for any reason at all, you need to attend to it and respect the participant's wishes.

Significant wandering. However, the participants may be communicating something other than avoidance; the wandering may in the end make significant sense. This is discussed in greater detail later in the section on interpretation, but, for now, note that often there is great meaning in what is concealed. So, we are not only listening to what is said, but what is not said and also to where the participant goes to seek meaning, to another narrative. Moving into a more conversational mode allows the researcher to gently probe as to the meaning of what is said. Saying something like, "Please go on, what are you thinking?" if the participant should fall silent is good for the conversation. Once again, remember how important you are to this process. A good phenomenological researcher has heightened consciousness, focuses intently, and is continuously attentive to self and to the participant. If you, the researcher, find yourself wandering in thought, you must be vigilant and bring your attention back to the dialogue. Make a quick mental note about where you wandered when you might have thought yourself to be distracted. This, too, may have significance in regard to its association.

B. Reflect on personal experiences and expressions.

Phenomenology begins with the personal, the subjective world in which you are present, a part of, and connected to in your own situated context, life worlds, and different contingencies, which all contribute to you as a person. You begin your phenomenological study with self-reflection. Record this self-reflection in a journal. Because this kind of inquiry reflects a coming and going, a back-and-forth between and among parts of the study and the whole, your own personal experiential journey will change you. Your self-reflection includes analyzing your life world, situated context, and the contingencies, which bring you into relation to this human experience. Why do you, as a person, want to study this experience? How did you become interested in this experience, in meaning, in understanding?

This part of the study is ongoing, and your journal should reflect a deepening of "thinking," a "giving over" to the study, as well as your frustrations, surprises, and questions as your study evolves. Sarah Lauterbach (2007) shares with us her own experience with what she is studying. I refer you back to previous editions of this text as to her enriching work on perinatal loss of a twin and the meaning in the present moment and over time. She is intricately involved and at once "knows for herself" but puts that in abeyance to see the meaning for others. This often raises the implication of the researcher having had the experience that he or she is studying. Such questions are addressed in *Revisioning Phenomenology*, so in the interest of space I refer you to that book because this component is an important one to think about. The assurance that this personal expression section is being done well is that others who read your study understand in an authentic manner who you are in this study, your experiential perspective, and how and why you are engaged in studying the experience.

C. Provide experiential descriptive expressions: The experiencer.

This step pertains to experiences that may have a clinical component. Clinical means the experience was in some way related to health care and the nursing domain or the nursing care of individuals living through specific experiences. This is very broad and not limited to individuals who are currently in a clinical setting, but who have had an experience that has a clinical aspect. Examples could be experiences of physical, psychological, or psychosomatic illnesses, diagnoses, and the emotional and physical responses: worry, fear, hope, disorientation, loneliness. Though this step is focused on the experiencer we must always be cognizant that the person is always in interaction with others. This enriches your study and gives additional material for interpretation. Here is a concrete example: In a study related to Sarah's, a doctoral student also studied the same experience with mothers. She also asked the meaning or the experiences of the nurses caring for the mothers and found, as did Sarah, that many nurses did not have an awareness of the grief of the mother who had also experienced perinatal loss of a twin. A pragmatic defense seemed to be part of the nurses' and others' reactions to the experience. The belief that the mother had one healthy child for which she should be grateful overrode in almost all descriptions the belief that the mother had a need to mourn. Some "others" were even intolerant of such an idea. Now we find through Sarah's study that this mourning continues and is part of the dailiness of having the surviving twin. The surviving twin is a reminder of the one who died. We have also found out something critical about the attitude of others (Lauterbach, 2007).

These kinds of studies also remind us of the importance of phenomenology as a critical philosophy and that we need to go beyond interpretation to critique. One can also see that an orthodox data collection of 10 transcribed interviews could not provide the depth and breadth of the existential material. Sarah, I believe, has a real interest in studying the experiential descriptions found in art, literature, music, photography, and other aesthetic works. This interest has increased her focus on that dimension and someday could become a study of its own. One should note how a program of research could be had for those doing phenomenology, and a very meaningful one as the study branches out and continues to shed light on the many facets of an experience. When doing phenomenology, we need to be vigilant of when we find ourselves looking to the rules for research of the scientific method. We do not have the limitations of operational definitions; nor do we have the limitations of linear steps. We are searching for a full-of-meaning-and-detail narrative of experience, which contains whatever adds to meaning. This is a simple and liberating criterion. If something contributes to the meaning of our understanding of an experience, one need not argue whether it belongs or not; of course, it belongs. The material enriches our understanding.

In this step you begin to collect material from individuals who have experienced the phenomenon of interest in your study. *Revisioning Phenomenology* presents structural ways in which you can select themes and essences from transcribed interviews. I refer you to that book for more detail if you believe you need more structure to enable you to elucidate themes. If you feel as though you can listen with "the third ear" (Chapter 1), asking individuals if they would be willing to share with you their experience in more than one sitting, then you might not need to tape the dialogue, but it is good practice to write immediately afterward as much as you can remember of what was said. Laptops make this a bit easier today.

Some information about interviews. In hermeneutic phenomenological human science, the interview serves very specific purposes: 1) it may be used as a means of exploring and gathering experiential narrative material that can serve as a resource for developing a richer and deeper understanding of a human phenomenon, and 2) it may be used as a vehicle to develop a conversational relation with a partner (interviewee) about the meaning of an experience (van Manen,

1990, p. 66). In our evolution of the past 10 years or so, our phenomenological studies often relied primarily on interviews. Researchers often asked the following questions:

- What question should I ask?
- How many people do I need to interview?
- How do I keep people focused?
- What do I do with all this material (transcripts)?

As discussed earlier in this chapter, we must be careful in framing our question. The "what is it like" approach is fine, understandable, and concrete. Asking people to tell you about their lived experience of being cared for might prompt different responses from asking people what it is like to feel cared for: the first is asking for examples, and the second is asking for descriptions. There is no need here for either/or; both are fine. Because of individuals' infinite differences, I find interactive dialogue, as conversation, to be very important. Additionally, stories, anecdotes, pictures, and any writing that the individual may be willing to share with you will enrich your study. I find the idea of being in dialogue to be one of a relation between two human beings. In this type of conversation, the unknower is seeking understanding of something from the speaker and not vice versa. It certainly is not a demographic interview, and though often tempting, it does not seek affirmation of your beliefs. Researchers sometimes find themselves saying:

- Don't you think . . . ?
- Did you find that . . . ?
- Do you think it was because they were . . . ?

Such questions may appear harmless, but they have the potential to structure a person's story. They are the kind of questions through which you might be seeking to substantiate some of your own beliefs. The following lead-ins help explicate the person's unfolding of the experience.

- Could you give me an example of that?
- Do you remember how that made you feel (assuming there's a reason for a feeling question)?
- What did that do for you?
- (After a sentence) Go on. . . . Could you elaborate more on that?
- (After a period of silence, ask) Can you tell me what you are thinking about?

And never underestimate the "umm . . ." One student, after conducting some of her first interviews, told me that her mouth was sore from smiling. Although you might smile, it is certainly not a requisite and would sometimes be inappropriate. Try to follow the mood of the person you are interviewing. Also be aware of the participant's body, posture, intonation of words, and being. Because the interview has sometimes assumed preeminence in the phenomenological approach, other considerations need to be made:

- If you have never interviewed people before in the form of a dialogic conversation, then you need to practice. Practice with someone who has a background in psychiatric nursing, psychology, or psychoanalysis. In their disciplines, listening is elevated to an art. In phenomenology, listening also becomes an art.

- Listening is an art. Try to hear just what is being said. Try not to be anticipating what comes next. Let there be pauses and silence. Silence is important. An individual says something. You listen. There is a pause. You are both reflecting. The pause will often yield additional reflection. Becoming comfortable with a silence or a pregnant pause enables the storyteller to probe deeper within. Let the silence remain until you intuit that a prompt might be helpful.

- Many studies are a result of one-time interviews. As I have suggested elsewhere, two to three interviews with the same person may be more helpful. More "reflected upon" material is usually forthcoming, as is interpretation of what was said in previous interviews. A practitioner or researcher who ends a single interview with, "Is there anything else you might like to add?" is asking the question for that moment. Often, in the week that follows, more reflection occurs and the person desires to tell more about the experience.

- Imagine yourself in the interviewee's place. What might he or she be thinking about? Another reason that I strongly recommend additional interviews is that there is so much to process in the first encounter. You may need to use the first interview to establish trust and rapport, depending on what you are discussing. That effort will ensure the integrity of the material forthcoming.

- I believe it is critical to conduct these interviews/conversations where the participant is most comfortable. Sometimes to find participants, you first need to go to where the experience is located; for example, a school, office, clinic, or church.

- Be aware of your participant's holistic condition. You do not need to stop an interview because of crying or anger (as long as the interviewer knows whether it is therapeutic). However, you need good judgment. Even though informed consent ensures that the interviewee can stop the interview at any time, sometimes the interviewer needs to recognize that it is time to relax and change direction. Relief time, perhaps a little casual talk, may be comforting. Our intention here is not psychotherapy or nursing intervention. Our role must be clearly known, and we must act accordingly (discussed in Chapter 20). We need to be cognizant and attuned to our participant's psychological condition. Again, follow-up interviews help protect the psychological comfort of interviewees and demonstrate our genuine interest in them as persons.

Also include in your notes other observations that you or your participant have made. Phenomenology is not only the language of words but also the language of semiotics, the symbols and signs in our environment that "speak" to us and tell us what is going on in this environment. They speak to your participants and are other sources of meaning as participants attempt to make "meaning sense" out of their experience. Your participant will most likely describe his or her own examples or observations, but you as a healthcare provider can also incorporate your own for comment and feedback. Again, this is an example of the "coming and going," the varying of examples, the varying of perspectives, and the looking upon a reflection with another reflection. This is what makes doing phenomenology so rewarding and worthwhile. The descriptions and interpretations attempt to be as inclusive as is feasible in the study, so as not to present a shallow description but a deeply embroidered tapestry of meaning.

The way you can be assured this step is accomplished is to bring your descriptions and reflections to your participants. If your descriptions and interpretations of the meaning of the experience resonate with the participants, then you can be assured that you did indeed tell the meaning of their story. Now does everyone share the same meaning? Of course not. So, first you go to the person with whom you have had several conversations to see if you captured his or her meaning. At the conclusion of your study, you will have reflected on all the material and will have begun to write a description and interpretation of your study. When that is completed, you once again return to your participants with the material woven into one narrative. Listen to the responses of your participants. Many will read an interpretation and remark that they did not have that experience or share that meaning. This returns us to the reason for separate stories and why it is critical to have in your narrative the similarities and differences found in the meaning of the same experience.

Some studies are written so that it seems that everyone in a particular study experienced the phenomenon in a similar manner. However, I need to stress once again that when you write a phenomenological narrative, you must heed the differences in meaning as well as the similarities. One needs to be careful not to collapse the data as an aggregate. Phenomenology is not interested in generalizability. It is interested in how various individuals interpret the meaning of experience in their own individual ways. The example used in Chapter 1 about palliative care demonstrates the meaning of that experience and the danger in making assumptions that apply to all.

D. Provide experiential descriptive expressions: "others engaged in the experience."
In this section, your interviews/conversations are with individuals who have
lived through an experience in which you are interested but from another perspective. They have not experienced the phenomenon itself but have relationally interacted with the experience. For example, the previously mentioned
doctoral student also interviewed the nurses who cared for mothers who had
lost one of their twin babies. These individuals become an additional source
of material; the material gathered will help vary the examples, provide different perspectives, and actually provide a source for another study or a furthering of one's study.

If you have the desire to broaden the depth of your study, you can talk to
those individuals, as in a "going back and forth," to see if you can capture the
various meanings from different individuals who may not be "directly" having
the experience but who are "directly" involved in the experience. Observing,
once again, the language and semiotics of the "others" around the experience
at hand is another source of material. The recognition that "others" play a role
in phenomenological study comes from the belief that being in experience
does not occur in isolation. Imagine yourself painting a picture that is rich in
detail and uses different colors and hues. The picture tries to capture, in the
expression of individuals, their feelings and thoughts, which is an attempt to
let the viewer know the meaning of an experience for those in the picture. Oftentimes, in a museum or elsewhere, individuals gaze at a painting. This is like
the phenomenological gaze—searching for something in the picture that will
speak to us, to tell us the meaning of this work of art. That is actually what
you are doing when you lay out all the pieces of your study, always remembering that it is the pieces, and the individuals themselves, that have provided the
meaning in interaction.

In the end, your phenomenological writing will try to make sense of the experience in the many ways in which it has appeared or been concealed; and varying the material will enrich the text and fuse it with meaning. Perhaps the lack
of looking beyond interviews with the participants has led to findings that consist of lists of themes described in one or two sentences. We have moved beyond
that phase of doing phenomenology, and I believe we should be allowing ourselves to "do" phenomenology in various ways, using various guiding philosophers, and experiencing the freedom to do what makes sense. Rather than
being restricted by method, we are guided. We are not closed off from the appearance or concealment of some "thing" because the method allows us to look
there. The method is different in intent from the methods of science in that the
scientific method's delimiting steps must be respected or we will have a flawed
experiment. With phenomenology, if we do not go where participants lead us
or where the experience leads us, then we distort our findings. We will be sharing only some of the meaning, a limited part, grounded in rules about what to

include and what to exclude. In this existential investigation, if you the researcher have found some material that is not covered in Figure 5-3, you need to include it, if it helps you understand the meaning of the experience.

Researcher in Interaction

When nurses do phenomenology, it is not with the same aim, say, as that of a philosopher. We can say very directly that we are conducting a study with the aim of understanding the meaning of experience for our clients or other individuals relevant to our professional purposes. We can acknowledge our values; that is, that we want to improve the quality of life of those we serve, or the quality of life of the caregivers, who may be nurses. So it is different. Nurses are interacting with "beings," and they are "being-in-the-world" in a service profession. Understanding meaning is the best way of designing interventions. I must add, if interventions are called for, better they be designed in consideration of the patient's perspective of the experience than from the caregiver's assumptions (again, see the palliative care example in Chapter 1). One could argue that it is here where theory development must begin. Before all else, one needs a phenomenological baseline to describe, explain, predict, and control, if that is what is needed in specific circumstances. The argument could be furthered with the observation of how poorly individuals often "comply" with directions or education. If directions, interventions, and education are not derived from understanding what individuals experience and the meaning that they attach to their experiences, we have missed opportunities to be more effective.

Individuals in experience are the ones to inform us of what it is they need, how we could be more helpful, and how we could assist in improving the quality of their health. Only from an understanding of the "other" in experience can we develop theory from "the individuals themselves." Theory needs to be grounded in the authentic experience of what is to be theorized, not from what an authority believes it should be. "Should be" theories usually lead to all sorts of "deficits"; the ideals are not grounded in the everyday lives of individuals.

I would suggest that what is before us and what often cries out for our attention and seeks understanding at the deepest levels is the human experience. I would go even further and say that we have an ethical and moral imperative to use phenomenology to foster the highest and most humanistic standards of care. Wherever, then, you as researcher are able to hear, see, or touch material that has relevance to your study, remember that you are not bounded by rules. Your search is for as much experiential material as is available to you so that your original aim is full of "life." And real life is what nurses are engaged in with others, and our lives are all wonderfully intertwined. We mutually unfold in experience.

E. Provide experiential descriptive expressions: The arts and literature review.
This step embodies the experience that you are studying, in coming into contact with others who have explored it either purposely or tangentially in aesthetic work. The arts are poised to offer us a wealth of understanding if we engage in the search. Leaving yourself open to the experiential appearance, whether by accident or deliberate action, will often capture your imagination in ways that will literally excite you. I say this because I have watched countless students, colleagues, and myself act as though we have found gold when we come upon a film, a novel, biography, paintings, photographs, diaries, or other aesthetic works that announce themselves to us through the experience that we are studying. We are open to appearance. We are also aware of what may be concealed. So we come to these works and keep narratives of them, quotations, verse, a copy of a painting or photograph, lines from films and plays to illustrate the meaning of the experience. We begin to understand more and sometimes stand in awe in regard to where our study has taken us. We stand with the work or we view the film for the third time, we reread the play or the novel, and we search for deeper layers of meaning. This is what we do when we return to an individual for the third time or maybe more. The researcher collects this material or records meaning and understanding gathered from these sources in his or her journal. The process becomes a way of being. You can be assured that you have engaged in this process when you have found representations of the experience under study in the form of the various arts. If you find a paucity of material in this realm, begin to write verse, take photographs, or paint to represent what you have heard from your participants or from your own soul and spirit.

Reading the literature. Regarding experiential material in theoretical literature, you might think of the familiar literature review but, in phenomenology, it is used for a different purpose from a hypothesis. Rather than reading all that is known about an experience in the literature or in theories so as to support a hypothesis, you seek experiential descriptions of the experience or the meaning of the experience that may have been written from different perspectives. The intent is also different in that this step is considered part of your existential investigation, your gathering of material to deepen your understanding of these other perspectives.

Although it has been suggested that you delay this step until after you have had interviews/conversations with your participants so as not to overlay the literature on your "decentered self," literature about the experience may appear when you least expect it. In that case, it is a good idea to read it; just as with other existential descriptions, the content contributes to meaning and understanding.

In phenomenological research, material directs you to areas that you would not have thought of at the beginning of your study. As with all existential material, it shows itself to the researcher to be seen, to be read, to be touched, "as it is" within the life worlds of the participants. "As it is" for the participants and what is described in the literature at times are very similar and other times very different. What is not in the literature is as important as what is in the literature and in many instances more important. The question of the literature reflecting, contrasting, and/or refuting what you have come to find in your analysis and interpretation is of critical importance to the advancement of understanding and our knowledge base. Often our literature or theories are grounded in the knowledge base of the expert. If that knowledge base is deduced from other literature, from scientific observation of the scientific method mode, and from the perspective of the expert of "knowing," we may find an entirely different account of experience when we "go to the persons themselves." Who can better tell us the nature, the meaning, and the "whatness" of an experience than the person who has had the experience? The question enlarges as previously described when we allow others engaged in different ways with the experience to voice what is going on, what it means, and how they perceive it.

It actually is preferable to postpone the experiential description in the literature until after you have completed your interviews/dialogues with your participants. It can assist you in staying as close to the participant's narratives as possible, without the influence of a literature review. However, as you progress in sophistication with the processes and the interview/dialogue becomes more conversational, you could introduce to the participant something that you have read and ask what the participant thinks about the material. This once again enriches the study, broadens its scope, and provides another perspective. Whatever happens with this step, it should not appear under "literature review" in a research proposal. If you "must" have a literature review, the literature review should be of the philosophy of phenomenology and how you are planning to follow its underpinnings and suppositions. Your "literature review" of the phenomenon under study is part of your existential investigation.

More about decentering. Here is an important point to clarify. Phenomenological inquiry does have suppositions. The suppositions are clearly articulated in the foundation of the phenomenological approach to being-in-the-world. We do not decenter ourselves from phenomenology; in fact, it guides us through the entire study. What we do decenter from are presuppositions, beliefs, values, knowledge, thoughts, and ideas about the experience that we are studying and attempting to understand without the overlay of prior knowledge. Doing a literature review at the outset only serves the purpose of obtaining additional knowledge from which to separate ourselves. You can be assured that you have accomplished this review when you have gone to the literature on the experience that interests you and have obtained a good description of what is currently in the literature or in theories. This review is another narrative to describe and interpret as it relates to your own findings and understanding of the experience.

F. Provide anecdotal descriptive expressions: As experience appears.

This process step is one that requires a consciousness of the experience or meaning of the experience when you are not necessarily expecting its appearance or concealment. The material appears in a serendipitous manner. You might be engaged in a conversation with a friend or neighbor who begins to talk about the experience without your prompting. You may hear about this experience at a conference in a formal presentation or in questions that people bring up in various formats. The more commonplace your experience is, the more often this will occur. This type of serendipitous appearance can be a very important source of material because sometimes people, without knowing it, become participants though not formally. They begin to converse with you about how "it is" with them to either be in this experience or to know of someone who is in it and how they are responding to that situation. This is anecdotal and not within the formal frame of your study. You did not expect it; nor did you ask for it. If you wish to pursue this with any one person and engage him or her in the study as a participant, then you must ask his or her permission and follow the same process of informed consent as when you have identified volunteer participants. Informed consent is discussed further in Chapter 20.

Other interesting sources of material for your study are people's responses to the subject. Just their reactions can be fascinating. I recall once discussing with a colleague the study of anger, and she angrily replied to me, "I don't ever get angry," apparently concealing to herself how she does experience anger. Your colleagues can provide feedback on how you are doing with your study and also material from the perspective of their own initial responses to the experience. They may also be potential participants. Again, as you become more familiar with this kind of inquiry, you will find yourself more awake to all experiences and engaging in the world in a different manner. Sometimes it seems to me that "everything" said or seen has potential for a study, that I can collect material and write about "things" that I am not studying at the moment. I feel sometimes as though phenomenology has made me "always" a student of our everyday world. Establishing a phenomenological perspective toward the world at hand stimulates attentiveness to the "everydayness" of life, experiences, and objects, and you begin to see and articulate the taken-for-grantedness of much experience. This attentiveness will further enrich your study with the addition of unforeseen appearances of material reflective within your experience.

You can be assured this process step has been accomplished by evaluating the material that you came upon in a serendipitous way. Serendipitous material comes about because of the aforementioned attentiveness by which a phenomenological study takes up residence within you.

G. *Record ongoing reflection in your personal journal.*

This process step is ongoing from the very first day of your study or from the time you begin thinking about your study. I cannot overemphasize the importance of almost daily entries in your journal. After a conversational interview, the participant's material, your responses, thoughts, associations, what you were feeling, and what you thought the other person was feeling should be written into your journal. This is your phenomenological journal and situates you in the life world of your study.

What happens to you during this time also should be included. If you don't write as often as possible, you will lose this material; it will naturally be forgotten in the rush of your everyday life. When you embark on description and interpretation, the material in this journal will most likely reflect a greatly enlarged view of the experience and a greatly changed "you," as far as perspective and understanding are concerned. That is why you would never want to lose a record of your own personal growth. Most likely you will see that you have enlarged your perspective in depth and breadth and have become much more sensitive and alert to the "taken for grantedness" of individual people and experiences.

In your phenomenological journal, go beyond description and try to incorporate the meaning of "what is going on" and the meaning of the various experiences that you may be having in the course of this study. All phenomena within this study—the interactions, the responses, the good and the woeful times—will reflect in a back-and-forth way on your study. My journals during studies reflect this back-and-forth, both in tearful entries and in spontaneous "aha" entries. If you are a student doing a phenomenological study for a dissertation, you may have many tearful entries. Stay with it.

Another promise: you will have traveled a journey to becoming more humanistic and sensitive than you thought possible. And your world will be enlarged because of it. Your journal will read like a book when you are completed, and I think you will marvel at the richness of your own text as well as your own growth in awareness of meaning and of being human. You will be assured this process step is completed if the preceding sentence rings true!

IV. Phenomenological Contextual Processing

This process step parallels the process step of existential inquiry and processing. In this step you present your thoughts about the material gathered in step III. It is here where you write for the reader, describing the situated contexts of all who take part in the study, where participants are located in the various life worlds, and the contingencies of those in the study, including the researcher.

The experience is not separated from the participant, so that context needs to be articulated as well.

A. Analyze emergent situated contexts.

This concept is actually quite literal. It refers to the situation in which you and others currently are with all the contingencies that exist at the moment and as you progress in the study. Heidegger (1962) uses the term "thrownness" to express the perspective that the person is always "situated." The person is in context in his or her "being-in-the-world." From what we know thus far, we are without prior consultation, born into a historical time period, a culture, a family with a specific worldview and language. Other parts of the situated context are the experiences that we sometimes choose and other times do not choose. Because of our situated context, some choices are not available to us, and others are not choices but are required within the situated context.

B. Analyze day-to-day contingencies.

Contingencies are most often the reason for our action or inaction, decisions or avoidance of decisions, and voluntary or involuntary change. Whatever the contingencies of one's life, they are within one's situated context and, in actuality, unify with the life worlds. This unity exerts tremendous influence on the meaning of experience and a person's understanding of that meaning. A person's situated context allows certain actions and simultaneously limits other actions. To truly understand another person, the researcher must engage in hearing and seeing that person by processing the material gathered through the lens of that person's situated context.

C. Assess life worlds.

The four existential life worlds are other dimensions from which we need to process phenomenological material to give meaning a perspective that tells us more about it. It is critical to understand that the life worlds shown in Figure 6–4 are a unity and reflect the interconnectedness of all four life worlds. Contemplating the spatiality, corporeality, temporality, and relationality furthers our understanding of the person in the world.

Spatiality refers to the space in which we are, our environment, which can assume different meanings for different experiences. The phenomenological material needs to be processed once again through the lens of the environment. In regard to my study on women's anger, spatiality was a very important world to discuss in many instances. The home environment for many of these women, especially those living in domestic-violence situations, needed to be part of the interpretation of anger. An experience does not exist alone. It is always embedded and connected.

Corporeality refers to the body that we inhabit and is also referred to as embodiment. Rather than the idea that we have bodies, we think now that we *are* our bodies. Because we often speak as though our bodies and minds are separate, we know that the mind is embodied in this wonderful access to experience, the body. There are times that it is not such a wonderful experience. For this reason, the researcher must contemplate the connectedness of embodiment with experience. Body intelligence is what experiences phenomena. We negotiate experience through the unity of mind and body. Perceptions are created through the mind and body in addition to the contingencies of our lives, and therefore become the starting point of meaning. In the example of anger and domestic violence, not only is a woman's physical body shattered or damaged, but her whole perception of self can be shattered and damaged. The woman's embodiment is severely threatened, and readers familiar with the effects of this life world understand the many different meanings of this experience for a woman. This is how all these ideas are interconnected. I write "as if this, then this" and need to occasionally focus on the interconnectedness of all these phenomena. Meaning and experience cannot exist in isolation.

Temporality is the time in which we are living. We are always living through this concept called time. Our embodied bodies occupy a space and that space is located in time. Our participants often bring up the life world of time, as is illustrated in Sarah's study (Lauterbach, 2007). The passage of time, the temporal life world, did little to ease the mourning process. Many readers of her study may express surprise, which is a sign of an excellent study. Sarah succeeds here in "liberating" some readers from their preconceptions. The perception of time is another important concept to contemplate when listening to participants and interpreting phenomenological material. The perception of time passing varies, often in incredible ways, with experience and is very meaningful. "Losing track of time" and "the time seemed endless" are phrases that the researcher needs to process with the participant. Actual interventions can be suggested by understanding the meaning of life worlds in experience. You might recall intensive care unit patients who were diagnosed as being disoriented because they did not know the time and day. They were in rooms without windows, so the orienting dark and light cycles were not present, not to mention that their space lacked clocks that could be seen. This is what might be called "everyday" experience for these patients. I believe the outcome of being in the world in a phenomenological way can lead a nurse to explore the space and time dimensions and arrive at a very practical solution: place large clocks showing time of day and the day of the week where patients can view them. Make sure that they indicate A.M. or P.M. Some would say that it is obvious. Yes, and understanding experience can result in the most obvious solutions. Yet, for years, patients who didn't know the time and day were labeled as "disoriented."

Critical to temporality is history. We not only occupy a place in time, but we are located in a historical period with its particular contingencies. That period is extremely influential in regard to our behavior, attitudes, beliefs, and where we are located (spatiality). The country and city or town is a critical influence, as is the family.

Relationality refers to the world in which we find ourselves in relation to others. When studying phenomenological material, you need to contemplate the relationships within the experience being studied and as articulated by participants or found in other existential material. The importance of ourselves in relation to others is not just the phenomenologist's interest. This life world seems to dominate popular culture in all of its manifestations. What is critical to phenomenologists is the recognition that the self is self-interpreting. We now can add "for interpretation" to "to the persons themselves": "to the persons themselves for interpretation"! For example, returning to the subject of women and domestic violence, we as researchers or healthcare professionals could interpret their situations from all the literature available. There are numerous interpretations, and to adopt the wrong interpretation could be very harmful. To understand a particular woman in this situation, we must ask her for her interpretation. Otherwise, we further violate her unique life world of relationality.

In this process, the researcher begins to contemplate and look for meaning in all the materials gathered in the existential inquiry. Individuals provide meaning in their experiences through the expression of their feelings, thoughts, intentions, reflections, motives, desires, and emotions. These same expressions can be described by using many other existential modes of inquiry. This concurrent contextual processing allows for integration of experience within context. The researcher is beginning to think in a narrative style, there is a wholeness to it, a story with many different expressions of meaning. What is critical is to transcend the natural tendency to generate common emotions, themes, essences, categories, or meaning units. The narratives need to reflect one person's description of the experience with his or her own interpretation of his or her situated context. Where researchers in phenomenology can divert from the philosophy of phenomenology is in the normal inclination to look for similarities, clusters, or themes. This is what has led critics to say that many of our studies are reductionistic. Of course, this reflects the dilemma, discussed earlier, of how to understand individuals. Do we study the parts, in this case, the themes, and then put them back together as a "whole"? We have long rejected the premise that a person is the "sum total of his parts" and have adopted the view that a person is "greater than the sum of his parts." Of all places, then, it is in phenomenology that we need to remember that people are greater than the sum of their themes. This is particularly true when we put them in aggregates or categories. This is demonstrated in studies that have as findings for a group of people (an aggregate) a list of themes, which seem to describe the nature of an experience and how it is lived through the perceptions of our sample of individuals reported as a group. This is the principle used in quantitative research and, as challenging as it may be to phenomenology, we need to use our imaginations to report meanings that acknowledge the individual in experience, not a synthesis of meanings. I would venture to say that, in Western culture, that remains the most challenging task of doing phenomenological research.

So, in this step, because it does not have the full richness of depth and breadth until it is combined with the next process step, we need to include in narrative each individual's description and interpretation of the meaning of the experience. The researcher's main task is to choose very carefully from the participant's very long narrative the centrality of meaning that has been communicated and then to integrate the narrative with the life worlds. One cannot exist without the other, if an authentic meaning is to be the outcome. This is a subjective process in which our own assumptions, prejudices, and predilections can confuse an authentic delineation of what is most significant in one person's story. We cannot do this alone, without our participant's agreement with our much shorter version of the meaning of the experience that was communicated. People do not think or feel in terms of themes and essences, for the most part. That is what researchers have been doing with phenomenological descriptions.

This method varies from the practice of categorization and asks the researcher to search through the material and to begin writing narratives reflective of each participant's experience. The interviews/conversations that you have had with individuals are in verbal form, which by nature is much longer than descriptive summaries in written form. Recall that such narrative summation cannot take place until you have dwelled with the narrative and the memories of the interviews/conversations and have contemplated the meanings that were communicated to you. However, narrative summation takes considerable practice so as not to be writing through your own assumptions and frameworks, and it needs to be returned to the participant as a written narrative with the question, "Does this reflect our conversations (interviews)?"

In the next process step, we will answer the question, "Why did we ever think we could find out the meaning of experience as though there was 'one' meaning?" Although there are common perceptions of experiences, they are quite different from common meanings. These differences depend on each individual's interpretive interaction.

V. Analysis of Interpretive Interaction

A. Integrate existential investigation with phenomenological contextual processing. This step returns us to step IV, "Phenomenological Contextual Processing." This step needs intensive integration with your existential experiential expressions, or those descriptions will lack authentic meanings. Contextual processing, as described, calls on the researcher and the participant to be historical, political, cultural, and social; in other words, being-in-the-world as it is in a specific time and place. Meaning cannot be found in an acontextual place or in an ahistorical time, if such notions even exist. However, in some descriptions, they have been completely ignored, and meanings gleaned from those studies are without the essentials that create and contribute to meaning.

In this interpretation of the interaction of the situated context in which individuals find themselves while in experience, we can arrive at a meaningful, holistic, simultaneous interpretation of an experience. Each participant in our study brings a personal biography and has already formed an interpretive system from which they will give voice to their experience. Each already has his or her own way of interacting with the larger world. Each has different situations in the life worlds. Particular contingencies will influence his or her description, interpretation, and formulated meaning of experience.

B. Describe expressions of meaning (thoughts, emotions, feelings, statements, motives, metaphors, examples, behaviors, appearances and concealments, voiced and nonvoiced language).

This analysis of the situated context gives the thoughts, feelings, and emotions a horizon, a context, knowledge, and a biography; in other words, a thick web of relational interactional processes that contribute to who the individual "is" among others and that enable the researcher to capture meaning encapsulated in context. In this process of interpretive interactionism, it is critical once again not to move into thinking in aggregates, categories, themes, or essences. Because two people were born in the same year or in the same family, town, or society does not mean sameness. We would be guilty of reductionism if we were to think in that manner. In quantitative terms, they are just variables, devoid of meaning. Only in interaction with all the other contingencies of individual life worlds can we approximate phenomenological meaning. This is so complex that it is always an approximation of meaning. I have viewed groups agreeing on a meaning of some "thing," only later to realize how divergent the agreed-upon meaning actually is.

C. Interpret expressions of meaning as appearing from integration.

To reemphasize, it is critical to understand the meaning of being human within context. From these understandings, we can give others the things that will assist them in generating further meaning, the "interventions" that they may need to increase the quality of life or minimize suffering. Such understanding enables us to individualize our approaches to individuals and enlarges our consciousness to a phenomenological way of being with others. We no longer have only one approach to an experience. We recognize that meaning for the individual is how we individualize care. Meaning should be at the core of our care, of what we do and plan with others. One might ask,

"Then how can we have procedures, policies, treatments, and prescriptive theory?" We can have them, but we need to know why they often fail or meet with "complications," or why we have a high rate of "noncompliance."

There are many reasons why such acontextual, homogeneous approaches do not work. One of them is that large groups of people were reduced to "one" person, whether in a qualitative or quantitative study. The "one" person is a synthesis of many people and, in actuality, *the "one" person does not even exist.* This is critical to keep in the forefront as you do phenomenological inquiry; that is, you are not homogenizing differences. What you are attempting to do is to have your participants and yourself interpret the interactions of their context with the experience at hand and to write a rich description of their experiences. Process steps III & IV combined lead to existential, experiential expressions. Proceeding in this manner, you will have fulfilled many of the philosophical underpinnings of phenomenological inquiry. You will undoubtedly have varied examples, varied interpretations, and varied meanings. In nursing, we espouse phenomenological beliefs and values in our nursing philosophies. We believe individuals are unique organisms in interaction with their environment and then paradoxically attempt to have a nursing care model that fits all. Why this does not work has already been discussed, so let us proceed to the next step and see if it affords us better opportunities to generate knowledge that is more particular than general.

VI. Writing the Phenomenological Narrative

A. Choose a style of writing that will communicate an understanding of the meaning of this particular experience.

In this activity, an analysis of each individual's experiential expressions and interpretive interaction is narrated as one life world, vivid in description and detail. The narrative is reflective of the complexity of the interconnectedness of all the expressions that were spoken or that "showed themselves" as evidence of the deeper contexualized meaning of experience. There are many different ways to present your findings. For exemplars, I refer you to two books: one by James Hillman (1997), called *Emotion: A Comprehensive Phenomenology of Theories and Their Meanings for Therapy*, and another by Robert Coles (1991), titled *Spiritual Life of Children*. These two books show the variation of presentations, for which there is no formula. Writing is a creative activity, and your subject and content should inspire your own presentation, sparked by your imagination.

The introduction in Hillman's (1997) book is quite good: it presents phenomenology as method and describes how Hillman used the method to write this book on human emotions. It is an example and also provides an interpretation of phenomenology as a method. Coles (1991) states in his introduction that his book is a phenomenological text. It contains one narrative after another about individual children talking about their spiritual life. Each chapter is one child's story. Coles finishes with a critique of spiritual life for children and its implications for our society. The book is a good example of presenting narratives for individuals and then doing a critique of the meaning of the study, which is the seventh step of this method. Also, volumes 1 and 2 of *In Women's Experience* (Munhall, 1994b, 1995) contain 21 different phenomenological writings by different authors. As you read them, you will see a wide variation in style and creativity.

B. Write inclusively of all meanings, not just the "general" but the "particular."
In this method, there is a moving away from the idea of synthesizing experience into one-narrative-fits-all. Surely, there may be similar meanings voiced by individuals, but, when they are contextualized, the interpretations may be different. Perception of experience is always grounded in the historical, political, social, and personal background. One might ask, "Is this not several one-case studies placed together?" There are fundamental differences and they are articulated in phenomenological philosophy, the aim of phenomenology, and the method. The knowledge base of a person conducting phenomenological studies must be sophisticated, and the researcher needs to develop many different practices. The outcome of existential experiential expressions, within a deeply contextual world, produces a narrative that describes and interprets 1) the heterogeneity of responses, which a case study does not do; 2) the heterogeneity of meanings, which case studies do not do; and 3) some similarities, which a case study does not do. However, because this method is phenomenological, we do not want to be reductionistic in "listing" those differences and similarities in the narrative. Once we do that, we have removed the deeply embedded contextual interpretations. In the narrative, similarities and differences will "show" themselves. So in contrast to a case study where one person or situation is described and interpreted, in a phenomenological study we have an array of interpretations, each with its own significance. We come to know, respect and act from the different meanings individuals give to experience.

C. Write inclusively of language and expressions of meaning with the interpretive interaction of the experience of the situated context.
What we produce in these vivid life world descriptions of our participants' meanings in experience are the possibilities of being-in-the-world for us to consider when we attempt to understand another individual. In casual conversations, "We are more alike than different" can often be heard. Even if we were to base our theories on such an observation, the differences are probably the most important characteristics to consider when approaching patients, planning patient care, and developing nursing research ideas and projects. The similarities are easy to incorporate, if indeed there are such entities. The differences are what challenge us and make all the difference in meeting the needs of patients. The differences are paramount in our endeavor to understand individuals in their multiple realities, subjective worlds, life worlds, and individual contingencies.

D. Interpret with participants the meaning of the interaction of the experience with contextual processing (steps III and IV).

This is a process that has been ongoing in your research endeavor and can be referred to as co-interpretation of all the phenomenological material. The best sources the phenomenological researcher has are the participants and the other existential material that he or she has amassed. The researcher goes, as before, back to the participant and asks, "In this narrative am I interpreting correctly the meaning of this experience for you?" This is the "mirror," the capturing of the whole: the participant's experiential descriptive expressions of the meaning of the experience and the participant's situated context. I cannot overemphasize the influence of the situated context on the meaning of an experience for an individual. It contributes to the complexity of understanding experience, but without complexity, a contextual meaning emerges that is essentially meaningless. Every life world contingency has an influence on the interpretation of meaning of an experience. We do an injustice to individuals by minimizing their life worlds in our interpretations of experience or the meaning of being human. From an inclusive interpretation will emerge the material for your own interpretive critique, which can be used for direction for theory, practice, and change. The critique will be enriched if you ask your participant about ways the experience can become more meaningful, tolerable, understood, and how healthcare professionals can demonstrate understanding of participants' meanings. It is critical to act from the perceptions and meanings that individuals have in specific experiences. They are in essence the one who know: the knowledge holders.

E. Narrate a story that at once gives voice to actual language and simultaneously interprets meaning from expressions used to describe the experience.

How you capture this complexity in writing about meaning and understanding, I believe, is by narrating the experiences in the language as told to you, in the material that appeared to you, and in the realization of the things that were concealed from you. The researcher's task is to reflect accurately, as if a mirror, using words in the interpretive analysis of interactions that have given meaning to experience. The integration of all material is essential to the wholeness of experience. The researcher reconstructs from the existential inquiry and contextual analysis a narrative that captures the contingencies and meaning in which individuals have socially constructed for this experience. The researcher narrates findings that were discovered and uncovered in the course of the study. New and unexpected meanings of experience are significant findings and lead to new possibilities of "being."

Discovering. Discovering the meaning in experience fosters the emergence of authentic encounters with one another. We come to understand the role of perception. We come to question our assumptions. And, often, we take phenomenology as not only a way to do research but also a way of being-in-the-world, in our everyday lives. After becoming phenomenologic, we often develop an entirely new worldview, an entirely new understanding of how to encounter our existence and the existence of others.

VII. Writing a Narrative with Implications on the Meaning of Your Study

In this final descriptive and interpretive piece, as nurses, we have a moral and/or ethical imperative to fill. We are ultimately in a profession that has aims and goals to assist others in attaining a better quality of life by enhancing awareness of how life might be lived in a way that has meaning for the individual, in finding meaning in an individual's situated context, and by enabling individuals to understand who they are as persons. Our final research narratives of description and interpretation need to have implications for the profession. What does this meaning have for nursing practice? What does this meaning have for nursing theory? Does the final narrative contain implications that critique current practice? Does the interpretation introduce us to new ways of understanding experience? Does it free us from preexisting suppositions? In this way, does it liberate us from a way of thinking about an experience or its meaning that is no longer evident as evidenced from our inquiry? I do not believe that we can do phenomenology without answering these questions about its relevance. Relevance must extend beyond listing essences and themes, especially when they are acontextual. We have come a long way in our phenomenological thinking and savvy, and we are more critical of our efforts, which is a sign of confidence and growth in our own understanding. In the final analysis, if we are studying meaning, the ultimate paradox would be if our study did not have meaning. Be sure you have included the significance of your study!

A. Summarize the answer to your phenomenological question with breadth and depth.
For the purposes of this section, you take the narrative from the previous phenomenological writing and condense it into a summary of major interpretations. Here, it is a good idea to once again return to participants and ask them to read the summary. Explain that the summary is not the complete narrative of their experience, that it does not contain that kind of detail, but that it will be used to look for meanings or direction for change in thought or practice.

B. Indicate how this understanding, obtained from those who have lived the experience, calls for self-reflection and/or system reflection.
In the evaluation of your study, ask whether the study itself has meaning and what is that meaning. Ask interpretive interaction questions. Make sure your study is embedded in the situated context in which individuals and experiences are located. Be able to articulate clearly the meaning for nursing that

your study has explicated and interpreted. Unveiling the meaning of experience contributes to human understanding. We need to remember that this does not lend itself to predictive theory since we are so aware of the many different contingencies of individual lives. If we were to entertain the thought that the study may lead to descriptive theory, we would have to include many qualifications. The theory would have to be explicit to specific cultures, contexts, and contingencies. The development of grounded theory has to keep this in the forefront. Recall that we want to avoid reductionistic formulations; we want to call attention to differences in interpreting realities. Yet, at the same time, usefulness becomes apparent in the realization of similarities.

C. Interpret meanings of these reflections to small and large systems with specific content.
The outcome of phenomenological description and interpretation can have different purposes, as heretofore mentioned. We cannot lose concentration or the ability to reflect on what we are doing. Even as I write, I reflect and can see another possibility. If you have tolerance for uncertainty, are able to feel a bit unbalanced, and have a philosophical leaning to understand the meaning of experience, phenomenology will enrich your professional life and your personal life as well. It becomes a way of being-in-the-world. Being-in-the-world, from a phenomenological perspective, calls for wide-awakeness and attentiveness. From our phenomenological narrative, we must ask, "Are there implications for change in our situated context?" "Do our narratives contradict prevailing norms, or beliefs, and/or theories?" If we are in agreement that critique should be an intricate part of phenomenology, we must interpret the narratives to find their implications for social, cultural, political, health care, and educational change and approaches.

D. Critique this interpretation with implications and recommendations for political, social, cultural, health care, family, and other social systems.
The meaning question asked at the end of a study is, "So what?" We must be prepared to answer this question from a critical perspective. In a previous example, we have considered research about domestic violence. If we ended a phenomenological study with a narrative on the experience of domestic violence as it is experienced by women or men who have been victimized, and then provided an understanding of the meaning of that experience, I believe the study is not yet completed from a moral-ethical perspective. We stand on higher ground if we critique the implications derived from the descriptions and interpretations and state them as direction for change and recognition. A call to action is sometimes the most appropriate conclusion of a phenomenological study. A call for specific research on recommendations gives impetus for improving quality of care. All too often, because a critique is not highlighted or narrated, a "very good" study does not fulfill its potential and becomes a

narrative without consequence. In a field dedicated to improving the quality of life for members of all societies, we have a mandate to listen, beyond the participant's descriptions and interpretations, to how we can make this a better experience. We do this because in the meaning of our study lies an authentic caring about individuals in experience. We do this kind of research ultimately to shed light on what might otherwise be hidden and then to find ways to act on narratives that include direction and implications for change toward quality experiences characterized by caring. Perhaps there are fields of study that do not require a response to the meaning of the study. However, we do a disservice if we encourage individuals to share the meaning of their experiences if we do not act on what they themselves critiqued. In a very big way, it was the narratives of individuals, which passed healthcare reform in this country in 2010. This is the power and significance of phenomenology.

Coming to an End, for Now

Phenomenology questions our consciousness, how we are in the world, how we experience the world, and how we give meaning to experiences. Meanings and interpretations emerge from our situated context and provide for heterogeneous perspectives on life events. This chapter presents interpretations of how you might do a phenomenological study. It may be flawed in many ways. There are always questions to ask about a claim, and so I must let you know that all claims made herein are tentative. I hope that the method discussed here answers the questions students most frequently ask and clarifies the process of conducting phenomenological inquiry. Research guided by this philosophy seeks to unveil meanings and reveals to us the multiplicity of individual perspectives of our multi-storied world. For example, using the method in this chapter with the prerequisite skills of "unknowing," "decentering," and developing essential listening skills should guide you in the uncovering of what is not yet known. From that place, you provide a critique with suggested changes that foster a better quality of life for our patients and selves, thus fulfilling the purpose of phenomenological research in a human science.

Aren't There a Lot of Steps in This Method?

That is an excellent question. How come there seem to be so many "steps"?

What is presented here is more a multifaceted process that occurs simultaneously and that is impossible to describe without categorizing it into what appear to be linear steps. My intent is to take you step by step through the philosophical process of gathering material, interpreting it, and presenting it with a critique. I have attempted to answer common questions and concerns along the way.

The "steps" can be collapsed and thought of as a process after you have become familiar with phenomenological thinking and being. It will come quite naturally. Take what looks here like a very detailed method and see it as a guide to enable your study to flow from phenomenological philosophy in a systematic way that will satisfy your research "method requirements." Each step leads to a place where you have accumulated "more," in this instance, more understanding, more meaning of a phenomenon, more substance, more significance from a critique. Because I do not believe the journey ends there, you will reach a place that illuminates a focus for the continuation of your next study.

Our Hope for Understanding

As a philosophy, phenomenology is our hope for understanding in this world.

If we were to understand the meaning of events and experiences to people, we could approach people in a way that reflects understanding of them specifically, not of theory reflecting aggregates of individuals or the non-existent person. Our theories can acknowledge the many ways of being and that one way is not the best or the only way to be-in-the-world. The healthcare provider cannot be the author of or the authority on much of patient care. Until the meaning of experience for a patient is known, an intervention is acontextual and then often ineffective.

"Noncompliance," I believe, results from not understanding the patient and the meaning of a behavior to the patient. Because nurses are often concerned in a caring way about behavior that may be detrimental to a patient, family, or community, they need to understand meaning. At the meaning level, we can offer to patients our understanding, and perhaps this generalization is well grounded: we all wish to be understood.

Phenomenology resists homogenizing responses to experiences, categorizing individuals, and placing them in stages. Unfortunately, individuals are viewed as atypical or, worse, abnormal if they deviate from the "mean" of a statistical equation or the goals of a theory. That mathematical "mean" might be the non-existent person. In contrast, researchers following the path of phenomenology are interested in the "particular" of experience, while recognizing that there are similarities. However, they see the meaning of the experience, the context in which the experience occurs, and the contingencies affecting the individual as being integrated and critically influential. With this, there is no attempt at generalizing. The phenomenologist bears witness to individual consciousness and the consciousness of the same event perceived quite differently.

In the end, phenomenological studies raise and expand our consciousness and enable us to understand that at the central core from which all life experience evolves is meaning. The interpretation of the meaning allows for congruency in communication and in nurse–patient interaction. There is optimism in phenomenology, in its wide-awakeness to experience, in its reverence for differences and the subsequent possibilities, and in its ability to liberate us from our preconceptions and emancipate us from presuppositions that no longer work. Sadler (1969) using much of the language in this chapter aptly summarizes:

> Our experience is not less than an existential encounter with a world which has a potentially infinite horizon. This human world is not predetermined, as common sense or physicalist language would indicate; it is a world that is open for discovery and creation of ever-new direction for encounter, and hence open to the emergence of as yet undiscovered significance. Because our experience is a creative and thoroughly historical encounter in a lived world, one that is alive with our encounter of it, it is potentially open to new possibilities of significant existence. (p. 20)

References

Allen, D., Benner, P., & Diekelmann, N. (1986). Three paradigms for nursing research: Methodological implications. In P. Chinn (Ed.), *Nursing research methodology issues and implementation*. Rockville, MD: Aspen.

Anderson, K. (2009). The avenging amateur. *TIME, 8*(10), 68.

Atwood, D., & Stolorow, R. (1993). *Structures of subjectivity: Explorations in psychoanalytic phenomenology* (Psychoanalytic Inquiry, vol. 4). New York: Routledge.

Beattie, A. (1989). *Picturing Will*. New York: Random House.

Benner, P. (Ed.). (1994). *Interpretive phenomenology: Embodiment, caring, and ethics in health and illness*. Thousand Oaks, CA: Sage.

Cohen, M. (1987). A historical overview of the phenomenological movement. *The Journal of Nursing Scholarship, 19,* 31–34.

Coles, R. (1991). *Spiritual life of children*. Boston, MA: Houghton-Mifflin.

Crotty, M. (1996). *Phenomenology and nursing research*. South Melbourne, Australia: Churchill Livingstone.

Dreyfus, H. (1972). *What computers can't do: A critique of artificial reason*. New York: Harper & Row.

Heidegger, M. (1962). *Being and time*. San Francisco: Harper & Row. (Original work published 1927.)

Hillman, J. (1997). *Emotion: A comprehensive phenomenology of theories and their meanings for therapy*. Evanston, IL: Northwestern University Press.

Lauterbach, S. (2007). Longitudinal phenomenology: An example of "doing" phenomenology over time; phenomenology of maternal mourning: Being-a-mother "In Another World (1992) and Five Years Later (1997)." In P. Munhall (Ed.), *Nursing research: A qualitative perspective* (2nd, 3rd, and 4th editions). Sudbury, MA: Jones & Bartlett.

Merleau-Ponty, M. (1962). *Phenomenology and perception*. (C. Smith, Trans.). New York: Humanities Press.

Munhall, P. (1993). Unknowing: Toward another pattern of knowing. *Nursing Outlook, 41,* 125–128.

Munhall, P. (1994a). *Revisioning phenomenology: Nursing and health science research.* Sudbury, MA: Jones & Bartlett.

Munhall, P. (1994b). *In women's experience* (Vol. 1). Sudbury, MA: Jones & Bartlett.

Munhall, P. (1995). *In women's experience* (Vol. 2). Sudbury, MA: Jones & Bartlett.

Munhall, P. (2001). *Nursing research: A qualitative perspective* (3rd ed.). Sudbury, MA: Jones & Bartlett.

Munhall, P., & Oiler-Boyd, C. (Eds.). (1993). *Nursing research: A qualitative perspective* (2nd ed.). Sudbury, MA: Jones & Bartlett.

Newman, M. A. (1986). *Health as expanding consciousness.* St. Louis, MO: Mosby.

Parse, R. (1987). *Nursing science: Major paradigms, theories, and critiques.* Philadelphia: Saunders.

Paterson, J., & Zderad, L. (1976). *Humanistic nursing.* New York: Wiley.

Paterson, J., & Zderad, L. (1988). *Humanistic nursing* (rev. ed.). New York: National League for Nursing.

Ray, M. (1990). Phenomenological method for nursing research. In H. Chaska (Ed.), *The nursing profession: Turning points.* Orlando, FL: Grune & Stratton.

Reeder, F. (1987). The phenomenological movement. *Image: The Journal of Nursing Scholarship, 19,* 150–152.

Sadler, W. A. (1969). *Existence and love: A new approach in existential phenomenology.* New York: Scribner's.

Schutz, A., & Wagner, H. (1970). *On phenomenology and social relations.* Chicago: University of Chicago Press.

Smiley, J. (1989). *Ordinary love and good will.* New York: Random House.

Spiegelberg, H. (1976). *Doing phenomenology.* The Hague, Netherlands: Martinus Nijjhoff.

van Manen, M. (1984). *"Doing" phenomenological research and writing.* Alberta, Canada: University of Alberta Press.

van Manen, M. (1990). *Researching the lived experience.* Albany, NY: SUNY Press.

van Manen, M. (1998). Phenomenological workshop. International Institute for Qualitative Methodology Conference, Edmonton, Canada.

Watson, J. (1985). *Nursing: Human science and human care: A theory of nursing.* Norwalk, CT: Appleton-Century-Crofts.

Additional Resources

Allen, D. G. (1995). Hermeneutics: Philosophical traditions and nursing practice research. *Nursing Science Quarterly, 8*(4), 174–182.

Allgood, M. R., & Fawcett, J. (1999). Acceptance of the invitation to dialogue: Examination of an interpretive approach for the science of unitary human beings. *Visions: The Journal of Rogerian Nursing Science, 7,* 5–13.

Anderson, W. (Ed.). (1995). *The truth about the truth: De-confusing and re-constructing the postmodern world.* New York: Tarcher/Putnam.

Annells, M. (1999). Phenomenology revisited. Evaluating phenomenology: Usefulness quality and philosophical foundations. *Nurse Researcher, 6*(3), 5–19.

Anzul, M., Downing, M., Ely, M. & Vinz, R. (1997). *On writing qualitative research: Living by words.* London: Routledge.

Ashworth, P. D. (1997). The variety of qualitative research (Part 2): Non-positivist approaches. *Nurse Education Today, 17*(3), 219–224.

Asp, M., & Fagerberg, I. (2005). Developing concepts in caring science based on a lifeworld perspective. *International Journal of Qualitative Methods, 4*(2), article 4.

Astedt-Kurki, P. (1994). Phenomenological approach in nursing research: Experiences of health, well-being and nursing are studied from the point of view of clients and nurses. *Hoitotiede, 6,* 2–7.

Atwood, G., & Stolorow, R. (2001). *Faces in a cloud: Intersubjectivity in personality theory.* Northvale, NJ: Jason Aronson.

Baker, C., Norton, S., Young, P., & Ward, S. (1998). An exploration of methodological pluralism in nursing research. *Research in Nursing and Health, 21,* 545–555.

Barnard, A., McCosker, H., & Gerber, R. (1999). Phenomenology: A qualitative research approach for exploring understanding in health care. *Qualitative Health Research, 9*(2), 212–216.

Bishop, A., & Scudder, J. (1990). *The practical, moral and personal sense of nursing: A phenomenological philosophy of practice.* Albany, NY: SUNY Press.

Bruner, J. (1992). *The acts of meaning: Four lectures on mind and culture* (Harvard-Jerusalem Lectures). Cambridge, MA: Harvard University Press.

Cerbone, D. R. (2006). *Understanding phenomenology.* Montreal: McGill-Queen's University Press.

Charalambous, A. (2010, March 10). Interpreting patients as a means of clinical practice: Introducing nursing hermeneutics. *International Journal of Nursing Studies Online.*

Conroy, S. (2003). A pathway for interpretive phenomenology. *International Journal of Qualitative Methods, 2*(3), article 4.

Corben, V. (1999). Phenomenology revisited. Misusing phenomenology in nursing research: Identifying the issues. *Nurse Researcher, 6*(3), 52–56.

Davis, S. F., & Finlay, L. (1999). Applying phenomenology in research: Problems, principles and practice. *British Journal of Occupational Therapy, 62*(9), 424.

Denzin, N. (1994). The art and politics of interpretation. In N. Denzin & Y. Lincoln (Eds.), *Handbook of qualitative research* (pp. 500–515). Thousand Oaks, CA: Sage.

Finlay, L. (1999). Applying phenomenology in research: Problems, principles and practice. *British Journal of Occupational Therapy, 62*(7), 299–306.

Flood, A. (2010). Understanding phenomenology. *Nursing Research, 17*(2), 7–15.

Forbes, D. A., King, K. M., Kushner, K. E., Letourneau, N. L., Myrick, A. F., & Profetto-McGrath, J. (1999). Warrantable evidence in nursing science. *Journal of Advanced Nursing, 29,* 373–379.

Frankl, V. E. (2006). *Man's search for meaning.* Boston, MA: Beacon Press.

Gademer, H. G., Weinsheimer, J., & Marshall, D. G. (2005). *Truth and method* (2nd rev. ed.). New York: Continuum.

Gearing, R. E. (2004). Bracketing in research: A typology. *Qualitative Health Research, 14*(10), 1429–1452.

Grace, S., & Higgs, J. (2010). Practitioner-client relationships in integrative medicine clinics in Australia: A contemporary social phenomenon. *Complementary Therapies in Medicine, 18*(1), 8–12.

Hamil, C. (2010). Bracketing—practical considerations in Husserlian phenomenological research. *Nursing Research, 17*(2), 16–24.

Hammond, M., Howarth, J., & Keat, R. (1991). *Understanding phenomenology.* Cambridge, MA: Basil Blackwell.

Irving, J., & Klenke, K. (2004). Telos, Chronos and Hermeneia: The role of metanarrative in leadership effectiveness through the production of meaning. *International Journal of Qualitative Methods, 3*(3), article 3.

Kelly, J. S., Langdon, D., & Serpell, L. (2009). The phenomenology of body image in men living with HIV. *AIDS Care, 21*(12), 1560–1567.

Koch, T. (1995). Interpretive approaches in nursing research: The influence of Husserl and Heidegger. *Journal of Advanced Nursing, 21*(5), 827–836.

Koch, T. (1999). Phenomenology revisited. An interpretive research process: Revisiting phenomenological and hermeneutical approaches. *Nurse Researcher, 6*(3), 20–34.

Lauterbach, S. (1993). In another world: A phenomenological perspective and discovery of meaning in mothers' experience with death of a wished for baby: Doing phenomenology. In P. Munhall & C. Oiler-Boyd (Eds.), *Nursing research: A qualitative perspective* (2nd ed.). Sudbury, MA: Jones & Bartlett.

LeVasseur, J. J. (2003). The problem with bracketing in phenomenology. *Qualitative Health Research, 13,* 408–420.

Laverty, S. (2003). Hermeneutic phenomenology and phenomenology: A comparison of historical and methodological considerations. *International Journal of Qualitative Methods, 2*(3), article 3.

Levin-Rozalis, M. (2004). Searching for the unknowable: A process of detection—abductive research generated by projective techniques. *International Journal of Qualitative Methods, 3*(2), article 1.

Locke, J. (1975). *An essay concerning human understanding.* Oxford, England: Oxford University Press.

Lopez, K., & Willis, D. (2004). Descriptive versus interpretive phenomenology: Their contributions to nursing knowledge. *Qualitative Health Research, 14*(5), 726, 735.

MacLean, L. M., Meyer, M., & Estable, A. (2004). Improving accuracy of transcripts in qualitative research. *Qualitative Health Research, 14*(1), 113–123.

Marques, J., & McCall, C. (2005). The application of interrater reliability as solidification instrument in a phenomenological study. *Qualitative Report, 10*(3), 438–461.

Merleau-Ponty, M. (1999). *The phenomenology of perception.* London: Routledge. (Original work published 1962.)

Moerer-Urdahl, T., & Creswell, J. (2004). Using transcendental phenomenology to explore the "ripple effect" in a leadership mentoring program. *International Journal of Qualitative Methods, 3*(2), article 2.

Moran, D. (2000). *Introduction to phenomenology.* London: Routledge.

Moustakas, C. (1994). *Phenomenological research methods.* Thousand Oaks, CA: Sage.

Munhall, P., & Fitzsimons, V. (1995). *The emergence of women into the 21st century.* Sudbury, MA: Jones & Bartlett.

Munhall, P., & Fitzsimons, V. (2000). The *emergence of family into the 21st century.* Sudbury, MA: Jones & Bartlett.

Norlyk, A., & Harder, I. (2010). What makes a phenomenological study phenomenological? An analysis of peer-reviewed empirical nursing studies. *Qualitative Health Research, 20*(3), 420–431.

Parse, R. (1990). Parse's research methodology with an illustration of the lived experience of hope. *Nursing Science Quarterly, 3*(1), 9–17.

Paterson, M., & Higgs, J. (2005). Using hermeneutics as a qualitative research approach in professional practice. *Qualitative Report, 10*(2), 339–357.

Picard, C. (1997). Embodied soul: The focus of nursing praxis. *Journal of Holistic Nursing, 15*(10), 41–53.

Pink, D. (2005). *A whole new mind: Moving from the information age to the conceptual age.* New York: Riverhead Books.

Polifroni, C., & King, M. (Eds.). (1999). *Perspectives on philosophy of science in nursing: An historical and contemporary anthology.* Philadelphia: Lippincott.

Power, E. (2004). Toward understanding in postmodern interview analysis: Interpreting the contradictory remarks of a research participant. *Qualitative Health Research, 14*(6), 858–865.

Proctor, S. (1998). Linking philosophy and method in the research process: The case of realism. *Nurse Researcher, 5*(4), 73–90.

Ray, M. A. (1994). The richness of phenomenology: Philosophic, theoretic and methodologic concerns. In J. M. Morse (Ed.), *Critical issues in qualitative research methods* (pp. 117–133). Thousand Oaks, CA: Sage.

Rehorick, D. A. (2009). *Transformative phenomenology: Changing ourselves, lifeworlds, and professional practice.* Lanham, MD: Lexington Books.

Rorty, R. (1991). *Essays on Heidegger and others.* New York: Cambridge University Press.

Sandelowski, M. (2002). Reembodying qualitative inquiry. *Qualitative Health Research, 12*(1), 104–115.

Seymour, J., & Clark, D. (1998). Issues in research. Phenomenological approaches to palliative care research. *Palliative Medicine, 12*(2), 127–131.

Smaling, A. (2003). Inductive, analogical and communicative generalization. *International Journal of Qualitative Methods, 2*(1), article 5.

Stubblefield, C., & Murray, R. L. (2002). A phenomenological framework for psychiatric nursing research. *Archives of Psychiatric Nursing, 16*(4), 149–155.

Thorne, S. E., Kirkham, S. R., & Henderson, A. (1999). Ideological implications of paradigm discourse. *Nursing Inquiry, 6*(2), 123–131.

Wolcott, H. F. (2002). Writing up qualitative research . . . better. *Qualitative Health Research, 12*(1), 91–103.

Endnotes

[1] I acknowledge that many religions have attempted to teach what the meaning of being is, or why we are here. In this text, I take this question out of the religious context while maintaining utmost respect for peoples' religious beliefs.

[2] Perhaps you might think I am overemphasizing this, but once into doing phenomenological research, you will understand this readily!

*Visually, the more interaction, the larger the shared perceptual space.

6

Exemplar: In the Eye of the Storm: A Phenomenological Inquiry of the Parallel Experience of Victims of Katrina and Nurses Who Cared for Them: Exemplar of Linguistic Transformation in Phenomenology and Exemplar of Longitudinal Phenomenology

Sarah Steen Lauterbach and Deborah L. Frank

Acknowledgments

This chapter is based on findings of a phenomenological investigation of lived experience of nurses involved with disaster care along the Gulf Coast during the hurricane season of 2005. The research was completed in 2006 by Professor Deborah Frank, PhD and Linda Sullivan, DSN (2008), both of whom were nursing faculty at Florida State University School of Nursing. A review of data and reflection on original thematic findings from the research was completed by Sarah Steen Lauterbach. The review included a reflection on nurses' lived experience using van Manen's phenomenology, nurse researcher Patricia L. Munhall, and Lauterbach's previous research and writings.

The original research uncovered an often overlooked need in disaster care services. It uncovered and articulated care needs of nurses and others who respond to disasters. This is especially timely as there seems to be an increasing occurrence of catastrophic environmental disasters worldwide. This chapter hopes to articulate a need for more attention to the care needs of those who provide emergency relief—the first responders, nurses, doctors, healthcare providers, volunteer citizens, and other professionals—and for institutional support to hospitals, organizations, and companies. These are often the hidden victims of disasters.

177

The authors acknowledge the contribution of researchers, nurses, health-care providers, rescue workers, and volunteers who cared for Katrina victims and especially nurses who participated in the research.

Abstract

Using the findings of a phenomenological inquiry which investigated nurses' lived experience of caring for victims of the 2005 hurricanes along the Gulf Coast of the United States this chapter aims to create a greater depth and breadth of understanding. In order to accomplish this, it transforms the findings of an inquiry into narrative form and articulates nurses' stories of the experience. The transformation of research findings into narrative is called a linguistic transformation by van Manen (2002) and other phenomenologists. This retrospective review identified a central overarching theme within the original research. It is described as nurses' parallel experience of disaster while caring for victims of disaster. The descriptions of nurses' experience have been constructed into narratives and "stories," and transformed into hypothetical cases and examples. The purpose of this chapter, like the original study, is to capture the "essence" of nurses' lived experience through narrative. It also identifies care needs of nurses as well as victims of Katrina. Ultimately, the purpose of this chapter is to inform disaster care so that timely, informed, relevant, and supportive disaster care protocols are facilitated and developed.

As a review on the original research and findings, this secondary reflective processing revealed that nurses, along with disaster workers and first responders, experience the ravages of disaster while serving as care providers. Further, it highlights the importance of caring for caregivers and disaster workers while caring for needs of the population experiencing disaster. From this reflection, nurses' needs were similar to needs of victims of disasters during the acute period and in the following months and perhaps years after disaster. Further, this analysis highlights the inadequate supportive care system available to nurses as well as to the population in the Gulf Coast region during and after the 2005 hurricane season.

At the time of this writing, one only has to look at the ravages of the Haiti earthquake to realize that disaster care is still in need of attention, and an institutional system and resources for care are needed. Further, there is a need to coordinate local, regional, national, and international policy with adequate institutional resources. The World Health Organization is currently involved in articulating and addressing the increased needs for disaster preparation and resource management for Haiti. Member nations have made pledges to assist in the rebuilding of Haiti. An international and institutional memory with a significant commitment to disaster care and intervention is also needed.

Introduction

Findings from the qualitative, phenomenological investigation by Frank and Sullivan (2008) of nurses' experience following hurricane Katrina are discussed in this chapter. In addition, a secondary analysis and interpretation of the original findings are shared. Additionally, the findings have been transformed into hypothetical narratives or "stories" reflecting the meaning(s) discovered in nurses' experience. The stories and hypothetical narratives describe nurses' experience of caring for victims of Katrina, while, at the same time experiencing the disaster themselves.

Narratives have been constructed from the original data with a retrospective secondary analysis of findings and using the methodology and phenomenological process of investigation provided by van Manen (1997, 1990). Additionally, nurse researcher, Munhall's (1986, 1993, 2001, 2007) phenomenological writings and the articulation of the life worlds within human experience provides the reflective framework for this chapter. The narratives and "stories" of nurses' experience describe nurses' parallel experience of disaster, while caring for victims of Katrina.

Where this study uncovered the needs of Katrina nurses, it points to similarities in care needs for victims of disaster and for first responders and volunteers who assist with disasters. When watching the news and programs of recent earthquakes in Haiti and Chile in January 2010, or following the Tsunami in Myanmar (Burma), or the earthquake in China several years ago, one is struck by the level of concern and the magnitude of the human response of volunteers and first responders. Findings from the Katrina study are relevant to other disasters.

Responding to disaster is traumatic for first responders, for volunteers, and for professionals who also through volunteering experience the disaster up close and personal, not unlike members of the population under stress. There is a need to conceptualize, plan, and care for those who are called upon to answer the call for assistance, whether the disaster is natural, geographic, or man made.

The authors are interested in using phenomenology to uncover and identify human phenomena that often are hidden, or that reside in silence, or phenomena that are just under the radar and often go unnoticed and unattended to. In this study of Katrina nurses, which focused on lived experience of nurses providing disaster care, nurses' experience and needs mirrored needs of the population.

There is a need for organizations and volunteer groups to care for caregivers and first responders, during and following the disaster experience. Follow-up care is needed for victims, and for those who care for victims of disaster. This need often is unrealized as everyone focuses on the priority of meeting victims' needs. Hopefully, the research by Frank and Sullivan (2008) and this reflection will bring needed attention to needs of responders. Care for responders' needs can be anticipated and intervention planned in protocols that focus on disaster care. Organizations and agencies need to address the volunteer care needs and begin intervention when they first solicit and prepare volunteers to answer the call for help.

According to van Manen (2002; 1997; 1984) and nurse researcher, Munhall (2007), phenomenologic writing assists the reader in gleaning an interpretation of experience. The transformation of research findings into narratives and stories is referred to in this chapter as a linguistic transformation. With the recent experience of the earthquakes in Haiti and Chile, experiences of care givers and disaster workers through news and personal testimony strikes a familiar note to the experiences of nurses caring for victims of Katrina. While many Katrina nurses from the surrounding area volunteered and provided care in shelters and hospitals, many were also resident victims themselves. Nurses who responded from other areas of the country, such as California, and other volunteers experienced the need for personal care. Nurses experienced a parallel experience of the people of the region as Katrina simply overwhelmed public disaster relief organizations and healthcare facilities.

The purpose of the original research of Frank and Sullivan (2008) and of this transformative narrative is to capture the "essence" of nurses' lived experience in order to more fully understand the needs of all involved when disaster strikes. As stated in the original research proposal, "By understanding the experience of these nurses, it was anticipated that healthcare providers could better prepare for future episodes in similar situations where nursing services will be required" (Frank & Sullivan, 2008, p. 2).

The purpose of this chapter in a research text is to demonstrate the potential outcomes of using phenomenology as a research method. Whether exploring disaster or another phenomenon, phenomenology has potential to create a greater depth and breadth of human understanding of experience. Thus, needs can be more adequately addressed and interventions can emerge from "knowing" and understanding.

Intervention in disaster and crisis situations needs to meet the following criteria:

- It needs to be informed in that it is based in research and human experience.
- It needs to be timely and available when the need first presents and as long as needed.
- It needs to be relevant and informed by understanding and caring.
- It needs to be provided with significant, relevant, supportive assistance at the time of need and beyond (Lauterbach, unpublished manuscript).

From the first author's previous research with mothers' experience of perinatal infant death, it was found that mothers' mourning develops, changes, and evolves over time. Mothers found that participating in research informed them as they led their families through the acute grief and mourning experience. Mourning care needs to be available as mothers continue to reflect and process the experience of loss and mourning over time (Lauterbach, 2007).

Similarly, nurses who participated in this research, most likely found that participation in research assisted in their coping with their own experience of disaster and in developing meanings in the experience over time. Where this has not been verified one-on-one with nurses in this study, informal conversations with nurses who provided disaster relief care reflect similar effects of supportive care received simply from participating in research and discussing the experience with other nurses. Similarly, in the many presentations of this author's research on perinatal loss, people from the audience shared that being the recipient of research findings was also helpful in understanding personal and professional experiences with infant death. From the elder women's study, this was a common experience. Several elder women had never discussed their experiences with anyone. One woman revealed that she had never "forgotten" the infant, and she often felt guilty that she had not "done right" by her baby. For her, participation in research provided welcomed relief.

Thematic Findings by Frank and Sullivan

The following thematic groupings of nurses' experience were identified by Frank and Sullivan (2008) through interviews of nurses: chaos, reality check, reorganizing, stabilizing, and planning for the future. The research used van Kaam's phenomenology method. This method is a little different from van Manen's and Munhall's, but it is quite compatible in that there was a continual reflection on meanings and descriptions of experience.

Initially, nurses experienced complete chaos. Initially, the chaos was completely disorienting. Thereafter, at varying times during the storm and following the storm, chaos was a prevailing theme embedded within nurses' experience. Over time the chaos abated, but even now, several years later, chaos is still present in descriptions of people who lived through Katrina. As with many crises, an acute, intense level of stress is difficult to withstand. Within a relatively short time, chaos gave way to a reality orientation, even though the new-found reality was quite different from before, and perhaps not always the "real" reality. The reality was a perception which changed rapidly. However, the new-found reality was grounding and helped to reorder and orient people to the tasks and problem solving needed for survival and beyond. It was exhausting to be in constant chaos and crisis.

When the intensity of crisis and chaos subsided a little, a kind of order emerged as nurses, relief workers, and the population coped. In the period following Katrina there was constant organization and reorganization. One still often experiences change and a semblance of the original chaos today along the coast, even though it is not as palpable and visible. The landscape has been tidied, but there are areas of people's lives that continue to be in disorder. Over time a semblance of order has been achieved, but it is an order very different from before Katrina, with a more short-lived, present focus. Following the themes of order and reality check, organization, and reorganization, a feeling of stability was achieved during the enormous and incredible changes ushered in by Katrina and other storms. In time people were better able to meet personal and family needs. But, the feelings of chaos persist. People, including the nurses needed to do more than just survive. There was a need for people, including Katrina nurses, to plan for the future.

Retrospective Reflection on Findings

When reflecting on the research findings and rereading transcripts 2 years after interviews with Katrina nurses were completed, there seemed to be an overarching theme present, which was not as explicit when the original research was conducted. Katrina nurses experienced a "parallel experience" with victim survivors. The reflection on findings over time was extremely helpful as this theme was not explicit during the original analysis of date. Similarly, a longitudinal perspective was found to be very informative when the first author completed her doctoral research with mothers who had experienced perinatal loss. Now, several years following the analysis of Katrina nurses, a reflection on original findings is informative. Further, viewing findings through using a different phenomenological method, is informative. The experience and conceptualization of longitudinal phenomenological perspectives was thus used in uncovering nurses' parallel lived experience of Katrina. Findings from this study can be relevant when considering the recent earthquake disasters in Haiti and Chile. First responders, disaster workers, nurses, and other medical providers may experience similar care needs to Katrina nurses.

In the review of transcripts and findings from Frank and Sullivan (2008), the overarching theme found retrospectively in nurses' lived experience was that nurses experienced a parallel experience with victim survivors. Munhall's (1986, 1993, 1994, 2001, 2007) phenomenological writings that focused on "life worlds" in human experience provided the framework for the articulation of meanings surrounding Katrina nurses' experience.

The following sections articulate the overarching themes of nurses' experience through these dimensions of human experience:

1. Embodiment—lived experience
2. Temporality—lived time
3. Spatiality—lived space and time

4. Relational—lived within relationships and connections
5. Lived context—multiple, changing, dynamic meaning contexts experienced and lived over time, with others, within time, within spatial proximity (Lauterbach, 1993)

These dimensions of experience are intimately related and are described along with Frank and Sullivan's (2008) thematic findings.

Embodiment—Lived Body

Embodiment is a phenomenological concept which refers to the way humans experience life, and how they, we, live "with" experience. In the perinatal research (Lauterbach, 1992, 1993, 2000) mothers discussed in detail their experience of acute grief and mourning following the death of a wished-for baby. They described their aching arms, full breasts, the inability to breathe, a feeling that a weight was on their chests, and their inability to go about simple daily life and difficulty with completing daily tasks. Acute grief and mourning have physical, psychological, and cognitive symptoms.

Similarly, Katrina nurses experienced the hurricane and its effects and embodiment in their own lives. They found it difficult to manage their lives, while at the same time providing expert care for victims in hospitals and shelters. Meeting basic self-care needs for sleep, rest, nutrition, and respite was difficult. They found the experience of nursing during disaster to be liberating since they were able to practice at the level they were prepared for—at the level of expertise. They had to be creative and innovative continuously to meet the demands of care needs for victims.

Nurses also described how consumed they were with their own survival at the same time they were filled with concern for their families, friends, and neighbors. They described the difficulty of caring for patients in hospitals and shelters in unbelievable heat and humidity, where air conditioning, power, and electricity were out. They also described the healing effects of a good night's sleep in a cot, still warm from the nurse who had just slept there for a few hours before returning to her duty station. Cots and sleeping bags were used 24/7 and were kept warm by nurses' heat, as they took turns relieving each other for shift changes. They described the healing effects of a good meal. In addition, the descriptions of experiencing exhaustion from working for 21–24 hours a shift, day after day, over several weeks, were universal. Nurses stated that they had never been so tired, while at the same time, so filled with a satisfaction in their work. They described the experience of being able to make decisions without hospital red tape and protocols, which often delay meeting needs of patients.

Katrina nurses were empowered to work at a level they felt competent and prepared for, without a lot of interference. The mental satisfaction of doing a job well, in actually practicing up to their level of expertise was empowering, physically, mentally, and professionally. This is interpreted as the experience of providing *embodied care*. It propelled nurses to continue giving as much as humanly possible. They also discussed the ultimate fatigue from providing consuming, relentless, embodied care with little respite. They worried about their ability to continue the pace as the days wore on, knowing that they, themselves, and others would not be able to continue the level of care and commitment needed.

Katrina nurses' experience is similar to nurses and others who experience burnout from caring too much, too long, without support, respite, or acknowledgment. Similarly, the demands of providing disaster care for too long, without adequate support, without respite, and without personal care needs being met, set the stage for the nurses to experience burnout. This phenomenon is relevant to the previous work by the first author and a colleague that focused on reflective practice (Lauterbach & Becker, 1998, Lauterbach & Hentz, 2005a; Lauterbach, 2006). While nurses cared for victims, they too were experiencing devastation and destruction, loss of property, and massive changes to a way of life as a result of the disaster, and they too needed care. The transformation narratives focus on nurses' experiences and human needs when they answer a call for disaster service. While caring for others, nurses needed care, support, and ultimately needed more commitment and attention to self-care. Katrina nurses had spent their lives caring for others without caring for themselves. This seems to be a universal phenomenon for caring professionals.

Temporality—Lived Time

The immediacy of care for and needs of the residents of the Gulf Coast region was compounded by the large-scale environmental disaster and disruption of services. This continued for weeks, months, and the couple of years that followed. Emergency and crisis care were needed for months. Many people are just now feeling a sigh of relief that they survived. For most residents of the region, life, work, and recreation along the coast changed dramatically forever. Many say that Katrina completely devastated the institutional supports in place at the time, and in the years that followed. The recovery is still in process. In addition, the inadequacy of response elevated the population's level of anxiety about life in general. Personal, family, and institutional resources were overwhelmed. Basic needs for shelter, housing, nutrition, safety, and protection were of paramount importance and continue to be needed to this day.

The experience of living through Katrina is still very fresh, especially for residents who survived and for many who provided care and emergency assistance to the region. Over time, recovery and reorganization, chaos and confusion, diminished in kind and quality. At times nurses still experience post-traumatic–like memories of Katrina. One nursing faculty member from the region, who lived in a Federal Emergency Management Agency (FEMA) trailer for almost 2 years, recently expressed to the author that she only needed to close her eyes to visually remember. She often experiences a familiar fear and anxiety about "something not being right." While she has more control now, she also stated that she "did not want to forget, that memories will help her cope in the future," She is convinced that having survived Katrina will be useful, again. She has included more emphasis on disaster care and crisis intervention strategies in teaching nursing courses. She also stated that the "nation has seemingly forgotten people of the region, and that many people still need tremendous support and assistance." The 24-hour news organizations have long ago left the Gulf Coast, just as is seen as time passes since the earthquake in Haiti, even though the quake event occurred relatively recently. Over time the interest and intensity diminishes and the aftermath of devastation is less visible. There were many people in Mississippi, Louisiana, and Alabama who were displaced during Katrina to northern Mississippi and other areas of the country. Dealing with loss and anxiety will continue for many people for years, and even though it will change in quality or immediacy, other storms and environmental events will probably precipitate familiar feelings to those felt during Katrina. As with mothers' experiences of grief and mourning in the months and years following infant death, anniversary events stimulated responses of loss all over again. For Katrina survivors, new environmental disasters, storms, tornados, and hurricanes will be reminders of the tremendous chaos, devastation, loss, and anxiety they experienced.

Context—Historical, Dynamic, Lived, Evolving Contexts and Meanings of Being and Living Situated in the Eye of the Storm

Hurricane Katrina came ashore on the Mississippi coast on August 28, 2005. It devastated the whole northern Gulf coastal region, including New Orleans, Louisiana, Mississippi, and Alabama. In the beginning, the warnings sounded like many other hurricane warnings. Hurricane warnings had become a way of life for people who lived, worked, and played along the Gulf Coast. In the 1990s, people along the coast had become accustomed to the growing intensity and frequency of storms. Today, many have very vivid memories of the devastation following hurricane Camille in the late 1960s. This author went to a folk festival in Louisiana after Camille and remembers the coastal devastation well. However, a drive along the Gulf in 2007 revealed that the coastal destruction to this same route caused by Camille was simply nothing compared to Katrina. The topography and visual image of the coastal region after Katrina was a reminder of the hurricane's force, leaving complete and utter destruction—large mansions completely gone, with only the foundations left;

huge 100-year-old oak trees lining the coastal highway completely uprooted; FEMA trailers in places mansions had been. The region looked like a war zone.

Hurricane warnings preceded Katrina and were noted, but did not seem "out of the ordinary" that day, as people went about their daily lives. People of the region got used to warnings during hurricane season. Most people did a cursory job of preparing for hurricanes, which included stocking up on batteries, water, and nonperishable food supplies. But, no one really imagined before Katrina, that this would be "the big one" and that it would completely overwhelm families' and residents' abilities to go about their ordinary lives.

Yet, the predictions and warnings about the gravity of this storm turned out to be accurate. Katrina was the worst hurricane recorded in history along the Gulf Coast of Mississippi and Louisiana. It is noted by many as the "storm of all storms." In many ways, it represents the "perfect storm" when considering the inadequate and incapable disaster-relief system available. It completely overwhelmed all local, state, and federal systems available to deal with disaster. No one could really imagine how unprepared rescue and emergency response agencies were to deal with such a large-scale disaster. The level of devastation and disaster had simply never been imagined by the people of the region, by the agencies who deal with disasters, and by the nation as a whole. In retrospect, batteries, food supplies, and emergency kits, the things that the news and media marketed, would have been completely inadequate had the whole population prepared. The hurricane incapacitated all disaster planning resources and agencies. It took the healthcare system almost completely by surprise. No one had imagined what devastation would accompany a large-scale disaster in the region. Even though the Gulf Coast had experienced many hurricanes, it had not experienced a hurricane on the scale of Katrina.

In order to deal with such a storm, providing the emergency and basic needs for the whole population to survive, a plan of significant magnitude, including emergency evacuation of whole communities and groups of vulnerable people, was needed. Large-scale relief efforts for the people remaining in the area were also necessary. During Katrina and in the aftermath, there were many people who were literally stuck in their homes and hospitals, who simply had no means to leave; or, they were too ill or disabled to leave. There were many who had trouble walking away from their homes, and belongings, even if they could have left. They could not bear to leave their homes, belongings, and pets. Those who were able and chose to leave walked away from their lives with great sadness and despair, often feeling they had physically survived, but "for what?"

The whole region and states that bordered the Gulf and areas to the north in central and northern Mississippi, Tennessee, and Kentucky, experienced a degree of devastation and disaster due to Katrina that previously had not been imagined. Erosion and flooding completely and permanently changed the topography of the region. It forever changed the demographics of the area.

Where New Orleans was incredibly devastated, other communities, such as Waveland, Mississippi, were completely obliterated. The Mississippi, Alabama, and Louisiana coasts were changed forever by their location in the hurricane belt. The whole region was in the eye of unforgiving, relentless storms that year.

Emergency Response to Katrina and Its Aftermath

Prior to Katrina, people who lived and worked in the Gulf coastal region had slowly gotten used to extreme weather and an increasing intensity of hurricanes. However, following hurricane Andrew in Florida in the early 1990s, most people assumed that there was a federal emergency response to disaster in place which included coordinated relief.

It was simply assumed by most people, including the governmental agencies and FEMA, that there would be an adequate, rapid response to any disaster. And, it had been assumed by the population in the country that the ability to purchase home owner's insurance provided residents, homeowners, and businesses some protection. Many of these assumptions were simply not true. Now, years later, many of the conditions and causes of suffering and tragedy following Katrina, still have not been corrected. Mary's story highlights this unpreparedness later.

Katrina has raised the anxiety of the whole population living in vulnerable areas, in the country, and in the whole world. No one is spared anxiety in general about security, protection, assistance, and one's personal ability to recover from a catastrophic disaster. As the research by Frank and Sullivan (2008) portrayed, nurses who were providing disaster medical services experienced the storm in two ways, personally and as nursing crisis providers.

Now several years later, what began as an acute crisis during and immediately after has, for some people, turned into a state of chronic anxiety, fear, loss, and unease regarding one's ability to cope and to trust that authorities and agencies will be able to handle another major disaster. The efforts to rebuild and restore essential services and businesses since Katrina have been in a constant state of exacerbation between crisis and recovery, between people coping and not coping with the new reality. To the visible eye much has been cleared away, but pockets still exist in New Orleans and along the coast that look like disaster or war zones. Hurricane Katrina has continued to take its toll on the coping resources of people of the region—one person, one family, one community at a time. Where stories of hope and recovery have emerged, there are also many poignant experiences and stories of despair, loss, disparity, and untold, continued, human suffering.

Even though life had changed forever, many people found a new resilience and opportunity emerging from chaos and disaster. However, coping with the level of change has remained quite challenging. Many displaced people in other areas of the country, including northern Mississippi and Tennessee, continue to be unable to return home. Katrina changed lives forever. Change in life and location is often perceived as loss. Plus, dealing with lost loved ones, pets, way of life, lost belongings, and as some have termed, "lost history," has required a resilience and hardiness that often people were unaware they possessed. Others have incorporated the loss into their narratives, to live as best they can, with what they have. There are many survivor experiences and many tragedies that come from living "with" and "through" disaster. However, the vulnerable are most at risk in disasters.

Relational—Lived Relationships and Human Connections

Nurses' experience of providing disaster care to Katrina victim survivors was an experience that was intimately lived with other nurses, with the people who were victims, and within their own lives. Those who lived in the region experienced the hurricane up close, in their personal and professional lives. They were in the eye of the storm, while at the same time, providing emergency care and relief to others. Nurses who worked in hospitals and institutions in the area, experienced the effects of the hurricane in their own lives, while trying to provide for themselves, friends, and family while at the same time answering the call to nursing duty, often 24 hours a day. Transportation to and from work was almost impossible, so many had to rely on family or neighbors to supervise children and keep loved ones safe. Intimate care relationships were established with those who were brought in for emergency care. There was a personal understanding and sharing of the experience of loss, trauma, disruption, and of surviving the untoward consequences of disaster.

Katrina brought home aspects of nurses' professional work and relationships that often go unacknowledged in nursing services—the pettiness that nurses sometimes exhibited in relationships with colleagues prior to Katrina. Recently, a faculty member stated that she hoped she learned a lesson about what was important and what was trivial following Katrina. Nurses' experience of horizontal violence and aggressiveness with each other following Katrina seemed to take on a new perspective. Back biting, gossiping, griping about details of work, and difficulties with coworkers seemed, in retrospect, so "silly" and immature, and served to defeat the care objectives of nursing work. Many made a commitment to change this destructive regressive pattern of behavior.

Nurses took the opportunity in the new-found awareness of relationship pettiness, to engage in reflective assessment of work and other relationships. Many found that they needed to value and develop more meaningful relationships, professionally as well as in personal and intimate domains, family, friendship, and community. Coming to terms with and making a commitment to improve the quality of relationships and connections to others and to important values and goals occurred for nurses. Nurses have long known that they had needs for self-care, but many had not really practiced this. The storm brought many personal health and relational issues to the foreground for assessment, reflection, and renewed commitment.

Linguistic Narrative Construction

The linguistic narratives, constructed through the reflective process using data from transcripts and nurses' experience described in the earlier research by Frank and Sullivan (2008), are shared here. The qualitative outcomes (Lauterbach, 2006) found through the reflection on these transcripts of nurses' narratives describe the lived experience of nurses. Narratives uncover and highlight needs of nurses who provide nursing services and care following disasters. There is need for development of a structured, formal program and institutional system of support and care for nurses, caregivers, volunteers, and others involved in disaster relief and care. Further, needs for caregiver and disaster worker support should begin with the planning phase, continue through disaster care experience, and be maintained over time, to go beyond the immediate disaster relief experience and into the aftermath.

Finally, descriptions of Katrina victim survivors' lived experience is found to be embedded within nurses' survival experience. The relevance of this chapter focusing on Katrina nurses' needs for care is evident when examined within the global context. The writing of this manuscript has also occurred during times of increased attention to disasters worldwide. The following international events have heightened attention to the need for improved disaster planning: earthquakes in Haiti and Chile at the beginning of 2010; in the continuing incidence of Pacific earthquakes and southern California; and even in the West Virginia coal mining accident. When this manuscript was first begun the world's attention was drawn to Myanmar (Burma) and China.

The following linguistic narratives describe nurses' experience of caring for victims of hurricanes and particularly, Katrina, from the up-close-and-personal vantage. Nurses experienced a professional call to action to serve the people of the region, as well as to assist family, friends, and neighbors personally. They have coped with effects of hurricanes in their own lives, while caring for others. Two nurses' stories have been constructed from nine nurses' lived experience caring for hurricane and Katrina victims. Themes discovered in Frank and Sullivan's (2008) research have been used to construct and transform the narrative, or "story," into a possible nursing experience.

The first story is about Kay, hypothetically constructed, to be a nurse in a hospital in New Orleans. The second constructed story is about Mary, a nurse, who was working in an ER in a hospital in Gulfport, Mississippi. Where the experience was unique for each of the nine nurses in the study, who served in varying facilities throughout the coastal area, there were common themes of meaning(s) in their experience. The constructed stories describe how nurses coped with Katrina themselves, while caring for victim survivors.

Kay's Story

Another hurricane was coming. This was the news in that early morning on August 26, 2005, as Kay headed to work in the NICU at Tulane. She had just dropped off her daughter, a second grader, at her mom's house so she could take her to school that morning. *Maybe I should have called out today*, she thought. Then, remembering, that another nurse had called out sick, she realized that it had not even crossed her mind. But, now with the hurricane coming, *Maybe I should have.* Her thinking continued, *It is a constant struggle as a single parent, with a young school-aged child. What is a legitimate reason for calling out?*

Kay had intended to stop at the grocery the previous evening, but she was dead tired after working her day shift and an evening shift for another nurse, who had called out sick at the last minute. She had pulled a double shift. *It always happens when I am low on food*, she thought. *I know I should stay on top of grocery buying during hurricane season.* But, she was scheduled for work today at 7:00 A.M. which really meant 6:45! Also, she was hoping, *Maybe Mom will pack Kayla a lunch today.*

With the hurricane coming, Kay felt a growing anxiety accompanied by an increasing wave of guilt: *I will do better, and I promise myself that I will buy a 2-week supply of nonperishable food, with this next paycheck, before I am too short.* Now, since it was the end of the month, there had simply not been enough money last week to stock up. *Hurricanes are always inconvenient, but this, one, too, is probably overreported. I wonder if there is a conspiracy between the weather forecasters and businesses marketing items for the hurricane*, she thought. *This will probably be another false alarm.*

In the days that followed, Kay hoped against hope that it had been just "another false alarm." When Katrina hit on August 28, the whole region was literally brought to a standstill. What followed were weeks of power outages; flooding; loss of life; people clinging to rooftops; abandoned elders; nursing home residents who were not evacuated; overcrowded shelters; temperatures above 100 degrees; and damp hospitals and shelters, with humid linens and paper products and an overpowering stench throughout. Many people who could afford to, or had transportation, evacuated when it was known that Katrina was not just another hurricane, but one of horrendous proportions. Kay's house was intact. She was one of the lucky ones. She lived on the edge of the French Quarter.

A cycle of guilt accompanied by tremendous relief continued to intensify for Kay in the weeks following Katrina. She experienced relief that she still had her home, and mother and daughter Kayla were safe. They had been able to go stay with another relative who lived in Jackson, Mississippi. Still, she had had to leave her home vacant in order to work around the clock many days providing nursing services and care to Katrina victims.

Leaving her home to evacuate to the hospital had been tremendously difficult—leaving her belongings, not knowing when she would be able to return, or if there would be anything to return to. *What do I take? What do I leave?* Kayla had been born and lived in her small New Orleans style house for her whole life. Thankfully, her mom, also alone since her dad died, was nearby. But, now, with her mom and Kayla in Jackson, she felt isolated and alone while working in the midst of a crowded hospital with a tremendous workload. She felt more vulnerable, with an anxiety mixed with worry, like nothing she had ever experienced. And, there was fear—fear that she might be in harm's way, from the continued effects of the hurricane winds and flooding, as well as threats from others. She worried about leaving her home and belongings. People in need are desperate. She had seen that already. She needed to stay focused on her nursing work, which luckily was absorbing. Worries of the rumors and stories of vandalism, theft, robbery had to be pushed aside.

Luckily, Kay did not have access to the 24-hour news that the rest of the world watched during the days following Katrina. It would have scared her to death. But, at least her mom and Kayla were "safe" or, "safer." However, Jackson experienced tremendous hurricane damage, wind, and flooding, so even though it was 150 miles north of New Orleans, there was no truly "safe" place in the region. She was probably safest in New Orleans in the hospital. Hattiesburg and Jackson were flooded and experienced extensive damage to homes, and had power outages for several weeks. The flood of coastal residents into the city overwhelmed its facilities and services. (There were nursing faculty at the University of Southern Mississippi at the Gulfport campus who were still in FEMA trailers, at the writing of the Frank and Sullivan study in May, 2008.)

Kay had been asked to stay at the hospital and work, which she loved. "Yes, I get fed up with hospital policy at times, but I always leave work feeling I have done something meaningful." She could not anticipate what work would be like. She was not aware that there would be many days of working around the clock, with little sleep, without a shower, and without a clean change of clothes. Days ran into nights and then days. It was hard to keep track of the day of the week, time of day, or the date. It was hard to know when to eat or when to sleep. Usually, sleep came when there was a spare cot and when she simply could not do anything else. The hospital generator was problematic, since there was no air conditioning and 100-plus-degree heat and humidity. The impact of the temperature was unbearable to the people who were everywhere—in corridors, waiting rooms, stairways, or anywhere they could find space. The staff of the hospital also had families—some of whom were evacuated, but many whose whereabouts and well-being were unknown. Many staff members were not able to be in touch with their families because of power outages and cell phone towers being overwhelmed.

Many months later, these images remained as visual and fresh as they were at the time they were experienced. Sometimes they intruded on Kay's daily activities, or they would just pop up when passing a particular landmark or hospital corridor. Post-traumatic–like experiences were also common with many of Kay's friends. Sometimes she and her friends would find themselves crying for no apparent reason. The feelings of loss and desperation were common, though often hidden and seemingly unrelated to what was currently going on. They talked a lot about it. They learned that the disturbing images become more infrequent and that taking care of self really helped. Self-care is critical in healing and helped ward off despair. *Loss and change are forever,* Kay realized when thinking about the New Orleans where she had lived. Her mom and daughter have since returned and now live with Kay in her New Orleans row house.

Back to the time after Katrina hit

The hospital and all of New Orleans were in a state of crisis and chaos following Katrina. However, amazingly, the work was almost easier, the paperwork less oppressive, and decisions, independent. She felt in some way that she was really using her knowledge and skills as a nurse, with less bureaucratic hassle. The hallways were full of the injured, infirm, ill, and exposed; there were refugees from the stadium, and those who had been plucked from rooftops. All of the people flooding the hospital were overwhelmed, anxious, and fearful, much as she had felt. But, they also were in need of personal care, a hot meal, and rest. Many did not know where other family members were, or if they were alive, or needing rescue. Later, the nurses, along with the Katrina victims talked about the restorative effects of a hot meal and a good night's sleep.

Kay felt lucky, too, because the Louisiana Nurses Association had asked her to stay and work in her hospital rather than at a shelter or the stadium. She had several nurse colleagues and friends who were sent to the stadium; Kay's friend, Mary, was at an emergency room in a hospital in Gulfport, Mississippi. Kay was glad that she could work around familiar people, knowing the hospital's ins and outs, having supplies and some protection from the wrath of Katrina. She was needed here and could work with greater efficiency in a place she knew.

Kay felt that the hospital provided personal safety. Safety was an issue that was described by nurses who were assigned to some of the community shelters. Kay and other nurses took turns sleeping on cots in the staff room. She found she needed no privacy or quiet to sleep. She just needed to be able to lie down and close her eyes. After a few hours of sleep, she would awaken, feeling rested, find something to eat, and start her work routine all over.

In retrospect, one of the things Kay appreciated so much, were her relationships with grateful, appreciative patients and families for whom she cared. Never before had she paid that much attention to how her patients felt and what they thought about her relationship with them or her care. The gratitude was incredibly heart warming and restorative. It validated her work and her commitment to stay behind when asked to help out with Katrina victims after her mother and daughter left for safer ground. She knew without a doubt that she made a tremendous difference in the lives of the people she served and cared for. It was her finest nursing moment and experience!

In addition, Kay found that she and other nurses were quite capable of improvisation, that creative solutions were easily identified to handle issues and problems that arose. She thought she functioned in the *ultimate* nursing role. Kay also experienced feeling much more at ease with the nursing role of Advanced Registered Nurse Practitioner (ARNP in Florida). The role, interestingly, had been elusive before. She was able to practice fully in the role for which she was prepared. She was able to make collaborative and independent decisions that she was clearly capable of making, without some of the red tape and/or limitations of hospital regulations. If she needed a medication from the pharmacy, she would simply go get it. There was no red tape, no worry about hospital protocol, no worry about legal ramifications of her practice, nor worry about whether insurance would cover a patient's treatment and care. She knew what was within her practice repertoire, what she needed to consult about, and who to go to for help.

Kay experienced camaraderie with staff, from housekeeping to the physicians, that had never been present to that degree in her work. She relied on patients' families to do what they could to help relieve patient suffering, and gave them needed instruction and information about care. She felt fully appreciated by everyone with whom she worked, including administration, who pitched in with what was needed including cleaning toilets and washing equipment. Often, she had not felt that her work was noticed or fully appreciated by administration, but this was not the case during Katrina. Finally, she was considered by others as well as herself to be able to practice up to her ability as an ARNP, which made her think to herself, *This is the essence of nursing.*

Mary's Story

Mary, a nurse for 36 years, had just moved from northern Mississippi to the coast, a place she had always longed to live, which was also closer to her elderly parents. As she anticipated retirement, with adult children who had their own lives, she decided to move near Waveland, Mississippi, a small year-round community with relatively reasonable real estate. She transferred from her position as nurse manager in Jackson, to a local hospital emergency room. She loved the Mississippi coast as it was still relatively undeveloped. Highway 90 runs right along the beach, so there is a stretch of the Gulf to which the public has almost total access. This area is unlike much of the emerald coast along the Gulf in that it has areas that are undeveloped and, in her opinion, "unspoiled." Anyone, regardless of one's station in life, can park a car or bike and simply walk out onto the sandy beach and wade in the aquamarine, magical, salty water of the Gulf of Mexico!

Mary did her daily walk along the beach, but today it was not sunny as is usual in the late afternoon. She loved the low-lying sun prior to setting behind the water. *The gulf, sand, water, and sun are part of my soul,* Mary thought as she walked along, looking for shells and thinking about the day. It was her day off. How she loved living here after years of hoping to be able to live on the coast. But, today, the sky looked just a little foreboding. It was a little cloudy and overcast, not real dark, but darkish with a little yellowish, greenish tint. There was not the bluish green water as usual, and the waves broke with white caps as they approached the shore. It was August 23, 2005. *My grandfather could tell when a storm was brewing. I wonder if that is what is happening now. I must look at the weather forecast this evening.*

Having lived in Mississippi all of her life, Mary was quite accustomed to being in what everyone called, "hurricane alley." But, since hurricane Georges in the late 1990s, there had not been significant damage from hurricanes. Georges had just hovered along the Gulf for several days, created much rain, but little wind damage. In 2003, a hurricane named Ivan created much damage in Pensacola, Florida, and Mobile, Alabama, about 50 miles east of Gulfport. When Mary was a child, hurricane Camille hit the coast and came ashore in the Biloxi and Gulfport area. Camille was a significant storm that caused significant damage to homes and businesses along Highway 90.

After a brisk walk, concerned about the sky and what was in store for the weekend, Mary returned home. That coming Saturday she was planning to go to a beach party that her unit was sponsoring, a clam bake. This would be her first party since arriving and she was anxious to meet people and socialize with work colleagues. She looked forward to making new friends and had already enhanced her wardrobe with an appropriate outfit for a beach party. She turned the news on and the weather forecast confirmed her suspicion that a storm was in the Gulf. She hoped that, *just maybe it will move toward Mexico, since it is several days away and is only just a tropical depression now.*

In the several years since the late 1990s, storms seemed to be occurring with more frequency and more force. People along the coastal areas were warned continuously, and advised to buy supplies for emergencies. But, rarely did it seem necessary afterward. Camille had seen people ignore the warnings, and, in spite of warnings, often had "hurricane parties." One such party was devastating and several party attendees died. Since then, the hurricane party was not "the thing to do" even though it is known that some parties develop when a hurricane is forecasted. Actually, people along the coast often experienced hurricane warning fatigue, and did not always heed warnings, since often the disaster did not occur.

There was no way of knowing if this hurricane would develop or reach the magnitude of a category 3 hurricane as predicted. "What is a category 3 hurricane anyway, when 5 is the strongest?" This was the thinking of many coastal residents prior to Katrina before it moved and sounded like a freight train over the whole Gulf coastal region. Perhaps it was denial, perhaps wishful thinking, or perhaps just part of the fatigue which accompanies living near the Gulf. Regardless, everyone was mistaken.

When Katrina actually hit on August 28, Mary's life and other's lives completely changed. Katrina devastated the Gulf Coast, utterly obliterating communities. Waveland, a small community, was completely devastated. Mary had bought a small house close to Waveland. She was lucky—the house still stood, sustaining minimal damage. The shore where Mary had walked shortly before Katrina, while looking forward to the unit beach party, was not recognizable after Katrina. Debris littered the area for months. Whole structures, were completely washed away; foundations were washed out from under hotels; huge 100-year-old oak trees that had lined the properties north of Highway 90, were uprooted; the large, upscale homes along the way were simply gone.

Nine months later Mary was still shell shocked when she drove along the place she had usually walked. Occasionally, FEMA trailers were seen on sites where homes once stood. Foundations survived, but houses had vanished. If trees still stood, they held debris from people's homes—clothes were still hanging in trees; debris was all over the place; people who had lived in the upscale homes and dressed in designer clothes, now visited the food bank or were still in shelters; no one, even those who had homes, property, or money had anything; the rich and poor were all reduced to sharing basic necessities. However, the poor were the hardest hit and would be stuck in shelters, indefinitely.

One day Mary met a woman on her walk along the beach 6–8 months after the storm. She stated, "I came home to get a few things. Then, I came back later and everything was gone." Mary stood there and she pointed to the different areas of the concrete foundation, "This is where I had these big plants; this was my kitchen; my couch was here; my bed was here; I can't find anything. I cannot find any of my stuff."

Mary described to the interviewer what people experienced during and after Katrina. The images were constant; it was hard to get them out of her mind. She also hoped she would never forget. It helped her clarify what is important and what is not. Her valuing and priorities had shifted, probably, forever. "And, this was not a bad thing," she said, continuing:

> It is hard to imagine that six months later—that they still have nothing. I even got lost because the streets were gone and I could not find any landmarks. When I hit 90, I started crying because that is the first time I had really seen the coast. There is nothing really left. I have seen the coast grow and become wall-to-wall casinos and restaurants. Restaurants that I had been to—they are still closed or, they are gone. For me, it just totally changed how I looked at things. We all do, we all look at the things you worry about . . . they are very minimal to what these people have gone through and are still facing. It makes your heart go out to them, because you try to give to them. And, then you still need to give to them a year later. Those who are still there a year later are still trying to fix their houses up. I have family and friends that this has affected. My parents were without power for three weeks. I have had minimal damage to my house and yard—my parents did, too. We were the lucky ones.

Mary went on to tell the interviewer:

> I was in the ER. For the most part, I was there constantly that first week. The conditions were horrible . . . unbelievable heat, humidity, long, hard hours of meeting all kinds of medical needs. I basically do ER nursing. We had patients that came in anywhere from, "I had to leave and I don't have my medicine," to "I only have 5 days of medicine," "I don't have my diabetic supplies." Or, they were on Coumadin and were diabetics. We had people who said, "I was supposed to have heart surgery the day of the hurricane and it got cancelled. What do I do? The hospital is destroyed." We saw everything from that to fractures after the cleanup. Then, just the regular, "I cannot breathe. We don't have electricity and my oxygen is running out. I need oxygen." I also went to the airport to pick up and triage patients there, and get them in from the airplane. Seeing them come off the plane . . . Even now I cannot really talk about it without tearing up. That was just a vision that will probably never leave me. They looked like POWs. Their clothes were torn, they had on dirty clothes, or a pajama bottom or shirt that they were given. Or, their clothes were torn or ripped. Some had cut their pants off because it was so hot. They had shoes on, and I know that when they left that was all they had. The look on the faces was of sadness and defeat. From then on, I guess that is what has the most emotional effect on me. I still have moments when I relive it. It is not bad, but can really take the joy out of a birthday, for example. I think, I am lucky to be a year older, rather than, gosh, I hate getting older.

Discussion

Anxiety, helplessness, fear, frustration, anger, sadness, guilt, and a sense of feeling totally overwhelmed by the devastation and loss were only some of the emotions experienced by the nurses and the people they cared for. Nurses and many victims tried to cope by pulling together and providing support to others as best they could. It may be that because nurses had a body of knowledge to draw upon and a role to play, they could marshal their coping skills to be effective in meeting the needs of those around them, despite the environmental conditions. Nurses could derive professional sense of meaning from the trauma of their work (Frank & Sullivan, 2008).

The after effects of the hurricanes—with nurses verbalizing experiences of post-traumatic distress symptoms, being unable to forget the images, having the realization that everything has changed and nothing will be the same as it had been—are human responses to natural disaster and are likely prevalent among many who experienced Hurricane Katrina. Nurses talked to each other and found support from each other. They worked through their feelings after the crisis period had passed, and some communities were also able to pull together to rebuild and move forward. Yet, for nurses and victims directly involved in the destruction wreaked by Katrina, as well as the general population who was not directly involved, Katrina has revealed the weaknesses in their emergency response system that were never anticipated. It has forced nurses and the general population to reassess their value system as well as their own plans for disaster preparedness. It has changed this population forever.

Epilogue

As this narrative and reflection on findings from the Katrina nurses' experience was first begun, and while the coastal area was still in Katrina's wake, Myanmar (Burma) was hit with a cyclone on May 3, 2008. Thousands of people were without water, food, and shelter. The United Nations estimated at the time that 100,000 people died. Many more died from lack of timely assistance. As many as 1.5–2.5 million people still needed assistance when this chapter was first begun. Thousands were predicted to die within a very short time if rescue, clean water, food, and medical care were not made available. Many were still missing, and thousands of people were at risk of exposure and disease. As in Katrina, the children, sick, elderly, and the poor were among the most vulnerable.

Another cyclone threatened the same region the week after this chapter was begun. In addition, a total of 7,000,000 people live in the delta and coastal region. The military junta in rule in Myanmar had been refusing international aid initially; visas for aide agency volunteers were not being approved; 4 weeks later supplies and people were finally being allowed in to assist the population, but were not allowed to go into the remote areas, where the devastation was thought to be greater. People suffered unimaginable conditions.

The earthquake in January 2010, which devastated Haiti, the Chile earthquake, and the earthquake in southern California are reminders that disaster care is becoming more and more relevant. It is of interest that the writing of this chapter has coincided with other large-scale disasters around the world. Findings from this Katrina study when considered alongside news reports of the Haiti disaster demonstrate that people continue to suffer from the devastation of earthquakes and disasters long after the initial event. News and personal stories describe incredible conditions of survival and disaster. The level of poverty in Haiti, including living conditions, in good times was often difficult for the people. Following the quake disaster, the human suffering has been almost indescribable. Billions of dollars in aid have been pledged by nations to rebuild Haiti, but clearly more supervision and direct involvement are needed to ensure that aid does reach those who need it the most. Political issues in areas of disasters often confound the process.

Similarly, socioeconomic factors are involved in disasters. At the time of Katrina, many of the federal, state, and local emergency resources had been deployed to Iraq. This was particularly significant for the National Guard, who often responded to domestic needs. The inadequate response of agencies to Katrina was tossed about in the media as related to the Iraq War and necessary deployment of equipment, supplies, and personnel. Additionally, in the back of the public's mind was knowledge of the simple fact that the National Guard numbers were low, since many had been deployed to Iraq along with emergency equipment and supplies.

For the Gulf region, Myanmar, China, Haiti, and Chile, political issues continue to be involved in protection and recovery responses. There has been less public focus on Chile, perhaps since it is viewed as a resource-rich country. Abuses of power and politics often become more visible in disasters. The uncovering of need, following disaster is opportunity for local, regional, and global responses and activism. The poor, marginalized, and often forgotten, vulnerable people are most at risk in disaster. In addition, first responders and care givers are in need of care, attention, and continuing support following the immediate crisis resolution.

Similar to uncovering disparities in New Orleans following Katrina, the disparities in poverty and plight of the Haitian people are more visible following the earthquake. While the Presidential palace was destroyed in Haiti, built during a time when American contributions to the Haitian government were high, it is clear that American money was not distributed adequately to provide services and care for Haitian people. The earthquake uncovered a grossly inadequate infrastructure and service system. As the rainy season in Haiti is just beginning following the destruction of millions of homes and shelters, it is predicted that more death, disease, and human suffering will occur as basic needs are not met.

In the Haitian recovery and rebuilding phase ahead, it is clear that human needs and human rights issues need to be addressed. There are often hidden issues involved in providing relief and aid to underdeveloped countries following catastrophic disaster. Katrina and the 2005 hurricanes exposed tremendous economic and ethnic disparities in human life, human rights, poverty, and vulnerability, along the Gulf coastal area, and particularly, in New Orleans. Such weakness will likely continue to be uncovered in future disasters in unprepared areas.

The 2008 earthquake in China similarly was accompanied with devastation of proportion, which had been unimagined. Even though China was later receptive to aid, it initially rejected aid from other countries. Clearly the country and world were caught with grossly inadequate preparations. The lack of a timely response to aid further impoverished the population. In the last few years, China had undergone a massive building program. However, the quake has exposed inadequate, faulty construction practices, which, in a region of frequent earthquakes, put the very large population in extreme danger. Large lakes caused by the earthquake threatened hundreds of thousands of people with flood waters. Additionally, the vulnerability of the nuclear plants in China's Chengdu province threatened another disaster. One questioned at the time if construction of nuclear plants had also been compromised during the massive building phase.

When this chapter was first begun, there were more than 80,000 people confirmed dead in China and the number climbed every day, with more than 23, 000 still missing. There were 59,000 rescue workers, and reports from news agencies indicated that rescue workers were in dire need of sleep and respite care.

Just as Katrina nurses' need for personal care underpinned their ability to care for others, there was a need for support and protective efforts aimed at assisting all rescue workers in the handling of difficult work caring for victim survivors. The stress of caring for people who have experienced such devastating losses is significant for caregivers. Katrina nurses talked about the restorative effects of a good meal and a night's sleep.

Katrina exposed poverty with ethnic and cultural overtones. The earthquake in China has exposed the need for building codes and standards that are earthquake worthy. The cyclone in Myanmar exposed a military junta that was prohibiting aid from reaching the people. The Haiti earthquake exposed gross injustices in standards of living among the leaders and population, among those with resources and adequate housing, and those who had not. The United Nations has convened a humanitarian resolution to intervene in the rebuilding of Haiti and has billions of dollars from nations that have pledged for the purpose. Natural disasters expose issues of local, regional, national, and international concern, especially in the increasingly global economy and politic, with 24-hour news and the increasing journalistic accounts of citizens with cell phones with video and picture capability. Today, if one watches national news, one simply cannot be unaware and uninformed of impending disaster. Video and personal accounts of experience are compelling and facilitate understanding of disaster and need.

Compared to Myanmar, or the quake in China, considering the vast resources of the United States, the response of the emergency and care systems was completely, surprisingly, overwhelmed by the storms of 2005 and Katrina. The storm brought into public scrutiny that there had been a lack of funding and support for levee construction in New Orleans; the system was not able to withstand a category 5 hurricane as advised by the Corps of Engineers.

Now, years later, the memory and plight of New Orleans and the coastal people is fading. Following Katrina, the demographics of New Orleans and the Gulf region changed forever. The storm exposed the condition and plight of the poor and disadvantaged in a city where, although officials and the public were somewhat aware, these issues had previously been hidden. It was not completely unknown, because the crime rate and level of disrepair in poor neighborhoods like the Ninth District attracted attention from time to time. During the storm and afterwards, the storm exposed the disparities existing in New Orleans relating to poverty, wealth, and opportunity.

Summary and Reflection on Practice

Natural disasters are local, national, and global events and are occurring at a seemingly increasing intensity in recent years. These events expose the strengths as well as the weaknesses within populations and the response systems. Statistics are very useful in determining the magnitude of a health phenomenon or disaster. However, it is also important to realize that each statistic represents a human consequence, and that each person is connected to many others, including family, community, work group, and more. Often the human consequence is not made explicit in statistics. In qualitative research it is possible to humanize the use of statistics, rates, and the like through descriptions of human experiences.

Regardless of the cause of the destruction and need, where or when it occurs, nurses and volunteer workers are greatly needed and appreciated in order to achieve a timely, appropriate, effective, and meaningful response in caring for people experiencing crisis and disaster. Nurses and other disaster workers have to cope with their own responses personally and professionally while caring for people affected by disaster and devastation. Understanding lived experience of nurses in caring for victims of Katrina provided insight into the needs of nurses, caregivers, and other disaster workers.

It is evident from examining the experience of Katrina nurses, that more attention is needed in planning care for the caregivers and disaster workers during and after disaster, regardless of when and where they occur. This finding and outcome of this research is gleaned from a retrospective review of the original transcripts with Katrina nurses regarding their experience. In addition to being accessible to the international nursing audience, the findings from the phenomenological study and this linguistic transformative reflection need to be made public so that each community can include as disaster care protocol a critically important, *caring for the caregiver plan.*

Since the mid to late 1990s, there has been an increasing development of literature focused on reflection in nursing practice. In the 1970s and 1980s attention to nursing work increased. It is assumed that many nurses experience difficulties in dealing with the stress of caring, and many experience a high potential for burnout. Menzies's (1970) classic study completed while at the Tavistock Institute of Human Relations concerned nursing service in a London hospital. Menzies looked at strategies and staffing patterns developed by nursing administration to deal with the stress of nursing. She pointed out that many of the shift and staffing patterns developed to help nurses deal with stress often create more stress. Nearly 2 decades later, Wolf's (1988) qualitative dissertation described nursing work as encompassing elements of the sacred and the profane. Her reflection on nursing rituals has been especially meaningful.

In the 1990s and early 2000s, reflective practice has been addressed in international professional nursing literature. Several works on reflective practice and becoming a reflective nurse practitioner have been particularly informative (Hentz & Lauterbach, 2005; Lauterbach, 2005a, 2005b, 2008; Lauterbach & Becker, 1996, 1998). The studies' authors, who are educators and colleagues, found that many registered nurses who were returning to educational programs to complete a baccalaureate degree were either close to burnout or contemplating leaving the profession. Nurses needed to develop self-care strategies in order to help prevent burnout and to deal with the stress of nursing care.

The reflective and scholarly work on caring for self is especially relevant to the Katrina nurses' needs and experience. There is a need to address the needs of disaster workers during and following disaster work. There is a need for development of more involved support programs than the simple debriefing sessions described by several of the nurses. Some had no debriefing whatsoever. Rather, there is a need for recovery support, identifying and caring for nurses' and disaster workers' needs. While the restorative effects of a good meal and a good night's sleep were identified, disaster care needs to be developed more fully. There is a need for a more involved follow-up with nurses over time. Needs, like meanings in experience, continue to be evident and change over time (Lauterbach, 2005a).

Nurses expressed their appreciation for the opportunity to talk with researchers and described the healing effects of talking about the experience and for contributing to knowledge by participating in research. Therapeutic effects were described by nurses simply as a result of participation in research. Several participants were also interested in learning about the findings from the study. Nurse researchers Frank and Sullivan (2008) made attempts to call and talk with nurses who participated. They provided nurses with opportunities to explore continuing needs for support, in addition to exploring new thoughts and reflections on their experience. Over time, meanings change and continue to evolve as they become more visible. It is important to follow up research which focuses on difficult or traumatic experiences, with opportunities for participants to process and reflect (Lauterbach, 2005b).

References

Frank, D., & Sullivan, L. (2008). The lived experience of nurses providing care to victims of the 2005 hurricanes. *Online Journal of Nursing Research, 8*(3).

Hentz, P., & Lauterbach, S. S. (2005). Becoming self reflective: Caring for self and others. *International Journal for Human Caring, 9*(1).

Lauterbach, S. S. (1993). In another world: A phenomenological perspective and discovery of meaning in mothers' experience of death of a wished-for baby. In P. L. Munhall & C. Oiler (Eds.), *Nursing research: A qualitative perspective.* New York: National League for Nursing Press.

Lauterbach, S. S. (1998). In another world: "Essences" of mothers' mourning experience. In P. L. Munhall (Ed.), *In women's experience* (pp. 233–293). New York: National League for Nursing Press.

Lauterbach, S. S. (2000). In another world: Five years later. In P. L. Munhall (Ed.), *Nursing research: A qualitative perspective.* Sudbury, MA: Jones & Bartlett.

Lauterbach, S. S. (2003). Phenomenological silence surrounding infant death. *International Journal of Human Caring, 7*(23), 38–43.

Lauterbach, S. S. (2005a, May 11–13). *Reflective nursing education: Caring for self, the process, the experience, with qualitative outcomes.* Presented at Qualitative Methods Conference, Utrecht, The Netherlands.

Lauterbach, S. S. (2005b, May 11–13). *Uncovering silence, discovering, and creating meanings in experience over time: Qualitative outcomes and therapeutic process in phenomenologic research.* Qualitative Methods Conference, Utrecht, The Netherlands.

Lauterbach, S. S. (2006). *Qualitative outcomes and therapeutic process in Phenomenologic research.* Isabel Stewart 2006 Research Conference, Nursing Alumni Association (NEAA) Teachers College, Columbia University, New York, NY. April 21, 2006.

Lauterbach, S. S. (2007). Meanings in mothers' experience with infant death: Three phenomenological inquiries: In another world; Five years later; and What forever means. In P. L. Munhall (Ed.), *Nursing research: A qualitative perspective* (pp. 221–227). Sudbury, MA: Jones & Bartlett.

Lauterbach, S. S. (2008, April 18). *Reflective nursing education: Caring for self, the process, the experience, with qualitative outcomes.* Exhibit at Epsilon Pi Chapter Research Conference, Valdosta State University.

Lauterbach, S. S., & Becker, P. (1996). "Caring for self: Becoming a self reflective nurse. *Journal of Holistic Nursing Practice, 10*(2), 57–68.

Lauterbach, S. S., & Becker, P. (1998). Caring for self: Becoming a self-reflective nurse. In K. E. Guzetta (Ed.), *Essential readings in holistic nursing* (pp. 97–107). Gaithersburg, MD: Aspen.

Lauterbach, S. S., & Hentz, P. (2005). Journaling to learn: A reflective nursing education strategy to develop the nurse as person and person as nurse. *International Journal for Human Caring, 9*(1).

Menzies, I. P. (1970). *The social system as a defence against anxiety.* London: Tavistock.

Munhall, P. (1994). *In women's experience.* New York: National League for Nursing Press.

Munhall, P. (2001). *Nursing Research: A qualitative perspective.* (3rd ed.) Boston: National League for Nursing.

Munhall, P. (2007). *Nursing research: A qualitative perspective.* (4th ed.) Sudbury, MA: Jones & Bartlett.

Munhall, P. & Oiler, C. (1986). *Nursing research: A qualitative perspective.* Norwalk: Appleton-Century-Crofts.

Munhall, P., & Oiler, C. (1993). *Nursing research: A qualitative perspective.* Sudbury, MA: Jones & Bartlett.

Sullivan, L., & Frank, D. (2008, February 21). *The lived experience of nurses providing care to victims of the 2005 hurricanes.* The Southern Nursing Research Society Annual Conference (SNRS) Podium Presentation, Birmingham, AL.

van Manen, M. (1984). *"Doing" phenomenological research and writing.* Alberta, Canada: The University of Alberta Press.

van Manen, M. (1990). *Researching lived experience: Human science for an action sensitive pedagogy.* New York: SUNY Press.

van Manen, M. (1997). *Researching lived experience: Human science for an action sensitive pedagogy.* (2nd ed.) Ontario, Canada: The University of Ontario.

van Manen, M. (2002). *Writing in the dark: Phenomenological studies for interpretive inquiry.* London, Ontario: The University of Western Ontario.

Wolf, Z. R. (1988). *Nurses work, the sacred and the profane.* Philadelphia: The University of Pennsylvania Press.

7

Exemplar: Grief Interrupted: The Experience of Loss Among Incarcerated Women

Holly M. Harner, Patricia Hentz, and Maria Carmela Evangelista; Corresponding Author: Holly M. Harner

*Qualitative Health Research OnlineFirst
Copyright 2010 by SAGE, Reprinted by
Permission of SAGE Publications, Inc.*

Incarcerated women face a number of stressors apart from the actual incarceration. Nearly half of all women in prison experience the death of a loved one during their incarceration. Our purpose for this study was to explore the experience of grief and loss among incarcerated women using a phenomenological method. Our study approach followed van Manen's method of phenomenology and Munhall's description of the existential life worlds. Our analysis revealed four existential life worlds: temporality: frozen in time; spatiality: no place, no space to grieve; corporeality: buried emotions; and relationality: never alone, yet feeling so lonely. Our findings generated from this study can help mental health providers as well as correctional professionals develop policies and programs that facilitate the grief process of incarcerated women within the confines of imprisonment.

The number of women in prison has increased by more than 800% in the last 3 decades (Greene, Pranis, & Frost, 2006). In 2008, there were more than

---

Originally published in Qualitative Health Research (QHR).

115,000 women who were imprisoned in state and federal institutions in the
United States, representing a 3% annual increase (West, Sabol, & Cooper,
2010). Incarcerated women, most of whom have significant mental health
and medical problems that predate their imprisonment, face a number of
stressors apart from the actual incarceration (Keaveny & Zauszniewski, 1999).
The death of a loved one is one stressor that nearly half of all women in prison
experience during their incarceration. For incarcerated women, poor health
coupled with the limited social supports and restrictions imposed by incarceration can have a significant impact on the grieving process. Because of the
paucity of knowledge on inmates' experience of loss in prison, the purpose of
our phenomenological study was to explore the experience of loss of a loved
one. Although grieving is a normal universal experience, grieving in prison is
met with additional challenges, placing these women at high risk for unresolved or complicated grief. Understanding their experience has important
implications for the women themselves, mental health and medical services,
correctional staff, and the larger community of taxpayers who support the
state correctional health system. Finally, we provide recommendations for future research, practice, and policy.

Evolution of the Study

Our study aim was to describe the experience of losing a loved one through
death while incarcerated. Our research assumption was that much of the available data on grief and adaptation to loss did not fully address the effect of incarceration on the experience of loss. The first author's experience working
with women in a maximum security women's prison prompted the current
study. At that time the work involved implementing an exercise intervention
program. As the women became comfortable, they shared more personal aspects of their lives. It began with one of the participants discussing her
mother's failing health and impending death. She expressed guilt, powerlessness, and lack of control. Her sharing led to other women sharing the pain of
having a family member die during their incarceration. Another inmate whose
mother had died had a picture of her mother taped to her uniform. The wrin-
kled photograph showed her mother smiling and surrounded by several generations of children. Next to the picture was taped a Mass card. The woman
tearfully shared that her mother had died and she was unable to attend any of
the funeral or memorial services because they were out of state. She was unsure of the cause of death because family members had told her only "bits and
pieces" over the phone. Although family members sent her pictures of her
mother in the casket, she said, "It doesn't look like her." Placing the picture of
her mother and the Mass card on her uniform was her way of remembering
her mother and showing her respect for her life. This action also signaled to

others, including other inmates, correctional staff, and healthcare profession-als, that she was grieving. Together, these women expressed that grief in prison is often experienced without the support of family and without witness to rit-uals surrounding death. It is important to understand the experience of los-ing a loved one while incarcerated in order to meet the mental health needs of this vulnerable population.

Justification and Significance

Although almost half of all women in prison report experiencing the death of a close friend or family member while incarcerated, scant data exist that elucidate the experience of grief and loss among female inmates. Our pur-pose was to explore the phenomenon of loss using a phenomenological ap-proach. We interviewed women incarcerated in a minimum security prison located in the Northeastern part of the United States. It is hoped that knowl-edge gained from this investigation can help correctional nursing, mental health, and medical staff better anticipate the health needs of women during this difficult time. Findings from this investigation might also help Depart-ments of Correction (DOC) respond appropriately to inmates during their times of loss while still maintaining pertinent security protocols. Because loss of a loved one is a universal experience, findings from this work may also help generate knowledge about the experience of loss among other popula-tions of women who are left to grieve alone in similarly constrained situa-tions, including women in the military, women in shelters, and women separated by migration.

Review of the Literature

Grief is a term commonly used to describe the emotional response to the loss of a loved one through death (Stroebe, Hansson, Schut, & Stroebe, 2008). Grieving involves a process of diverse psychological and physical elements, which occur differently among individuals (Stroebe et al., 2008). Mental health symptoms of grief include depression and anxiety, anger, suicidal ideation, and post-traumatic stress disorder (PTSD; Stroebe, Schut, & Stroebe, 2007). Although grief is an unavoidable and universal experience, for some the experience is much more intense, leading to what has been described as unresolved grief, pro-tracted grief, traumatic grief, or complicated grief and symptoms similar to PTSD ("Complicated grief," 2006).

There is an abundance of research and theory in the distinct yet related areas of grief, death, mourning, and suffering. A common consensus that dominates the literature is that in order for individuals to achieve a resolu-tion and experience a degree of acceptance, a state of peace with the loss must be reached (Cutcliffe, 1998). The work of Kübler-Ross and Kessler (2005) on the experience of death and dying lists five stages that characterize a normal grieving process: denial, anger, bargaining, depression, and acceptance. Bowlby (1980) described three phases of mourning beginning with the preoccupation with the lost person, followed by a second phase that focuses on the pain of the experience, and then a final phase of reorganization characterized by a return to normal functioning. In the reorganization phase, memories and experiences of the pain of loss might still occur with associations to the memory.

Gorle (2008) noted the importance of ceremonies, rites, signs, symbols, and rituals in assisting individuals to cope with crisis and change in the grieving process. Gorle illustrated his point, writing, "The act of sprinkling or shoveling earth onto the casket in the grave is a poignant 'ceremony' within the funeral 'ritual' that speaks to the finality of death. It is the action in and of itself that is the 'ceremony.'" Gorle also explained that rituals like funerals, wakes, and services allow for the freedom of expression of feelings surrounding loss due to death of a loved one and that these rituals have the potential to assist in navigating the tasks and stages in the grieving process.

Not all individuals experience uncomplicated grief. Parkes and Weiss (1983) identified three patterns of abnormal grieving: unanticipated grief, complicated grief, and chronic grief. Raphael (1983) similarly highlighted three patterns of pathological grief: distorted grief, chronic grief, and absent, delayed, or inhibited grief. Parkes (1998) discussed the potential effect of unresolved grief in individuals—like the incarcerated—who are prevented the experience of grief either by internal or external factors. These individuals are more likely to experience sleep disorders, depression, and hypochondriac symptoms. Unresolved grief can result in a number of complicated grieving processes. Among them is disenfranchised grief. It is characterized by the inability to grieve due to external restrictions (Gilbert, 2007) and ultimately results in grief that is not allowed to be publicly expressed (Young, 2003). The resulting transitions lead the individual to perceive the loss as ambiguous or lacking a sense of clarity (Gilbert, 2007), which doubly complicates the grieving process.

The concept of suffering, as outlined by Morse (2001), encompasses two behavioral states: enduring and emotional suffering. The concept of suffering informs our work on grief in several ways. Enduring behaviors, which include suppressing emotions and focusing on the present, allow sufferers to survive, to live, and, in some cases, to die. The second type of enduring, enduring to live, is voiced by those suffering as the need to "just get through the day." This need to "pull it together" can be seen in many stages of the grief process as an individual "recognizes that he or she must function in order to survive or get through the situation" (Morse, 2001, p. 52). This functioning might include writing obituaries, making funeral arrangements, and comforting others. Although the trajectory of suffering is not linear in nature, behaviors associated with emotional suffering include releasing emotions and publically displaying suffering (crying, sobbing, moaning, etc.). Morse postulated that emotional suffering is necessary for healing as it allows individuals to work through their suffering until they have "suffered enough" (p. 51). Subsequently, individuals slowly reformulate their future, set realistic goals, and move forward. For some individuals, however, the nature and context of their life and situation might require prolonged periods of endurance. As a result, they must internalize their emotions. Though their emotions are guarded and their suffering hidden from others, their suppressed energy might be released as angry outbursts often directed at something unrelated to the actual cause of suffering.

Loss and Grief Among Incarcerated Women

Incarcerated women are disproportionately women of color; they are primarily from low-income families with fragmented family histories and are survivors of sexual and/or physical abuse as children or adults (Browne, Miller, & Maguin, 1999; Greenfeld & Snell, 1999; Harlow, 1999). Almost half have high school degrees or passed the General Educational Development (GED) test and most have limited vocational training or work experience. Many have significant substance abuse problems and mental health issues (Covington, 2007). The Bureau of Justice Statistics reported in 2006 that 73% of the women in state prisons and 75% of women in local jails have symptoms of mental health disorders, compared to 12% reported among females in the general population. Among the inmates who had mental health issues, three-quarters also met the criteria for substance abuse and dependence (James & Glaze, 2006). All of these factors may further complicate the experience of grief and loss.

Ferszt (2002) succeeded in describing the lived experiences of inmates with regard to the loss of loved ones. The investigator used qualitative methods based on in-depth interviews with three participants and suggested that women who lost a loved one through death during their incarceration suffered unresolved grief and a lack of integration and resolution. Furthermore, Ferszt described the circumstances surrounding the experience of loss by women in prison as marked by absence of support, relatives, and counseling; lack of time spent with the deceased as a consequence of incarceration; and prohibitions to attending the funeral. Gaps were also seen in the process of informing the inmate and creating provisions for a supportive environment for grieving. Uninhibited expression of grief was hindered by the fear of disciplinary action from supervisors.

Phenomenological Perspective

The process of uncomplicated grief has been well documented with stages and tasks to facilitate the accommodation of the loss. Although the exact timeline for grieving varies among experts, it is a process that transitions from acute grief toward an integration of the loss and a return to the everyday world. From a phenomenological perspective, human behavior is understood as it occurs in the context of relationships to things, people, events, and situations in what Merleau-Ponty (1989) referred to as embodiment (Boyd, 1993). Based on this concept, people are tied to their worlds, and perception is more than what is thought—it includes the mind and body.

Thoughts, feelings, and emotions are deeply embedded in the participant's life, or life world (Munhall, 2007). Thus, understanding the experience of loss for incarcerated women needs to take into count their spatial, corporeal, temporal, and relational life worlds (Munhall, 2007). Spatiality involves exploring the space or environment and its meaning related to the lived experience. Specifically, we understand the experience by taking into consideration the "situated context." Corporeality or embodiment refers to experiencing the phenomenon as lived through one's body, which is described by Munhall (2007) as body intelligence. Temporality relates to the element of time and the perception of time as it relates to the phenomenon. Relationality is the connection to self and others in the world. Finally, each of these life worlds is connected and overlaps.

Methods

We obtained approval from the Institutional Review Board (IRB) and the DOC's Research Division in fall 2005 and placed a flyer asking for participants in the dayroom of the prison. The flyer was written at the Flesch-Kincaide Grade level 4.5 (passive sentences = 0%; Flesch reading ease = 85.7; Flesch, 1948). Women who were interested in the study gave their names to the registered nurse located in the Health Services Unit. The first author contacted women who were interested in participating, described the study, and obtained informed consent. Because of the high rate of illiteracy in prison populations, the informed consent document was read aloud to all potential participants. Women who spoke and understood English, but did not read and write, were enrolled in a study by "making their mark" on the consent document (Food and Drug Administration, 2009).

Many of the participants were aware that in addition to the first author's role at the university, she also practiced as a nurse practitioner in the facility. The first author was aware of the power differential and attempted to "create a welcoming, nonthreatening environment" (Karnieli-Miller, Strier, & Pessach, 2009, p. 280) as well as diffuse any perceived coercion using several strategies. First, flyers regarding the study were not posted near the Health Services Unit.

Next, as noted, women interested in participating did not give their name to the first author, but rather to the registered nurse in the Health Services Unit. During the course of the informed consent, as well as during the actual interview, participants were provided an opportunity to ask questions. Furthermore, they were informed that participation in this investigation would have no impact on their sentence length, sentence structure, parole, or their access to health services. No incentives to participate, including money, time out of work, or other prison groups/programs, were given. Participants were advised that they were free to end the interview at any point in time without fear of reprisal. Participants were made aware that the first author was a mandated reporter and would report to the designated medical/mental health professional any indication of suicidal or homicidal ideation. Last, participants were informed that the function of the interview was investigatory in nature and that in order to receive mental health care or counseling, they should seek immediate care through the registered nurse located in the Health Services Unit.

We invited women to participate in the audio taped interview if they had served at least 3 months in prison (for their current sentence) and had experienced the death of a loved one (as defined by the participant) during their current confinement. Loved ones included, but were not limited to friends, family members, partners, and children. Women who had lost more than one loved one while incarcerated were able to discuss whichever loss/losses was/were the most significant to them. Although the length of time since the death was noted, no discrimination was made on how recently the loss was experienced. Because the investigation was qualitative in nature, thus requiring ongoing dialogue between the participant and the first author (who speaks English), only women who spoke English were included in the investigation. Women who had suffered a miscarriage as their only loss during incarceration were ineligible. Women who had suffered the death of a pet were not included.

Women who participated in the study were asked to describe the experience of losing a loved one while incarcerated. Specifically, the interview was opened with one specific question, "Please tell me, in your own words, about the experience of losing your (mother, grandmother, etc.) while you were incarcerated." The word "loss" was chosen as it reflected the common vernacular used by women at the study site ("I lost my mom"). Every attempt was made to allow the participant to continue speaking without interruption. However, probing questions were used if clarification was needed, or if the participant needed prompting. These in-depth interviews lasted 1–2 hours. Interviews were audio taped and transcribed verbatim. The third author took notes during the interviews, recoding the participant's body language and emotions (such as crying). Written field notes were recorded after each interview was conducted, identifying relevant concepts and ideas that were beginning to emerge as well as pertinent issues that developed related to the prison facility itself.

Data Analysis

The second author's expertise in phenomenology was instrumental in guiding the analysis of the data. As stated by van Manen (1990), phenomenology aims at a deeper understanding of the nature or meaning of our everyday experiences. "Meaning is found in the transaction between the individual and a situation" (Munhall, 2007, p. 162). We approached this study using van Manen's (1990) method of phenomenology with four concurrent processes involving 11 steps. The first process, turning to the nature of the lived experience, involved orienting to the phenomenon, formulating the phenomenological question, and explicating assumptions and pre-understandings. Using purposive sampling, 15 incarcerated women who had experienced a loss of a loved one agreed to be interviewed. The second process, the existential investigation, involved exploring the phenomenon. We used Munhall's (2007) description of the existential life worlds in the data analysis with specific attention to the four existential life worlds: temporality, spatiality, corporeality, and relationality. Work by Hentz (2002) was also used in the development of themes and the organization of the existential life worlds. The third process, phenomenological reflection, relates to the thematic analysis, the process of reflecting on the lived experience of these women. Our aim was to uncover the essence of the experience for each participant as well as the common themes. We explored how words were used and how common patterns and essential themes related to the experience. The fourth process was phenomenological writing that involved creating phenomenological descriptions in order to sensitize the reader to the "deeper significance or structure of the lived experience being described" (Munhall, 2007, p. 162; van Manen, 1990).

Findings

A total of 15 women responded to the flyer. The age range of the 15 participants was 23–67 years (X = 39, SD = 11.5). Among the respondents, three of the participants were African American, four were Hispanic, and eight were White. The length of their current sentence that had been served ranged from 4 months to 11 years (X = 4.1, SD = 3.7). The themes we uncovered have been organized around the four existential life worlds; temporality, spatiality, corporeality, and relationality.

Temporality: Frozen in Time

The grieving process for the women who participated in our study gave the appearance of being suspended in time. For some it had been years since the loss of a loved one, but they felt that they could not really grieve the loss until they were out of prison. Women spoke of not having closure because they did not participate in the funeral or see the gravesite. Although they all acknowledged that death was real, there was an element of disbelief—a sense that it was not real until they could actually see it for themselves. As one woman expressed,

> So I think I was still in shock. It was only a year and I don't think I have dealt with it yet. Like I have to go home and see, go to the cemetery and see for myself. I think that's what I need. I am not in denial that she is dead because I know she is dead. It's just seeing it that I think will be the moment that I will probably break down.

Women expressed that the time to grieve would be when they returned home. It would be a process that they would be doing alone because all their family had already finished their grieving. Indeed, the timeline for grieving was suspended while incarcerated. One woman expressed how she will be completely alone in her grieving:

> I could not grieve them the way you'd normally do if you were on the outside. Like pay your respects, go the family's house, and stuff like that, and it's hard because like when I go home, it's been months since this happened. I don't feel like going to the family's house now and me rehashing the pain for them because they've already gone through the process.

Only a few women were permitted to leave the prison to attend their loved one's viewing. One woman whose son died was given 15 minutes at the funeral home to see her son's body. For her it was not enough time to bring closure and begin grieving.

> I saw him there to say goodbye. I think that maybe if they had given me a few extra minutes. . . . I just need to have some kind of closure so that we can move on. People need more than 15 minutes. The 15 minutes is cruel. Fifteen minutes . . . just isn't long enough, unless you are like some kind of dangerous psycho escapee, you know, someone who is a real threat. But you know they wouldn't even let you go if you were like that. People need more time than 15 minutes. So I think I'm not going to start grieving until I leave here. When I can go to the cemetery. It's going to be strange to go home after all this time.

Spatiality: No Place, No Space to Grieve

For these women, prison was not the *place* to grieve, and there is no personal *space* for grieving. There is no privacy in prison. Participants voiced that there are always people around but not ones who truly cared. Women spoke of the lack of privacy and that many of them were informed in front of other inmates that their loved one had died. Women yearned for a place where they could be alone to grieve without others witnessing their distress. And for most, facing the reality of the loss and being able to grieve was associated with being out of prison and at home. The lack of privacy and space is recounted in this woman's experience:

> Right in front of everybody. They made me call in front of everybody. It was horrible. The experience just sucked. I used the admissions phone and there was new people coming in and there were officers everywhere. And the officers, they didn't even really give a shit. They were just looking at me like just another day.

Some women expressed that they were not in their real life—"out of sight" and "out of mind"—and that their grieving would begin when they got back home. Prison was no place to grieve:

> It just doesn't seem real because I am not in my real life right now. I'm not in the environment I'm in. I'm not in the state of mind that I'm normally in at home. I'm not in a routine that I'm in. I am stuck away locked up. Nothing here is normal.

Even when women were given a physical space to meet with loved ones, the space was no place to express loss or sadness. One woman recounted her experience of visiting with her father in the prison visiting room shortly after her mother had been buried. She said:

> My father came to visit me the next week, he just buried my mother. I said, "My dad's coming. My mother just passed last week and he just buried her, could we maybe sit in the corner over there by ourselves?" Because I knew we were going to cry. They said, "No." So we had to sit in this visiting room with all these people hugging and crying and trying to do it quietly.

During the interview, one woman discussed how comforting and peaceful it was in the private interview space, stating:

> I wish I had someplace to go where I could just be. Just not be stressed by outside factors, a roommate who doesn't want to have you in the room. I just wish I had somewhere where I could just go and get some peace. I wish that I could just stay in this room. Just sleep on the floor under that chair. That's how I feel. I am just so desperately tired and so desperately in need of something. In need of peace. I can't get a bit of peace.

Corporeality: Buried Emotions

One comes to more fully understand an experience through the body's experience of the phenomenon. Munhall (2007) described it as the starting point of meaning. These women experienced an acute response to the loss followed by an urgent need to block their emotional responses. Many of the women shared that it was too risky to show their feelings. Being emotional and crying in front of other inmates made them look weak and vulnerable. So too, excess displays of emotion could be interpreted by correctional officers as being a potential suicide risk. Women did not want to be locked up in a room for suicide precautions so they concealed the expression of emotions and in doing so also blocked their grieving.

Denying the body its expression contributed to the suspension of the grieving process for these women. They were not in denial of the loss, but they indeed denied themselves the ability to express their grief. The emotional expression was controlled but the emotional pain and anguish were buried deep inside. For these women the pain of the loss lived in their bodies. Merleau-Ponty (1989) wrote, "[the] haunting of the present by a particular past experience is possible because we all carry our past with us insofar as its structures have become 'sedimented' in our habitual body" (p. 33). Thus, these women carry their unresolved grief. The following story was common among these women; it illustrates the initial response and then the control of emotions:

> So when my mother told me, I just broke down in pieces. . . . It was a lot of emotions. I think that it just was very devastating. . . . I could not stop crying. I mean I was constantly crying. . . . I couldn't drink water. I couldn't eat. I am always trying to be in control of my feelings and not let them overwhelm me because of the long time I have to do here and I was always scared to get put in one of those rooms you know because they think you're going to do something to yourself and I always try to be okay. Everything is okay. I talk to myself and try to handle my feelings. People never see me crying that often. I wanted to die because I couldn't handle the pain. I felt that the pain was so bad. . . . People cannot express their true feelings. I wanted to cry and cry and cry but I couldn't cry the way I wanted to because I was scared I was going to be put in a room with no clothes on and have somebody look at me 24/7.

Women spoke about the lack of concern even when someone experiences the death of a loved one. They discussed how they needed to control their expression of grief for fear that they would be seen as weak by the other inmates. These women described the need to put up walls in order to be able to deal with things. They became immune to feeling. Showing too much emotion, they believed, placed them at risk for being locked up for suicide precautions. As one woman stated:

> If you cry too much or if they see that you're having a hard time, maybe adapting, they'll put you back behind the wall and I don't want that to

happen. So I continue to try to pick myself up every morning. I try to preoccupy my mind . . . I really do not want to be around people. My biggest thing is that I just have to stay out of my room because if they see me isolating and crying too much they will ship me back over there.

In addition to sadness, women spoke of anger, "feeling so damn mad," as an emotion that needed to be buried inside and controlled, even hidden from mental health providers. The desire to physically act out their anger was tempered by fear of getting "locked up." As one woman, who did seek mental health care shortly after learning that her father died, said:

All they cared about was whether I was going to hurt myself or anybody else and once I said "No," they went, "Well there's really nothing we can do," and I got pissed and I said, "Well then what the hell did you call me down here for?" "Well, we have to check." I was so damn mad I wanted to kick her. You didn't call down to see if maybe you needed to talk? Take something to rest? Anything? Would you like a journal to write down how you feel? There was nothing there.

Relationality: Never Alone, Yet Feeling So Lonely

Relational life world refers to the world in which we find ourselves in relation to others (Munhall, 2007). It also relates to the relationship to one's self, how we define ourselves and how we are defined by those around us. The concept of *self* for incarcerated women takes on new meaning after entering prison. As many women recounted, "You are an inmate. They don't see you as human." Expressions of kindness, empathy, and compassion are all but a memory for many women. The occasional expression of kindness was sparse. These women also expressed how they needed to be different while in prison, and how they could not be their true selves. They needed to keep their emotions to themselves, knowing that they could not trust anyone. With family ties distant and for many inaccessible, women lacked the comfort and support they so desperately needed to help them through the grieving process. Painfully absent was the comfort of human touch. Women spoke about how they felt they needed to be held and comforted when they learned of their loss. The following responses speak to the experience of being alone and losing a part of self.

You don't have nobody to reach out to. You're completely alone. It's bad for anybody to have to go through this even on the outside but at least you got family, you got loved ones out there that you can be around. In here, you don't have nobody. You don't have nobody to hold you, to talk to, or anything like that.

I know these women are different when they're out of here, but while in here, they're not our friends and I can't trust anybody with my feelings.

That's a big thing and any woman will tell you that. You become some-body else when you come in here just to protect yourself because we're so sensitive that it's easy to be hurt. . . . So we build these walls in all dif-ferent aspects and trust is a big one here. I want to interact, I want close-ness. It just doesn't happen here. I protect myself here and there, but I'm not going to harden up because that's just not who I am.

Though the prison is a setting in which you are never alone, it is a setting that is inherently structured to limit the development of relationships that foster human connection. Opportunities to show kindness and compassion are few and often ignored. One woman described how she was informed that her aunt, who had served as her primary caregiver for most of her life, had passed away:

The sergeant just called me. I was out on the sidewalk. She didn't tell me in a building or anything. "Oh by the way, your aunt passed away." It was so cold. They're so cold. So that was so cold and she was mean. I could have fallen on the ground when she told me. That was cold.

For many women in prison, the emotional distance was amplified by physical distance. Without the physical connection at the time of loss, women were placated with writing letters to express "the worst situation you'd want to be in." As one woman noted:

There was absolutely nothing I could do. Write and call. But you need hugs and to see a person's face. A lot of families are closer by. But my oldest daughter lives like 5 hours from here. . . . And a letter is nice but it just doesn't do it.

Relationships with other women in the prison, although at times well inten-tioned, were not able to replace the sense of human connection and connec-tion to the lost loved one that so many women needed; it is just not the same. Lack of trust resulted in relationships of limited depth and limited potential:

Your family can't hug you. You have complete strangers that don't even have a clue about who died hugging you and I mean, you want a hug, but it's just not the same. I'm not close to anybody. I have wicked trust issues. . . . I'm close to one certain girl here. I talk to her about all my stuff, but I don't give her my all because I don't know. That un-known is the scariest part of any part of your life. Only when I feel like I can trust you with every bit of my life will I talk to you. All these women they're going to leave and you'll never see them again. It's not like I'm gonna call up another inmate and say, "let's hang out" be-cause if they're in jail, they obviously have issues and I have issues. Two sick-ees don't make a well-ee, you know what I mean?

Relationships with mental health providers were viewed by many as "useless" and, as one woman noted, "I don't really feel like she's listening to me or has an opinion." Indeed, women voiced that getting appointments with mental health providers was difficult and were angered that their main concern related to suicide risk:

> Who the hell would I talk to about that here? They'll ask you "Do you want to speak to somebody?" But I mean why do you want to speak to someone that half the time it's like a hassle to get them to talk to you? And then it's like "Okay, are you going to hurt yourself? Okay do you want meds?" I don't know, that's not what I need.

Discussion

The accounts that women provided resonated with what Morse (2001) described as "enduring to live" as prison was not a safe place for them to suffer, to release their emotions, or lose control. Demonstrating what Morse (2001) described as "tast[ing] emotional suffering" (p. 52), many participants found, at least for a brief moment, a safe space to move from enduring to actually expressing emotional suffering. In fact, almost every woman who participated in the study expressed some form of emotional release (crying, sobbing, etc.), often at the start of the interview. Participants in this study found comfort in sharing their experiences. For most of the women it was the first time since their loss that they really talked about it. They also shared how that felt and that it was the first time that they had someone who really cared, listened, and understood their experience and needs. As one woman described, "I am glad that you are doing this. It's a tough crowd around here. It felt good to talk about it, too." Through this investigation, the women had control over when and if they would display their emotions. They signed up voluntarily, knew when and where the interview would take place, and some even brought Mass cards and pictures to touch and share during the interview. As one woman noted, "I knew I was going to get upset, but I have been looking forward to talking about this with you."

The mental health needs of these women, by their own accounts, were not addressed, placing them at increased risk for complicated grief and an increase in psychiatric symptoms. These data support accounts from other incarcerated women and additionally support the need for a change in institutional protocols when an inmate loses a loved one. In response to the distrust of and limited access to mental health services in prison, incarcerated women deal with the loss by suppressing and hiding their grieving. Indeed, it is unclear if the majority of women returned to enduring the suffering after completing the interview. According to Morse (2001), flipping between enduring and emotional suffering is largely based on "energy level, context, and available support" (p. 52).

Women in this study expressed that they had a desire to help other women who have experienced a loss during incarceration. Additionally, there was overwhelming interest in a support group for women who have lost a loved one while incarcerated. The typical distrust toward other inmates was not extended to other women experiencing a loss; the desire for a support group was expressed by almost all of the women in the study.

The women clearly expressed that they needed compassion and support during their time of loss. They also needed privacy within the constraints of the prison environment. Mental health services are needed that provide support beyond medication management or emergency evaluation for suicide/homicide risk. Most female inmates are convicted of nonviolent drug-related crimes and are not "hardened criminals." They just want to be treated "like a human being." Indeed, if facilitating the grieving process for even individuals who have committed the most heinous of crimes can result in improved public safety and a better institutional milieu, might this be an important component of social justice, both for the perpetrators and their victims (Waldram, 2007)?

Understanding the effect of the experience of grief on this large vulnerable population has important implications for the women themselves, mental health and medical services, correctional staff, and the larger community. Women are released back to their communities with little transitional support or access to services that address their substance abuse and mental health issues (Bloom & Covington, 2008). Unresolved grief can complicate this transitional process. In order to decrease the impact on incarcerated women, their families, and communities, it is beneficial to facilitate the grieving process prior to release.

Facilitating proper grieving and allowing for healing is a goal itself, but it can also help to create a path to seek help with other mental health issues, substance abuse and past physical and sexual abuse. Treatment for any/all of these issues can help these women, their families, their community, and the larger community of taxpayers by reducing substance abuse and the resulting crimes. As one woman said, "hopefully . . . for the time that I'm here I can express myself like this to you and get it out so that it's not something that I want to cover up with drugs and alcohol again when I get out of here." Our study supports previous accounts of women's experience of grief during incarceration (Ferszt, 2002). It also offers new insight into the specific attitudes toward mental health services in dealing with a crisis. Our results can be used by mental health providers and prison staff to facilitate the grieving process for female inmates. By resolving some of their grief, women might be less likely to return to the community and utilize unhealthy coping mechanisms such as drugs or alcohol.

Limitations

Given the state of the science, our investigation was necessarily qualitative in nature. As such, our sample size was limited and thus limits the ability to show causal relationships. As noted previously, because the first author was also employed as a nurse practitioner at the facility, participants might have felt obligated in some way to volunteer for the study. It is also possible that participants might have believed that their answers could negatively impact them and were, therefore, providing socially desirable responses. However, we employed several strategies in an effort to minimize perceived coercion as a result of the obvious power differential. Another limitation of the study is that the demographics of the participants are not representative of the national profile of female inmates. Selection bias is also possible because of the voluntary nature of recruitment.

Recommendations

Research

Future research is needed in other prisons of various security levels and geographic locations to explore the experience of loss among persons in prison. Additionally, while we chose the word "loss" to convey the experience of the death of a loved one, rephrasing the question to simply "death of someone you know/knew" might generate different findings. For example, the death of a past abuser/perpetrator might result in different reactions, including relief, anger over not being able to confront the abuser before their death, grief over the loss of closure, and guilt over being thankful that the abuser is dead (Violence Against Women Net, 2010). For some women, the death of their abuser may result in memories, both old and new, and flashbacks of their victimization. Our study has raised additional researchable questions: What is the grieving experience of these women after they leave prison? What is the long-term impact of suspended grief on mental health? On physical health? And what is the impact of supportive interventions on grieving? While this work focused on women who were incarcerated, the experience of loss is universal. Other environments and situations, though not intended to be punitive or "prison-like" in nature, may also impose limits on the expression of grief. For example, women serving in the military, women in shelters, or women who migrate away from their home countries may feel similar constraints on their ability to express their grief. Future research should also address grief in the context of these extraordinary situations.

Practice

In light of practice, we hope that the knowledge gained from this study will help nurses, mental health providers, and medical staff anticipate inmates' needs when losing a loved one. Offering inmates the opportunity to provide feedback to the medical and corrections staff is a rare occurrence. Based on the results of this study, we suggest that facilities provide grief counseling to women who have lost a loved one. This counseling could take the form of a support group, as requested by the majority of the women in this study. There is evidence that group therapy is beneficial for women in creating connection to others (Bloom & Covington, 2008), which is precisely what these female inmates are lacking. A support group for grieving women could be a cost-effective intervention in an environment of scarce resources. Other therapeutic modalities, such as art therapy (Ferszt, Hayes, DeFedele, & Horn, 2004) or participation in groups that address psychosocial and spiritual well-being (Ferszt, Salgado, DeFedele, & Leveillee, 2009), might also be useful.

Policy
Other recommendations include providing training in grief work and basic counseling topics for the correctional professionals and implementing protocols regarding the delivery of notification of a death to an inmate. It is clear that many people in general, regardless of the setting, might be uneasy discussing death with someone grieving. We suspect this discussion must be especially conflicting for correctional officers as they must balance their institutional responsibilities with their own desire to help ease another human being's suffering. Policy changes that could improve inmates' experiences with grief and loss include allowing for semi-private visitation and/or phone communication when an inmate has recently lost a loved one. Creating a protocol surrounding the death of a loved one would be beneficial to the incarcerated women, corrections professionals, medical staff, and the families of the inmates.

Acknowledgments

The first author acknowledges the support of Sandy Mott, Sage MacLeod, and the Center for Health Equity Research at the University of Pennsylvania School of Nursing.

Author's Note

A poster presentation of the data was presented at the International Council of Women's Health Issues (ICOWHI) conference on April 7, 2010, in Philadelphia, Pennsylvania.

Declaration of Conflicting Interest

The authors declared no conflicts of interest with respect to the authorship and/or publication of this article.

Funding

The authors disclosed receipt of the following financial support for the research and/or authorship of the article: This work was supported by a Research Expense Grant from Boston College.

References

Bloom, B. E., & Covington, S. S. (2008). Addressing the mental health needs of women offenders. In R. Gido & L. Dalley (Eds.), *Women's mental health issues across the criminal justice system.* Columbus, OH: Prentice Hall.

Bowlby, J. (1980). *Loss: Sadness & depression. Attachment and loss trilogy* (Vol. 3). New York: Basic Books.

Boyd, C. O. (1993). Phenomenology: The method. In P. L. Munhall & C. O. Boyd (Eds.), *Nursing research: A qualitative perspective* (2nd ed., pp. 99-132). New York: National League of Nursing.

Browne, A., Miller, B., & Maguin, E. (1999). Prevalence and severity of lifetime physical and sexual victimization among incarcerated women. *International Journal of Law and Psychiatry, 22*(3-4), 301-322.

Complicated grief. (Cover story). (2006). *Harvard Mental Health Letter, 23*(4), 1-3.

Covington, S. S. (2007). Women and the criminal justice system. *Women's Health Issues, 17*(4), 180-182.

Cutcliffe, J. R. (1998). Hope, counselling and complicated bereavement reactions. *Journal of Advanced Nursing, 28*(4), 754-761.

Ferszt, G. G. (2002). Grief experiences of women in prison following the death of a loved one. *Illness, Crisis & Loss, 10*(3), 242-254.

Ferszt, G., Hayes, P. M., DeFedele, S., & Horn, L. (2004). Art therapy with incarcerated women who have experienced the death of a loved one. *Art Therapy: Journal of the American Art Therapy Association, 21*(4), 191-199.

Ferszt, G., Salgado, D., DeFedele, S., & Leveillee, M. (2009). Houses of healing a group intervention for grieving women in prison. *Prison Journal, 89*(1), 46-64.

Flesch, R. (1948). A new readability yardstick. *Journal of Applied Psychology, 32*(3), 221-233.

Food and Drug Administration. (2009). *Guide to informed consent.* Retrieved June 20, 2010, from http://www.fda.gov/ScienceResearch/SpecialTopics/RunningClinicalTrials/Guidances InformationSheetsandNotices/ucm116333.htm

Gilbert, K. R. (2007). *Unit 9—Ambiguous loss and disenfranchised grief: Grief in a family context.* Retrieved June 20, 2010, from http://www.indiana.edu/~famlygrf/units/ambiguous.html

Gorle, H. (2008). *Unit 14—Ceremonies and rituals for connection and change: Grief in a family context.* Retrieved June 20, 2010, from http://www.indiana.edu/~famlygrf/units/ceremonies. html

Greene, J., Pranis, K., & Frost, N. A. (2006). *The punitiveness report. HARD HIT: The growth in the imprisonment of women, 1977-2004.* Retrieved June 20, 2010, from http://www. wpaonline.org/institute/hardhit/HardHitReport4.pdf

Greenfeld, L., & Snell, T. (1999). *Women offenders.* Retrieved June 20, 2010, from http://bjs. ojp.usdoj.gov/content/pub/pdf/wo.pdf

Harlow, C. W. (1999). *Prior abuse reported by inmates and probationers.* Retrieved June 20, 2010, from http://bjs.ojp.usdoj.gov/content/pub/pdf/parip.pdf

Hentz, P. (2002). The body remembers: Grieving and a circle of time. *Qualitative Health Research, 12*(2), 161–172.

James, D., & Glaze, L. (2006). *Mental health problems of prisons and jail inmates.* Retrieved June 20, 2010, from http://bjs.ojp.usdoj.gov/content/pub/pdf/mhppji.pdf

Karnieli-Miller, O., Strier, R., & Pessach, L. (2009). Power relations in qualitative research. *Qualitative Health Research, 19*(2), 279–289.

Keaveny, M. E., & Zauszniewski, J. A. (1999). Life events and psychological well-being in women sentenced to prison. *Issues in Mental Health Nursing, 20*(1), 73–89.

Kübler-Ross, E., & Kessler, D. (2005). *On grief and grieving: Finding the meaning of grief through the five stages of loss.* New York: Scribner.

Merleau-Ponty, M. (1989). *Phenomenology of perception* (M. M. Langer, Trans.). Tallahassee, FL: Florida State University Press.

Morse, J. (2001). Toward a praxis theory of suffering. *Advances in Nursing Science, 24*(1), 47–59.

Munhall, P. L. (2007). A phenomenological method. In P. L. Munhall (Ed.), *Nursing research: A qualitative perspective* (pp. 145–159). Sudbury, MA: Jones & Bartlett.

Parkes, C. M. (1998). Coping with loss: Bereavement in adult life. *British Medical Journal, 316,* 856–859.

Parkes, C. M., & Weiss, R. S. (1983). *Recovery from bereavement.* New York: Basic Books.

Raphael, B. (1983). *The anatomy of bereavement.* New York: Basic Books.

Stroebe, M., Hansson, R., Schut, H., & Stroebe, W. (Eds.). (2008). *Handbook of bereavement research and practice.* Washington, DC: American Psychological Association.

Stroebe, M., Schut, H., & Stroebe, W. (2007). Health outcomes of bereavement. *Lancet, 370*(9603), 1960–1973.

van Manen, M. (1990). *Research lived experience.* New York: SUNY Press.

Violence Against Women Net. (2010). *When an abuser/perpetrator dies.* Retrieved June 20, 2010, from http://new.vawnet.org/category/Main_Doc.php?docid=836

Waldram, J. B. (2007). Everybody has a story: Listening to imprisoned sexual offenders. *Qualitative Health Research, 17,* 963–970.

West, H. C., Sabol, W. J., & Cooper, M. (2010). *Prisoners in 2008.* Retrieved from http://bjs.ojp.usdoj.gov/content/pub/pdf/p08.pdf

Young, V. C. (2003). Helping female inmates cope with grief and loss. *Corrections Today, 65*(3), 76–79.

8

Grounded Theory: The Method

Judith Wuest

Grounded Theory: The Method

I became captivated by grounded theory as a graduate student. I was interested in family disruption when children have chronic middle ear disease and I had been struggling throughout my course work to locate a theory suitable for guiding my thesis research. The most likely match seemed to be stress and coping theory with a specific focus on uncertainty, but I felt uneasy about framing family experience this way. Then, during the qualitative methods course taught by Phyllis Noerager Stern, I encountered grounded theory. Here, *at last*, was an approach that would permit studying the problem from the perspective of the families without force fitting it into an existing framework. Additionally, the research process felt consistent with my community health background and my way of thinking. Although I began a course assignment that required collecting and analyzing three interviews with trepidation, I became so engaged that my fears vanished. Since then, each grounded theory project has afforded me opportunities to reflect on and reach new understandings of this versatile research approach and its usefulness for generating nursing knowledge.

Barney Glaser and Anselm Strauss in their 1967 text *The Discovery of Grounded Theory* presented grounded theory as a new approach to research developed in their study of dying. Grounded theory is a research approach that results in the development of middle range theory at a substantive or formal level (Glaser, 1978). This explicit goal of theory development makes grounded theory unique among qualitative methods. A grounded theory approach demands that the researcher move beyond description of the domain of study towards a theoretical rendering that identifies key explanatory concepts and the relationships among them. The challenge of theoretical analysis and theoretical writing is frequently daunting, especially to novice qualitative researchers. Grounded theory has been embraced by nurses since Glaser and Strauss introduced the method to graduate students at the University of California, San Francisco in the early 1970s (Stern & Covan, 2001). Grounded theories are useful for directing nursing practice because they are explanatory theories of human behavior within social context. Nonetheless, nurses have found the sociological writing of Glaser and Strauss (Glaser, 1978; Glaser & Strauss, 1967; Strauss, 1987) unfamiliar and have written many articles and books to demystify the method and explicate its contribution to knowledge generation (Artinian, Giske, & Cone, 2009; Beck, 1999; Benoliel, 1996; Chenitz & Swanson, 1986; Hutchinson & Wilson, 2001; Morse, Stern, Corbin, Bowers, Charmaz, & Clarke, 2009; Schreiber & Stern, 2001; Stern, 1980; Stern & Pyles, 1986; Wuest, 1995, 1997a, 2000, 2001; Wuest, Berman, Ford-Gilboe, & Merritt-Gray, 2002; Wuest & Merritt-Gray, 2001).

Grounded theory has evolved since its introduction almost 40 years ago. For me, the original texts (Glaser, 1978; Glaser & Strauss, 1967; Strauss, 1987) continue to provide the best overview. Strauss's approach to grounded theory altered over time and this shift was captured in his books written with Corbin (Corbin & Strauss, 2008; Strauss & Corbin, 1990, 1998). Glaser (1992) took exception to Strauss and Corbin's more prescriptive approach to analysis.[1] However, Glaser's more recent writings demonstrate his own evolution (Glaser, 1998, 1999, 2002, 2004).[2] Such shifts in thinking, I believe, are to be expected as any method is used over time within a changing social context. Researchers, therefore, are obligated to disclose their own orientation to the method. In the 1990s when the differences between the two originators of the method were being widely discussed, this was achieved by identifying one's grounded theory approach as Straussian or Glaserian. However, such identification is insufficient in light of the continued evolution of each of those traditions (Glaser, 1998, 1999, 2002, 2004; Strauss & Corbin, 1998), and the efforts of second-generation grounded theorists (scholars who studied with Glaser, Strauss, or both) to articulate their approaches to grounded theory (Artinian et al., 2009; Charmaz, 2006; Clarke, 2005; Corbin & Strauss, 2008; Morse et al., 2009). In 2007, Jan Morse organized a "Grounded Theory Bash," a one-day symposium sponsored by the International Institute for Qualitative Methodology to celebrate the contributions of Glaser and Strauss. The rich discussion of the evolution of grounded theory by second-generation grounded theory scholars provides a valuable perspective for grounded theory researchers (Morse et al., 2009). The evolution of grounded theory is the legacy of multiple mentors;

grounded theory is not a static approach but changes in the process of being taught (Covan, 2007).

My own approach to grounded theory is rooted in the earlier writings. Phyllis Noerager Stern, a student of Glaser, supervised my master's research and, as a mentor and colleague, continues to support my development as a grounded theorist. Marsha Cohen, a student of Strauss, supervised my doctoral work, and challenged me to critically consider how my approach fit with the shifting traditions of grounded theory. I have argued elsewhere for the utility of combining feminist theory with grounded theory (Wuest, 1995) and have also wrestled with a more critical participatory approach (Wuest et al., 2002). Thus, my way of doing grounded theory has evolved but remains close to the early work; the text that continues to be most useful to me is *Theoretical Sensitivity* (Glaser, 1978).

In the following chapter, my goal is not just to provide an overview of my understanding of grounded theory and its theoretical underpinnings, but also to discuss strategies for handling some of the more common challenges faced by researchers in moving beyond description to theoretical analysis. My intent is not to be prescriptive, since each of us finds her/his own path to theoretical thinking, but rather to offer some tools that may or may not work for any single researcher. I suggest guidelines to assist novice grounded theorists in evaluating emerging theory. Finally, I will briefly discuss the evolution of grounded theory and its paradigm location.

Philosophical Underpinning of Grounded Theory

While other researchers have discussed symbolic interactionism as the basic underpinning of grounded theory (Bryant & Charmaz, 2007a; Chenitz & Swanson, 1986; Crooks, 2001; Hutchinson & Wilson, 2001; Milliken & Schreiber, 2001), Glaser and Strauss (1967) wrote comparatively little. Strauss (1987) briefly addressed the philosophical traditions that informed the development of grounded theory, noting the influence of pragmatism and the Chicago School of Sociology. He delineated the underlying assumptions: 1) change is a feature of social life that needs to be accounted for through attention to social interaction and social process; and 2) interaction, process, and social change are best understood by grasping the actor's viewpoint. Glaser, in his 1992 writing, explicitly stated that an assumption of grounded theory is that people actively shape the worlds they live in through the process of symbolic interaction and that life is characterized by variability, complexity, change and process. These assertions by the founders of grounded theory suggest that two key underpinnings are symbolic interactionism and pragmatism. More recently Glaser (1998, 2004) argued that symbolic interactionism is not inherent in grounded theory. His critique is not of symbolic interactionism as a philosophical orientation underlying the method, but rather of symbolic interactionism as a dominant theoretical code to guide analysis. I agree that data is not analyzed through the theoretical code of symbolic interactionism. But my understanding of grounded theory suggests that symbolic interactionism and pragmatism inform the underlying assumptions of the method.

Symbolic Interactionism

Blumer (1969) identified three assumptions of symbolic interactionism: 1) people act toward things and people on the basis of meanings they have for them, 2) meanings stem from interaction with others, and 3) people's meanings are modified through an interpretive process used to make sense of and manage their social worlds. Snow (2001) expanded these tenets, reframing the principles of symbolic interactionism as *interactive determination, symbolization, emergence*, and *human agency*. *Interactive determination* suggests that phenomena exist only in relation to each other and can only be understood by considering interactions and interactional contexts. Because interactions are problematic, they are worthy of observation and analysis. *Symbolization* refers to the process of ascribing meaning to things, people, events, etc. such that they elicit particular feelings and actions. Such meanings become "embedded in and reflective of existing cultural and organizational contexts" (p. 371). Snow asserted that the question then is not how people act in terms of the meanings they ascribe but rather 1) how do meanings become taken-for-granted or routinized; 2) what contexts, relationships or structures support such acceptance; and finally 3) are those embedded meanings as a basis for action problematic?

Such questioning leads to *emergence* as a principle (Snow, 2001). By focusing on what is going on in particular social contexts, symbolic interactionism allows for the identification of social, emotional, or cognitive change as it emerges. The final principle of *human agency* refers to the "active, willful nature of human actors" (p. 373). Social actors make choices or decisions about their actions while taking into account the social or cultural constraints or expectations. Snow argued that the influence of these constraints is often unacknowledged until a disruption makes them visible. At that point, *human agency* drives people toward some sort of corrective action.

Pragmatism

Pragmatism refers to theoretical perspectives that emphasize the practical, giving primacy to usefulness over theoretical knowledge; as such the goal is transformative (Seigfried, 1998). From a pragmatist perspective, truth cannot be arrived at through deductive reasoning from a priori theory but rather must be developed inductively with constant empirical verification. Truth is modified in light of new discoveries and is relative to time and place. "Pragmatic reflection begins with experience as an interactive process involving individuals and their social and natural environment" (p. 51). Knowledge development is not value free and is historically contextualized. Situated perspectives of the marginalized are seen as more legitimate because they know the limits of the dominant interpretation of reality better than others, but even these perspectives must be reflectively validated. Differences in perspectives are valued and provide a basis for reciprocal problem-solving, drawing on existing knowledge and resources, and ongoing revisions of understanding. Under pragmatism the goals of inquiry are judged in terms of their usefulness for making change and thus values are an inherent part of pragmatism.

Summary

Symbolic interactionism directs grounded theorists to assume that meaning is made and constantly changed through interaction and becomes embedded in social context. Both meaning and social context influence the ways that human agency is enacted. Pragmatism supports seeking revised understandings for the purpose of making useful change through inductive exploration of diverse situated human experience with reflexive confirmation and use of applicable existing knowledge. Thus, pragmatism and symbolic interactionism are the source of foundational assumptions of grounded theory.

Grounded Theory Approach

"The goal of grounded theory is to generate a theory that accounts for a pattern of behavior which is relevant and problematic for those involved" (Glaser, 1978, p. 93). Data analysis occurs concurrently with data collection and the specific research focus or problem emerges as the analysis proceeds. Data analysis involves coding data on a line by line basis, asking "What is this a conceptual indicator of?" and constant comparison of various indicators for similarities and differences. Informal hypotheses and concepts are derived inductively from the data, but then deductively checked out and modified as new data is collected so that evolving concepts fit the collected data. Throughout the analysis process, memos are written to capture emerging ideas about concepts and their relationships.

Sources of data are selected for what they can contribute to the emerging theory and may include formal or informal interviews, field observation, or written data. This process of collecting data to develop the hypotheses and further identify properties and relationships among concepts is called theoretical sampling (Glaser & Strauss, 1967). Exceptions or extreme cases identified through constant comparison generate new categories that are further developed through theoretical sampling. The emerging theory is further integrated by theoretical coding, a process of examining the data in theoretical rather than descriptive terms (Glaser, 1978). Diagramming relationships among concepts increases the level of abstraction. As data collection and analysis proceed, a core category that explains most of the variation in the behavior pattern is identified (Glaser, 1978). Core categories may be basic social processes if they have at least two stages that "differentiate and account for variation in the problematic pattern of behavior" (Glaser, 1978, p. 97). Once the core variable is identified, extant theory and literature are theoretically sampled for what they can contribute to the developing theory. The final grounded theory report is generally written as a theoretical discussion (Glaser & Strauss, 1967). An important characteristic of grounded theories is their modifiability as new data is generated. Grounded theories may be constantly recast to reflect new variations.

When Is Grounded Theory an Appropriate Approach?

Because a grounded theory captures social process in social context, the grounded theory research approach is most useful when the goal is a framework or theory that explains human behavior in context (Glaser & Strauss, 1967; Glaser, 1978). Stern (2007) noted that an essential quality of grounded theory is that it makes sense. Thus, human behavior related to health issues, developmental transitions, and situational challenges is well suited to grounded theory research in nursing.

Grounded theory is particularly useful when little is known about the area to be studied, or when what is known is from a theoretical perspective that does not satisfactorily explain what is going on. For example, I carried out a study of women's caring/caregiving using grounded theory because the conceptual understandings of caring (burden and stress [Farran & Keane-Hagerty, 1991; Given & Given, 1991] or fulfilment, satisfaction, and life enhancement [Bevis, 1988; Ray, 1988, Roach, 1992]) that guided this large body of research were conflicting and failed to account for clinical observations of women caring for family members.

The Research Question

Unlike other research methods, the starting point in grounded theory is not a focused research question, but rather exploration of a domain of human behavior. Symbolic interactionism informs the underlying assumption that people in the domain under study share a common social psychological problem, of which they are normally unaware at a conscious level. The researcher will construct both the problem and the way it is processed through inductive and deductive analysis of data.

Thus, rather than a list of research questions or hypotheses, the researcher begins with a statement of purpose, such as "The purpose of this study is to develop a substantive theory of family behavior when a child has chronic middle ear disease (OME)." Due to the constraints of funding agencies and the requirements of graduate programs, researchers may be forced to articulate more specific objectives or research questions. The key challenge here is doing so without making assumptions about what will be most problematic for people in the study domain, and without using theory-laden language. The problem that emerges during data collection and analysis may not be what the researcher had anticipated. I had a hunch from my practice that the key problem for families whose children had chronic OME would be related to speech development. The problem that emerged from the data was the family's relationship with the healthcare system (Wuest & Stern, 1990). Theory-laden language in the statement of purpose or objectives may also derail a study. Had I written my purpose "to discover how families *cope* with children with chronic OME," I would have situated the study in a well-established body of theoretical knowledge (stress and coping theory). Avoiding language that may link the study to dominant extant theory at the outset is important.

A common way of framing the grounded theory study focus is in terms of finding a *particular* process. This can be problematic because one does not know which process will be discovered. For example, if in my study of women's caring, I had stated that the study goal was "to discover the process of caring/caregiving for family members", readers would have expected an explanatory theory of how women care for family members. Rather I stated my study focus as the "domain of women's caring". The resultant theory of *precarious ordering* (Wuest, 1997a, 1997b, 2001) did not capture the process of caring, but rather the process of addressing the negative health consequences that stemmed from the problem of competing and changing caring demands. While this may seem a subtle difference, it is noteworthy. A challenge for novice grounded theorists is distinguishing the situational trajectory of the domain of study from the basic social problem/process. For example, in a study of women having myocardial infarctions (MI), initially the problem might be seen as the MI, and the situational trajectory, is *having symptoms, seeking treatment, being treated,* and *recovering.* This sort of trajectory will always be in data, and may be a condition or context, but it is usually NOT the social-psychological problem/process being sought.

Review of the Literature

The review of the literature is a frequent source of contention in grounded theory studies. According to Glaser (1992), the literature is reviewed after the core variable is generated. The rationale for not conducting an extensive literature review earlier is to avoid beginning the study with pre-conceived ideas. Stern and Covan (2001) recalled that their doctoral dissertation proposals were 10 and 5 pages respectively, a far cry from the lengthy literature reviews expected today. From my perspective, an initial literature review is necessary in grounded theory research in order to justify to the thesis committee or research funding agency that a grounded theory study is needed. Additionally, knowledge of what is known in the domain under study allows the researcher to understand how the generated theory is similar to or different from what is known (Morse & Richards, 2002). Through a literature review, the researcher demonstrates a broad grasp of the strengths and limitations of the theoretical and empirical knowledge in the domain under study. If little is known, the literature review is fairly straightforward. On the other hand, if the broad domain has been well studied, a case must be developed for why existing theoretical perspectives are inadequate, and why a grounded theory approach is needed. Thus, dominant theories are critiqued for their limitations. Empirical research is reviewed broadly and organized by concepts to highlight the complexity of the domain of study. A detailed critique of individual studies as normally required to provide the groundwork for a theory-testing study is unnecessary. The literature review is completed with a summary in which an argument for the proposed study is made. By summarizing the inadequacies or absence of theoretical frameworks to explain what is going on in the proposed area of study, the researcher builds a case for a grounded theory study. Once the data is collected and the core variable identified, the researcher will then theoretically sample the literature relevant to the emerging theory. Most frequently this involves seeking new bodies of literature previously not explored.

Regardless of how the literature review for the proposal is handled, critique is likely. If a scant literature review is carried out, reviewers may say the researcher has failed to demonstrate knowledge of the field or justification for the research. If a thorough literature review is carried out, reviewers more familiar with the grounded theory approach may argue that such a review violates a basic premise of grounded theory and biases the researcher. Be prepared to defend this assertion. Two foundational elements of grounded theory, *constant comparison* and *theoretical sensitivity* may inform the counter argument. A key element of the analytic is *constant comparison*. Data are analyzed through coding, that is breaking the data into bits (phrases, sentences or paragraphs) that are judged to be indicators of a code, inductively named from the data. Each data bit is compared to each other data bit that is an indicator of the same code for similarities and differences and for what theoretical property of the code it suggests. In this way, a full range of properties of the code are developed and the name given to the code evolves to fit those properties. One source of data is literature which is compared in the same way. So long as the principle of *constant comparison* is respected and the codes evolve to fit all data, knowledge from extant theory will not dominate, and the emerging theory will be grounded in the data. Thus, exploration of the literature in advance will not derail the research process, and the phenomenological strategy of *bracketing* is not necessary (Wuest, 2000).

Knowledge of theoretical literature also has relevance for a researcher's *theoretical sensitivity*. "The root of all significant theorizing is the sensitive insights of the observer" (Glaser & Strauss, 1967, p. 251). Theoretical sensitivity refers to an individual's ability to "render theoretically their discovered substantive, grounded categories" (Glaser, 1978, p. 1). Thus, theoretical sensitivity is the researcher's personal capacity to have theoretical insights related to the conceptualization of data and the relationships between concepts based on personal experiences, vicarious experiences, and knowledge of theoretical constructions in many disciplines (Glaser, 1978). Some of this capacity comes from researchers' knowledge of their own disciplinary theories. However, understanding theoretical literature in other fields is also useful for expanding insights regarding what is theoretically possible. Thus, Glaser (1978) advocates reading widely outside the substantive area under study to increase familiarity with theoretical codes. "Theoretical codes are conceptual models of relationships that are discovered to relate the substantive codes to each theoretically" (Glaser, 1992, p. 27). Let me be clear that this does not mean that one takes an extant theoretical framework and uses it to name and organize concepts. Rather the theoretical codes gleaned from disciplinary knowledge, reading widely, or from using Glaser's (1978) coding families are templates that help the researcher to recognize theoretical properties and relationships among categories. Glaser's coding family, the 6 C's, commonly sensitizes researchers to the way codes may be related as cause and consequence. Knowledge of feminist theory means that I bring to my analysis a sensitivity to how dominant social structures such as gender, race, and class may be conditions that influence social process (Wuest, 1995; Wuest & Merritt-Gray, 2001). This does not mean that I code for these factors, only that if there are conceptual indicators for them in the data, I am more likely to see them. Thus, when reviewing the literature for the literature review, paying attention not only to the findings but also to the ways that the findings are theoretically organized may strengthen the researcher's understanding of which theoretical relationships are possible.

Theoretical Sampling

Sampling in grounded theory studies is theoretical. Initially the researcher makes choices about where and how to collect data based on his/her judgment of the best sources of observational, interview, and/or document data for the domain of study. While I have come to understand this as part of theoretical sampling, Morse (2007) described grounded theory sampling as shifting from initial convenience sampling to purposeful sampling for maximum variation in emergent concepts, then to theoretical sampling. In theoretical sampling, codes are generated inductively from the data and deductive decisions about where next to collect data are based on what is needed to clarify the properties of and relationships among emerging concepts (Glaser, 1978). Theoretical sampling takes place by seeking answers to questions or hypotheses that arise during analysis by interviewing new participants who are likely to have relevant experiences, looking for comparisons in data already collected, returning to participants to ask new questions, participant observation, consulting policies or documents, and looking at literature.

Specifying the sample in advance and developing a sampling plan is difficult. Yet, on a practical level, research ethics boards, granting agencies, and institutions expect that the sample will be specified both in terms of population and number, and are becoming increasingly intolerant towards proposals that refer to emergence as the rationale for not doing so. A strategy for addressing this challenge is to consider broadly the range of people who may offer insight into the domain of study and prepare the proposal inclusively. If the study domain is caregiving for family members with Alzheimer's Disease (AD), the researcher might designate the initial sample as English-speaking men and women over 19 years of age who are providing care to a family member with AD. This could be followed with a statement indicating that based on initial theoretical analysis, data may be collected from others such as family members, home support workers, and healthcare professionals who have knowledge of family caregiving for persons with AD. Including these groups in the initial proposal does not mean that data must be collected from them. Rather, if theoretically it is necessary to seek data from these sources, the researcher is positioned to do so without gaining additional ethical approval. Prepare consent forms and letters of information in language that will make them applicable to all potential participants. Considering potential sources for theoretical sampling is an informed judgment call and, unquestionably, analysis may send the researcher in directions previously unimagined. Nonetheless, some potential sources are obvious and including them in the proposal may save time later.

Sample size

In grounded theory, sample size should not be an issue. Researchers collect data by theoretically sampling until theoretical saturation is achieved; that is, no further theoretical variation in a concept emerges from the data being analyzed (Glaser & Strauss, 1967). The focus of theoretical sampling is discovery, not verification. Saturation is not judged by the number of times similar properties of a concept are identified, but rather by whether a full range of variation in conceptual properties is identified. To some extent, how rapidly saturation occurs depends on how narrowly the study domain is defined. If, in an AD study, the domain studied was constrained to family caregiving when the caregiver is male, lives in a specific community, and is a member of a support group, saturation would most likely be achieved more quickly than if the domain included all family caregivers. While Glaser (1978) cautioned that demographic variables such as age, gender, location etc. must earn their way into the data and do not necessarily influence variation, some undoubtedly will. Breadth and diversity of study domain is significant when considering time and costs of achieving theoretical saturation.

Still, reviewers, thesis committees, and review boards struggle if no sample size is specified. Morse (1994) suggested that 30–50 interviews are needed in a grounded theory study. In my experience, a grounded theory in a narrow domain such as that carried out by masters students usually can be achieved from interviews with 10–15 participants. In the case of a broader domain, interviews with about 40 participants are manageable and allow for theoretical saturation. However, much depends on the quality of data collected; these are only estimates to assist with proposal writing. Researchers need to be prepared to be guided by the demands of data for theory building.

Recruitment

The initial recruitment focuses on ways to access participants who are judged to have good knowledge of the study domain. A specific organization (support group, community agency) or person (physician, clinical nurse specialist, public health nurse) may be approached to give information letters to persons who meet the initial sample criteria. Broader recruitment takes place by putting an advertisement in the newspaper or posters in various community sites. To avoid being deluged by initial volunteers, limit the initial recruitment effort to circulating a small number of letters of information, or one newspaper advertisement. When screening participants for inclusion in the study, record demographic characteristics that may influence variation in the study domain as a basis for later theoretical sampling. For example, in the proposed AD study, age, gender, geographic location, ethnicity, help being received, stage of AD, length of time caregiving, and relationship to care recipient might conceivably be salient. This demographic information facilitates later theoretically sampling, if these characteristics emerge as salient.[3]

By limiting initial recruitment, subsequent recruitment can take place purposefully to collect data that are likely to allow hypotheses about properties of, or relationships among, concepts to be confirmed or refined thus moving analysis towards theoretical saturation. In our study of women leaving abusive partners, we initially recruited women who had been out of the relationship for at least a year (Wuest & Merritt-Gray, 1999). As our understanding of the concept of *leaving* shifted from singular act to multiple acts of breaking free, we sought help from lay and professional helpers to recruit some women who were in the process of leaving, in order to illuminate the variation in the ways and timing of breaking free.

Data Collection

Much has been written about the interview process in grounded theory (Swanson, 1987; May, 1991; Hutchinson & Wilson, 1994; Wuest, 1995). The matrix operation of grounded theory is very difficult if the person collecting the data is unfamiliar with the evolving analysis. Thus the researcher must be fully engaged in the data collection and analysis process. If a research assistant is employed, I suggest that he/she collect no more than half the data and be involved fully in the analysis. An interview protocol that includes participant tracking forms, processes for screening participants for eligibility, routines for making and confirming interview times and locations, standard interview packages and equipment, and finally a safety protocol for data collectors and participants (Paterson, Gregory, & Thorne, 1999) is important for taking the guess work out of the data collection process.

Familiarity with recording equipment and access to a power outlet and an extension cord is advisable if interviews are to be recorded. Glaser (2004) argued against audio-recording interviews, saying that field notes are more useful because they contain only relevant data. Transcripts of audio-recorded interviews often include much data that ultimately is not used because it is not salient to the core variable. Stern (2007) recalled that Glaser and Strauss claimed that essential information (the cream) from an interview would rise to the top in field notes. She cautioned that emphasis on accuracy of interview transcriptions puts researchers at risk of emphasizing a rich description of the social scene and neglecting the theoretical rendering. However, unless a novice researcher has solid training in ethnographic traditions of recording field notes during and following interviews, audio-recording may be advisable. Even experienced investigators may benefit from listening to recorded interviews to capture the most salient ideas. Whether interviews are captured by audio-recording or field note, field notes are important for capturing the researcher's reflections on the data collection process (Montgomery & Bailey, 2007).

Interviews are most fruitful in a setting where the participant feels safe and comfortable, and when there are no interruptions. While there are diverse opinions on whether fees should be paid to participants, compensating for transportation and/or dependent care is respectful and facilitates recruitment. An information sheet of relevant accessible resources provided at the end of the interview is a useful way to thank participants while providing them with information they may not have.

Grounded theory interviews are semi-structured in that the researcher normally has an overview question with some follow-up probes. In our study of *caregiving for a family member with AD*, we asked participants to tell us what it was like for them to care for their family member (Wuest, Ericson, & Stern, 1994). In general, if the domain of study is importance to the participant, the general overview question is a catalyst for participants to share their experience in detail and few additional probes are required from the researcher. If the domain of study seems inconsequential to the participant, then the researcher may need to use the prepared follow-up probes more purposefully. In our study of *health promotion in single-parent families after leaving,* women and children were hesitant in responding to a broad question related to how they attended to their health; specific follow-up probes were essential (Ford-Gilboe, Wuest, & Merritt-Gray, 2005). As data collection and analysis proceeds, the interview process shifts in light of the emerging theory. While I continue to begin with the initial overview question, follow-up probes change; some may prove irrelevant to the developing theory, and new ones are needed to check out theoretical hunches. Analysis sensitizes the researcher to compare what is being said during the interview with what is emerging from the analysis, leading to spontaneous probing or theoretical sampling to obtain further clarification. In order to confirm, expand, or refine the properties of the emerging concepts or the relationships among them, researchers ask more focused questions as the study progresses. In our *leaving an abusive partner* study, workplace support emerged as instrumental in fortifying women for leaving, leading us to theoretically sample by probing new participants and old data about how the workplace influenced leaving. In order for theory development to proceed most effectively, the interviewer builds on data analysis with each subsequent interview.

Novice researchers often struggle with letting participants respond to the overview question in their own ways, often believing at first that they are not getting good data and that they need to focus the interview more. I would caution that we do not know what is salient early on, so give participants latitude. Interviews that are staccato, that is many questions followed by short answers, are less likely to yield rich data. Each of us upon reading our interviews is struck by our obvious errors in interviewing such as interrupting a discussion line, asking a totally unrelated question or failing to encourage elaboration. Phyllis Stern (personal communication, 1989) asserted that participants are very forgiving, replying politely to our off-base inquiries and then returning to what they really want to talk about. Participants disclose important information once they know their words are no longer being recorded, often as the researcher is on the way out the door. Always ask whether this information can be used, and if the answer is affirmative, take a time later to dictate this information, along with any observations, at the end of the recording so that it becomes part of the transcription.

While transcribing interviews take a great deal of time for everyone except skilled typists, the benefit is that the researcher comes to know the data very well. If someone else transcribes, more time will be needed to listen to the recording while reading the transcription. Transcriptions need to be accurate and without identifying data, particularly names and locations. I replace names with the relationship of person named to the participant (DAUGHTER,

PHYSICIAN, FRIEND) and location with a more general classification (NEAR-BY CITY, VILLAGE). Format transcripts such that they are single spaced with a double space between speakers. Set margins so that text extends only half the page width, leaving room for coding. Finally, number the lines in the interview for easy referencing of conceptual indicators (Int 2: Line 423–445).

Data Analysis

Analysis in grounded theory is aimed at generating a theoretical, as opposed to a descriptive, account of patterns of behavior in the study domain. Analysis begins through inductive identification of substantive codes to name what is happening in the data, often with more than one code being assigned to a particular data segment (phrase, sentence, paragraph). Eventually codes are grouped into more abstract categories that reflect the domain of study at a descriptive level. Analysis shifts to a more theoretical level largely through theoretical coding, diagramming, and reduction. Theoretical coding is the process of examining data through the theoretical lens of the coding families (Glaser, 1978). Theoretical properties of categories are identified. Reduction occurs as categories are collapsed into more abstract concepts and linked. The central problem and core variable, which may be a basic social process, are identified. Categories unrelated to the core variable are dropped from the analysis. Additional data is collected through theoretical sampling to further saturate concepts and further clarify the relationships among them. In this process, concepts may be renamed, additionally collapsed, or linked differently. Literature is also theoretically sampled as data to support the emerging theory. Theoretical memos are written to capture the conceptual development throughout this analytic process and become the basis for the final report.

Descriptions, such as this, fail to do justice to the complex and infinitely messy process of grounded theory analysis. The process is far from linear, and the analyst is perpetually moving back and forth from the substantive line-by-line coding, to theoretical consideration, to memoing, and then back to the substantive data. Doing grounded theory is a process of inductively deriving codes, developing hunches about properties and relationships, checking out those hunches deductively in old and new data by theoretically sampling, and developing yet another inductive theoretical hunch. This process is captured by writing memos about developing concepts and their interrelationships: "If data are the building blocks of developing theory, memos are the mortar" (Stern, 2007, p. 119). Two recent discussion of memoing (Lempert, 2007; Montgomery & Bailey, 2007) provide valuable direction for the novice. Glaser (1978) also recommended diagramming the theory. Diagramming has always helped me capture how categories fit together theoretically. Artinian and West (2009) extend this process to *conceptual mapping* as a means of displaying theoretical relationships.

One aspect of analysis rarely discussed is the need to alternately consider the data at both a macro and micro level. By macro level, I mean considering the larger picture by reading and listening to entire transcripts, asking "What is going on here with regard to the domain of study?", "What is the problem?", and "What is being done in response to the problem?" This macro level analysis is important to keep the researcher focused on identifying the core problem and core variable related to the study domain. Data normally includes much information that may be background, but not central, to the domain studied. For example, Enman (2004) studied help-seeking behaviors of caregivers of spouses with AD. Her data contained considerable information about caregiving processes. Hence, she had to focus on her domain by asking "What is the basic problem *related to help seeking*?" Looking at the bigger picture must go hand-in-hand with the micro-level analysis of line-by-line open coding. Open coding involves focusing on each data bit, asking what it is an indicator of and assigning a code or label (Glaser, 1978). As codes recur in the data, the researcher compares data bits, asking how they are the same or different and what accounts for the variation. As properties are identified, memos are written separately tracking theoretical development. Substantive codes are then reviewed for grouping into categories. Throughout the analytical process, the researcher moves back and forth from the micro to the macro level, staying grounded in the data, but thinking about how it is related to the domain of study. In this way, the problem related to the study domain is eventually identified.

Open coding
While open coding seems straightforward, at the beginning it is daunting. Each of us is trying to measure up to an elusive "right way" and thus feels like an impostor. The goal of open coding is to generate as many conceptual codes as possible to fit the data. As coding continues, and the researcher compares incidents, some codes recur more than others, others collapse, and categories begin to develop. Often in the initial data, researchers are unable to see indicators of particular codes until later when they emerge in other data. Thus, theoretically sampling of previously coded data is important; subsequent discoveries influence how old data is seen. Expect to code and recode data, particularly initial interviews. At first it may be difficult to discern what is relevant and what is "filler" (Stern, 2007, p. 118); however as coding and categorization proceeds, this will become more obvious. When selecting words for coding, stay close to the data, choosing words that reflect what is going on. *In vivo* codes, that is, words of the participants that are particularly apt sometimes may be the best code. Avoid words that are theory-laden such as "stress," "resilience," and "denial." Metaphors and analogies are risky to use for coding because they can begin to drive the analysis, rather like a theoretical framework (Glaser, 1978;

Sandelowski, 1998).[4] As open coding continues, codes are constantly compared and gradually grouped together into more abstract categories.

Theoretical coding

The process of theoretical coding is challenging and little is written about how to do it. In the following paragraphs, I offer my approach to ensuring that I shift from open to theoretical coding in my analysis. Theoretical coding often begins during open coding with constant comparison when the researcher recognizes that a segment of data is a conceptual indicator of a condition, or a consequence of another code. I write memos to track the theoretical development and gradually group the codes into categories. Nonetheless, after approximately 8–12 interviews (the number depends on the richness and variation in the data), I find myself swimming in evolving codes and categories. I feel as though I have lost control and need to stop data collection temporarily and focus on analysis.

I list all substantive codes and through constant comparison, group them into 15–20 categories named with a label that best fits the codes combined. Remember these categorical groupings and their labels are still very provisional, and as data collection and analysis proceeds, they will expand and shift to *fit* the data. Some of these categories will be processes and will have labels that are gerunds (words ending in "ing"); others will have labels that are nouns, and will be more likely to be conditions or context or the problem. I then recode all of the data collected to date in terms of the categories I derived from inductive analysis. The next step is to sort all data by categories. Recoding and sorting can take place in one of several ways: 1) using a computer program focusing on qualitative analysis; 2) coding, cutting up and sorting hard copies; or 3) cutting and pasting in a word processing program. I use qualitative analysis computer programs for preparing numbered interview transcripts, coding my data categorically, and generating sorted hard copy output for each category. However, for all of my initial open coding and categorizing, I work with pencil and printed transcripts.

Once the data is sorted by category, I reflect on the big picture by considering how each category is related to each of the others, and what each tells me about the basic social problem and how it is being processed. Glaser's (1978) 18 coding families are the basis for theoretical coding and offer diverse lenses for helping researchers see how categories may be related to one another. Having a working knowledge of all of the coding families such as the foundational 6 Cs (cause, consequence, condition, context, covariance, and contingency), process, degree, dimension, strategy, and type allows researchers to consider the relationships among, and the properties of, each category.[5] In short, the coding families act like a template of possible theoretical relationships that assist the analyst to move to a more abstract level, away from descriptive understandings.

The researcher may select codes from various coding families that work to explain theoretically what is going on in the study domain. Diagramming is helpful for visual thinkers to see how concepts relate to one another. This macro level consideration of categorical relationships helps me to consolidate my hunches related to naming the basic social problem and the core variable, although this remains quite preliminary. Memoing is important to capture theoretical ideas at this point.

My next step is to take one category, preferably a process category that seems important, and examine the data related to it through the lens of theoretical codes. I begin with a large piece of paper, writing the category name in the middle. One at a time, I read each segment of data that has been sorted for this category, asking, "What does this segment tell me about the theoretical properties of this category? Is there anything here about the cause or consequences, the conditions under which it happens, strategies for how it happens, conditions that might influence the degree or frequency or how it happens? I systematically consider the data through a range of theoretical codes. As I generate theoretical properties from the data, I name and organize them according to whether they are conditions, causes, consequences, strategies, processes, turning points etc., always noting data location (interview and line number). In my study of women caring, the following data segment had been categorized as "asserting":

Int 2
I knew what I wanted. I felt comfortable with my decisions about breastfeeding and if somebody wanted me to do something that I didn't agree with I would say no. But I was 30 when I had my first child and older and more mature for my other two.

These data indicated that a *cause* of asserting is "someone wanting me to do something I didn't agree with," *conditions* for asserting are knowing what you want (possibly from past experience), being comfortable with your decision, and maturity. A *strategy* for asserting is saying no. As I systematically examine each data segment of a category through the lens of the coding families, and record the findings in terms of their theoretical properties and relationships to one another, the page is gradually filled. Each indicator is compared with others, and the various causes, consequences and so on are grouped conceptually. A range of theoretical properties are recorded. When the theoretical coding of the category is completed, I write an extensive memo that captures this detailed theoretical analysis. I try to pay close attention to Glaser's (1978) dictum to write about the concepts, not about the people. It is good practice for the final report writing, and is part of shifting from the descriptive to the theoretical level. I begin by specifying the meaning of the concept: "Asserting is a process of . . ." This conceptual specification is derived from the theoretical analysis as opposed to an *a priori* definition (Glaser, 1978). I discuss the theoretical properties of the concept such as the antecedents, the strategies, the consequences. Of particular importance is identifying the conditions that influence the variation in timing, intensity or duration of the process. As I finish one category, I move on to theoretical coding and writing memos about the next category. Often I discover that some categories are actually conditions or consequences of categories I have already theoretically coded. These discoveries help me reduce the number of concepts, and integrate the developing theory. When theoretically coding categories that are not processes, the coding families of type, degree, and dimensions may be more helpful. For example, the basic problem for caring women was caring demands. Analysis of the category labeled "demands" focused on the theoretical codes of *types* (competing or changing), and *dimensions* (pervasive, arising daily, simultaneous). Glaser (1978) suggested using typologies (qualitative cross tabulation) to clarify variation according to the presence or absence of dimensions.[6] For example, in the study of women's caring, "caring options" was a condition of the process of "negotiating". By creating a typology or cross tabulation based on the *dimensions* of "suitability" and "availability" of caring options, variation in caregiver's negotiation with the healthcare system was explicated: resources are available but not suitable (constantly shopping for other options), resources are available and suitable (satisfied, not negotiating), resources are suitable but not available (taking risks to make suitable options available), resources are neither suitable nor available (no indicators of this in the data, so left blank) (Wuest, 2001). While unquestionably the construction of typologies is based on an artificial presence/absence of dimensions (some resources may be somewhat suitable), the strategy nonetheless helps the analyst to identify how dimensions make a difference. The analyst may then apply the theoretical code of "degree" to consider further variation when dimensions are somewhat present.

After theoretically coding and memoing for each category, it is important to reflect on the bigger picture again. At this point, the concepts of the emerging theory can be diagrammed, the basic problem named, and the core category provisionally identified. The core category links categories together, explains what is going on, and accounts for variation (Glaser, 1978). Reflection on how well this provisional framework works for explaining the domain of study in terms of the data collected then takes place by a selective theoretically sampling of data to check out whether the relationships hypothesized between concepts hold across cases. I reread transcripts through the lens of my emerging theory, reflecting on data that informed my conceptual construction. When relationships do not hold, I am forced to reconsider my conceptualization, asking what factors account for the variation, and how I might increase the level of abstraction to include all data. A second point of reflection is considering which categories are not saturated and which relationships among concepts need confirmation or further development. This reflection continues with conceptual elaboration, that is, systematic deduction from the data of theoretical possibilities in the form of hypotheses that lead to further theoretical sampling and constant comparative analysis (Glaser, 1978).

Theoretical sampling and integration

Based on these reflections, I begin to recruit new participants or seek out other salient data such as documents. Importantly, in these new interviews, the researcher continues to begin with the broad overview question. However, as the researcher attends to the participant, he/she is listening through the lens of the emerging theory, seeking further clarification and expansion of concept properties, conditions that influence variation in process, and relationships among concepts. When new conceptual indicators emerge that are not accounted for by the emerging theory, the researcher again must modify the concept such that it "fits" the data; this normally means increasing the level of abstraction. Data that do not fit the emerging theory contribute to theoretical expansion; they do not disprove the emerging theory (Glaser, 1978). Thus, theory development is a continual process of modification and refinement such that the emerging theory fits the data. Because the researcher is consciously theoretically sampling, he/she is more focused on data salient to theoretical development. Similarly, if returning to participants a second time, the researcher normally has some theoretical purpose. Usually during second interviews, I give the person the opportunity to tell me about what has happened since I last saw them, and then I tell them about what I am learning, asking them further questions. I do this by bringing a diagram of the emerging theory, and talking about each concept or process, briefly explaining how the participant's data contributed to their development (Wuest & Merritt-Gray, 2001). Such discussion normally results in additional data that further saturate or refine the concept.

Analysis of data from these continuing interviews is focused to purposefully develop and integrate the theory. Concepts are expanded, sometimes shifted to higher levels of abstraction to account for new data, sometimes collapsed together. Linkages among concepts and conditions that influence variation are more fully saturated. Memos document the ongoing theoretical analysis. By labeling memos according to relevant concepts, including the location of salient data, and keeping them within the conceptual boundaries of the emerging theory, they provide a useful basis for report writing. Problem, process, and concept names evolve to fit the additional data. Diagrams are revised to reflect the more fully integrated theory. The theory generated at this point may be quite different to the initial framework. Data collection continues until data being collected are not producing new variation in the emerging theory. Unquestionably, the researcher has some control over this in terms of how broadly he/she theoretically samples.

Once the core process is identified, I begin theoretically sampling the literature well beyond the original literature review. This sampling is guided by the emerging theoretical concepts and extends across disciplines. As I read, I consider the literature as data to expand and densify concepts. I constantly compare for similarities and differences with the emerging substantive theory, and memo so that I can readily retrieve salient literature for the final report. Sometimes, concepts in extant theory through constant comparison are identified as fitting with the concept specified from the data. In this case, the researcher may decide to adopt the extant theoretical concept through this constant comparative process of emergent fit (Wuest, 2000). However, when this occurs, the researcher acknowledges within the research report that emergent fit has taken place and provides exemplars. In this way, deduction is always in service of induction within the grounded theory process (Glaser, 1978).

At this point, preparation for writing begins. The starting point is to sort previous memos by concepts and to diagram the relationships among the concepts.

Writing the Report

The grounded theory report is a theoretical account of the study domain identifying the basic problem and discussing how the core category addresses the basic problem. Writing theoretically is almost as challenging as theoretical coding. Glaser (1978) urged, "The dictum is to *write conceptually*, by making theoretical statements about relationships between concepts, rather than writing descriptive statements about people" (p. 133). Yet many grounded theory reports are written only at a descriptive level, with cursory naming of concepts or processes, supported by numerous compelling quotes from data. May (1986) cautioned that researchers "lapse into pure description and present these data in detail because they are 'too good to throw away'" (p. 148). Pure description can be the result of simply not engaging in the systematic theoretical coding and constant comparison needed to tease out the properties of concepts, and the theoretical relationships among them. On the other hand, even after putting extraordinary work into this analysis, some researchers have difficulty carrying their analysis through the writing process such that the end product is written at a theoretical level. This may be related to poorly developed theoretical sensitivity, or to not having access to a mentor or expert in grounded theory methods.

What are the indicators of a grounded theory report written at a theoretical level? Normally the findings section of the report will begin with an overview of the theory in which the basic social problem and the basic social process and its core concepts are named and conceptually specified (Glaser, 1978). Conceptual specifications are operational meanings derived from the data, and not from the dictionary, disciplinary usage, or extant theory. They have evolved through constant comparison as the theory is developed. The theoretical linkages among concepts are delineated. Often a diagram is provided to capture the basic social process, particularly movement between stages. This summary of the theoretical scheme provides a map that guides the researcher in the writing of detailed discussion of the theory (May, 1986). When the process identified is somewhat linear, another helpful tool, for both the researcher and the reader, is a chart of the stages in the process. While many grounded theorists infer rather than specify the problem, I urge researchers to stipulate the problem. Because the theory accounts for what takes place in response to the problem, naming and conceptually specifying the problem helps to keep the researcher focused as the theory is written. Sometimes this is a brief section, other times it is lengthy, leading to a published paper such as our discussion of *intrusion*, the basic problem for health promotion after leaving an abusive partner (Wuest, Ford-Gilboe, Merritt-Gray, & Berman, 2003).

Continue the write up with a detailed discussion of key theoretical concepts and their properties. At this more detailed level, concepts are conceptually specified, the theoretical properties of the concepts and the conditions that influence their variation are discussed, conceptual indicators are provided from the data, and literature to support the emerging theory is used as data. A limitation of many grounded theories is their failure to explain variation in the substantive concepts or in the basic social process. The theory is written homogeneously, implying that all people move through the basic social process in the same way. Conditions that influence variation may be named but not conceptually specified; nor is the effect of the condition on the timing, duration, intensity or range of the behavior well developed. Yet a major strength of grounded theory for the discipline of nursing is its capacity to account for variation in behavior. Understanding the conditions that produce variation in the process is often the starting point for nursing intervention or practice change.

In capturing variation, focus beyond how the core variable is affected by the presence/absence of specific conditions and consider how the degree or type of a condition or the interaction among dimensions of a condition makes a difference. Envisioning the variation in this way often moves the theory to a higher level of abstraction. Some conditions influence all stages of the process. The dimensions of these conditions may be described in a separate section. Other conditions are salient only to one subprocess or concept, and may be discussed when that subprocess is being explained. But naming and conceptually specifying conditions is not enough. In the detailed discussion of theory, the way that these conditions affect variation in the basic social process or core variable, particularly with regard to degree, duration, and timing, must be delineated and supported with data as conceptual indicators.

Many novice grounded theorists view analysis and writing as separate activities and are shocked to discover how much analysis takes place in the writing process. It is only through writing a coherent storyline about the basic social process or core variable that the inconsistencies in the scope and relationships among concepts emerge, forcing the analyst ever back to the data to confirm and refine through further constant comparison, theoretical sampling, and reduction. Moreover, although one begins writing with an overview of the theory, often the detailed articulation of the properties and relationships among concepts yields further insights that force the researcher to revise the initial overview, moving closer to a clear and parsimonious theory. Some researchers who struggle with getting beyond description, find a good starting point is to prepare an outline of key concepts and properties, a procedure similar to preparing overheads for a presentation. Decisions regarding what to include and the words to use in each bullet help the researcher to determine what is core and to reduce the categories to key concepts, thereby increasing the level of abstraction.

One way to avoid writing descriptively is to write the first detailed draft without including conceptual indicators from the data or the literature. Glaser warned, "The *credibility* of the theory should be won by its integration, relevance, and workability, not by illustration used as if it were proof" (1978, p. 134). Writing without data forces the researcher to write about concepts, not cases. Once satisfied with a conceptual discussion of the theory, the researcher can write a second draft inserting salient data as conceptual indicators. Data or descriptive statements about the data are used only for "illustration and imagery" (Glaser, 1978, p. 134). Data, particularly that collected by talking to people about their experiences, is often beguiling. Hence researchers are reluctant to abandon rich and detailed narrative in service of theory construction. Consequently, many first drafts, and all too many final papers, of grounded theory studies consist of lengthy direct quotes strung together to tell the "story" of a particular experience. Unlike other qualitative research methods such as narrative analysis, the goal of grounded theory is not to accurately describe an individual's experience. Rather it is to construct a middle range theory that explains how the basic social problem is processed. The researcher takes responsibility for constructing this theory which reaches far beyond the understanding of any single participant (Pyett, 2004). While the resulting theory will resonate for the participant, it will not describe the detail of their personal journey. A strength, in fact, of a grounded theory is that the theoretical framework often provides the participant with a new or fuller perspective. Another hazard of being immersed in the data is that researchers may have difficulty using data judiciously. Because the data are so compelling, the researcher may include a lengthy quote in which the conceptual indicator is buried. Select the best indicator of the concept and check that the connection to the concept is readily apparent.

A third writing of the theory focuses on adding in literature. Literature is theoretically sampled and added as supporting data for the theory, or to demonstrate how this conceptualization differs from the current state of the knowledge. A challenge in integrating the literature into the write up, as opposed to dealing with it in a separate discussion chapter, is ensuring that it does not take over. Be succinct and discriminating. Many novice researchers struggle with using literature as data, commonly integrating it "backwards." What I mean by this is that they discuss how their findings support the research or theoretical perspectives of others. Rather, the literature should be discussed as data to support the emerging theory. The researcher handles the literature as other data, theoretically sampling, constantly comparing, and integrating what adds to the emerging theory.

Having written, and rewritten the grounded theory adding data exemplars and then literature, the researcher normally has a dense and parsimonious theory. The strength of theory construction is that the outcome can be applied to nursing practice as a lens to interpret people's experience or to direct actions and interventions. Completing the write up with a section discussing implications helps others to understand the significance of the theory. Often, novice grounded theorists return exclusively to the descriptive data when explaining the implications of their study findings, thus nullifying the power of the explanatory theory. Framing implications of the study in terms of the theoretical process or concepts, demonstrates the significance of the framework, and offers direction for application. Thus, when writing this final section, consider how this theoretical rendering of the study domain contributes new knowledge to the discipline, and how it might be useful for practice and policy.

But Is It Grounded Theory?

How does a researcher know whether the grounded theory generated is credible? Most qualitative research studies are evaluated in terms of broad criteria for rigor that mirror the post-positivist criteria of validity and reliability. The most broadly referenced are Lincoln and Guba's (1985) guidelines of trustworthiness and authenticity (Whittemore, Chase, & Mandel, 2001). Because these guidelines are broadly applicable to most qualitative methods, the researcher may follow them rigorously and produce a report that is not grounded theory. Glaser's (1978) criteria of *fit* (concepts must evolve to fit the data), *grab* (captures interest because it resonates), *work* (usefulness for explaining, interpreting, and predicting), and *modifiability* (capacity to change in response to new data) are specific to grounded theory. Both Lincoln and Guba's and Glaser's criteria offer more direction for rigor in doing grounded theory than for evaluation of the final product. Over the past decade, I have been increasingly challenged to articulate and justify how I evaluate a qualitative research report that is put forward as grounded theory. Working with graduate students who are learning the method has forced me to begin to consider, not just what is wrong with beginning drafts, but also what has to be done to produce a thesis that is defensible as grounded theory. Similarly review activities for journals, granting agencies, and graduate schools have assisted me to develop clear benchmarks for what constitutes a grounded theory. Those benchmarks have guided the forgoing discussion of how to write the grounded theory report. I am aware that articulating criteria for judging whether a qualitative report is grounded theory may be considered dogmatic given the diversity of grounded theory approaches; however, I believe the following benchmarks will stand regardless of the approach used.

Broadly my benchmarks for grounded theory are as follows:

1. The theory is written at a theoretical level.
2. The conditions that account for variation in the basic social process or core variable are delineated and demonstrated in the discussion of the theory.
3. Primacy is given to inductively derived concepts/processes in the substantive theory which are conceptually specified from the data.
4. Emergent fit is delineated when concepts/processes are labeled as existing theory-laden concepts already well developed in the literature.
5. Data, particularly direct quotes, are used judiciously to demonstrate theoretical properties and variation.
6. Existing theory and research is used to support the substantive theory and its uniqueness, as opposed to substantive theory being used to support extant theory.
7. The implications of the study are written in terms of the substantive theory, not in terms of the descriptive data.

Where Does Grounded Theory Fit in the Paradigm Debate?

Benoliel (1998) in a letter to Pam Brink, editor of *Western Journal of Nursing Research* observed, "Within nursing . . . the notion of qualitative research has been approached as a way of *doing* more than as a way of *thinking* (p. 238). She further argued that "the 'hows' of doing research are embedded within basic assumptions about the nature of knowledge and knowing and the paradigms or formats through which the investigator designs and implements specific proposals" (p. 238). These observations resonate for me because in my development as a researcher, I focused initially more on doing than thinking. Yet, I now understand that the way I do grounded theory is influenced greatly by my paradigm orientation. Increasingly, qualitative researchers are expected to be clear about their paradigms or worldviews—that is, assumptions regarding the nature of reality, what can be known, and how it can be known (Guba & Lincoln, 1994). My initial introduction to worldviews was in the first edition of this text (Munhall & Oiler, 1986) where worldviews were presented as received (traditional mechanistic) and nonreceived (holistic humanistic) and were, in my mind aligned with quantitative and qualitative methods respectively. I classified grounded theory with the nonreceived view. Subsequently, Guba and Lincoln identified four paradigms: positivist, post-positivist, constructivist, and critical. To my surprise, they located grounded theory in the post-positivist paradigm which is informed by the assumptions that 1) a single reality exists that can only be imperfectly apprehended, 2) objectivity is a regulatory ideal, and 3) findings are confirmed through replication and fit with existing knowledge.

In my judgment, grounded theory is more consistent with the constructivist paradigm. Glaser and Strauss in their early writings (Glaser, 1978; Glaser & Strauss, 1967; Strauss, 1987) discussed how their research approach challenged verification of extant theory, the dominant research approach at that time in sociology. They questioned the dominant grand theories of their day, suggesting that these theories were not sufficient to explain relevant social issues. In contrast to grand theory, substantive middle range theories, called grounded theories, explain focused areas of sociological inquiry. Grounded theories are generated by first discovering inductively what concepts and hypotheses are relevant to the area being studied. Strauss (1987) asserted that a key assumption of grounded theory is that social phenomena are complex. He observed that a major limitation of much social research is to ignore complexity and study phenomena in isolation, assuming that complexity would be dealt with later. Grounded theory "emphasizes the need for developing many concepts and their linkages in order to capture a great deal of the variation that characterizes central phenomena studied during any research project" (Strauss, p. 7). Glaser and Strauss (1967) also broke with the dominant research tradition of that time by asserting that the researcher is not "a passive receiver of impression" but rather is actively hypothesizing and checking out hunches to generate theory (p. 39). "Grounded theory is developed in intimate relationship with data, with researchers fully aware of themselves as instruments for developing that grounded theory" (Strauss, 1987, p. 6). How the researcher actively engages in shaping the research process depends in part on the researcher's theoretical sensitivity. This acknowledgment of the researcher as an active participant in the construction of the research outcome was a significant departure from the objectivist position.

A criterion for judging grounded theory is whether it works; that is, interprets what is happening, explains what did happen, and predicts what will happen (Glaser, 1978). While the notion of prediction is somewhat post-positivist, Glaser recognized the partial perspective offered by a grounded theory, arguing that grounded theory is modifiable and can be recast as new data is collected and compared. Nonetheless, the language that Glaser and Strauss used in their various writings (Glaser, 1978, 1992; Glaser & Strauss, 1967; Strauss, 1987) is rooted in the positivist tradition of their research training in the mid-20th century. Critics of grounded theory often focus on this language, sometimes ignoring the significant shifts of thinking that align the approach more with what is often called the constructivist paradigm.

Charmaz (2000) wrote extensively about constructivist grounded theory. "Constructivism assumes the relativism of multiple social realities, recognizes the mutual creation of knowledge by the viewer and the viewed, and aims toward interpretive understandings of the subject's meanings" (p. 510). "Causality is suggestive, incomplete, and indeterminate in constructivist grounded theory" (p. 524). She argued that all data are narrative reconstructions of experience, not indicators of an external reality. The constructed theory does not constitute participant reality; rather it is a theoretical rendering, "one interpretation among multiple interpretations of a shared or individual reality" (p. 523). Charmaz presented her perspective as if it were a total departure from the original position of Glaser and Strauss, failing to give the originators credit for the ways they did challenge dominant positivist thinking. This is particularly evident in the discussion of the epistemology. Charmaz argued that Glaser assumed that "we gather our data unfettered by bias or biography" (p. 592). Yet Glaser and Strauss (1967) were clear that the researcher's theoretical sensitivity influences data collection and analysis and that the researcher is an active participant in generating theory. Thus, Charmaz's strong assertion that the theory is shaped and constructed by the researcher and that coding is an interpretive process, is consistent with that of the originators. Glaser (1978) used the language of emergence and discovery, but I understand emergence as a process of researcher generation which is consistent with constructivism. Charmaz moved beyond Glaser and Strauss in offering important direction conducting constructivist grounded theory when she called for exploration of values, and establishing relationships with participants so that they may tell their stories their way, preferably through a sustained relationship rather than once only. This direction expands the approach to doing grounded theory and supports the constructivist location. More recently, Bryant and Charmaz (2007b) have written extensively about the epistemology of grounded theory, acknowledging the contribution of the early writings to challenging the approaches to theory development of the time, and recognizing that within Glaser and Strauss's early writings exist hints of a different underlying epistemology.

In recent years, I have debated whether grounded theory could legitimately be located in the critical paradigm (Wuest et al., 2002). Benoliel (1996) noted that while most grounded theory studies result in practical knowledge based on interpretive understanding, "some findings provided an *emancipatory* focus in that they point to interactional and environmental constraints on the freedom and well-being of individuals with health problems" (p. 417). Emancipation and critique are the explicit goals of research in the critical paradigm. The ontology is historical realism; that is, reality has been shaped over time by dominant social, political, cultural, economic and ethnic factors and ultimately crystallized (Guba & Lincoln, 1994). The investigator and the investigated engage in a dialogic interaction that is value mediated and intended to challenge what has been taken for granted as real. Although Glaser (1978) argued that grounded theory is a starting point for change, change is not normally an explicit goal of the research process. In the development of a program of research focusing on health promotion in single parent families after leaving an abusive partner (Wuest et al., 2003; Ford-Gilboe, Wuest, & Merritt-Gray, 2005), we theoretically sampled data related to policy and services to expand our conceptual understanding of how these social structures influenced the basic social process. Within the critical paradigm, the test of the emerging theory is not just in how it explains what is happening but also in how it opens up alternatives for thought and action about how things could be (Kvale, 1995). We hoped our research would influence policy and services for families and reasoned that change would be more likely to take place as part of the research process if we shared our emerging theory derived from interviews with the families as a starting point for our discussions with policymakers and service providers (Wuest et al., 2002). Our discussions were dialogues that allowed for generation of theory based not only on the perspectives of the family, but also on those of the providers and policymakers.

Similarly, Kushner and Morrow (2003) proposed a critical feminist grounded theory methodology arguing that the conscious use of feminist and critical theory with grounded theory supports "the integration of social structural analysis in the generation of explanations of human interaction in the social world" (p. 41). Clarke (2003) also positioned grounded theory in the critical paradigm with her assertion that grounded theory is postmodern. Interactionist grounded theory, according to Clarke, has always had the capacity to reveal perspectives in ways that are congruent with the postmodern situated knowledges. Clarke argued that new methods needed to address the complexity and heterogeneity of a postmodern world "should be epistemologically/ontologically based in the pragmatist soil that has historically nurtured symbolic interactionism and grounded theory" (p. 555). "The methodological implications of the postmodern primarily require taking situatedness, variations, complicatedness, differences of all kinds, and positionality/relationality very seriously in all their complexities, multiplicities, instabilities, and contradictions" (p. 556). Grounded theory, by virtue of producing substantive theory, may be seen as imposing a universal narrative that entrenches a singular viewpoint, rather than encouraging situated knowledge. Grounded theory especially when conducted from a feminist perspective allows for the inclusion of difference in the development of explanatory frameworks (Wuest & Merritt-Gray, 2001). Although the core variable or basic social process reflects the commonality of the experience, conditions are identified that influence the variation in the way the theory is enacted. Clarke observed that most methodological approaches in the post-modern center on giving individual voice through narrative and other biographic strategies that neglect social context. In contrast, grounded theory has the capacity to capture complexity within the social context, and thus is an important research approach for the postmodern.

Researchers are using grounded theory across paradigms. Using grounded theory from different worldviews does not violate the intellectual roots of the method. The paradigm in which the grounded theory project is located will influence the relationship between the researcher and the participants, and the broad goal of the project (explanation, understanding, or transformation). Thus, sorting out the paradigm location may be helpful for designing the research study.

Final Words

Grounded theory is a versatile research approach useful for generating explanatory substantive theory of human behavior in social context. Thus the research problem must be one that will be illuminated by understanding social psychological process in the study domain. Moreover, grounded theory is only an appropriate method when the researcher intends to go beyond description of the study domain, toward a theoretical rendering. Choosing to use grounded theory is not a decision that should be taken without considerable forethought. A critical issue is the individual researcher's capacity to think theoretically. Most researchers have a sense of their capacity to handle quantitative research approaches from their education and life experience related to mathematics and basic statistics. Background in qualitative analysis is less common. In my experience, most novice researchers handle initial open coding well. However, moving from open coding to theoretical coding and theory construction is much more challenging. Working with experienced researchers on an ongoing grounded theory project or engaging in a small pilot project with guidance from an experienced grounded theorist is invaluable in helping researchers determine whether grounded theory is a suitable approach for them. For some, descriptive understanding is much more meaningful and the shift toward conceptualization is painful. Learning that *before* embarking on a grounded theory project is wise.

Doing grounded theory requires persistence, tolerance of uncertainty, abstract thinking, ability to make connections, facility with words, and willingness to live with an emerging theory always in the back of one's mind. Indeed, often it is when it is in the background, that the most useful theoretical thoughts arise. Grounded theory is also hard work. Open coding, categorizing, theoretical coding and writing memos all require methodical, diligent effort if the outcome is to be a parsimonious and well-integrated theory. Grounded theories do not magically appear; they are generated from the data, one step at a time.

Sometimes the process is slow and tedious, but when theoretical concepts and linkages begin to come together researchers can experience what Glaser (1978) called a "drugless high". Researchers find the emerging theory interesting and recognize its usefulness. Work on conceptual specification and theory integration is stimulating and exciting as the theory begins to take shape.

In summary, grounded theory research is all about fit: 1) fit between the research problem and the grounded theory product, 2) fit between researcher capacity and the grounded theory method, and 3) fit between the data and the evolving theoretical construction. The first fit can be determined before getting started. The second can be partially determined in advance through some training experience. The last is up to the researcher once the project is underway.

References

Artinian, B., Giske, T., & Cone, P. (2009). *Glaserian grounded theory in nursing research: Trusting emergence*. New York: Springer.

Artinian, B., & West, K. (2009). Conceptual mapping as an aid to grounded theory development. In B. Artinian, T. Giske, & P. Cone (Eds.), *Glaserian grounded theory in nursing research: Trusting emergence* (pp. 27–34). New York: Springer.

Beck, C. T. (1999). Grounded theory research. In J. Fain (Ed.), *Reading, understanding, and applying nursing research* (pp. 205–225). Philadelphia: Davis.

Benoliel, J. Q. (1996). Grounded theory and nursing knowledge . . . presented at a symposium sponsored by the College of Nursing, University of Rhode Island in October 1994. *Qualitative Health Research, 6*(3), 406–428.

Benoliel, J. Q. (1998). Letter to the Editor. *Western Journal of Nursing Research, 20*(2), 238.

Bevis, E. O. (1988). Caring: A life force. In M. Leininger (Ed.), *Caring: An essential human need* (pp. 49–60). Detroit: Wayne State University Press.

Blumer, H. (1969). *Symbolic interactionism: Perspective and method*. Englewood Cliffs, NJ: Prentice Hall.

Bryant, A., & Charmaz, K. (2007a). Introduction: Grounded theory research: Methods and practices. In A. Bryant & K. Charmaz (Eds.), *The Sage handbook of grounded theory* (pp. 1–28). Los Angeles: Sage.

Bryant, A., & Charmaz, K. (2007b). Grounded theory in historical perspective: An epistemological account. In A. Bryant & K. Charmaz (Eds.), *The Sage handbook of grounded theory* (pp. 31–57). Los Angeles: Sage.

Charmaz, K. (2000). Grounded theory: Objectivist and constructivist methods. In N. Denzin & Y. Lincoln (Eds.), *Handbook of qualitative research* (2nd ed., pp. 509–535). Thousand Oaks, CA: Sage.

Charmaz, K. (2006). *Constructing grounded theory: A practical guide through qualitative methods*. London: Sage.

Chenitz, W. C., & Swanson, J. (1986). *From practice to grounded theory: Qualitative research in nursing*. Menlo Park, CA: Addison-Wesley.

Clark, A. (2003). Situational analyses: Grounded theory mapping after the postmodern turn. *Symbolic Interaction, 26*(4), 553–576.

Clarke, A. (2005). *Situational Analysis: Grounded theory after the postmodern turn*. Thousand Oaks, CA: Sage.

Corbin, J., & Strauss, A. (2008). *Basics of qualitative research* (3rd ed.). Thousand Oaks, CA: Sage.

Covan, E. K. (2007). The discovery of grounded theory in practice: The legacy of multiple mentors. In A. Bryant & K. Charmaz (Eds.), *The Sage handbook of grounded theory* (pp. 58–74). Los Angeles: Sage.

Crooks, D. (2001). The importance of symbolic interaction in grounded theory research on women's health. *Health Care for Women International, 22*(1–2), 11–27.

Enman, A. (2004). *Help seeking in spousal caregivers of those with Alzheimer's Disease and related disorders.* Unpublished Master of Nursing Thesis Proposal.

Farran, C., & Keane-Hagerty, E. (1991). An interactive model for finding meaning through caregiving. In P. Chinn (Ed.), *Anthology of caring* (pp. 225–238). New York: National League for Nursing.

Ford-Gilboe, M., Wuest, J., & Merritt-Gray, M. (2005). Strengthening capacity to limit intrusion: Theorizing family health promotion in the aftermath of woman abuse. *Qualitative Health Research, 15,* 477–501.

Given, B., & Given, C. (1991). Family caregiving for the elderly. In J. Fitzpatrick, R. Taunton, & A. Jacox (Eds.), *Annual Review of Nursing Research* (Vol. 9, pp. 77–99). New York: Springer.

Glaser, B. (1978). *Theoretical sensitivity.* Mill Valley, CA: Sociology Press.

Glaser, B. (1992). *Basics of grounded theory analysis.* Mill Valley, CA: Sociology Press.

Glaser, B. (1998). *Doing grounded theory: Issues and discussions.* Mill Valley, CA: Sociology Press.

Glaser, B. (1999). The future of grounded theory. *Qualitative Health Research, 9*(6), 836–845.

Glaser, B. (2002). Conceptualization: On theory and theorizing using grounded theory. *International Journal of Qualitative Methods, 1*(2), 23–38.

Glaser, B. (2004). Remodelling grounded theory. *Forum: Qualitative Social Research, 5*(2). Retrieved June 22, 2010, from http://www.qualitative-research.net/fqs-texte/2-04/2-04 glaser-e.htm

Glaser, B., & Strauss, A. (1967). *The discovery of grounded theory.* Chicago: Aldine.

Guba, E., & Lincoln, Y. (1994). Competing paradigms in qualitative research. In N. Denzin & Lincoln, (Eds.). *Handbook of qualitative research.* (pp.105-117). Thousand Oaks, CA: Sage.

Hutchinson, S., & Wilson, H. (1994). Research and therapeutic interviews: A post-structuralist perspective. In J. Morse (Ed.), *Critical issues in qualitative research methods* (pp. 300–315). Thousand Oaks, CA: Sage.

Hutchinson, S., & Wilson, H. (2001). Grounded theory: The method. In P. Munhall (Ed.), *Nursing research: A qualitative perspective* (3rd ed., pp. 209–244). Sudbury, MA: Jones & Bartlett.

Kushner, K., & Morrow, R. (2003). Grounded theory, feminist theory, critical theory: Toward theoretical triangulation. *Advances in Nursing Science, 26,* 30–43.

Kvale, S. (1995). The social construction of validity. *Qualitative Inquiry, 1,* 19–40.

Lempert, L. B. (2007). Asking questions of the data: Memo writing in the grounded theory tradition. In A. Bryant & K. Charmaz (Eds.), *The Sage handbook of grounded theory* (pp. 245–264). Los Angeles: Sage.

Lincoln, Y., & Guba, E. (1985). *Naturalistic inquiry.* Thousand Oaks, CA: Sage.

MacDonald, M. (2001). Finding a critical perspective in grounded theory. In R. Schreiber & P. N. Stern (Eds.), *Using grounded theory in nursing* (pp. 113–158). New York: Springer.

May, K. (1991). Interviewing techniques: Concerns and challenges. In J. Morse (Ed.), *Qualitative nursing research* (pp. 180–201). Newbury Park, CA: Sage.

May, K. A. (1986). Writing and evaluating the grounded theory research report. In W. C. Chenitz & J. M. Swanson (Eds.), *From practice to grounded theory: Qualitative research in nursing* (pp. 146–154). Menlo Park, CA: Addison-Wesley.

Milliken, P. J., & Schreiber, R. (2001). Can you "do" grounded theory without symbolic interactionism? In R. Schreiber & P. Stern (Eds.), *Using grounded theory in nursing* (pp. 176–190). New York: Springer Publishing.

Montgomery, P., & Bailey, P. (2007). Field notes and theoretical memos in grounded theory. *Western Journal of Nursing Research, 29,* 65–79.

Morse, J. (1994). Designing funded qualitative research. In N. Denzin & Y. Lincoln (Eds.), *Handbook of qualitative research* (pp. 220–235). Thousand Oaks, CA: Sage.

Morse, J. (2007). Sampling in grounded theory. In A. Bryant & K. Charmaz (Eds.), *The Sage handbook of grounded theory* (pp. 229–244). Los Angeles: Sage.

Morse, J., Stern, P. N., Corbin, J., Bowers, B., Charmaz, K., & Clarke, A. (2009). *Developing grounded theory: The second generation.* Walnut Creek, CA: Left Coast Books.

Morse, J., & Richards, L. (2002). *README FIRST for a user's guide to qualitative methods.* Thousand Oaks, CA: Sage.

Munhall, P., & Oiler, C. (1986). *Nursing research: A qualitative perspective.* Norwalk, Conn: Appleton-Century-Crofts.

Paterson, B., Gregory, D., & Thorne, S. (1999). A protocol for research safety. *Qualitative Health Research, 9,* 259–269.

Pyett, P. (2004). Validation of qualitative research in the "real world". *Qualitative Health Research, 13,* 1170–1179.

Ray, M. (1981/1988). A philosophical analysis of caring within nursing. In M. Leininger (Ed.), *Caring: An essential human need* (pp. 25–36). Detroit: Wayne State University Press.

Roach, Sister S. (1992). *The human act of caring.* Ottawa, Ontario: Canadian Hospital Association.

Sandelowski, M. (1998). Writing a good read: Strategies for re-presenting qualitative data. *Research in Nursing & Health, 21,* 375–382.

Schreiber, R., & Stern, P.N. (2001). *Using grounded theory in nursing.* New York: Springer Publishing.

Seigfried, C. H. (1998). Pragmatism. In A. Jaggar & I. Young (Eds.), *A companion to feminist philosophy* (pp. 49–57). Malden, MA: Blackwell.

Snow, D. (2001). Expanding and broadening Blumer's conceptualization of symbolic interactionism. *Symbolic Interaction, 24,* 367–377.

Stern, P. (1980). Grounded theory methodology: Its uses and processes. *Image, 12,* 20–23.

Stern, P. N. (2007). On solid ground: Essential properties for growing grounded theory. In A. Bryant & K. Charmaz (Eds.), *The Sage handbook of grounded theory* (pp. 114–126). Los Angeles: Sage.

Stern, P. N., & Covan, E. (2001). Early grounded theory: Its processes and products. In R. Schreiber & P. N. Stern (Eds.), *Using grounded theory in nursing* (pp. 17–34). New York: Springer.

Stern, P. N., & Pyles, S. (1986). Using grounded theory methodology to study women's culturally based decisions about health. In P. N. Stern (Ed.), *Women, health, and culture* (pp. 1–24). Washington, DC: Hemisphere.

Strauss, A. (1987). *Qualitative analysis for social scientists.* Cambridge: Cambridge University Press.

Strauss, A., & Corbin, J. (1990). *Basics of qualitative research: Grounded theory procedures and techniques.* Newbury Park, CA: Sage.

Strauss, A., & Corbin, J. (1998). *Basics of qualitative research: Techniques and procedures for developing grounded theory.* Thousand Oaks, CA: Sage.

Swanson, J. (1987). The formal qualitative interview for grounded theory. In W. C. Chenitz & J. Swanson (Eds.), *From practice to grounded theory: Qualitative research in nursing* (pp. 66–78). Menlo Park, CA: Addison-Wesley.

Whittemore, R., Chase, S., & Mandle, C. L. (2001). Validity in qualitative research. *Qualitative Health Research, 11,* 522–537.

Wuest, J. (1995). Feminist grounded theory: An exploration of congruency and tensions between two traditions in knowledge discovery. *Qualitative Health Research, 5*(1), 125–137.

Wuest, J. (1997a). Fraying connections of caring women: An exemplar of including difference in the development of explanatory frameworks. *Canadian Journal of Nursing Research, 29,* 99–116.

Wuest, J. (1997b). Illuminating environmental influences on women's caring. *Journal of Advanced Nursing, 26,* 49–58.

Wuest, J. (2000). Negotiating with helping systems: An example of grounded theory evolving through emergent fit. *Qualitative Health Research, 10,* 51–70.

Wuest, J. (2001). Precarious ordering: Toward a formal theory of women's caring. *Health Care for Women International: Special Volume, Using Grounded Theory to Study Women's Health., 22,* 1–2, 167–193.

Wuest, J., Berman, H., Ford-Gilboe, M., & Merritt-Gray, M. (2002). Illuminating social determinants of women's health using grounded theory. *Health Care for Women International, 23*(8), 794–808.

Wuest, J., Ford-Gilboe, M., Merritt-Gray, M., & Berman, H. (2003). Intrusion: The basic social problem identified in a grounded theory study of family health promotion among children and single mothers after leaving an abusive partner. *Qualitative Health Research, 13*(5), 597–622.

Wuest, J., Ford-Gilboe, M., Merritt-Gray, M. (2005). Strengthening capacity to limit intrusion: Theorizing family health promotion in the aftermath of woman abuse. *Qualitative Health Research, 15.*

Wuest, J., Ericson, P., & Stern, P. N. (1994). Becoming strangers: Changing family relationships in Alzheimer's Disease. *Journal of Advanced Nursing, 20,* 437–443.

Wuest, J., & Merritt-Gray, M. (1999). Not going back: Sustaining the separation in the process of leaving abusive relationships. *Violence Against Women, 5,* 110–133.

Wuest, J., & Merritt-Gray, M. (2001). Feminist grounded theory revisited. In R. Schreiber & P. Stern (Eds.), *Using grounded theory in nursing* (pp. 159–176). New York: Springer Publishing.

Wuest, J., & Stern, P. (1990). The impact of fluctuating relationships with the Canadian health care system on family management of *otitis media* with effusion. *Journal of Advanced Nursing, 15,* 556–563.

Endnotes

[1] For an excellent comparison of the approaches of Strauss and Corbin (1990) and Glaser (1992), see MacDonald (2001, pp. 138–153)

[2] See the Grounded Theory Institute http://www.groundedtheory.com/

[3] See Wuest (2001) for an explicit depiction of theoretical sampling in a study of women's caring.

[4] See Sandelowski (1998) for an excellent discussion of the hazards of metaphor.

[5] See Glaser (1978) Chapter 4 for a full discussion of coding families

[6] See Glaser (1978) pp. 65–70 for a discussion of typology construction

9

Exemplar: Teetering on the Edge: A Second Grounded Theory Modification

Cheryl Tatano Beck

Postpartum depression is a major public health problem (Wisner, Chambers, & Sit, 2006). Up to 19% of new mothers suffer from depression during the first 3 months after birth (Gavin et al., 2005). Undiagnosed postpartum depression can plunge mothers into the depths of despair, rob them of the joys of motherhood, and turn their first months after birth into blackness. Up to 50% of all cases of this crippling mood disorder can go undetected (Ramsay, 1993).

Long-term sequelae of postpartum depression on cognitive and behavioral development of children are being reported. At 11 years of age children whose mothers had suffered from postpartum depression were 4 times more likely to develop psychiatric disorders than children of nondepressed mothers (Pawlby, Sharp, Hay, & O'Keane, 2008). Anxiety disorders in 13-year-old adolescents of mothers who had developed postpartum depression were also found to be elevated compared to the group whose mothers had not been postpartum depressed, regardless of the occurrence of subsequent maternal depression (Halligan, Murray, Martins, & Cooper, 2007). Children, age 11 and 16 years, of mothers who experienced postpartum depression also have significantly lower IQ scores; this is especially apparent in boys (Hay, Pawlby, Waters, & Sharp, 2008).

Background

One question that has been debated over the years is whether postpartum depression is a Western culture-bound syndrome. Stern and Kruckman (1983) hypothesize "that the negative outcomes of depression and baby blues in the U.S. result from the relative lack of (1) social structuring of postpartum events, (2) social recognition of a role transition for the new mother, and (3) instrumental assistance to the new mother" (p. 1036). They list the following six components of postpartum activities which provide social support for new mothers and help to buffer or prevent postpartum depression (p. 1039):

- Structuring of a distinct postpartum time period
- Protective measures of rituals reflecting the presumed vulnerability of the new mother
- Social seclusion
- Mandated rest
- Assistance in tasks from relative and/or midwife
- Social recognition through rituals, gifts, and so forth after new social status of the mother

The works of Seel (1986) and Bhugra and Gregoire (1993) support Stern and Kruckman's (1983) hypothesis. Seel (1986) purports that rituals and customs surrounding birth and the postpartum period are critical for a woman to feel that her new role is valued by her culture and that a supporting network of family and friends surrounds her. Bhugra and Gregoire (1993) described four themes within these protective rituals: 1) isolating and secluding the new mother, 2) intensive caring and support of the new mother, 3) behavioral proscriptions on the women such as "doing the month" among the Chinese (Pillsbury, 1978) or dietary restrictions, and 4) suspending of social roles and protecting from previous demands. Seel (1986) referred to these childbirth rituals as "rites de passage"; when incomplete, as in Western society, these rites are associated with an increase in postpartum depression. Seel argued that in the Western society the mother and father are left in limbo. New parents have to fend for themselves as they can. Without these rituals, mothers are stripped of protective layers. This cultural stereotyping is dangerous, however, because of the possibility that postpartum depression in non-Western culture may go unrecognized (Kumar, 1994).

Since the 1990s, findings from transcultural research on postpartum depression have accumulated evidence that the prevalence of this postpartum mood disorder is fairly consistent around the globe. Oates et al. (2004) examined whether postpartum depression was a universal experience with common attributes and how it was described by women. The research occurred in 11 countries: France, Ireland, Italy, Sweden, United States, Uganda, United Kingdom, Japan, Portugal, Austria, and Switzerland. "Morbid unhappiness" (postpartum depression) was recognized by women in all 11 countries as a common experience after delivery.

Internationally, rates of elevated postpartum depressive symptoms were found to be 13.8% in China (Gao, Chan, & Mao, 2009), 14.5% in Greece (Giakoumaki, Vasilaki, Lili, Skouroliakou, & Liosis, 2009), 16.4% in South Africa (Ramchandani, Richter, Stein, & Norris, 2009), 22% in Bangladesh (Gausia, Fisher, Ali, & Oosthuizen, 2009), 23.4% in Italy (Monti, Agostini, Marano, & Lupi, 2008), 33.2% in Turkey (Ege, Timur, Zincir, Geçkil, & Sunar-Reeder, 2008), and 37.1% in Iran (Kheirabadi et al., 2009).

A grounded theory study of postpartum depression, called "Teetering on the Edge," was first developed by Beck in 1993. At the time that study was conducted, there were only two other qualitative studies on the topic that had been published (Beck, 1992; Nicolson, 1990). Neither of these studies used a grounded theory design. The grounded theory of "Teetering on the Edge" was first modified (Beck, 2007) to increase its scope to include the behavior of postpartum-depressed women from other countries than just the Caucasian women in the United States who composed the original sample (Beck, 1993). In that first modification, data from the following 10 qualitative studies were included: Hmong women in the United States (Stewart & Jambunathan, 1996), Canadian women (Berggren-Clive, 1998), Middle Eastern women in Australia (Nahas, Hillege, & Amasheh, 1999), Australians (Holopainen, 2002), women in Ireland (Lawler & Sinclair, 2003), women in India (Rodrigues, Patel, Jaswal, & deSouza, 2003), Black Caribbean women in the United Kingdom (Edge, Baker, & Rogers, 2004; Templeton, Velleman, Persaud, & Milner, 2003), African-American women in the United States (Amankwaa, 2003), and Hong Kong Chinese women (Chan, Levy, Chung, & Lee, 2002).

Five years have passed since that first grounded theory modification. Since that time 17 new transcultural qualitative studies of postpartum-depressed women have been published and have been included in this second modification of "Teetering on the Edge" (**Table 9–1**). These 17 qualitative studies of postpartum depression included data from mothers in the following countries: Canada (Ahmed, Stewart, Teng, Wahoush, & Gagnon, 2008; Morrow, Smith, Lai, & Jaswal, 2008; Sword, Busser, Ganann, McMillan, & Swinton, 2008); Sweden (Edhborg, Friberg, Lundh, & Widström, 2005), Australia (Barr, 2006; Barr & Beck, 2008; Buultjens & Liamputtong, 2007), New Zealand (McCarthy & McMahon, 2008), United Kingdom (Chew-Graham, Sharp, Chamberlain, Folkes, & Turner, 2009; Hall, 2006; Hanley, 2007; Hanley & Long, 2006); Indonesia (Andajani-Sutjahjo, Manderson, & Astbury, 2007), the Democratic Republic of Congo (Bass, Ryder, Lammers, Mukaba, & Bolton, 2008), Ethiopia (Hanlon, Whitley, Wondimagegn, Alem, & Prince, 2009), United Arab Emirates (Ghubash & Eapen, 2009), Taiwan (Chen, Wang, Chung, Tseng, & Chou, 2006), and Japanese mothers in the United States (Taniguchi & Baruffi, 2007). In 8 of these 17 studies the samples consisted of immigrant women.

TABLE 9–1 Seventeen New Transcultural Qualitative Studies on Postpartum Depression included in the Second Grounded Theory Modification

Author/Year	Sample	Country Where Research Conducted	Qualitative Research Design	Data Collection
Bass, Ryder, Lammers, Mukaba, & Bolton/2008	41 women with postpartum depression who had given birth within past 2 years	Democratic Republic of Congo	Mixed Methods Descriptive, Qualitative	Interviews semi-structured
Morrow, Smith, Lai, & Jaswal/2008	18 first generation immigrant women and 1 second generation immigrant woman. 7 women born in Hong Kong, 5 born in China, 4 born in India, 1 in Taiwan, 1 in Uganda, 1 in Canada	Canada	Ethnographic narrative approach Thematic Analysis	Semi-structured interviews
Hanlon, Whitley, Wondimagegn, Alem, & Prince/2009	25 women interviewed in depth and 53 women in focus groups	Ethiopia	Descriptive Qualitative Thematic Analysis	In-cepth interviews & 5 focus groups
Ghubash & Eapen/2009	19 women of childbearing age	United Arab Emirates	Descriptive Qualitative Thematic Analysis	Key informant interviews & Focus groups
Chen, Wang, Chung, Tseng & Chou/2006	23 postpartum depressed women	Taiwan	Grounded Theory	Interviews 10–12 weeks postpartum

TABLE 9-1 Seventeen New Transcultural Qualitative Studies on Postpartum Depression included in the Second Grounded Theory Modification *(continued)*

Author/Year	Sample	Country Where Research Conducted	Qualitative Research Design	Data Collection
Taniguchi & Baruffi/ 2007	45 Japanese women born & raised in Japan living in Hawaii within 1 year postpartum	United States	Mixed Methods Descriptive, Qualitative (Content Analysis)	Telephone interviews (semi-structured questions)
Hanley/2007	10 Bangladeshi mothers who were brought up within Muslim community who resided in Wales	United Kingdom	Descriptive Qualitative Thematic Analysis	Focus group interviews
Ahmed, Stewart, Teng, Wahoush & Gagnon/2008	10 immigrant mothers with elevated postpartum depressive symptoms: 2 from China, 2 from India, 1 from Pakistan, 3 from S. America, 1 from Egypt & 1 from Haiti	Canada	Descriptive Qualitative Thematic Analysis	Telephone interviews, semi-structured, 12 to 15 months after birth.
Edhborg, Friberg, Lundh, & Widström/ 2005	22 women with elevated postpartum depressive symptoms between 67–125 days postpartum	Sweden	Grounded Theory	Interviews Constant Comparative Method

(continues)

TABLE 9-1   Seventeen New Transcultural Qualitative Studies on Postpartum Depression included in the Second Grounded Theory Modification *(continued)*

Author/Year	Sample	Country Where Research Conducted	Qualitative Research Design	Data Collection
Hanley & Long/2006	10 women with postpartum depression	United Kingdom	Interviews Content Analysis	Case Study
Hall/2006	10 women with postpartum depression	United Kingdom	Interpretive Phenomenology	Interviews Thematic Analysis
Barr/2006	11 women diagnosed with postpartum depression from 2–11 months postpartum	Australia	Phenomenology Hermeneutic	In-depth interviews
Andajani-Sutjahjo, Manderson, & Astbury/2007	41 women at 6 weeks postpartum	Indonesia	Descriptive Qualitative	Interviews Thematic Analysis
Buultjens & Liamputtong/2007	10 women within 12 months postpartum	Australia	Descriptive Qualitative	In-depth interviews Thematic Analysis
Chew-Graham, Sharp, Chamberlain, Folkes, & Turner/2009	28 women diagnosed with postpartum depression	U.K.	Descriptive Qualitative	Interviews Thematic Analysis
Barr & Beck/2008	15 women diagnosed with PPD & were within 12 months after birth	Australia	Hermeneutic	Interviews Thematic Analysis
McCarthy & McMahon/2008	15 women diagnosed with PPD & who had taken antidepressants	New Zealand	Descriptive Qualitative	Interviews Modified Analytic Induction

Research Design

Details of the original grounded theory research design of "Teetering on the Edge" can be found in Beck's works (1993, 2007). In grounded theory, modification never stops (Glaser, 2001). As new data come in, the substantive theory is modified to accommodate the varying conditions to increase the theory's power and completeness. "All is data" in grounded theory (Glaser, 2001, p. 145). Whatever is happening in the research scene are data no matter the source. As new literature is discovered, it is simply compared as additional data (Glaser, 1998). Constantly comparing this new literature yields new properties of the categories. The theory is modified as the data-literature is woven into it.

The scope of a substantive theory can be carefully increased and controlled by making conscious choices of groups for comparison (Glaser & Strauss, 1967). It must be remembered, however, that persons are not categorized, but the behavior persons engage in is (Glaser, 1998). Maximum differences among these groups are sought so that comparisons can be made on as many relevant differences and similarities in the data as can be found. Maximizing differences among comparative groups is a powerful method for enhancing the generation of theoretical properties and extending and saturating the theory.

Modification of a grounded theory happens with conceptual saturation, theoretical sampling, and with integration of concepts. It does not occur by testing but instead by conceptual generation: "The power of abstraction is shown clearly in modification" (Glaser, 2001, p. 58). By continually modifying a grounded theory, it is generated to a higher level of theoretical completeness. By comparison of new data and the resulting modification, the existing substantive theory is kept "close to the data, yet abstract of it." (p. 57)

Results of the Second Modification

Loss of control was the basic social psychological problem in postpartum depression (Beck, 1993). Women lacked control of their emotions, thought processes, and actions. This is demonstrated by Taiwanese mothers who shared that "they had lost control, even control of themselves" (Chen et al., 2006, p. 453). The basic social psychological process of postpartum depression is the process of teetering on the edge, which refers to walking the fine line between sanity and insanity. As discovered in the original "Teetering on the Edge" grounded theory, women suffering from postpartum depression attempted to cope with the problem of loss of control through a four-stage process (**Figure 9–1**). The stages that emerged from the data included 1) encountering terror, 2) dying of self, 3) struggling to survive, and 4) regaining control. With the help of data from the 17 qualitative studies published since the first modification (Beck, 2007), **Figures 9–2** through **9–5** illustrate the

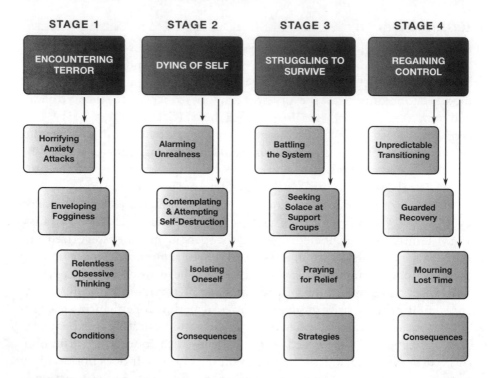

FIGURE 9–1 The Four-Stage Process of Teetering on the Edge.
Reprinted with permission from Beck, C. T. (1993). Teetering on the edge: A substantive theory of postpartum depression. *Nursing Research*, 42, p. 43.

continuing modifications made in this second grounded theory modification. Under each of the categories in these figures are listed the countries, other than the United States, where the qualitative research studies had been conducted and mothers had endorsed the categories. These lists include countries from both the first and second modifications.

Stage 1: Encountering Terror

In the initial stage, women were hit suddenly and unexpectedly by postpartum depression. The syndrome can begin within the first few weeks after delivery or can be delayed until 6 months or more after birth. Five conditions of encountering terror can occur during this first stage:

- Emotional lability
- Horrifying anxiety
- Relentless obsessive thinking
- Enveloping fogginess
- Somatic expressions

In this second modification two new categories were added to Stage 1— emotional lability and somatic expressions.

Emotional lability

In the original "Teetering on the Edge" grounded theory (Beck, 1993), emotional lability had been subsumed under the basic social psychological problem of loss of control; specifically loss of control of mothers' emotions. Because so many women from across the globe reported suffering from distressing emotions they could not control, it was decided to pull this out as a separate category to bring more attention to it.

In Australia, for example, one mother vividly described anger that she could not control:

> You are so angry it's like a rage, it's all consuming, like a fury, like a volcano, you know, when it erupts. You feel like the lava as it starts at your feet and flows through your veins, rushing, and you can't stop it. It's so frightening and you can't stop it. (Barr & Beck, 2008, p. 1717, e3)

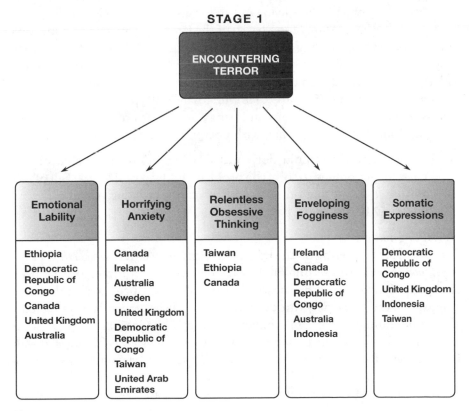

FIGURE 9–2   Second Modification of Teetering on the Edge: Stage 1.

In Indonesia a mother revealed, "I felt that I could not take good care of my baby. My mother did everything for me. I did not have the patience. I often got angry with the baby" (Andajani- Sutjahjo et al., 2007, p. 111). Another woman in Indonesia described how pervasive her irritability was and how she could not control her anger which was compounded by her frequent crying:

> Feeling *pegel* [Javanese: a feeling of being upset, which can be expressed as anger] and dizziness. I often felt sad, I was unhappy and often cried . . . I blamed myself almost all the time . . . because I don't think I am capable of doing anything . . . I often get *pegel* with my child, sometimes I even hit her . . . my baby has difficulty going to sleep. I felt *pegel* with my husband when he did not help me. Almost every single day I fight with him, I even hit him. When I asked him to help, he did not pay any attention, he just kept on day dreaming. (Andajani-Sutjahjo et al., 2007, p. 114)

Forty-two percent of mothers in India reported anger and irritability which negatively affected their relationships with their children and husbands (Rodrigues et al., 2003). Hmong mothers living in Wisconsin reported crying spells (Stewart & Jambunathan, 1996). More than half the Hmong women in this study reported mood swings—feeling happy one moment and sad the next. One Hmong mother tried to explain this: "When I'm happy, I'm really happy. And when I'm sad, I'm very depressed. And that causes me to have headaches, and I can't sleep and tears keep coming" (Stewart & Jambunathan, 1996, p. 325).

Loss of control over emotions and behavior was also reported in mothers living in Hong Kong. One woman with postpartum depression admitted,

> I suffered greatly. I could not control my emotions and behavior. I have no idea of how to solve the problem. In the past, I was so full of confidence, but at that time I lost all my abilities to cope. (Chan et al., 2002, p. 574)

Horrifying anxiety

In the original "Teetering on the Edge" this category was termed *horrifying anxiety attacks*. Now in this second modification, the title of this category has been changed to *horrifying anxiety*. The word "attacks" was dropped so that the more pervasive nature of anxiety throughout the daily lives of women is reflected.

As one immigrant Indian woman living in Canada shared, "I felt that something bad was going to happen. I didn't know why I was feeling that way. I didn't even talk to my husband about it. I felt scared that something was going to happen" (Morrow et al., 2008, p. 601).

An immigrant Chinese mother also living in Canada revealed:

> There was a change in me when I just gave birth. I thought, 'what am I to do with this little thing?' I was afraid that I would drop her and

cause her harm. I felt I couldn't bear such a heavy responsibility. I was emotionally very unstable in these days. I felt I could not look after her. (Morrow et al., 2008, p. 601)

In Bangladesh a woman admitted, "I couldn't sleep and worried about everything" (Hanley, 2007, p. 36).

Common anxiety symptoms in mothers suffering from postpartum depression in the Democratic Republic of Congo were described as "restless/agitated heart, worry and lack of peace" (Bass et al., 2008, p. 1537). Two mothers from the United Arab Emirates described symptoms of anxiety in their lives: "Nervous and tense, stressed, worried about the safety of the baby" (Ghubash & Eapen, 2009, p. 133).

Relentless obsessive thinking

Women from the following four countries have endorsed suffering from relentless obsessive thinking in this second modification of the "Teetering on the Edge" theory: the Democratic Republic of Congo, Taiwan, Ethiopia, and Asia. A mother in Taiwan stated, "I couldn't sleep. There was no way to put my brain at ease. My entire brain was completely focused on something worrisome. Then I would keep on worrying and worrying" (Chan et al., 2006, p. 453).

For some women their obsessive thoughts were often unthinkable—specifically, thoughts about harming their infants. Mothers could not control these horrific thoughts. An Australian mother vividly recalled:

How I imagined hurting the baby was awful . . . you really don't want anyone to know . . . if they did, they would want to put you away or take the baby away. [pause] I mean to say, why would you leave a baby with a mother who is thinking about putting him in a microwave. I used to see, in my mind, a pillow going over his head. So easy . . . the doctor says it's only thoughts. I get that, but what sort of a person am I to even imagine such things? . . . I have cried and cried over this. [pause] It was easier when I was numb and didn't feel at all. At least I didn't have these awful thoughts. (Barr & Beck, 2008, p. 1717.e3)

Enveloping fogginess

One Canadian mother reflected on her mental confusion during the time she experienced postpartum depression:

Well, it's terrible when you can't remember and I was getting to a point where, oh my God, am I forgeting important things like . . . I knew I wouldn't forget to feed the baby, you know, because she was always with me but my other kids. I would look at the clock and it was 2:00 and I haven't fed them lunch, oh my God, and they'd come to me and say "I'm hungry," which thank God they're old enough to do so. But my memory was just gone. (Sword et al., 2008, p. 1167)

A Japanese woman shared that "I can't count and forget often" (Taniguchi & Baruffi, 2007, p. 93). She experienced a weakening of her cognitive ability and memory. In Australia women reported their inability to start or complete tasks, such as housework. Being so indecisive was part of women's postpartum depression. For example this mother revealed,

> Decision making was something that I didn't do through that whole time . . . I never got around to doing anything. I would wake in the morning and I would think, *what am I going to feed you today*. I didn't know what to feed him and I didn't know how to plan ahead and I would be in tears. I didn't know what should be in his diet. (Barr & Beck, 2008, p. 366)

Somatic expressions

Somatic expressions is the second new category added to Stage 1 in this continuing modification of "Teetering on the Edge." Women in the Democratic Republic of Congo, Indonesia, Taiwan, Bangladesh, and India used somatic expressions when describing their postpartum depression. Indonesian mothers used such terms as *pegel* (Javanese: feeling upset in the heart; Anadajani-Sutjahjo et al., 2007). A 30-year-old mother in Indonesia experienced psychosomatic symptoms during the first 3 months after childbirth. She described not being able to bend her fingers and feeling itchy all over her body (Anadajani-Sutjahjo et al.). Another term used by Indonesian women to describe their postpartum depression was *sumpek* (tiredness in the heart). In the Democratic Republic of Congo new mothers complained of stomach pains and aches in the lower abdomen (Bass et al., 2008). Bangladeshi mothers living in England conveyed their depression using somatic terms of weakness, pain, and problems of the heart (Hanley, 2007).

In Taiwan a mother described her experience of postpartum depression:

> I lost strength in my arms. Then, I felt the strength also gone from my legs. I couldn't even stand on my own. My heart didn't seem to be working properly and all the muscles shrank together, my head ached, and I sweated all over. (Chen et al., 2006, p. 453)

Depressed mothers in Goa, India, commonly reported symptoms such as *bendant dukta* (lower back ache), *angar foddta* (body ache), and *potant dukta* (stomach ache).

Stage 2: Dying of Self

As a result of the conditions in the initial stage of postpartum depression, the dying of mothers' normal selves occurred during Stage 2. This stage consisted of the following three consequences: alarming unrealness, isolating oneself, and contemplating and attempting self-destruction. These three conse-quences were involuntary responses to the conditions in Stage 1.

Alarming unrealness
In this updated grounded theory, women from Canada, Taiwan, Japan, and Sweden reported this alarming unrealness. They experienced a loss of self. They did not recognize who they had become in the midst of their postpar-tum depression. Illustrating this is a quotation from one Japanese mother liv-ing in Hawaii: "It doesn't seem like me" (Taniguchi & Baruffi, 2007, p. 93). A Canadian woman shared, "I had called my mom to tell her like I'm not feel-ing and I was crying and stuff, she just like brushed it off... And I'm like no, this is really bad, like I don't feel like myself" (Sword et al., 2007, p. 1167).

Isolating oneself
Postpartum-depressed women from around the globe felt so isolated. Moth-ers from Australia, Canada, Sweden, Ethiopia, Democratic Republic of Congo, Asia, Japan, United Arab Emirates, and immigrants living in Canada all re-ported feeling lonely and isolated.

In Ethiopia the cultural ritual after childbirth adds to the woman's isolation:

> Because she is not allowed to go to other people's houses, talk with them, and share what she would like to share. Because this will give you pleasure and happiness. But if a woman is in the postnatal period, she has to stay at home. When she is in the house, she will be alone. So if she doesn't have anyone to talk to or someone near to her to send out for things she needs, this might change her mood and she will cre-ate arguments with others. (Hanlon et al., 2009, p. 1215)

Women living in countries other than their homeland had an additional layer of isolation to endure. Immigrant women living in Canada compared their ex-periences as new mothers being left alone with their infants all day to the post-partum customs in their country of origin where they would have been surrounded by family and friends following childbirth. The following are some quotations from immigrant women living in Canada:

> "Being surrounded by family and close friends is definitely a big help [to avoid feeling depressed]... obviously we are in North American cultures ... if I was back home my mother would be there. Having my mother there to help throughout, or after pregnancy would make me a lot hap-pier after the birth because I could take my mother's advice, and use it."

> "I think [what causes depression after childbirth] is loneliness. Just feeling lonely, because you feel empty."

> "[You feel depressed when] you're alone, with a baby, have no support, you feel isolated." (Ahmed et al., 2008, p. 298).

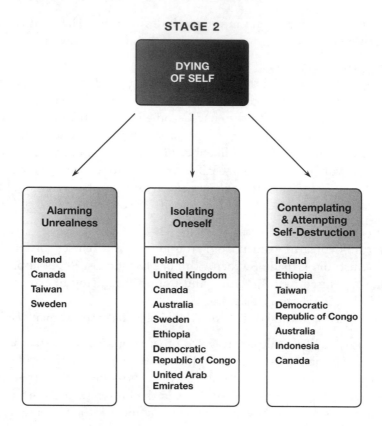

FIGURE 9–3   Second Modification of Teetering on the Edge: Stage 2.

Contemplating and attempting self-destruction

Quotes from women in Taiwan, Indonesia, and Australia illustrate the global nature of this most serious component of postpartum depression. A Taiwanese mother shared the depth of her suffering after childbirth: "During the tough time after the baby's birth, my bluest period, I thought about committing suicide. I kept wondering what people live in the world for." (Chen et al., 2006, p. 453).

In Indonesia a 22-year-old woman revealed:

> For a while, I even wished to die . . . it was just after giving birth . . . I could go a whole day without food. Looking at my child cured me. At times . . . I was like someone who had gone *edhan* [Javanese: insane]. (Andajani-Sutjahjo et al., 2007, p. 113)

At times for women who were contemplating ending their lives, infanticidal thoughts complicated their decisions. How could a woman leave her baby to grow up without a mother? How could children grow up knowing their mother killed herself because of their birth? These women bore a suffocating burden for being such "terrible mothers". One Australian mother painfully revealed:

> There were times when I thought I was such a terrible mother that he would be better off without me, and so I imagined him with someone else; and there were times when I thought that I would have to take him with me. I felt that it wasn't fair on [the baby] to have a terrible mother, but it also wasn't fair on him not to have a mother. And so, to take him with me was the only option. (Barr & Beck, 2008, p. 1717.e3)

In Ethiopia this woman shared:

> During that time I felt hopeless most of the time . . . I thought about everything. I even thought about ending my life or leaving everything and going somewhere else . . . Yes. At that time, had I been God or had I been the person who can do anything. I thought of killing her [her baby] and killing myself . . . Since I didn't have the guts to kill the baby or kill myself, I just thought about it. (Hanlon et al., 2009, p. 1215)

Stage 3: Struggling to Survive

In "struggling to survive," the third stage of "Teetering on the Edge," women employed the following three strategies: battling self and the system, praying for relief, and seeking support from multiple sources. The consequences in Stage 2 became conditions requiring strategies by the women. Consequences of one set of actions can become part of the conditions affecting the next set of actions occurring in a sequence.

Battling self and the system

In the original grounded theory of postpartum depression (Beck, 1993), this category was called "battling the system." For this second modification, this category was renamed to reflect data from a number of new qualitative studies that focused on women's help-seeking behavior for their postpartum depression.

To initiate their journey to regain control of their lives women not only had to battle the healthcare system but also themselves. Before seeking help from healthcare professionals, mothers had to overcome their fear of disclosing what they were feeling and thinking. There was incongruity between how motherhood was ideally portrayed and how it was in reality. For example, in Australia guilt and shame were experienced due to mothers' perception of their inability to cope (McCarthy & McMahon, 2008). Unrealistic, high expectations of how a "good mother" should perform added to the guilt. A Ugandan mother living in Canada shared:

> My husband would always really try to tell me to be more cheerful, but it would always seem impossible and of course it added to more guilt

on my part . . . And knowing that I should be really there for my daughter, that I should try to be happy, so I felt like a failure. There was more pressure because I thought I wasn't doing a good job to start off with, you know, before she was even born. (Morrow et al., 2008, p. 606)

Women also feared that if they disclosed their symptoms of postpartum depression, their children would be taken from them. In Australia one mother revealed her fears of disclosing to healthcare professionals:

My biggest fear was that I was going to be stereotyped as one of these mothers who just abused her children physically and mentally and verbally, and I was going to lose them and that was my biggest fear. I remember hearing people, because at the time I think there had been quite a few incidents, that a mother in Texas . . . had killed her children. (McCarthy & McMahon, 2008, p. 628)

This fear was echoed by women in a number of countries such as in Canada where this mother revealed:

Well, I was nervous about it at first. I didn't really want to go because I didn't want anyone to think I was crazy. And I know in postpartum depression some people get like postpartum psychosis and I was worried

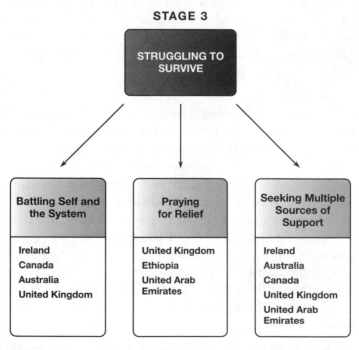

FIGURE 9–4   Second Modification of Teetering on the Edge: Stage 3.

that they would think that that was me or that they might take my kids from me if they knew I was depressed. (Sword et al., 2008, p. 1166)

In Australia a mother never told any clinicians about her thoughts of infanticide:

I had suicidal thoughts and plans for 3 weeks. I would think about it all day and I knew that was bad. I couldn't think what to do with the baby and so I thought I had to take the baby with me. Suddenly I knew there was something wrong with that picture. I knew I had to do something. But you know, you don't come straight out with it to your GP or your psychiatrist. I just say things are bad. (Barr & Beck, 2008, p. 1717.e3)

In the United Kingdom yet again fears of disclosing were reported:

There's still a stigma to it. I thought postnatal depression, God they just kill their children. That's all you see in the media, y'know drama of they're going to kill all their children in a horrible nasty way and then be put away for the rest of their life. That's what postnatal depression was, and that's what I thought if I told people, they'd be like, better watch her. (Hall, 2006, p. 258)

Another fear hindering disclosure was the fear of having to take antidepressants. This Canadian mother shared her fear: "That's all they have, GPs, and I just didn't want to go onto antidepressants, because obviously I've heard people get addicted to them and then you're stuck on them and you have a vicious circle" (Chew-Graham et al., 2009, p. 5). In Sweden these fears were echoed, "I didn't want to talk with anybody about it, I always had to pretend that I was doing just great . . . I thought that wasn't normal, that I was a bad mom who felt that way" (Edhborg et al., 2005, p. 264). Once overcoming these disclosure fears, immigrant women had an additional obstacle to seeking help for their postpartum depression: language barriers (Ahmed et al., 2008).

Praying for relief

In this grounded theory modification, mothers from four additional countries used prayer as one of their strategies to recover from postpartum depression. These women included Bangladeshi immigrants living in the United Kingdom, Ethiopians, Japanese immigrants living in the United States, and women of the United Arab Emirates. A Japanese mother living in Hawaii shared that she "felt reassured after praying to God" (Taniguchi & Baruffi, 2007, p. 93). Bangladeshi women living in the United Kingdom suffering from postpartum depression sought help from healers. For instance, while in England one mother attended a healer:

He prayed over an amulet and sealed it with wax. Why it works is because I believe it will work . . . In my home village they would do "house medicines"—specialized, then they tell you what to do—pray and that. (Hanley, 2007, pp. 36–37)

Another Bangladeshi mother revealed:

> I couldn't sleep and worried about everything. The doctor said I was suffering from "postnatal depression" and gave me some valium to take. My mother went to see a healer who gave me this amulet to wear around my neck. Within a few days I was better and I have worn this ever since. (Hanley, 2007, p. 36)

In the United Arab Emirates most women did not acknowledge postpartum depression per se as a mental disorder but instead it was due to Jinn, evil spirits. Jinn can come into a woman's body when she experiences mental problems. A religious healer is called in to exorcise Jinn (Ghubash & Eapen, 2009).

Seeking support from multiple sources

The theoretical sample from Beck's (1993) original grounded theory was obtained from women attending a postpartum depression support group. Consequently, the data regarding support concentrated on the solace mothers experienced within these groups. In this continuing grounded theory modification this original category of seeking solace at support groups was expanded based on the new data from the additional 17 qualitative studies. Women from around the globe shared the value of support, not only from support groups, but also from family, friends, and healthcare professionals in their struggle to overcome their postpartum depression. To reflect this, the category was renamed from "seeking solace at support group" to "seeking support from multiple sources."

These additional sources of support were especially needed by immigrant mothers living in a new country without close family surrounding them. Refugee, asylum-seeking, non-refugee, and immigrant new mothers living in Canada shared how helpful community support groups were. These groups were havens of caring and places to meet other women with whom they were able to share their feelings since the birth of their infants.

> I think that the thing that I looked most for [in a community service or support center] was something that allowed me to meet people, just get out of the house and meet others, like new mothers, people that I could speak to . . . people who are in the same position as myself, who are learning to be a new mom, dealing with the stresses of that, that's good. (Ahmed et al., 2008, p. 300)

Friends were an important source of support to help mothers cope with the difficulties they were experiencing due to postpartum depression. As one immigrant mother living in Canada revealed:

> My friends have been really, really great with me. I have mostly other Latin American women who are my family friends, who are mostly

also mothers, and they help me by, you know, meeting us in the park or coming to the playground, and I am able to talk to them and share stories. (Ahmed et al., 2008, p. 300)

Nurses were another important source of support for new mothers struggling with postpartum depression. In Canada, for example mothers reported encouragement given to them and the outreach and follow-up that nurses offered:

I felt good about it because she [the nurse] kept saying, you know, if you feel like anything gets worse or anything at all don't hesitate to call and we don't want anybody to slip through the cracks. She said that a couple of times, we don't want postpartum to slip through the cracks and don't suffer without you know telling us and don't be afraid to tell us. So it was, it was good. (Sword et al., 2008, p. 1169)

She [the nurse] has called on a couple of occasions. There was an appointment that I had missed that she was really concerned that I wasn't there, but I had forgotten about it. I guess they sort of worry if you're just not going because you don't want to, whatever. She's been good with following up with me and giving me possible options for help. (Sword et al., 2008, p. 1169)

In Australia this mother shared that:

It wasn't probably the advice that she [mental health nurse] gave me, it was just [that she] knew that someone else had been through what I had been through. I wasn't a weirdo, I wasn't a nutter, I wasn't a freak, I was just a normal person suffering what mums, some mums, suffer. And just to have that information from them just to hear her say it is okay . . . She [mental health nurse] is only seeing people with the same problem, and this is quite a good feeling just to know that I wasn't on my own. (McCarthy & McMahon, 2008, p. 630)

On the other hand, for some Asian women, their in-laws were not a source of this much needed support. The following quote from a woman from Hong Kong living in Canada illustrates this:

Yes I felt the pressure that I almost wanted to die, I felt the pressure mainly when I had to deal with my in-laws. I think my emotions would be calmer if they are not here . . . So I actually felt happy that they [parents-in-law] went back to Hong Kong when the baby was 3 months old. I felt relieved, because I can just make simple meals, I can wake up late, and I can ask my husband to feed the baby in the early morning, around 6 a.m. It would be reasonable to share the workload with him. If they were here, they would not be happy to see that I ask my husband to wake up and feed the baby in the early morning. (Morrow et al., 2008, p. 607)

This Taiwanese mother shared that:

> I can't get away from his [father-in-law's] confinement. It is like a net on me; I really want to rush out of it, but I can't unless I was no longer his daughter-in-law . . . divorced my husband and then escaped the authority of their entire family. But I can't. (Chen et al., 2006, p. 453)

A mother born in India and now living in Canada revealed:

> When I had the baby I wanted to spend some time at my parent's home. My in-laws took offense to this. My mother-in-law and my sister-in-law came on the day I was going to be discharged and their faces, they looked quite angry. They said that my mother had said that I was going to her house and that is where they were going to drop me off. They said a lot of things to me that were very upsetting, like this was an old tradition, they didn't know why some people were still living in the past. After having the baby, I spent time at my parents' home, about 13–14 days. My in-laws would not phone me or talk with me properly. I was very upset at that time. (Morrow et al., 2008, p. 608)

Stage 4: Regaining Control

Regaining control was the fourth and final stage of the substantive theory of "Teetering on the Edge." Regaining control was a slow process consisting of three consequences of the strategies used in the third stage: unpredictable transitioning, mourning lost time, and guarded recovery. The focus of the majority of the 17 qualitative studies included in this second grounded theory modification was on the experience of postpartum depression and women's help-seeking behavior. Only one of these studies concentrated specifically on the recovery process of postpartum depression, which is the behavior that is included in Stage 4 (Chen et al., 2006). Therefore, there were not much new data to use to modify this stage. The categories of unpredictable transitioning and mourning lost time were not modified. The category of guarded recovery was expanded to add data from Chen and colleagues' study of the recovery process of Taiwanese women suffering from postpartum depression.

Unpredictable transitioning

The process of recovery from postpartum depression was not sudden. Occasionally, among the bad days, there would be a good one. Gradually, the number of good days experienced would increase until only a few bad days cropped up here and there. These would be unpredictable. This erratic transition to regaining control is illustrated in the following quotation:

> When I got out of my severest depression, I had more good times than bad times. I had days where I felt like nothing bad ever happened.

I mean, I was normal. I really felt such intense love for my baby. I could have a relationship with my husband. Then the next day for no reason at all I'd wake up and just be off. (Beck, 1993, p. 47)

Mourning lost time
As the mothers progressed in their recovery from postpartum depression, they began to mourn the lost time that they would not be able to recapture with their infants: "I feel robbed of the first 6 months of my daughter's life. I never really got to hold her as a baby and I feel cheated."(Beck, 1993, p. 47)

Another mother repeatedly walked through the baby departments of stores in the mall looking at infants' clothes, mourning her baby's infancy that had been lost to her because of postpartum depression. Throughout the recovery period, the mothers needed to work through these feelings of being cheated of the opportunity to experience unique periods of their children's lives (Beck, 1993). Women in Ireland also described feeling cheated out of the joys of motherhood by their postpartum depression (Lawler & Sinclair, 2003).

Guarded recovery
Guarded recovery was the final consequence of the strategies used in struggling to survive. This occurred when the mothers felt they had essentially recovered from postpartum depression. Postpartum depression, however, left

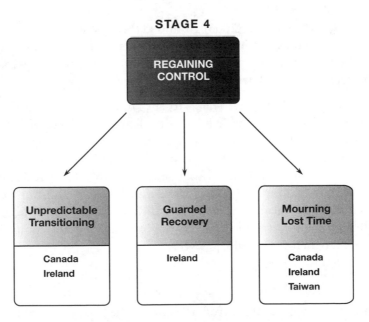

FIGURE 9–5 Second Modification of Teetering on the Edge: Stage 4.

an indelible mark on mothers' lives. Even after regaining control, women re-peatedly stated they still feared that at some point in the future they could be stricken with the depression again:

> Postpartum depression makes you very, very vulnerable. You still feel like you're on a fine line between sanity and insanity because when it first happened it came out of nowhere. You're normal and then the next thing you know you're crazy. (Beck, 1993, p. 47)

Canadian mothers agreed that coming through such a difficult time with postpartum depression left them with many scars. At the same time, however, surviving this ordeal became a source of strength for some women. As one woman expressed,

> I am a different person. Much stronger. I don't know how you could be the same person because so many things happen to make it differ-ent. Going through it was really terrible. I have the same family and a better understanding of myself. (Berggren-Clive, 1998, p. 114)

African-American mothers in the United States described their recovery as "feeling better" as they regained their strength and were able to function nor-mally again (Amankwaa, 2003). As one African-American mother shared at 11 months postpartum: "So I am back . . . I don't feel like my old self, but at this point I am—I am wondering if that's even realistic, because I am not the same" (Amankwaa, 2003, p. 308).

The focus of Chen et al.'s (2006) grounded theory was the recovery process of postpartum depression in Taiwanese mothers. Being reborn was the core concept. Regaining vitality was the last stage of the process. One mother in Taiwan expressed the following about her recovery:

> I am doing fine these days. That is to say, I have adjusted my attitude; I no longer feel that my child belongs to them. I mean, I originally ex-pected everybody in this house to come and help. But now I find I am the mother and that I am the one my child needs the most. I think about all of this in a different way. And I am what I am. It will be a blessing if the family members can lend me a helping hand, but if they don't, it's only natural. And I have a different feeling now because both my mental attitude and my way of thinking are completely changed. (Chen et al., 2006, p. 454)

Discussion

Teetering on the edge emerged from the data as the basic social process (BSP) in this grounded theory of postpartum depression. As Glaser (1996) claimed, "The practical implications of a BSP gives a transcending picture that helps practitioners access, evaluate, and develop desirable goals in a substantive area" (p. xv). The BSP suggests variables that yield interventions and the outcomes from such interventions. For practitioners, the BSP can be used as a guideline or framework for clinical practice to ground their efforts to assist patients in resolving their main problem or concern. In this case, the BSP of "teetering on the edge" can become the framework for clinicians working with mothers suffering from postpartum depression. The richness of the four stages described in this chapter can enable postpartum-depressed women to feel understood and to benefit from appropriate interventions tailored to whichever stage of their recovery process they are currently in.

This continuing modified grounded theory of postpartum depression gives women insightful ways to gain some degree of control over the situation in which they find themselves after the birth of their baby. It is a theory of process and addresses the problems postpartum-depressed mothers have to contend with in a language understandable to women. This second modified grounded theory now has wider applicability, because properties of its categories have been expanded from data from a number of cultural orientations.

Highlighted in this second modification of "Teetering on the Edge" are the daily struggles immigrant mothers suffering from postpartum depression have to contend with. Special attention needs to be given to immigrant mothers living in countries and cultures that are very different from those in which they were born and raised. The isolation these mothers feel is magnified as they try to cope with postpartum depression. Their longed-for comfort of being surrounded by family is nowhere to be found. Compounding this isolation for some of these women is a language barrier which also hinders their help seeking for their postpartum mood disorder.

The somatic expressions used by mothers in some cultures to describe postpartum depression have important implications for screening for this devastating mood disorder. Screening scales need to be developed with items that capture these somatic expressions in order for these instruments to achieve acceptable levels of sensitivity and specificity.

Summarizing

Teetering on the Edge: emerged from the substantive area of postpartum depression. A BSP helps to organize and transcend the literature in a field (Glaser, 1996). For example, in the healthcare industry and organizational change literature, teetering on the edge is also operating (Mycek, 1999). When discussing steering healthcare institutions, Mycek warned that there is a catch to teetering on the edge: "Venture too far and you're in complete and total chaos. Don't go far enough and you become stuck in monotony. The secret lies in operating on the edge" (p. 10). Teetering on the edge is linked to chaos theory. Irons (as cited in Mycek, 1999) proposed, "In chaos theory, you have to capitalize on trouble . . . It's when you walk on the edge of losing control that you make progress" (p. 11). Kaiser (as cited in Mycek, 1999) offers, "On the edge, you take responsibility for the creation of your preferred reality" (p. 13).

A BSP can also be used to address problems that are related to loss of control in a variety of substantive areas. Suggestions for future research can focus on elevating Teetering on the Edge to a formal grounded theory. Its exploratory potential need not be confined to postpartum mood disorders. Loss of control, the main problem this grounded theory helps to resolve, can be found through a range of human conditions, such as binge eating (Johnson, Boutelle, Torgrud, Davig, & Turner, 2000), pathological gambling (Toce-Gerstein, Gerstein, & Volberg, 2003), dementia (Gilmour & Huntington, 2005), nonvocal ventilated patients (Carroll, 2004), emergency patients with unexpected surgery (Pearson & Kiger, 2004), and alcoholism (Bartek, Lindeman, & Hawks, 1999).

Glaser's (1998) four criteria for judging grounded theory include workability, relevance, fit, and modifiability. He calls these criteria *product proof*. The proof of a grounded theory is in the outcome. In the nearly 2 decades that have passed since the original "Teetering on the Edge" was developed (Beck, 1993), the theory has 1) worked to explain the relevant behavior of women suffering with postpartum depression, 2) held relevance to the depressed mothers and health professionals working in that clinical field, and 3) fit the substantive area of postpartum mood and anxiety disorders. It is the fourth criterion for judging grounded theory, modifiability, for which this second modification of Teetering on the Edge has provided evidence. Teetering on the Edge was again readily modifiable with new data that emerged from the 17 qualitative studies of crosscultural experiences of postpartum depression published since the first modification in 2007.

References

Ahmed, A., Stewart, D. E., Teng, L., Wahoush, O., & Gagnon, A. J. (2008). Experiences of immigrant new mothers with symptoms of depression. *Archives of Women's Mental Health, 11*(4), 295–303.

Amankwaa, L. C. (2003). Postpartum depression, culture and African-American women. *Issues in Mental Health Nursing, 24,* 297–316.

Andajani-Sutjahjo, S., Manderson, L., & Astbury, J. (2007). Complex emotions, complex problems: Understanding the experiences of perinatal depression among new mothers in urban Indonesia. *Culture, Medicine and Psychiatry, 31*(1), 101–122.

Barr, J. A. (2006). Postpartum depression, delayed maternal adaptation, and mechanical infant caring: A phenomenological hermeneutic study. *International Journal of Nursing Studies, 45*(3), 362–369.

Barr, J. A., & Beck, C. T. (2008). Infanticide secrets: Qualitative study on postpartum depression. *Canadian Family Physician, 54*(12), 1716–1717.e1–5.

Bartek, J. K., Lindeman, M., & Hawks, J. H. (1999). Clinical validation of characteristics of the alcoholic family. *Nursing Diagnosis, 10*, 158–168.

Bass, J. K., Ryder, R. W., Lammers, M. C., Mukaba, T. N., & Bolton, P. A. (2008). Post-partum depression in Kinshasa, Democratic Republic of Congo: Validation of a concept using a mixed-methods cross-cultural approach. *Tropical Medicine and International Health, 13*(12), 1534–1542.

Beck, C. T. (1992). The lived experience of postpartum depression: A phenomenological study. *Nursing Research, 41*, 166–170.

Beck, C. T. (1993). Teetering on the edge: A substantive theory of postpartum depression. *Nursing Research, 42*(1), 42–48.

Beck, C. T. (2007). Exemplar: Teetering on the edge: A continually emerging theory of postpartum depression, In P. L. Munhall (Ed.), *Nursing Research: A qualitative perspective* (pp. 273–292). Sudbury, MA: Jones & Bartlett.

Berggren-Clive, K. (1998). Out of the darkness and into the light: Women's experiences with depression after childbirth. *Canadian Journal of Community Mental Health, 17*, 103–120.

Bhugra, D., & Gregoire, A. (1993). Social factors in the genesis and management of postnatal psychiatric disorders. In D. Bhurgra & J. Leff (Eds.), *Principles of social psychiatry*. Oxford: Blackwell.

Buultjens, M., & Liamputtong, P. (2007). When giving life starts to take the life out of you: Women's experiences of depression after childbirth. *Midwifery, 23*(1), 77–91.

Carroll, S. M. (2004). Nonvocal ventilated patients' perceptions of being understood. *Western Journal of Nursing Research, 26*, 85–112.

Chan, S. W., Levy, V., Chung, T. K., & Lee, P. (2002). A qualitative study of the experiences of a group of Hong Kong Chinese women diagnosed with postnatal depression. *Journal of Advanced Nursing, 39*, 571–579.

Chen, C. H., Wang, S. Y., Chung, U. L., Tseng, Y. F., & Chou, F. H. (2006). Being reborn: The recovery process of postpartum depression in Taiwanese women. *Journal of Advanced Nursing, 54*(4), 450–456.

Chew-Graham, C. A., Sharp, D., Chamberlain, E., Folkes, L., & Turner, K. M. (2009). Disclosure of symptoms of postnatal depression, the perspectives of health professionals and women: a qualitative study. *BMC Family Practice,* 10(7) doi:10.1186/1471-2296-1-7.

Edge, D., Baker, D., & Rogers, A. (2004). Perinatal depression among Black Caribbean women. *Health and Social Care in the Community, 12*, 430–438.

Edhborg, M., Friberg, M., Lundh, W., & Widström, A. M. (2005). "Struggling with life": Narratives from women with signs of postpartum depression. *Scandinavian Journal of Public Health, 33*(4), 261–267.

Ege, E., Timur, S., Zincir, H., Geçkil, E., & Sunar-Reeder, B. (2008). Social support and symptoms of postpartum depression among new mothers in Eastern Turkey. *Journal of Obstetrics and Gynecology Research, 34*(4), 585–593.

Gao, L-L., Chan, S. W., & Mao, Q. (2009). Depression, perceived stress, and social support among first-time Chinese mothers and fathers in the postpartum period. *Research in Nursing & Health, 32*(1), 50–58.

Gausia, K., Fisher, C., Ali, M., & Oosthuizen, J. (2009). Magnitude and contributory factors of postnatal depression: A community-based cohort study from a rural subdistrict of Bangladesh. *Psychological Medicine, 39*(6), 999–1007.

Gavin, N. I., Gaynes, B. N., Lohr, K. N., Meltzer-Brody, S., Gartlehner, G., & Swinson, T. (2005). Perinatal depression: A systematic review of prevalence and incidence. *Obstetrics & Gynecology, 106,* 1071–1083.

Ghubash, R., & Eapen, V. (2009). Postpartum mental illness: Perspectives from an Arabian Gulf population. *Psychological Reports, 105*(1), 127–136.

Giakoumaki, O., Vasilaki, K., Lili, L., Skouroliakou, M., & Liosis, G. (2009). The role of maternal anxiety in the early postpartum period: Screening for anxiety and depressive symptomatology in Greece. *Journal of Psychosomatic Obstetrics & Gynecology, 30*(1), 21–28.

Gilmour, J. A., & Huntington, A. D. (2005). Finding the balance: Living with memory loss. *International Journal of Nursing Practice, 11,* 118–124.

Glaser, B. G. (1996). *Gerund grounded theory: The basic social process dissertation.* Mill Valley, CA: Sociology Press.

Glaser, B. G. (1998). *Doing grounded theory: Issues and discussions.* Mill Valley, CA: Sociology Press.

Glaser, B. G. (2001). *The grounded theory perspective I: Conceptualization contrasted with description.* Mill Valley, CA: Sociology Press.

Glaser, B. G., & Stauss, A. L. (1967). *The discovery of grounded theory.* New York: Aldine de Gruyter.

Hall, P. (2006). Mothers' experiences of postnatal depression: An interpretative phenomenological analysis. *Community Practitioners, 79*(8), 256–260.

Halligan, S. L., Murray, L., Martins, C., & Cooper, P. J. (2007). Maternal depression and psychiatric outcomes in adolescent offspring: A 13-year longitudinal study. *Journal of Affective Disorders, 97,* 145–154.

Hanley, J. (2007). The emotional wellbeing of Bangladeshi mothers during the postnatal period. *Community Practitioner, 80*(5), 34–37.

Hanley, J., & Long, B. (2006). A study of Welsh mothers' experiences of postnatal depression. *Midwifery, 22*(2), 147–157.

Hanlon, C., Whitley, R., Wondimagegn, D., Alem, A., & Prince, M. (2009). Postnatal mental distress in relation to the sociocultural practices of childbirth: An exploratory qualitative study from Ethiopia. *Social Science & Medicine, 69*(8), 1211–1219.

Hay, D. F., Pawlby, S., Waters, C. S., & Sharp, D. (2008). Antepartum and postpartum exposure to maternal depression: Different effects on different adolescent outcomes. *Journal of Child Psychology and Psychiatry, 49*(10), 1079–1088.

Holopainen, D. (2002). The experience of seeking help for postnatal depression. *Australian Journal of Advanced Nursing, 19*(3), 39–44.

Johnson, W. G., Boutelle, K. N., Torgrud, L., Davig, J. P., & Turner S. (2000). What is a binge? The influence of amount, duration and loss of control criteria on judgments of binge eating. *International Journal of Eating Disorders, 27,* 471–479.

Kheirabadi, G. R., Maracy, M. R., Barekatain, M., Salehi, M., Sadri, G. H., Kelishadi, M., & Cassy, P. (2009). Risk factors of postpartum depression in rural areas of Isfahan Province, Iran. *Archives of Iranian Medicine, 12*(5), 461–467.

Kumar, R. (1994). Postnatal mental illness: A transcultural perspective. *Social Psychiatry and Psychiatric Epidemiology, 29,* 250–264.

Lawler, D., & Sinclair, M. (2003). Grieving for my former self: A phenomenological hermeneutical study of women's lived experience of postnatal depression. *Evidence Based Midwifery, 1,* 36–41.

McCarthy, M., & McMahon, C. (2008). Acceptance and experience of treatment for post-natal depression in a community mental health setting. *Health Care for Women International, 29*(6), 618–637.

Morrow, M., Smith, J. E., Lai, Y., & Jaswal, S. (2008). Shifting landscapes: Immigrant women and postpartum depression. *Health Care for Women International, 29*(6), 593–617.

Monti, F., Agostini, F., Marano, G., & Lupi, F. (2008). The course of maternal depressive symptomatology during the first 18 months postpartum in an Italian sample. *Archives of Women's Mental Health, 11*(3), 231–238.

Mycek, S. (1999). Teetering on the edge of chaos. *Trustee, 52,* 10–13.

Nahas, V. L., Hillege, S., & Amasheh, N. (1999). Postpartum depression: The lived experience of Middle Eastern migrant women in Australia. *Journal of Nurse-Midwifery, 44,* 65–74.

Nicolson, P. (1990). Understanding postnatal depression: A mother-centered approach. *Journal of Advanced Nursing, 15,* 689–695.

Oates, M. R., Cox, J. L., Nenna, S., Asten, P., Glangeud-Freudenthal, N., Figueiredo, B., et al. (2004). Postnatal depression across countries and cultures: A qualitative study. *British Journal of Psychiatry, 184*(suppl 46), 510–516.

Pawlby, S., Sharp, D., Hay, D., & O'Keane, V. (2008). Postnatal depression and child outcome at 11 years: The importance of accurate diagnosis. *Journal of Affective Disorders, 107*(1–3), 241–245.

Pearson, E., & Kiger, A. (2004). How emergency patients cope with their unexpected surgical event: An exploratory study. *Journal of Advanced Perioperative Care, 2,* 11–18.

Pillsbury, B. L. K. (1978). "Doing the mouth": Confinement and convalescence of Chinese women after childbirth. *Social Science and Medicine, 12,* 11–22.

Ramchandani, P. G., Richter, L. M., Stein, A., & Norris, S. A. (2009). Predictors of postnatal depression in an urban South African cohort. *Journal of Affective Disorders, 113*(3), 279–284.

Ramsay, R. (1993). Postnatal depression. *Lancet, 341,* 1358.

Rodrigues, M., Patel, V., Jaswal, S., & deSouza, N. (2003). Listening to mothers: Qualitative studies on motherhood and depression from Goa, India. *Social Science and Medicine, 57,* 1797–1806.

Seel, R. M. (1986). Birth rite. *Health Visitor, 69,* 135–138.

Stern, G., & Kruckman, L. (1983). Multi-disciplinary perspective on postpartum depression: An anthropological critique. *Social Science and Medicine, 17,* 1027–1041.

Stewart, S., & Jambunathan, J. (1996). Hmong women and postpartum depression. *Health Care for Women International, 17,* 319–330.

Sword, W., Busser, D., Ganann, R., McMillan, T., & Swinton, M. (2008). Women's care-seeking experiences after referral for postpartum depression. *Qualitative Health Research, 18*(9), 1161–1173.

Taniguchi, H., & Baruffi, G. (2007). Childbirth overseas: The experience of Japanese women in Hawaii. *Nursing and Health Sciences, 9*(2), 90–95.

Templeton, L., Velleman, R., Persaud, A., & Milner, P. (2003). The experience of postnatal depression in women from Black and minority ethnic communities in Wilshire, UK. *Ethnicity and Health, 8,* 207–221.

Toce-Gerstein, M., Gerstein, D. R., & Volberg, R. A. (2003). A hierarchy of gambling disorders in the community. *Addiction, 98,* 1661–1672.

Wisner, K. L., Chambers, C., & Sit, D. K. Y. (2006). Postpartum depression: A major public health problem. *JAMA, 296,* 2616–2618.

Endnotes

[1] For an excellent comparison of the approaches of Strauss and Corbin (1990) and Glaser (1992), see MacDonald (2001, pp. 138–153).

[2] See the Grounded Theory Institute http://www.groundedtheory.com/

[3] See Wuest (2001) for an explicit depiction of theoretical sampling in a study of women's caring.

[4] See Sandelowski (1998) for an excellent discussion of the hazards of metaphor.

[5] See Glaser (1978) pp. 65–70 for a discussion of typology construction.

10

Ethnography: The Method

Zane Robinson Wolf

Traditional Ethnography

Ethnographic research started with investigators who sought out and experienced worlds different from their own and then tried to understand the meanings of social action within cultures. Thus, the behavior of informants or insiders was translated into social action and represented descriptively in ethnographic reports. Understanding the symbols of cultures helped investigators with interpretation. Many ethnographers distinguished themselves by "going native," by living with, learning and speaking the language of, and participating in the cultures of the people being studied. They valued the life worlds of the "folk" who lived cultures dramatically different from their own. Through narrative descriptions, researchers revealed the social actions, beliefs, values, and norms of markedly different cultures from the viewpoint of an outsider, ideally keeping the perspectives of informants very much in mind.

Ethnographers have continued to make explicit the commonsense knowledge of the cultures by revealing what the social worlds mean for the persons within the worlds and what they mean as insiders acting within them. Traditional or classic ethnographies portray shared understandings of insiders' worlds. (See **Table 10–1** for selected types of ethnographic studies). Ethnographers study the processes of sense making that members of cultures use to create the social world and its factual properties (Leiter, 1980). Cultural rules inform, in part, human social behavior (Aamodt, 1982). Traditional ethnographies begin with investigators taking a somewhat naïve position about the

TABLE 10–1   SELECTED TYPES OF ETHNOGRAPHY

Type	Definition/ Description	Data Sources	Theoretical Perspective	References
Autoethnography	Study of awareness of self within a culture; identifying, thinking critically, and writing about a specific culture with which the writer has life experiences. Writer's subjective experience; insider ethnography; referring either to ethnography of one's own group or to autobiographical writing of ethnographic interest. Critique of self and society, self in society, and self as resistant and transformative force of society. Ethnographic analysis of personally lived experience; critical self-reflection.	Direct and participant observation of daily behavior; recording of life history; in-depth interviews; personal narratives; reflective journals.	Cultural	Alexander, B. K. (2005). Performance ethnography: The reenacting and inciting of culture. In N. K. Denzin, & Y. S. Lincoln (Eds.), The Sage handbook of qualitative research (3rd ed.) (pp. 411–441). Thousand Oaks, CA: Sage. Duncan, M. (2004). Autoethnography: Critical appreciation of an emerging art. International Journal of Qualitative Methods, 3(4). Retrieved from http://www.ualberta.ca/~iiqm/backissues/3_4/pdf/duncan.pdf

TABLE 10–1 SELECTED TYPES OF ETHNOGRAPHY *(continued)*

Type	Definition/ Description	Data Sources	Theoretical Perspective	References
Classical (holistic, traditional)	Description of culture; study of culture, subcultural group; humans understood in fullest possible context.	Fieldwork/field notes, participant observation, interview; thick description, event analysis, document analysis,	Ethnographic naturalism; culture as system of knowledge to interpret experience and generate behavior; linguistic expressions	Aamodt, A. M. (1991). Ethnography and epistemology: Generating nursing knowledge. In J. M. Morse (Ed.), Qualitative nursing research: a contemporary dialogue (rev. ed.) (pp. 40–53). Newbury Park, CA:
	Understanding people under study and activities in everyday life.	artifact analysis	used by informants during social interactions: symbolic interactionism	Sage.
				Boyle, J. S. (1991). Field research: A collaborative model for practice and research. In J. M. Morse (Ed.), Qualitative nursing research: A contemporary dialogue (rev. ed.) (pp. 271–299). Newbury Park, CA: Sage.
	"Grasping the native's point of view, his relation to life, to realize his vision of his world."			Malinowski, B. quoted in Sturtevant, W. C. (1968). Studies in ethnoscience. In R. Manners, & D. Kaplan (Eds.). Theory in anthropology (p. 476). Chicago, IL: Aldine-Atherton Press.
				Greckhamer, T., & Koro-Ljungberg, M. (2004, August 14). Paper presented to American Sociological Association. San Francisco, CA.

(continues)

TABLE 10–1   SELECTED TYPES OF ETHNOGRAPHY *(continued)*

Type	Definition/ Description	Data Sources	Theoretical Perspective	References
Cognitive	Study of cognitive processes that affect work carried out within a setting, recognizing effect of material world and social context on actions and meanings attributed within the setting.	Observation, interview	Distributed cognition	Cognitive ethnography. Retrieved from http://www.cs.st-andrews.ac.uk/~nh19/index_files/Page630.htm
	Focus on events carried out and meanings of social practices and absence of these to participants.			Marshall, C., & Rossman, G. B. (1989). Designing qualitative research. Newbury Park, CA: Sage.
	Study of how peoples of different cultures acquire information about the world (cultural transmission), how they process that information and reach decisions, and how they act so that information in ways that other members of their culture consider appropriate.			Bernard, H. R. (1994). Research methods in anthropology: Qualitative and quantitative approaches (2nd ed.). Thousand Oaks, CA: Sage.

TABLE 10–1   SELECTED TYPES OF ETHNOGRAPHY *(continued)*

Type	Definition/ Description	Data Sources	Theoretical Perspective	References
Critical (disrupted)	Conventional ethnography with political purpose, power relations and disempowerment, interpretation, critical historical analysis, reflexive presence of author, promotes cultural change. Focus on oppression, conflict, struggle, power; examine larger political, social, and economic issues.	Participant observation, key informants, interview	Marxism; neo-Marxism; poststructuralism; broad social movements; critical social; feminist	Greckhamer, T., & Koro-Ljungberg, M. (2004, August 14). Paper presented to American Sociological Association. San Francisco, CA. Hardcastle, M.-A., Usher, K., & Holmes, C. (2006). Carspecken's five-stage critical qualitative research method: an application to nursing research. Qualitative Health Research, *16,* 151–161. Koro-Ljungberg, M., & Greckhamer, T. (2005). Strategic turns labeled 'ethnography:' From description to openly ideological production of cultures. Qualitative Research, *5,* 285–306. doi:10.177/1468794105054456 Schwandt, T. A. (2001). Dictionary of qualitative inquiry (2nd ed.). Thousand Oaks, CA: Sage.

(continues)

TABLE 10–1   SELECTED TYPES OF ETHNOGRAPHY *(continued)*

Type	Definition/Description	Data Sources	Theoretical Perspective	References
Deconstructive (disruptive)	Concern about objectivity, positionality, and representation as postcritical; elements of multiplicity, fragmentation, and uncertainty added to cultural descriptions; representations of cultural systems created via complexities of language and under historical connections and influences; destabilized, multiply positioned subjectivity		Cultural theories analyze power, knowledge, and language of multiple political agendas embedded in particular cultures; critical social; feminist	Koro-Ljungberg, M., & Greckhamer, T. (2005). Strategic turns labeled 'ethnography:' From description to openly ideological production of cultures. Qualitative Research, 5, 285–306. doi:10.177/1468794105054456 Kincheloe, J. L., & McLaren, P. (2005). Rethinking critical theory and qualitative research. In N. K. Denzin, & Y. S. Lincoln (Eds.), The Sage handbook of qualitative research (3rd ed.) (pp. 303–342). Thousand Oaks, CA: Sage.
Disrupted (deconstructive, critical/feminist)	Disrupted ethnography includes critical/feminist and deconstructive types		Critical social; feminist	Koro-Ljungberg, M., & Greckhamer, T. (2005). Strategic turns labeled 'ethnography:' From description to openly ideological production of cultures. Qualitative Research, 5, 285–306. doi:10.177/1468794105054456 Greckhamer, T., & Koro-Ljungberg, M. (2004, August 14). Paper presented to American Sociological Association. San Francisco, CA.

TABLE 10–1 SELECTED TYPES OF ETHNOGRAPHY *(continued)*

Type	Definition/ Description	Data Sources	Theoretical Perspective	References
Focused	Study of small elements of one society, group, or culture; focus on distinct problem within a specific context among a small group of people. Some use short duration field visits seen as intensive data collection and analysis.	Participant observation, interview, evert analysis	Cultural	Roper, J. M., & Shapira, J. (2000). Ethnography in nursing research. Thousand Oaks, CA: Sage. Knoblauch, H. (2005). Focused ethnography. Forum Qualitative Social Research, 6. Retrieved at http://nbn-resolving.de/urn:nbn:de:0114-fqs0503440
Maxiethnography (classical, holistic, traditional)	Large, comprehensive study of general and particular features of a designated culture; holistic.	Participant observation, interview, event analysis, document analysis, artifact analysis	Cultural	Leininger, M. M. (Ed.). (1985). Qualitative research methods in nursing. Orlando, FL: Grune & Stratton.
Miniethnography	Small-scale, focused on narrow field of inquiry. Study of belief or behavior in limited timeframe.	Participant observation, interview	Cultural	Leininger, M. M. (Ed.). (1985). Qualitative research methods in nursing. Orlando, FL: Grune & Stratton.

(continues)

TABLE 10–1   SELECTED TYPES OF ETHNOGRAPHY *(continued)*

Type	Definition/Description	Data Sources	Theoretical Perspective	References
Microethnography	Study of social interaction; intellectual roots in content analysis; ethnography of communication interactional sociolinguistics; focus on proxemics and kinesics. Close-up view of a small social unit or an identifiable activity with the social unit.	Participant observation (audiotape and videotape of interactions)	Linguistics	Marshall, C., & Rossman, G. B. (1989). Designing qualitative research. Newbury Park, CA: Sage.
Performance	Presented as a performance text that one or more people write and read for an audience. Cultural study in which individuals are brought together with culture in an enacted manner; agency is revealed through the aesthetic which portrays the interactions, connecting politics, institutions, and experience. Ethnodrama.	Autobiographical stories, field notes, reflexive journal entities, memories of life events	Critical social	Smith, C. A., & Gallo, A. M. (2007). Applications of performance ethnography in nursing. Qualitative Health Research, 17, 521–528. Kincheloe, J. L., & Mclaren, P. (2005). Rethinking critical theory and qualitative research. In N. K. Denzin, & Y. S. Lincoln (Eds.), The Sage handbook of qualitative research aesthetic (3rd ed.) (pp. 303–342). Thousand Oaks, CA: Sage. Mienczakowski, J. (1996). An ethnographic act: The construction of consensual theater. In C. Ellis, & A. P. Bochner (Eds.), Composing ethnography: Alternative forms of qualitative writing (pp. 244–264). Walnut Creek, CA: AltaMira.

TABLE 10–1   SELECTED TYPES OF ETHNOGRAPHY *(continued)*

Type	Definition/ Description	Data Sources	Theoretical Perspective	References
Practitioner	Practitioner in field conducts study with direct application to practice; exploration of health and illness with practitioner participating in research process; member of the group being studied; lived insider/ observer balanced.	Participant observation, field notes, interview, archives, life histories, case studies, artifacts, reflexivity	Cultural; critical social	Barton, T. D. (2008). Understanding ethnography. Nurse Researcher, *15*, 7–18. Field, P. A. (1991). Doing fieldwork in your own culture. In J. M. Morse (Ed.). Qualitative nursing research: A contemporary dialogue (rev. ed.) (pp. 91–104). Newbury Park, CA: Sage. Simmons, M. (2007). Insider ethnography: Tinker, tailor, researcher or spy? Nurse Researcher, *14*(4), 7–17.
Reflexive	Ethnographer is not separate from object of investigation but viewed as unified subject of knowledge that can make hermeneutic efforts to establish identification between the observer and the observed. Who the researcher is, what is going on in themselves, and how a sense of self-consciousness can be put to use in an ethnographic context. Critical self-reflection.		Cultural; critical social	Kincheloe, J. L., & McLaren, P. (2005). Rethinking critical theory and qualitative research. In N. K. Denzin, & Y. S. Lincoln (Eds.), The Sage handbook of qualitative research (3rd ed.) (pp. 303–342). Thousand Oaks, CA: Sage. Aamodt, A. M. (1991). Ethnography and epistemology: Generating nursing knowledge. In J. M. Morse (Ed.), Qualitative nursing research: A contemporary dialogue (rev. ed.) (pp. 40–53). Newbury Park, CA: Sage. Schwandt, T. A. (2001). Dictionary of qualitative inquiry (2nd ed.). Thousand Oaks, CA: Sage. *(continues)*

TABLE 10–1 SELECTED TYPES OF ETHNOGRAPHY *(continued)*

Type	Definition/Description	Data Sources	Theoretical Perspective	References
Specialist	Social scientist conducts study; not necessarily practitioners in field; may have limited or no previous knowledge or experience of field	Fieldwork/field notes, participant observation, interview; thick description	Cultural; critical social	Barton, T. D. (2008). Understanding ethnography. Nurse Researcher, 15, 7–18.

culture and its insiders. They are described as exploratory and hypothesis-generating studies. Such ethnographic investigations characterize the traditional period or phase of qualitative research (Denzin & Lincoln, 2005).

Ethnographic research originated in the discipline of anthropology, caught the attention of the fields of sociology (Fox, 1959; Goffman, 1961; Liebow, 1993) and education, and appealed to nurse investigators in the 1960s and 1970s (Byerly, 1969; Germain, 2001; Pearsall, 1965; Ragucci, 1972). Later, nurse researchers (Robertson & Boyle, 1984; Thorne, 1991) emphasized the contribution of ethnographic research to nursing and pointed out what might be learned about health and illness phenomena studied in cultural contexts. The works of ethnographers who produced classics continue to influence researchers (Douglas, 1963, 1966, 1975; Douglass, 1969; Firth, 1936; Malinowski, 1922, 1948; Mauss, 1967; Turner, 1957; Turner, 1967) and have inspired ethnographers for decades (Spradley, 1970).

The classic ethnographic approach is a naturalistic, systematic, interpretive approach and relies on observation, interview, and description rather than statistics and experimentation (Ragucci, 1972). Descriptions of the culture studied were considered objective, consistent with the positivistic scientist paradigm (Denzin & Lincoln, 2005). Detailed descriptions of phenomena in context and insights gained through interpretation are hallmarks of traditional ethnography. Ethnographies rely on two forms of authority, the personal experience of the ethnographer, the research instrument (Atkinson, 1992), and the report, which combines factual writing (Richardson, 1988) and reflects field notes, methodological notes, theoretical notes, and investigator diaries or personal notes.

Culture, according to Sapir (1924), embraces:

> In a single term those general attitudes, views of life, and specific manifestations of civilization that give a particular people its distinctive place in the world. Emphasis is put not so much on what is done and believed by a people as on how what is done and believed functions in the whole life of that people, on what significance it has for them. (pp. 311–312)

Culture is also defined as the total way of life of a group and the learned behavior that is socially constructed and transmitted. Some questions of interest to ethnographers include what knowledge people use to interpret experience and mold their behavior within the context of their culturally constituted environment, what the nature of culture is, how culture emerges, how it is transmitted, and what the functions of culture are. Individuals in a culture hold common values and ideas acquired through learning from other members of the group. Traditional ethnographies describe the unique and distinctive processes of culture. Cultural phenomena, beliefs, values, rules, and norms are ethnographic emphases.

Traditional ethnography refers to a description of a culture or subculture. The term ethnography includes an account of the people of the culture and involves writing that depicts the culture. Many ethnographic studies differ from other forms of qualitative research by their focus on the cultural perspective. By generating cultural descriptions, ethnographic investigations examine what the world is like for people who have learned to see, hear, speak, think, and act in ways that are different from dominant cultures or not yet described. Ethnographers do not attempt to alter the lives of the natives, folk, insiders, or informants.

Concepts of structure, function, and symbol orient traditional or classic ethnographic studies (Fetterman, 1989). Structure indicates the social structure of the group, such as how various positions and job descriptions function on a patient unit. Function points to the social relationships and interactions among the members of the group. Symbol, as condensed meaning, operates like a "cognitive reflex" and evokes "powerful feelings and thoughts" (Fetterman, 1989, p. 36).

Often, investigators acquire skill in the research techniques of ethnography during apprenticeships. Nonetheless, in spite of learning the rules under the guidance of a seasoned fieldworker, the ethnographic process is personalistic because no ethnographer works just like another (Riemann, 2005). Also, one of the challenges for nurse ethnographers is the fact that nurses are also clinicians who study individuals in the circumstances of health and illness (Brody, 1981; Field, 1989). Research, not therapy, is the intent of ethnography. Nurse ethnographers always defer to the therapeutic imperative, however, when the welfare of patients is at stake, and data collection is suspended temporarily.

Disrupted Ethnography

Contemporary ethnography recognizes the work of traditional ethnographers as historical antecedents. Whether classified as post-structuralism, postmodernism, post-experimentalism, or *post-post*, contemporary ethnography has been labeled *disrupted ethnography* (Greckhamer & Koro-Ljungberg, 2004). The term *disrupted* suggests that many modern ethnographers frame studies with theories other than traditional ethnographic theory. For example, they may orient studies in constructivist, feminist, ethnic, Marxist, or critical theory approaches. Consequently, contemporary discourse about ethnography reflects a variety of approaches, all described as interpretive and illustrated by different types (Table 10–1). Contemporary ethnographies vary, oriented as critical, feminist, or post-structural. However, some contemporary ethnographers work in the middle of different paradigms, using multiple theoretical perspectives (Greckhamer & Koro-Ljungberg, 2004).

Disrupted ethnographic examples include interpretive case studies; ethnographic fiction; essays; stories; experimental writing; fables; dramas; historical, economic, and sociocultural analyses; cultural theory as criticism; and autobiography (Denzin & Lincoln, 2005, p. 24). Ethnographers continue to examine culture and socialization, yet look at culture using political and critical lenses.

Disrupted ethnographies signify a strategic turn in ethnographic investigation. One critique expresses the perspective that researchers completing traditional ethnographies failed to describe cultures in their complexity, having neglected issues of power and dominance (Carspecken, 1996). Sociologists, anthropologists, educational researchers, psychologists, and nurses have embraced disruptive ethnographic methods. They explore and describe human life and experience and are interested in social inequalities and positive social change (Carspecken, 1996). Critical social theory is the framework that dominates along with social and cultural criticism. "Criticalists find contemporary society to be unfair, unequal, and both subtly and overtly oppressive for many people. We do not like it, and we want to change it" (Carspecken, 1996, p. 7). They consider objective or neutral scientific findings subtly biased.

Purposes and Research Questions

The process of identifying the purposes of ethnographic studies is a complex one. Investigators often have a general idea of a topic that interests them and gradually realize that an ethnographic study might be the best strategy to discover the meanings and understandings of a cultural group or subgroup of society and a topic about which little is understood. They may investigate social action, subjective experience, and conditions influencing action and experience (Carspecken, 1996). A review of the literature might take researchers outside of their discipline as they recognize how few studies have been conducted on the topic by nurse investigators. Eventually, they focus the purpose(s) and research questions because it is not possible to study the topic to complete understanding of cultural groups. Four examples from nursing ethnographies follow:

> Purpose (traditional): A descriptive analysis of the nature of nursing rituals was the focus of the ethnographic study. Questions: (1) What actions, words, and objects make up nursing rituals? (2) What are the types of nursing rituals demonstrated by professional nurses caring for adult patients on a unit? (3) What explicit or manifest meanings do these rituals have to nurses, patients and their families, and to other hospital personnel, such as physicians, licensed practical nurses, and

nursing assistants? (4) What implicit or latent meanings are identified by the nurses, patients, and other hospital personnel, and by the investigator? (5) How are patients, physicians, licensed practical nurses, aides, and orderlies involved in these nursing rituals? (6) How are nursing rituals embedded within the context of the routines, procedures, and reports of the nursing unit? (Wolf, 1986, pp. 2–3)

The main question (traditional) to be answered was: How do elders survive in the midst of "drug warfare" in an inner-city community known for its dangerous streets and public spaces? (Kaufman, 1995, p. 231)

The purposes of this critical ethnographic study (critical) were to understand how mothers described and understood their experience of having a hospitalized, premature baby, including the mothers' actions in the NICU and the conditions affecting their descriptions, interpretations, and actions. (Hurst, 2001, p. 41)

The research (critical/feminist) aimed to explore and reveal common, different, unique and exceptional experiences that empowered, disempowered, and/or oppressed participants' personal, professional and corporate efforts towards their own empowerment, emancipation, and transformation. To reveal the ways in which women nurses empowered themselves in their work role and the network of power relations present in their practice settings. (Pannowitz, Glass, & Davis, 2009, p. 107)

Although the research questions and purpose of studies are central to investigations, ethnographers often discuss the evolving nature of the purpose as literature reviews are examined and participant observation and interviewing begins. Emergent decisions characterize ethnographies and are ongoing as investigators reflect on what has already been learned; often data collection and analysis run parallel. However, the members of institutional review boards, acting as guardians protecting human subjects from harm, demand specificity from proposals, such as the amount of time to be spent in the field; the expected number, gender, and race of informants; and how much time individual informants will be observed and interviewed. Although this is challenging, ethnographers must create a plan for data collection that best addresses how they intend to achieve the purpose of the study. They are called upon to notify institutional review boards of changes in data collection plans and sampling frames as issues emerge that warrant additional attention.

Ethnographic Methods

Ethnographic methods are distinctive because of use of self as an observer, on-site fieldwork, prolonged engagement in the fieldwork, interviews ranging from informal (unstructured) to formal (structured), event analysis, and document and artifact analysis. Fieldwork is considered a rite of passage for the "genuine" anthropologist, sociologist fieldworker, or ethnographer (Ward & Werner, 1984). Data collection is qualitative and inductive. The ethnographer creates a raw record during data collection that is written as text. The thick description (observing, recording, and analyzing a culture so that signs are interpreted to gain meaning and understanding within the culture; Geertz, 1973) produced by investigators takes a naturalistic stance in which the detailed patterns of cultural and social relationships are disclosed and placed in context. Interpretation is based on the meanings that actions and events have for members of the culture.

In contrast, disrupted ethnographies such as critical studies build primary (researcher's) records from observing interactions in a social site with field notes and audio and video recordings. Next, the primary record is reconstructed as the investigator examines social interaction patterns, their meanings, power relations, roles, interactive sequences, evidence of embodied meaning, intersubjective structures, and more. Cultural themes and systems factors are represented linguistically. Third, conversations with subjects generate data, and systems relations are examined. Finally, reasons are suggested for the study's experiences and cultural forms including class, race, gender, and political structures of society. Ultimately, the findings inform real social change (Carspecken, 1996, pp. 40–43).

Ethnographers' work with key informants, participants, or subjects leads to interpretations that cannot be separated from time, place, events, and actions of people. The phenomena to be studied through ethnography might be society, community, subculture, organization, group, work experience, hospitalization experience, gender relationships, or beliefs, rituals, events, routines, interactions, and any other aspect of human existence.

Participant Observation

Participant observation is defined as the method by which investigators join the insiders of a culture so that human relationships, events, patterns, and sociocultural contexts in which people live and work can be studied (Jorgensen, 1989). Traditional ethnographies use participant observation as a primary data source through field notes generated as investigators participate in the daily life of the members of the group. Participant observation, achieved through the experience of investigators' fieldwork, is a chief source of data (Bernard, 1994). Ethnographers are participant observers as they gather data during fieldwork by observing and interviewing. Through this involvement, they achieve on-site, temporary membership in the culture. Everyday life is studied and accessed through observations that are open-ended, flexible, opportunistic, factual, and situated in settings. The physical and social environment of the informants being studied provides the context. Total immersion in the culture, accomplished by living with the natives or insiders, is preferable for participant observers. However, disrupted ethnographies may not spend as much time in the field as traditional studies. This is also true for mini ethnographies and micro ethnographies. Furthermore, critical ethnographies "engage with their own participation within the ethnographic frame" (Tedlock, 2005, p. 467). Transparency results as investigators and participants gain the "outward gaze."

Some ethnographers use a team participant observation approach, whereas others conduct studies alone. Participant observation is useful for the study of alien, foreign, or exotic cultures; topics about which little is known; or everyday circumstances about which knowledge is assumed, but not necessarily examined. During participant observation, researchers learn the use of insider language and later seek clarification and understanding during interviews. Patience and openmindedness are required characteristics of ethnographers.

Participant observers may be strangers to the communities to be studied but can gradually and temporarily become members of the group (Stocking, 1983). They have been called "marginal natives" (Freilich, 1970). Shokeid (1988) disputes this idea and prefers the term *professional stranger*—one who develops closeness, detachment, indifference, and participation with informants. Developing face-to-face relationships is essential, and acceptance by the insiders, especially the gatekeepers, who may or may not be key informants, is crucial. Building trust and establishing relationships early in the first stages of the research are important aims. The quality of relationships is important as is the position and status of informants and investigators. In practitioner ethnographies, however, researchers are members of the group being studied (Simmons, 2007).

Participant observation is performed as a data collection strategy and helps ethnographers reduce the problem of reactivity. Fieldworkers formulate interview questions and probing questions based on what they learn over time. Participant observation enables investigators to answer research problems that are not easily answered by other methods. It takes time and requires ethnographers to learn the roles of informants, understand their language and experience, learn the functions and structures of the culture through explicit and implicit interpretation, build knowledge about the topic through increasingly focused participant observation, maintain curiosity and a naïve approach, and build the writing and analytic skills demanded by descriptive and analytic field notes and the ultimate product of the study, the ethnography.

Participant observation demands that investigators remain ethical by overt involvement, that is, with insiders' knowledge of their purpose. Covert investigations have been conducted; however, human subjects' considerations have ideally eliminated them. Overt participant observation demands observations to be direct, on site, and to return over an extended period of time. According to Spradley (1980), culture, the knowledge that people learn as members of a group, cannot be observed directly. However, the ethnographer directly observes the group of insiders. Cultural knowledge is gained through tacit and explicit understandings developed over the introductory, focused observation, and coding stages of projects (Keith, 1986). Coding consists of classifying and interpreting text for meaning. Inferences are developed by investigators. Observation is open-ended, and the surprises of fieldwork demand that investigators are flexible and opportunistic, following the inquiry where it leads. They frequently define sources of data and identify informants as the investigation progresses.

Junker (1960) describes participant observation roles of fieldworkers: participant as observer, observer as participant, complete participant, and complete observer. The complete participant may gradually become participant as observer. Another complete participant may never leave the role, however, and could remain completely ethnocentric and never become a social scientist. The complete observer may have a better chance of becoming a social scientist, emphasizes observation more than participation, and eventually moves to observer as participant. Although Junker's notions of the role seem somewhat artificial, they describe the dynamic nature of individual participant observers as they enter the field. Initially, fieldworkers observe more often. They gain the trust of informants, ask permission to observe, and gradually move among the various roles, depending on the situations and people at the center of attention. Thus, the idea of participant observer presents like a continuum of roles, where the movement from pure observer to pure participant depends on the social scene, how comfortable the ethnographer is at the moment, and which aspect of the culture calls for more study. Before the ideal participant observer role is achieved, investigators often find themselves explaining the purpose of the study repeatedly to potential informants. Furthermore, relationships with informants, once established, must be carefully maintained as everyday life is studied as unobtrusively as possible (Jorgensen, 1989). However, the more ethnographers participate, the less likely they are to observe, limiting access by restricting the time available for recording and analyzing events, actors, and everyday life.

In contrast to Junker (1960), Adler and Adler (1987) describe varying roles of membership involvement, peripheral membership, active membership, and complete membership. Peripheral membership is the most marginal, yet these ethnographers interact often and closely with informants through direct, first-hand experience. They do not assume functional roles within the group of informants. Active membership goes further, with the researchers becoming more engaged with the central activities of the group. They become co-participants in the research. Complete membership requires ethnographers to achieve equal status with informants. They are completely immersed in the field; some become the phenomenon, while others are more opportunistic (Adler & Adler, 1987). Similar to the point made about Junker's (1960) notions of participant observation, the nature of fieldwork demands movement among the various role classifications, with ethnographers ideally not frozen in one.

Typically, participant observers are outsiders who gradually gain insider knowledge of the culture. Often they transform to insider status and perform various roles over the course of the study. For example, in a study that took place on a nursing unit, one investigator (Wolf, 1986) transported laboratory slips, helped with patient care when a member of the nursing staff needed assistance caring for patients, and listened to the complaints of the staff about working conditions. Others assumed the "socially acceptable incompetent" (Lofland & Lofland, 1984, p. 38) position in which a nurse made beds, fetched and carried, and made tea (Hopkins, 2002) and provided comfort and emotional support (Varcoe, 2001). Such roles must fit within the scope of the investigators' expertise (Jorgensen, 1989) and are limited by the chief purpose that brought them to the field, the study. The "socially acceptable incompetent" position helps ethnographers to assume the role of the ones to be taught. It may be necessary to refuse to perform some duties, either because of human subjects' considerations consistent with restrictions of institutional review boards, awareness that the activity might blur fieldworkers' role with informants, or conflicts about threatened patient safety.

Fieldwork

Fieldwork is a disciplined mode of inquiry that engages the ethnographer firsthand in data collection over extended periods of time, particularly for traditional ethnographies. It combines art and science so that the accomplished ethnographer produces a narrative that offers insight and understanding of human social life to a "discerning audience" (Wolcott, 1995, p. 251). Traditional ethnographic fieldwork has a bias toward cultural interpretation, involves the study of people in social interaction, and aims to understand the culture from the native point of view (Bernard, 1994; Spradley, 1980; Wolcott, 1995). Fieldwork informs ethnographers about the cultures of groups. Doing fieldwork demands that observations are recorded in a systematic manner. It requires that ethnographers make a commitment to the individuals being studied; intimate, long-term acquaintances result. Fieldwork by participant observation is a hallmark of traditional ethnography (Stocking, 1983).

During fieldwork, ethnographers attempt to carry out the purpose of the study, although some of the subsequent questions asked, interviews conducted, and observations scheduled are emergent. Participant observation begins with performing broad descriptive observations, analyzing data, making focused observations, and conducting increasingly more focused interviews.

Through fieldwork, ethnographers gain primary data from informants in context, moving among various situations, crises, and events.

The 12-month standard of traditional ethnographic fieldwork has been accepted for many decades. However, this guideline is tempered by a judgment of the adequacy of the knowledge accumulated during uninterrupted or interrupted field encounters (Wolcott, 1995). Instead of specifying the length of time, some refer to the length of engagement as long-term immersion in the field. Alternatively, disrupted ethnographies may not rely heavily on fieldwork, for example, the engagement of micro ethnographies with the material may be extensive (Table 10–1).

Although the ethnographer's role of the "pure" participant observer is an ideal and must be visible to insiders, researchers benefit most when people carry out everyday activities so that fieldwork is conducted unobtrusively. Informants become so accustomed to the presence of investigators that investigators seem part of the typical surroundings of the settings for the study. This takes time. Ethnographers often try to conduct the study without having an impact on the lives of informants. Also of note is the fact that in spite of well-developed plans for data collection, fieldwork for all first-time ethnographers is learned by doing.

Because many ethnographers are strangers to informants, it takes time for ethnographers to establish themselves in the culture of the group. Courtesy and patience are required during participant observation. Ethnographers have to show up, day after day, so that people begin to learn their commitment to the study (Wolcott, 1995). They share stories and food and often develop rapport or friendships.

Fieldwork requires ethnographers to collect data using a variety of sources: structured and unstructured direct observations of events, including interaction analysis and situations; observation and recording of the characteristics of the physical environment through drawings, maps, photography, and video and audio recordings; social network analysis; unstructured, semistructured, and structured interviews with informants or subjects; document analysis; and artifact analysis.

Fieldwork taxes the energy of investigators and is intellectually challenging, particularly as data collection and analysis progress. The work that is accomplished between field notes and the readable prose generated at the completion of studies is significant (Agar, 1986). It is also stimulating and exciting as ethnographers illuminate taken-for-granted worlds and sensitize readers to commonsense knowledge and power relationships.

Fieldwork also demands making explicit what is implicitly or intuitively understood about what is going on in contexts. When rapport is established with members of the group, ethnographers learn to act with them. Next, they pull back to plan additional observations, write field notes, analyze data, think critically, and return for more interviews and observations. Cultural knowledge is gained on a daily basis during fieldwork; ethnographers often return to the field after dwelling with the data as the study goes forward.

Access to the Cultural Group and Informants, Participants, or Subjects

Ethnographers rely on gatekeepers to help them gain access to potential informants, participants, or subjects. For example, prominent administrators of a hospital or school and community leaders are approached to review proposals. They act as valuable consultants to the investigation and often give advice that benefits studies. They might sponsor the proposal during review by institutional review boards. Gatekeepers provide names of potential primary informants (DeSantis, 1990), and investigators use leaders' names to establish credibility within the group.

It may be very difficult to select and gain access to settings. Many ethnographers rely on personal acquaintances to review the potential fit of settings with the topic of the investigation (Jorgensen, 1989). In one ethnographic study (Wolf, 1986), a physician colleague suggested the hospital where he was employed as an ideal setting. Subsequent meetings with nurse administrators led the nurse investigator to realize the group's lack of commitment to nursing research and the proposed ethnography. Although political pressure could have been brought to bear on the nurse administrators, the investigator soon realized the futility of such efforts despite her disappointment. Later, a nurse administrator who was eager to support research within his hospital provided access and continued support for currently proposed and future investigations. Initial acceptance into the field by gatekeepers and later by informants, participants, or subjects is critical to the success of investigations.

Within the same study (Wolf, 1986), the investigator realized that some aspects of the nursing unit were more closed to fieldwork than were others. Whereas most of the nursing staff of the night shift welcomed her, two licensed practical nurses were suspicious of her motives and seemed to fear negative reports to supervisors. The investigator conducted fieldwork for a few nights and decided to rely on the permanent night nurse's talents as a key informant. Much of the data collection was visible to all staff, conducted front stage. Some participant observation episodes were private and backstage, such as witnessing nurses bathing patients and performing postmortem care.

Informants, actors, or insiders are members of the cultural or subcultural group. They are knowledgeable about topics and understand how things work in the culture. Informants must be willing to share knowledge with ethnographers by providing detailed explanations from insiders' points of view and providing the time and opportunity to be interviewed and observed. Key and other informants are crucial to the task of the ethnographer. Informants are chosen to share information about the research topic and the cultural group. Key informants are chosen after time is spent in the field during preliminary data collection. Each informant may or may not be able to explain subtleties of the culture. Different individuals serve different functions. Some are key, some are primary, and some are secondary. Ethnographers are informant-centered, and as such actively participate in the research process. Because interviews and participant observation are key data sources, the ethnographer must work to develop trusting relationships and collaborate with informants (Kleinman, 1988). It is through trust that informants allow ethnographers access to insiders' knowledge. Investigators often learn during fieldwork that informants ascribe their own interpretations to the nature of the research and form their own versions of the method. Many informants welcome investigators; however, at times a few do not. These few may remain suspicious over the course of data collection, seeing the study as an "I spy" opportunity for researchers that might situate informants at risk in the community or at work. This response is of increasing concern to investigators who conduct practitioner ethnographies (Table 10-1).

As the investigator conducts interviews and performs the work of participant observation, close relationships often develop. On the one hand, the intimate, meaningful, and trusting relationships among informants and fieldworkers are a privilege that investigators cherish for a lifetime. On the other hand, analysis forces ethnographers to stand back periodically and detach as coding and interpretation progress. It is wise to develop rapport with informants rather than friendships (Glesne, 1989). The time investigators are in the field enables them to develop relationships distinguished by confidence and trust. Rapport serves the interests of ethnographers in that they can acquire data easily while reducing the distance between informants and themselves, quieting informants' anxiety about being observed and described, and building trust. In contrast, friendships may hinder access to cultural knowledge because informants may over-identify with investigators. Some informants may be so preferred that data gathering is limited, or informants act in atypical ways or to impress researchers (Glesne, 1989). The distance between informants and fieldworkers arises chiefly because of theoretical reflections and analysis. However, understanding the life worlds of informants is achieved by entering into the subjectivity of their experiences during fieldwork (Adler & Adler, 1987). Intimate familiarity with the culture through a variety of data collection methods is a goal (Lofland, 1976).

The nature of relationships and the insider knowledge gained are protected by the ethical codes of investigators. It is not likely that the anonymity of informants is totally protected because the data collection period is prolonged and other study informants have also shared in the situations and events of the field research. However, to protect confidentiality, researchers use pseudonyms, limit access to data and records, secure records, and may eliminate or change small facts when writing the results of the study at informants' request or to protect disclosure of informants' identities that may place them at risk. Informants might become distrustful of members of their community if all possible protections are not used. Also, the uses of the study results may not be under the control of investigators (DeSantis, 1990). Nonetheless, ethnographers do their best to adhere to the strategies that protect human subjects and sites. Members of institutional review boards might have limited knowledge of ethnographic research so that prior to approval and entry into fieldwork, investigations may need to establish the legitimacy of the design (Reid, 1991).

One of the chief strategies that ethnographers use to protect informants is providing direct access to the narrative results prior to publication or public presentation. This is referred to as "member check" by Lincoln and Guba (1985). Informants might request that the investigator suppress or change findings, might refuse to permit the study to be published, or might restrict data collection (Hammersley & Atkinson, 1983). Investigators must protect informants' privacy and confidentiality and that of research locations (Christians, 2005).

Disruptive ethnographies, such as critical and autobiographical, modify participant observation by examining their participation. They seek interconnectedness, relationship, and performance—consistent with critical theory and feminist approaches—and invite others into the research and transform participants' views of themselves (Tedlock, 2005).

Investigators develop ongoing relationships with key or primary informants. Because of the close relationships that investigators develop with informants, it is necessary for ethnographers to maintain distance by being visible as researchers, by adhering to the focus of the study and the evolving nature of data collection, and by respecting the confidentiality of the people studied.

The number of informants varies according to the topic. A study of a nursing unit includes a more limited number of potential informants—who may all be included in observations and interviews—than a study of a community or large group does. Preliminary participant observation helps investigators to focus and restrict the number of informants. Some use purposive sampling to include the fullest range of informants, events, and situations being studied. This approach helps to obtain a more manageable number of interviews and observations. Theoretical sampling also accomplishes this outcome.

Field Notes

Ethnographers try to gain an inclusive and extensive picture of the group under study. Field notes are descriptive of the phenomena being studied (Bernard,

1994). How people act and the descriptions of activities are main sources of cultural knowledge and are gained through interpretation. Although it is not possible to gain understanding of the whole culture or group, ethnographers work toward understanding a holistic outlook of the purpose of the study. The main data source of ethnographic records is written field notes: "Field notes make 'the field' manageable and memorable" (Atkinson, 1992, p. 18). Field notes involve writing, in which observations and interviews are constructed and reconstructed, and reading the notes (Atkinson, 1992) when interpretation is performed. Field notes identify the dates, days, times, settings, and the names, status, and activities of informants being observed. They often combine native language and observer language. Ethnographers record in the language they use in everyday situations (Spradley, 1980). Accurate records of what informants say are documented through verbatim transcriptions of recorded interviews (either audio or video). When unstructured interviews are conducted, investigators paraphrase in field notes what informants say as soon as possible.

Field notes for ethnographies are written with a great amount of detail. Concrete language is used to reveal the physical and social details of each observational episode. Because initial field notes often are condensed and preferably recorded on the spot, ethnographers return to expand them as soon as possible. Computers have facilitated this process.

During fieldwork, ethnographers develop habits of recording observations through narrative records. Care is paid to identifying the informants as actors, identifying the location, date, and time of the episodes observed, as well as retaining duplicate copies of field notes and storing them in separate, safe locations. Field notes enable the published results to adhere to the "thick description" standard espoused by Geertz (1973). Field notes help investigators describe and analyze cultures; the data recorded are rooted in the realities of the episodes, situations, informants in action, and events witnessed by ethnographers. As they observe and record field notes, ethnographers think and reflect on social events, the use of space and artifacts, and informant conduct. Field notes begin with extensive detailed description with little evaluation or summary; they note language events, situations, leadership roles (formal and informal), and informants of importance. Next, they become more focused; tentative hypotheses may be stated about themes and patterns in observations. Ethnographers conduct more focused interviews, perform final coding, and may return to the field for more focused observations and field notes that are again coded to understand patterns in question. The finished product with the best "thick description" reveals the abstract and general patterns and traits of social life in cultures. Readers get a sense of the emotions, thoughts, and perceptions of informants. Carspecken (1996) provides an example of thick description.

It is wise for ethnographers to remind themselves to remain nonjudgmental about individual and cultural practices (Fetterman, 1989). Keeping personal notes separate from field notes might assist ethnographers to guard against biases and help prevent them from imposing their own culture on the one being studied.

During fieldwork, ethnographers make decisions about how to include and exclude events and informants, staying true to the research topic. Informants and their actions are observed along with the manner in which they interact with each other. Participant observation assists ethnographers in making choices about who to interview and which situations to witness. Interviews follow in which informants, as members of the group or culture, are asked to explain what they see and how they perceive what is going on, and to share their interpretations of events, rules, and roles. Systematic field notes, recorded by the ethnographer day after day, reflect what is learned through the perspectives of investigators. Regardless of whether the field notes record the events and actors during typical or atypical days, the ideal notes are characterized by "thick description." Such a narrative conveys the cultural scene, with details that other readers would appreciate almost as if they were witnesses. It is important that ethnographers pay attention to describing the language of informants and the language researchers select to depict each observation.

Field notes accumulate over time. Well-written field notes reveal the interplay of informants in natural contexts. The individuals, events, and situations change rapidly; crises occur. This results in ethnographers shifting attention to capture interaction. Field notes record the documentation of unexpected events. Precise control of factors is irrelevant. By capturing the stage or context, the actors, the behaviors involved in interaction, and the meaning and significance of the symbolic parts, field notes, and, later, analysis, help investigators gain understanding of the culture.

The physical depiction of the site is described in field notes, including photographs, drawings, and the use of space and time. Daily, weekly, and monthly time cycles frame events and behavior. The amount of field notes and other documents collected demands that investigators develop organized systems of data retrieval. Computer files, backup files, and scanned documents are stored in logical, indexed formats. They need to be organized initially and sequentially to facilitate data analysis. These files are arranged in an easily accessible manner and are augmented by other documents, photographs, maps, and available materials that expand the material on which data analysis depends.

Some investigators print field notes and organize them chronologically in loose-leaf binders. Backup printouts of field notes should be stored in a separate location. Backup file copies are stored on memory sticks and compact discs. Additional files that include demographic profiles of informants, institutional review board permission letter(s), signed consent forms, and a record of informant names with corresponding pseudonyms are also stored. Two indexes corresponding with field notes can be kept: 1) an index of the analysis or coding, and 2) an index of maps, drawings, photographs, and so forth. Video and audio recordings should be accurately labeled and files should be backed up. Verbatim transcriptions of interviews are either combined with field notes or filed in another chronologically organized, loose-leaf binder. "Field records must . . . be properly organized and preserved if their future research potential is to be realized" (Ruwell, 1985, p. 1).

Other Types of Records and Notes

Field notes are maintained separately from other ethnographic notes. Field journals are often kept by investigators. They serve as a calendar of events for the ethnography in combination with scheduled appointments with informants and gatekeepers. Field journals provide running, chronological records of fieldwork and serve as a history of studies.

Ethnographers' reflective journals contain personal reactions to stories, participant observation, and interviews. Thoughts and understandings are documented for reflection, exploration, and analysis (DeGraves & Aranda, 2008; Duncan, 2004). Journals help investigators record perceptions, assumptions, and judgments (Gillespie, Wallis, & Chaboyer, 2008). Reflective journals may also be labeled as diaries and personal notes.

Ethnographers often record personal notes, in which reflections, feelings, hunches, and speculations are documented (Wilson, 1989). "The personal experiences, anxieties, and fears are marginalized" (Richardson, 1988, p. 203) and sometimes have appeared in the memoirs of classic ethnographers. As personal reflections, they are introspective and also include mistakes, ideas, confusions, and epiphanies. It is preferable that personal notes are written as soon as possible. Paper records predominate because they are often recorded on site and are expanded later using computers to reflect ethnographers' insights. However, investigators might lose laptops to theft. Short notes work best in the field and can later be expanded and converted to electronic form as investigators reflect on what happened during a day's field observations.

Methodological notes help to describe how the study was conducted and to formulate additional plans for data collection as the study progresses. They remind ethnographers of the next steps in data collection. Methodological notes include analyses of cultural meanings, interpretations, and insights into the culture studied. Most of the tasks in the remaining steps involve detailed analysis and can be recorded in this category of field notes (Spradley, 1979, p. 76). Methodological notes assist ethnographers in writing final reports because they describe the methods used in studies.

Development of theoretical notes begins by coding field notes and interviews as codes or themes are identified and labeled. Investigators look for patterns and relationships among the facts of the data sources and may record interpretations and inferences in notes separate from the coding recorded directly on field notes. Theoretical notes could double as an index of codes that takes investigators back to specific pages in which thematic structures (themes, codes, categories, patterns, etc.) and indicators (chunks of data from field notes) are located. All notes can be organized and presented as part of the audit trail (Wolf, 2003).

Context

Because meaning changes with context, ethnographers are careful to orient observations into larger perspectives (Carspecken, 1996; Fetterman, 1989; Leiter, 1980). By contextualizing data and findings, researchers and readers of the study achieve greater understanding of final narratives. First, the physical context of the group being studied is detailed. This includes drawings, videotapes, or photographs for documentation. Multiple physical settings may be described, for example, meeting rooms, break rooms, patient rooms, classrooms, and dining rooms. These settings may also be placed in the larger context and physical description of a patient unit, school of nursing, or assisted living facility and community senior setting. Second, the social context requires attention and detailed description. For example, how the informants work together over the course of a 24-hour day, administer medications, manage patients' symptoms, care for patients with chest pain, and respond to a nursing professor during class or clinical assignments reveal the nature of the cultures being studied. Interactions and relationships are detailed as much as possible through field notes covering conversations. The elements of the context are constantly shifting, as does the meaning of the episodes and events being described (Leiter, 1980).

Interviews

Ethnographers depend on interviews to gain understanding of informants' worlds during participant observation opportunities. They are motivated by respect for insiders throughout the course of the study. Cultural understanding and interpretation are chief on the agenda for all types of ethnographic interviews. What people say and how they interact help investigators to understand cultural meanings. Ethnographers, working alone or with a team, carefully record the date, time, location, and names of informants in field journals as well as on verbatim transcriptions of audio-recorded or video-recorded interviews.

Carspecken (1996) characterizes interviews in relation to types of questions, ideal interviewer responses, and data analysis on transcripts. Additionally, interview questions vary (Spradley, 1979) from grand-tour questions that help to position subsequent questions to contrast questions that inquire about—for example, what happens if events go as planned or do not go as planned, what was good or bad about a crisis, or how to classify the benefits or detriments of a mistake. Grand-tour questions often present informants with "Tell me about . . ." leads. For example, an investigator might ask, "Tell me about what typically happens during your shift." More specific questions such as "What was going on then?", "What do you do when you administer medications?", and "What are the steps that you take when you determine that a patient has chest pain?" help to uncover cultural meanings. Questions are also described as open-ended and closed-ended.

Prior to scheduling formal ethnographic interviews, researchers take part in friendly conversations that help build rapport with insiders. Informal conversational interviews are open-ended and flexible (Patton, 1990). When the conversation shifts to a structured interview, the purpose of the conversation is explicit to informants and has been planned by interviewers (Spradley, 1979). Ethnographers remind insiders of the purpose of each interview and often record the session. Permission to record interviews is always asked whether consent is accomplished on a consent form, verbally, or electronically. If informants deviate from the purpose, ethnographers courteously bring them back to focus. Frequently, ethnographers interview key informants, or key actors (Fetterman, 1989), repeatedly over the course of data collection. By this time, ethnographers have realized who among the informants is best able to speak expertly about the cultural scene and to provide native explanations. On the other hand, ethnographers must avoid overreliance on one or two key informants. Not only could this lead to insufficient or inaccurate understanding, but it could isolate investigators from those informants who view the key informants jealously or adversarially.

Semistructured interviews are less formal than are structured ones. Investigators might start with a vague idea in mind, question informants, and follow the conversation to greater understanding as questions gradually become more focused. Probing questions or prompts are often used to augment interviews.

Investigators meet with informants during participant observations. They have already greeted each other casually and may be exploring various aspects of informants' concerns. At this time, ethnographers conduct unstructured interviews as topics present themselves suddenly and seem relevant to one of the various directions of the study. Interviewers follow leads, explore issues, and examine various points of view. Ethnographers allow their imagination and ingenuity to help them test hypotheses during the course of the dialogue (Becker & Geer, 1957). Different tactics and types of questions are used to help to gain explanations and descriptions of social interaction. However, it is important to consider how the presence of other informants influences the dialogue with a single informant (Weiss, 1994). Private interviews preserve informant confidentiality.

Event Analysis

Geertz (1973) suggests that ethnographies produce momentary examples of behavior. Nonetheless, during the process of participant observation, transient events take place that divert ethnographers to more focused observations. Event sampling and analysis evolve according to crises, chance occurrences, and planned observations. For example, in a study of nursing rituals (Wolf, 1986) in which postmortem care was considered an event that might evoke nursing rituals, the investigator realized that the recurrent context of postmortem care was events in which do-not-resuscitate decisions were made. She decided that when these decisions took place, she had to study such events along with postmortem-care events. Additionally, cardiopulmonary resuscitation events or codes were also witnessed and provided context. Describing events involves a description of the setting, artifacts, documents, actors or informants, and conversations.

Document Analysis

Documents are records collected by ethnographers that represent a broad range of cultural phenomena, such as technological, historical, demographic, and economic phenomena (Stocking, 1983). As sources of data or facts about a culture, they instruct ethnographers about what is going on and who is doing it. Documents include texts, such as journals, diaries, biographies, and histories; files; maps; charts; and other records that lead to a fuller understanding of the culture. Smyer and Chang (1999) included participant correspondence, medical records, nurses' notes, and hospital billing records in their study of consumers of institutional respite care.

Artifact Analysis

The way insiders use artifacts informs ethnographers about the culture. The use of objects in the contexts of physical settings and social interaction serves as another source of data. How the objects are used often assists investigators in comprehending tacit knowledge.

Emic/Etic Distinction

Emic perspectives, or those from the insiders' sense of the world around them, are valued in ethnographic studies more than etic perspectives, or the perspectives of the investigators. Emic understandings rely on understanding the culture, language, and situations of the insiders through the way members of the culture see their world. Emic is shortened from the word phonemic and is borrowed from linguists who used it to study native classificatory systems. Etic, from phonetic, originates in analyses produced by the investigators (Bernard, 1994; Leininger, 1987). The etic dimension originates in the intent of investigators to understand tacit knowledge, which is beneath the surface and hidden. It originates in outsiders' interpretation of experiences of the culture and social action. Etic dimensions include interpretation of meaning, theoretical explanations, and understanding of symbols.

Carspecken's (1996) five stages of critical qualitative research represent a method of identifying shared understandings about the study for the investigator and group. His representation of emic and etic strategies are to be used in "loosely cylindrical" manner; researchers may move from stage to stage and back to a previous state (Hardcastle, Usher, & Holmes, 2006).

Types of Ethnographies

Spradley (1980) places types of ethnographies on a continuum, from microethnography to macroethnography. His classification refers to the size and complexity of the social units studied. Cultures vary in complexity, for example, complex society, multiple communities, single community, multiple social institutions, single social institution, multiple social situations, and a single social situation. Omery (1988) concurs with Spradley, noting that macroethnography is the study of complex societies and is broad in reach. Miniethnography is limited to a subunit of a single institution, such as a nursing unit, and a focused topic.

Spradley further explains the distinct focus of studies, citing Hymes (1978). Comprehensive ethnography describes a total way of life. Topic-oriented or focused ethnography restricts the study to one or more aspects of life. Hypothesis-oriented ethnography is characterized by studies in process by which ethnographers engage in testing hunches about the way cultural practices might influence human development. Another classification for types of ethnographic studies is descriptive or conventional (traditional) ethnography and critical ethnography, in which power and hidden agendas are studied.

Ethnography may be holistic, wherein a society is described as a whole. This type is compared to focused ethnography, where the focus is on specific problems or situations within a larger social scene. Another example, cognitive ethnography, seeks to determine what things mean to participants and how those meanings are created. Often, students are assigned miniethnographies; these studies are small scale (Leininger, 1985) and can be conducted in a shortened time period, such as 6 weeks, with data collection on a single cultural practice taking place 1 day a week. Students are directed to the Human Relations Area Files (eHRAF), the detailed classification scheme and multicultural database.

eHRAF is unique because each culture or ethnic group contains a variety of source documents (books, articles, and dissertations) that have been indexed and organized according to HRAF's comprehensive culture and subject classification systems: the Outline of World Cultures and the Outline of Cultural Materials. These retrieval systems extend search capability well beyond keyword searching, thus allowing for precise culture and subject retrieval, even in a foreign language. The Development and Applications of the HRAF Collections can provide investigators with an extended overview of these resources (http://www.yale.edu/hraf/collections.htm).

Maxiethnographies are "comprehensive studies of general and particular features of a designated culture" (Leininger, 1985, p. 35). Comparative ethnographies are those whereby two societies are studied so that cross-cultural comparisons can be made. Other types of ethnographies have emerged as disciplinary boundaries have blurred; examples are autoethnography (Lahman, 2009) and reflexive ethnography (Ellis & Bochner, 1996). See Table 10–1 for selected examples of types of ethnographic studies.

Analysis

Many ethnographers record field notes using a great amount of detail. Field note construction has been facilitated by computers, scanners, digital cameras, and audio and video recordings. This contrasts markedly with the methods of early ethnographers whose notes were not always easily accessible, organized, or followed by other readers, for example, by peer reviewers asked to follow audit trails when assessing the rigor of studies.

The gold standard for field notes and completed studies is best expressed by Geertz (1973). "Thick description" refers to the characteristic of a study that is written artistically, like a story; the finished ethnography is so complex and descriptive that readers are able to see the social action in context. The thick description of field notes helps ethnographers recollect experiences in the field and provides sufficient data for analysis. The quality of field notes, transcribed interviews, document analysis, and other data sources strongly influences the quality of the study. The narrative of the finished ethnography must remain faithful to informants' perspectives in context. Additionally, Ward and Werner (1984) suggest a deeper analysis of data when discussing thick description: "Thick description is that description in which the ethnographer has made a full and conscious attempt to resolve (rather than adjudicate) the discrepancies among inconsistent data" (p. 233).

Data analysis is time and energy intensive as well as complex (Robertson & Boyle, 1984). The aim of data collection for ethnographic studies is to portray the culture as informed by the knowledge of the best informants. Analysis requires that ethnographers remain familiar with all of the data throughout the course of studies. It begins almost immediately as field notes are recorded and ends when researchers and participants or informants are satisfied with their interpretations and the written report. They make choices throughout the process and pay attention to the details and the larger contexts. Intuition also is important. As thematic analysis continues, themes are sorted and related to other themes. Critical thinking ability and skills in synthesis are important (Fetterman, 1989) as are persistence, writing, and rewriting.

To reflect informants' perspectives when writing drafts of final reports, ethnographers select indicators or extracts from field notes, such as examples, comments, phrases, or detailed descriptions to match the purpose of the investigation. This provides evidence of the skillful analytic techniques of investigators, because they make sense of cultures and beliefs, values, norms, structures, functions, and symbols. Commonsense knowledge and ethnographic descriptions produce impressionistic yet detailed accounts for readers that "reveal, rather than hide" their "context-dependent character" (Leiter, 1980, p. 91). From the start of fieldwork, data collection and analysis have interacted in the thoughts and records produced by ethnographers. The analytic cycle, described by Jorgensen (1989), involves data analysis in which research materials are broken up into units (themes, etc.); are sorted and searched for categories, patterns, or wholes; and are reconstructed in a meaningful and comprehensible way. The theories that emerge begin with thematic analysis and end as explanations appearing in the final record of ethnographies. Different disciplinary traditions use a variety of terms to describe units of analysis.

> A society's culture consists of whatever one has to know or believe in order to operate in a manner acceptable to its members. . . . It is the form of things that people have in mind, their models for perceiving, relating and otherwise interpreting them. . . . Ethnographic description . . . requires methods of processing observed phenomena such that we can inductively construct a theory of how our informants have organized the same phenomena. It is the theory, not the phenomena alone, which ethnographic description aims to present. (Goodenough, 1964, p. 36)

Ethnographers are active participants in both data collection and data analysis. Data analysis begins with the first field notes and continues throughout the time necessary for completion of ethnographic studies. Not only do ethnographers rely on themes or codes induced during content analysis, but they also rely on memory (Mulkay, 1985). According to Mulkay, ethnographic writing involves a reconstruction and produces a secondary text alongside the original text, a narrative that is superior to the original. Social worlds are reconstructed that depict tacit knowledge discovered by ethnographers and revealed as written into existence. The collective memory of the group (Halbwach, 1980) is disclosed, and a likeness of the original cultural model, the culture being studied, is produced.

Data analysis procedures for ethnographies involve content analysis of text. Cultural data, as recorded in field notes, are drawn from abstractions of behavior about what people do and what they say they do (Aamodt, 1982). Investigators keep the research purpose and questions in mind so that they adhere to the original focus of ethnographic proposals. At this juncture, they are familiar with field notes and return to them again and again. They read and review the text and begin the analysis. Each time analysis is performed, investigators read textual material to get a feeling for and make sense of the data. Coding assists researchers in identifying key words, themes, patterns, essences, conceptual models, indexes, concepts, social processes, and descriptive theories. Coding is accomplished by reading texts line by line and then identifying codes (category labels; Miles & Huberman, 1984) or themes (thematic structures) in margins of the field notes or other material. Next, significant statements (words, phrases, sentences, paragraphs) are extracted that correspond with the listed structures (themes).

Thematic or categorical analysis is accomplished through the process of coding. Coding is a process of classifying and interpreting data and reveals deep and surface structures. This suggests that meaning and symbols (deep structure, latent, hidden, symbolic, high inference, implicit) are identified as are explicit (surface structure, manifest, overt, explicit, descriptive, low inference) results. Whether major or minor themes (codes, categories), patterns (explanatory or inferential codes or meta-codes, also referred to as clusters or major themes), and clusters (grouped and conceptualized objects with similar patterns or characteristics, using comparison; Miles & Huberman, 1984) are identified, they serve to produce the narrative of reports along with theoretical formulations. Data analysis is typically etic, with consistent attention to emic dimensions, reflective of informants' cultural knowledge.

Software programs are used to facilitate the data analysis process. Qualitative software, such as NUD*IST (nonnumerical unstructured data indexing searching and theorizing), has been developed to assist in data management and analysis. Additionally, some ethnographers use Microsoft Office applications to create and manage all aspects of the study and produce the audit trail, from field notes to thematic analysis to the final product. Hahn (2008) presents ways to use Excel and Access to analyze material from qualitative studies.

Broad structures (categories, patterns, clusters) most likely exist in the thoughts of investigators as they begin data analysis early in fieldwork and continue throughout the study. The structures fit the research purposes and questions identified at the inception of the ethnography. Inference produces the themes and patterns that are labeled when analyzing textual accounts. Ethnographic inference helps ethnographers achieve coherence, linking different pieces of knowledge (field notes, transcribed interviews, etc.), and then connecting the knowledge to explanations of the culture being studied (Agar, 1986). Situations, informants, objects, actions, and goals can be connected through the inferences of ethnographers, thus generating greater clarity and understanding regarding aspects of the culture. A simple way to achieve inference and reveal part of the process is for ethnographers to create a table as a three-column organizer that helps them sort, compare, contrast, and synthesize indicators into themes and patterns. For example, the columns are labeled "Indicators," "Themes," and "Interpretive statements." In a table such as this, the indicators are selected from field notes and other data sources. They are considered to be facts or chunks of data when used in ethnographies as either a low-level inference (surface structure, descriptive, explicit) or a high-level inference (deep structure, symbolic, latent) to support an explanation. Symbolic meaning might be realized as investigators label and explain deep structures.

Inference and interpretation require investigators to make choices as they select data during analysis and disregard other material. The analytic processes of conducting ethnographic studies focus on generating themes (codes, categories), which are the structural features of the cognitive map of a society, and discovering relationships between these categories, such as describing how the structural features relate to one another (Aamodt, 1982).

Fetterman (1989) explores the idea of crystallization as thought processes—how "aha" moments propel ethnographers toward insights and conclusions during the course of data analysis. Whether it occurs as a mundane or extraordinary event, crystallization is the cohesion of themes into a pattern or category or a clear understanding of beliefs, values, or norms of a social group. Crystallization is a result of reflection, interpretation, and conscientious work. As studies are written, often the writing and revision process brings additional crystallizations as thoughts converge in meaning. Ethnographers might then return to field notes and other sources of raw data to locate confirmation of such insights with similar field note examples.

It is worthwhile for ethnographers to create a table of contents for all textual material generated during ethnographic studies in which field notes and other materials that show evidence of content analysis are organized into broad or main categories. The table of contents is further subdivided within those main categories into lists of themes with page numbers that correspond to the exact locations of those themes with significant words, phrases, and paragraphs, throughout the raw records (field notes, transcribed interviews, etc.).

Interpretation

All ethnographers interpret. Interpretation helps ethnographers create and uphold the factual character of the social and cultural world as represented in the ethnographic report. They use interpretation to translate the behavior of informants into meanings. Interpretation is framed by data analysis, the study's purpose and questions, the answers or report, the explanations (interpretations) produced, the data sources that are the evidence provided to accomplish the purpose and interpretation, and the organization of these elements (purpose/questions, data, interpretation) into an argument. Informants' words and actions are important for interpretation. Ideally, throughout the study, ethnographers have been immersing themselves in the data sources (Roper & Shapira, 2000). They are familiar with emerging themes, patterns, clusters, and explanations, and are sensitive to emerging meanings. Behavior is explained through socially constructed structures, functions, and processes of meaning.

Ethnographies are subjective as well as systematic, rigorous studies. The creativity of investigators as they analyze and interpret data is balanced with written explanations, supported by evidence and applied ethnographic methods (Whittemore, Chase, & Mandle, 2001).

Wolcott (1994) distinguishes ethnographic description from analysis and interpretation and proposes that they are the "three primary ingredients of qualitative research" (p. 49). He also notes that a balance must be achieved among all three with no particular combination or percentages of one to the others considered the best. He suggests that ethnographers might link interpretations to theory but cautions that such links might not be the best solution.

Findings of Ethnographic Studies

Ethnographic texts are written as stories that emerge from the data. Data have primacy; the theoretical framework is not predetermined by the data but derives from them. Ideally, ethnographic reports are artistically presented and accessible to more readers than the members of the discipline. As narrative presentations, they include straight and analytical description. Hypotheses about behavior, interpretive theories, concepts, constructs, associated theoretical definitions, taxonomies, and typologies might also emerge as findings.

When ethnographers begin to write the ethnography, they already have codes, categories, and patterns created when developing the rationales supporting their interpretations. Pieces of information are presented as objective reality through the raw data of field notes, recorded observations of subjects' words and behavioral actions, and verbatim transcriptions of audio- or video-recorded interviews. The pieces of information are empirical indicators of codes, themes, categories, patterns, and so forth.

Straight description is characterized by ethnographic details in which a situation might be revealed, including actors, their roles and behaviors, the artifacts used, conversations, and outcomes that were previously recorded in field notes and copied into the final product. As the writing of the report progresses, the text is then recontextualized to build understanding of the pattern of social and cultural action. There is a back-and-forth switch between the explicit/descriptive and the latent/symbolic.

Analytic description, also considered interpretive description, refers to the decontextualized narrative in which analysis and interpretation are exposed. The beliefs, norms, values, social structure, function, and symbols are revealed by the results of ethnographers' thoughts and creative insights.

Interpretive theories originate in themes or concepts and are built inductively from the raw material of field notes, transcribed interviews, analysis of documents, and the like. The interpretive theory of ethnography could be considered a descriptive formulation that is disciplined (Jorgensen, 1989). The explanations that are provided in ethnographic reports could be functional, associative, or causal. The explanations about a group's way of life provide a beginning and are never finished or absolute because cultures continue to develop and change.

Themes are repetitive, recurrent topics that emerge during analysis. Themes "cluster" or form patterns. Patterns are natural configurations of observations (van Manen, 1990). Concepts are abstract ideas generalized from the particulars revealed in the factual material of field notes, transcribed interviews, and the like. They may be equated with themes. Constructs are concepts constructed by the mental synthesis of ethnographers. Both concepts and constructs require theoretical definitions in which they are defined circularly, that is, a synonym or substitute for one or several words replaces the concept or construct name. For example, the following are circular definitions: ritual is patterned, symbolic action that refers to the beliefs, values, and goals of a social group; nursing ritual is patterned symbolic action that refers to the beliefs, values, and goals of a group of nurses (or nurses in general); therapeutic nursing rituals are symbolic actions that improve the condition of patients; and occupational nursing rituals (rites of socialization) are symbolic actions that facilitate the transition of professional neophytes into their professional role.

Hypotheses are conjectural statements about the relationships between two or more concepts. Ethnographic studies produce hypotheses inductively as data collection and analysis proceed. An example is this: the greater the nurse identification of a patient as temporary family, the greater the nurse's difficulty in performing postmortem care. Taxonomies are orderly classifications grouped according to presumed natural relationships; they are used to organize and interpret findings. Taxonomies include domains within the classificatory scheme. The domains are labeled (Powers, 2001). Taxon is the name given to a taxonomic group in a formal system of nomenclature. For example, the taxonomy for a code called in the event of cardiopulmonary arrest includes full code, no code, slow code, and almost no code (Wolf, 1986). Typologies are classification schemes and are useful in forming hypotheses and discovering themes.

Performance ethnographies and autoethnographies provide opportunities to make ethnographies available to different publics. As such they stand as examples of newer ways to share ethnographic findings with different publics.

Rigor, or Scientific Adequacy, of Ethnographies

It is important that ethnographers establish the rigor or scientific adequacy of ethnographic accounts. The methodological literature, although sparse initially (Ward & Werner, 1984), has been elaborated (Reid, 1991; Shokeid, 1988). Many ethnographers have followed the established methods of Lincoln and Guba (1985). Others take issue with their approaches.

To document the rigor of studies following Lincoln and Guba's (1985) strategies, investigators attempt to establish their trustworthiness. For the credibility criterion to be achieved, they engage in reading and reflecting on the material of studies, including field notes, transcribed interviews, documents, diaries, appointment records, and so forth. At the end of studies, they might attempt to achieve theoretical triangulation by matching published theories or concepts to the interpretive theories discovered in the study. They might request that a trusted, qualitative investigator review transcripts, field notes, essential themes, indexes, documents, and the ethnography. To achieve member check, investigators mail the results of the study to informants, meet with informants, or in other ways share drafts of studies and invite informants' assessment of the accuracy of the description and solicit their insights. Ethnographers look for transferability in nonstakeholder persons, those who were not informants but who share knowledge of the culture and can read and comment on the study.

To establish dependability, audit trails are made available for review by peer reviewers and other interested investigators. Data trails include field notes, documents, photographs, maps, drawings, personal notes, transcribed interviews (raw data), coding schemes, themes and indicators, and the text of the finished ethnography (data reduction and analysis products). Ideally, the results are confirmed through the manuscript as well as through implications and recommendations of the study. In contrast to Lincoln and Guba (1985), Whittemore, Chase, and Mandle (2001) reconceptualize validity in qualitative research, organizing criteria according to primary criteria, secondary criteria, and techniques.

Carspecken (1996) proposes an alternative conception of validity. Cultural categories in everyday contexts are successful in human communication and in the coordination of human action (p. 56). Achieving consensus is sought from the social group about the study's findings. Methodological procedures have to be followed so that people understand the claim:

> If a claim is made and supported in a way that meets its validity conditions, then it is to be regarded as "true" as long as it wins the consensus of potentially any cultural group. If groups disagree over the claim, then arguments should proceed that meet its validity conditions. (Carspecken, 1996, p. 57)

Reflexivity

Reflexivity is defined as the process by which researchers recognize that they are an integral part of the research and vice versa (Cutcliffe, 2003; Ellis & Bochner, 1996; Pellatt, 2003). Similar to other qualitative research, ethnographic studies achieve reflexivity when investigators are aware of themselves in relation to the informants, the data, and their own roles in the study (Lipson, 1989). Reflexivity recognizes the circularity of the relationship of investigators to the data; how and when different aspects of the interpretation emerge in the reports and in prior and various forms; how open investigators were to inducing breakdowns in their understanding of the data; and how their confidence in interpretations was challenged and tested over the course of study. They are aware of their role in the interpretation of the material and are sensitive to the meanings and patterns. The relationships and communication among researchers and informants, the influence of each in the knowledge produced in the study, as well as their reflections on the actions and observations in the field, are important. Reflexivity may be achieved when readers judge the validity of the researcher's work (Kahn, 1993).

Cutcliffe (2003) discusses different strategies used to establish reflexivity and ways to establish credibility of the study. He proposes that tacit knowledge/knowing are important for qualitative research and that it is difficult to explain investigators' flashes of insight. Cutcliffe encourages investigators to bring "creative, intellectual, and analytical processes to bear on any qualitative analysis" (p. 147) and to "let the magic happen" (p. 147). Allen (2004) discusses the dilemmas posed by the dual practitioner–researcher identity. However, the ethical codes of investigators help nurse ethnographers to always act on behalf of the welfare of patients when conducting studies. For example, if patient safety is threatened or if practitioners are behaving illegally, investigators must act, such as filing reports with administrators. While this might threaten the trust earned from informants, it is the best course.

Conclusion

Cultures are displayed in the writing of ethnographic studies. The process of doing ethnography is systematic and subjective and involves stating the purpose(s) and problem; collecting data through a variety of sources, chief of which are fieldwork, participant observation, and interviewing; and describing, analyzing, and interpreting the data. The best ethnographies display an interpretive understanding of social and cultural action in context. They are interesting to read and illuminate the worlds of informants. **Table 10–2** includes a selection of ethnographic studies conducted by nurses.

TABLE 10–2   EXAMPLES AND METHODS OF ETHNOGRAPHIC STUDIES BY NURSES

Citation	Type	Purpose	Participant Observation/ Field Notes	Interview	Document Analysis	Artifact Analysis	Time in Field	Findings
Allan, H. (2001). A 'good enough' nurse: Supporting patients in a fertility unit. Nursing Inquiry, 8, 51–60.	Focused critical	To describe two activities central to the nursing role in a fertility unit: caring and non-caring.	X	Semi structured			2 years	Taxonomy; definition; narrative description; analytic description
Brathwaite, A. C., & Williams, C. C. (2004). Childbirth experiences of professional Chinese Canadian women. JOGNN, 33, 748–755.	Focused	To provide detailed information about how Chinese culture influences the child-birth experience and how health care providers can support cultural expression and positive outcomes for these women, their children, and their families.	X	Structured; semi structured				Narrative description; analytic description
Cleary, M. (2003). The challenges of mental health care reform for contemporary mental health nursing practice: Relationships, power and control. International Journal of Mental Health Nursing, 12, 139–147.	Focused	The way mental health nurses interpret their practice in an acute inpatient psychiatric unit in light of the current challenges, demands, and influence brought about by service reforms.	X	Focused; discussion groups			5 months	Narrative description; analytic description

(continues)

TABLE 10–2 EXAMPLES AND METHODS OF ETHNOGRAPHIC STUDIES BY NURSES *(continued)*

Citation	Type	Purpose	Participant Observation/ Field Notes	Interview	Document Analysis	Artifact Analysis	Time in Field	Findings
Connelly, L. M., Keele, B. S., Kleinbeck, S. V., Schneider, J. K., & Cobb, A. K. (1993). A place to be yourself: Empowerment from the client's perspective. Image: Journal of Nursing Scholarship, 25, 297–304.	Focused	To describe the effects of chronically mentally ill consumer involvement in a client run, community support services, drop-in center.	X	Semi structured			5 weeks	Process domains; definition; model; narrative description; analytic description
Costello, J. (2002). Do not resuscitate orders and older patients: Findings from an ethnographic study of hospital wards for older people. Journal of Advanced Nursing, 39, 491–499.	Focused	To explore the way in which terminal care was provided to older patients; in the context of a larger study with the purpose: To explore the way in which DNR orders were a socially constructed part of the practices of both nurses and doctors.	X	Semi structured; unstructured	Medical notes (charts); nursing notes; field diary		9 months	Major themes; narrative description; analytic description

TABLE 10-2 EXAMPLES AND METHODS OF ETHNOGRAPHIC STUDIES BY NURSES *(continued)*

Citation	Type	Purpose	Participant Observation/ Field Notes	Interview	Document Analysis	Artifact Analysis	Time in Field	Findings
Cricco-Lizza, R. (2005). The milk of human kindness: Environmental and human interactions in a WIC clinic that influence infant-feeding decisions of black women. Qualitative Health Research, 15, 525–538.	Focused	To explore WIC's influence on the infant-feeding decisions of inner-city African American women enrolled in a New York metropolitan area WIC clinic.	X	Structured; semi-structured			18 months	Patterns; themes; narrative description; analytic description
DeGraves, S., & Aranda, S. (2008). Living with hope and fear—The uncertainty of childhood cancer after relapse. Cancer Nursing, 31, 292–301.	Critical	To explore with families their experiences following the relapse of the child's cancer.	X Reflective journals	In-depth			13 months	Patterns; themes; description; model
Gates, M. F., Lackey, N. R., & Brown, G. (2001). Caring demands and delay in seeking care in African American women newly diagnosed with breast cancer: An ethnographic, photographic study. ONF, 28, 529–537.	Focused	To describe the caring experiences in terms of the behaviors and demands of African American women newly diagnosed with breast cancer and to consider the influence of that caring on the women's decisions to delay prompt diagnosis and maintain continuing treatment.	X	Semi-structured	Journal; photographs			Themes; narrative description; analytic description

(continues)

TABLE 10–2   EXAMPLES AND METHODS OF ETHNOGRAPHIC STUDIES BY NURSES *(continued)*

Citation	Type	Purpose	Participant Observation/ Field Notes	Interview	Document Analysis	Artifact Analysis	Time in Field	Findings
Germain, C. P. (1979). The cancer unit: An ethnography. Wakefield, MA: Nursing Resources.	Holistic	Description of a community hospital adult oncology unit as a subculture.	X	Structured; unstructured			12 months	Narrative description; constructs
Gillespie, B. M., Wallis, M., & Chaboyer, W. (2008). Operating theater culture: Implications for nurse retention. Western Journal of Nursing Research, 30, 259–277.	Mini	To uncover the nature of organizational culture in an operating theater and how this culture was communicated and sustained.	X Reflective journals	Informal, in-depth focused			6 weeks	Themes; categories; thick description
Hall, J. M. (1994). Lesbians recovering from alcohol problems: An ethnographic study of health care experiences. Nursing Research, 43, 238–244.	Focused	To describe lesbians' experiences in alcohol recovery and identify barriers to help-seeking and recovery from their perspective.	X	Semi-structured				Themes; narrative description; analytic description
Haglund, K. (2000). Parenting a second time around: An ethnography of African American grandmothers parenting grandchildren due to parental cocaine abuse. Journal of Family Nursing, 6, 120–135.	Focused, micro	To examine the phenomenon of parenting grandchildren from the grandmothers' perspectives and to specifically investigate how parenting grandchildren affected the grandmothers' health.	X Logistics log, personal notes	In-depth	Letters, photographs, writings, newspaper articles, television special			Domains; taxonomies; themes; description

TABLE 10-2 EXAMPLES AND METHODS OF ETHNOGRAPHIC STUDIES BY NURSES *(continued)*

Citation	Type	Purpose	Participant Observation/ Field Notes	Interview	Document Analysis	Artifact Analysis	Time in Field	Findings
Hancock, H. C., & Easen, P. R. (2006). The decision-making processes of nurses when extubating patients following cardiac surgery: an ethnographic study. International Journal of Nursing Studies, 43, 693–705.	Focused	To explore the realities of research and evidence-based practice through an examination of the decision making of nurses when extubating patients following cardiac surgery.	X Analytic memos	Semi-structured			18 months	Categories; themes; description
Hessler, K. L. (2009). Physical activity behaviors of rural preschoolers. Pediatric Nursing, 35, 246–253.	Micro	To investigate the physical activity patterns of one group of northwestern rural preschoolers.	X	Individual, focus group (semi-structured)		Photograph	3 to 5 months	Major themes; patterns; categories; description
Hopkins, C. (2002). 'But what about the really ill, poorly people?' (An ethnographic study into what it means to nurses on medical admissions units to have people who have harmed themselves as their patients). Journal of Psychiatric and Mental Health Nursing, 9, 147–154.	Focused	To gain an understanding of what it means to nurses on medical admissions units to have people who have harmed themselves as their patients.	X	Semi-structured	Reflective fieldwork journal		1 month	Themes; narrative description; analytic description

(continues)

TABLE 10-2   EXAMPLES AND METHODS OF ETHNOGRAPHIC STUDIES BY NURSES *(continued)*

Citation	Type	Purpose	Participant Observation/ Field Notes	Interview	Document Analysis	Artifact Analysis	Time in Field	Findings
Hurst, I. (2001). Vigilant watching over: Mothers' actions to safeguard their premature babies in the newborn intensive care nursery. Journal of Perinatal Neonatal Nursing, 15, 39–57.	Critical	To understand how mothers described and understood their experience of having a hospitalized, premature baby, including the mothers' actions in the NICU and the conditions affecting their descriptions, interpretations, and actions.	X	Open-ended				Codes; exemplars; description
Kauffman, K. S. (1995). Center as haven: Findings of an urban ethnography. Nursing Research, 44, 231–236.	Focused	To describe how elders survive in the midst of "drug warfare" in an inner-city community known for its dangerous streets and public spaces?	X	Formal; casual conversations			3 years	Pattern; narrative description; analytic description
Kayser-Jones, J. (2002). The experience of dying: An ethnographic nursing home study. Gerontologist, 42, 11–19.	Focused	To investigate the process of providing end-of-life care to residents who were dying in nursing homes.	X Event analysis	In-depth			30 months	Themes; description

TABLE 10-2 EXAMPLES AND METHODS OF ETHNOGRAPHIC STUDIES BY NURSES *(continued)*

Citation	Type	Purpose	Participant Observation/ Field Notes	Interview	Document Analysis	Artifact Analysis	Time in Field	Findings
King, M., Munt, R., & Eastwood, A. (2007). The impact of a postgraduate diabetes course on the perceptions Aboriginal health workers and supervisors in South Australia. Contemporary Nurse: A Journal for the Australian Nursing Profession, 25(1-2), 82–93.	Critical	To identify the perceptions of an accredited Australian diabetes Educators Association course held by the health workers who had undertaken the course and the supervisors whose responsibility it was to oversee their clinical activities.	X	Semi-structured			12 months	Themes; sub-themes; minor themes; description
Ko, N-Y. (2005). Reproductive decision-making among HIV-positive couples in Taiwan. Journal of Nursing Scholarship, 37, 41–47.	Feminist	To address the need for better understanding of reproductive decision-making among HIV-positive couples in Taiwan.	X Observation					Story; stages; description
Lipson, J. G. (2001). We are the canaries: Self-care in multiple chemical sensitivity sufferers. Qualitative Health Research, 11, 103–116.	Focused	To describe the daily life experiences and ways of coping, Multiple Chemical Sensitivity sufferers' coping subcultures, current social/ cultural/political issues associated with this condition, dealing with negative reactions from health providers and others who do not believe in this illness, and self-care and medical treatment of MCS.	X	Semi-structured; chat rooms	Newsletters, news articles, TV programs		2 years	Categories; themes; narrative description; analytic description

(continues)

TABLE 10–2   EXAMPLES AND METHODS OF ETHNOGRAPHIC STUDIES BY NURSES (continued)

Citation	Type	Purpose	Participant Observation/ Field Notes	Interview	Document Analysis	Artifact Analysis	Time in Field	Findings
Miller, M. P. (1991). Factors promoting wellness in the aged person: An ethnographic study. Advances in Nursing Science, 13(4), 38–51.	Focused	To ascertain the factors contributing to well elderly persons' wellness state.	X	Semi-structured				Brief narrative; constructs
Neufeld, A., Harrison, M. J., Stewart, M. J., Hughes, K. D., & Spitzer, D. (2002). Immigrant women: Making connections to community resources for support in family caregiving. Qualitative Health Research, 12, 751–768.	Focused critical theory	To understand how Chinese and South Asian immigrant women caring for an ill or disabled family member gained access to support from community resources and identify the barriers to support that they experienced, including those arising from their social and material circumstances.	X	Semi-structured; focus group				Narrative description; constructs

TABLE 10–2 EXAMPLES AND METHODS OF ETHNOGRAPHIC STUDIES BY NURSES *(continued)*

Citation	Type	Purpose	Participant Observation/ Field Notes	Interview	Document Analysis	Artifact Analysis	Time in Field	Findings
Pannowitz, H. K., Glass, N., & Davis, K. (2009). Resisting gender-bias: Insights from Western Australian middle-level women nurses. Contemporary Nurse, 33, 103–119.	Critical/ feminist	The research aimed to explore and reveal common, different, unique and exceptional experiences that empowered, disempowered and/or oppressed participants' personal, professional and corporate efforts towards their own empowerment, emancipation and transformation; to reveal the ways in which women nurses empowered themselves in their work role and the network of power relations present in their practice settings; to reveal the ways in which women nurses empowered themselves in their work role and the network of power relations present in their practice settings.	X Critical reflective journaling	Semi-structured, critical conversations				Cultural discourses; themes; exemplars; description

(continues)

TABLE 10–2   EXAMPLES AND METHODS OF ETHNOGRAPHIC STUDIES BY NURSES *(continued)*

Citation	Type	Purpose	Participant Observation/ Field Notes	Interview	Document Analysis	Artifact Analysis	Time in Field	Findings
Pasco, A. C., Morse, J. M., & Olson, J. K. (2004). Cross-cultural relationships between nurses and Filipino Canadian patients. *Journal of Nursing Scholarship, 36,* 239–246.	Focused	To identify the culturally embedded values that implicitly guide Filipino Canadian patients' interactions in developing nurse-patient relationships.	X	Unstructured	Diary			Categories; types; model; description
Powers, B. A. (2001). Ethnographic analysis of everyday ethics in the care of nursing home residents with dementia. *Nursing Research, 50,* 332–339.	Focused critical	To critically examine ethical issues of daily living and to construct a descriptive data-based taxonomy.	X	Structured; semi-structured	Newsletters; activity calendars; daily care worksheets; in-service education calendars and teaching tools; annual reports; documents of ethics committee		2 years	Concept; taxonomy (4 domains); narrative description; analytic description

TABLE 10–2　EXAMPLES AND METHODS OF ETHNOGRAPHIC STUDIES BY NURSES *(continued)*

Citation	Type	Purpose	Participant Observation/ Field Notes	Interview	Document Analysis	Artifact Analysis	Time in Field	Findings
Reimer-Kirkham, S. (2009). Lived religion: Implications for nursing ethics. Nursing Ethics, 16, 406–417. doi: 10.1177/0969733009104605	Critical	How ethics and religion interface in everyday life by examining the negotiation of religious and spiritual plurality in health care.	X	Interview, discussion group				Themes (readings from patients' nursing; social standpoints); description
Smyer, T., & Chang, B. L. (1999). A typology of consumers of institutional respite care. Clinical Nursing Research, 8(1), 26–50. doi:10.1177/105477399922158133	Focused descriptive	To generate a typology of respite care users and to describe the process of adaptation to its use.	X Instruments	Informal, semi-structured	Participant correspondence, medical records, nurses' notes, hospital billing records		1 year	Categories; typology; description
Stevens, C. A. (2006). Being healthy: voices of adolescent women who are parenting. JSPN, 11(1), 28–40.	Focused	To explore how adolescent women who are parenting describe what "being healthy" means to them and how they define their health needs.	X	In-depth	Photovoice (photograph/ participant interpretation)			Concepts; sub-categories; description

(continues)

TABLE 10–2 EXAMPLES AND METHODS OF ETHNOGRAPHIC STUDIES BY NURSES *(continued)*

Citation	Type	Purpose	Participant Observation/ Field Notes	Interview	Document Analysis	Artifact Analysis	Time in Field	Findings
Varcoe, C. (2001). Abuse obscured: An ethnographic account of emergency nursing in relation to violence against women. Canadian Journal of Nursing Research, 32(4), 95–115.	Focused critical	To examine the relationship between the social context of practice and the ways in which nurses recognize and respond to the plight of women who have been abused.	X	Semi-structured; unstructured			2 years	Patterns; narrative description; analytic description
Wolf, Z. R. (1986). Nursing rituals in an adult acute care hospital: An ethnography. University of Pennsylvania School of Nursing. Ann Arbor, MI: University Microfilms.	Focused		X	Semi-structured; unstructured	Patient charts; nursing unit minutes; kardexes	Unit furniture; nursing care equipment; primary board	12 months	Patterns; narrative description; analytic description; taxonomy; definitions

Source: Adapted from "The Health of Teenagers: A Focused Ethnographic Study," by J.K. Magilvy et al., 1987, *Public Health Nursing 4*(1), 35–42.

References

Aamodt, A. M. (1982). Examining ethnography for nurse researchers. *Western Journal of Nursing Research, 4,* 207–221.

Adler, P. A., & Adler, P. (1987). *Membership roles in field research.* Newbury Park, CA: Sage.

Agar, M. H. (1986). *Speaking of ethnography.* Beverly Hills, CA: Sage.

Allen, D. (2004). Ethnomethodological insights into insider-outsider relationships in nursing ethnographies of healthcare settings. *Nursing Inquiry, 11*(1), 14–24.

Atkinson, P. (1992). *Understanding ethnographic texts.* Newbury Park, CA: Sage.

Becker, H. S., & Geer, B. (1957). Participant observation and interviewing: A comparison. *Human Organization, 16,* 28–32.

Bernard, H. R. (1994). *Research methods in anthropology* (2nd ed.). Thousand Oaks, CA: Sage.

Brody, E. B. (1981). The clinician as ethnographer: A psychoanalytic perspective on the epistemology of fieldwork. *Culture, Medicine and Psychiatry, 5*(3), 273–301.

Brody, E. B. (1989/2005). The clinician as ethnographer: A psychoanalytic perspective on the epistemology of fieldwork. *Culture, Medicine and Psychiatry, 5,* 273–301.

Byerly, E. L. (1969). The nurse researcher as a participant-observer in a nursing setting. *Nursing Researcher, 18,* 230–235.

Carspecken, P. F. (1996). *Critical ethnography in educational research: A theoretical and practical guide.* New York, NY: Routledge.

Christians, C. G. (2005). Ethics and politics in qualitative research. In N. K. Denzin, & Y. S. Lincoln (Eds.), *The Sage handbook of qualitative research* (3rd ed., pp. 139–181). Thousand Oaks, CA: Sage.

Cutcliffe, J. R. (2003). Reconsidering reflexivity. *Qualitative Health Research, 13*(1), 136–148.

DeGraves, S., & Aranda, S. (2008). Living with hope and fear—the uncertainty of childhood cancer after relapse. *Cancer Nursing, 31,* 292–301.

Denzin, N. K., & Lincoln, Y. S. (Eds.). (2005). *The Sage handbook of qualitative research* (3rd ed.). Thousand Oaks, CA: Sage.

DeSantis, L. (1990). Fieldwork with undocumented aliens and other populations at risk. *Western Journal of Nursing Research, 12,* 359–372.

Douglas, M. (1963). *The Lele of the Kasai.* London: Oxford University Press.

Douglas, M. (1966). *Purity and danger.* London: Routledge and Kegan Paul.

Douglas, M. (1975). *Implicit meanings: Essays in anthropology.* London: Routledge and Kegan Paul.

Douglass, W. A. (1969). *Death in Murelaga: Funerary ritual in a Spanish Basque village.* Seattle, WA: University of Washington Press.

Duncan, M. (2004). Autoethnography: Critical appreciation of an emerging art. *International Journal of Qualitative Methods.* Retrieved from http://www.ualberta.ca/~iiqm/backissues/3_4/pdf/duncan.pdf

Ellis, C., & Bochner, A. P. (Eds.). (1996). *Composing ethnography: Alternative forms of qualitative writing.* Walnut Creek, CA: Altamira Press.

Fetterman, D. (1989). *Ethnography: Step by step.* Newbury Park, CA: Sage.

Field, P. A. (1989). Doing fieldwork in your own culture. In J. M. Morse (Ed.), *Qualitative nursing research* (pp. 91–104). Newbury Park, CA: Sage.

Firth, R. (1936). *We, the Tikopia.* London: Allen and Unwin.

Fox, R. C. (1959). *Experiment perilous.* Philadelphia, PA: University of Pennsylvania Press.

Freilich, M. (Ed.). (1970). *Marginal natives: Anthropologists at work.* New York, NY: Harper & Row.

Geertz, C. (1973). *The interpretation of cultures.* New York, NY: Basic Books.

Germain, C. P. (2001). Ethnography: The method. In P. L. Munhall (Ed.), *Nursing research: A qualitative perspective* (3rd ed., pp. 277–306). Sudbury, MA: Jones & Bartlett, National League for Nursing.

Gillespie, B. M., Wallis, M., & Chaboyer, W. (2008). Operating theater culture: Implications for nurse retention. *Western Journal of Nursing Research, 30,* 259–277.

Glesne, C. (1989). Rapport and friendship in ethnographic research. *Qualitative Studies in Education, 2*(1), 45–54.

Goffman, E. (1961). *Asylums: Essays on the social situation of mental patients and other inmates.* Garden City, NY: Anchor Books.

Goodenough, W. (1964). Cultural anthropology and linguistics. In D. Hymes (Ed.), *Language and culture and society: A reader in linguistics and anthropology.* New York, NY: Harper & Row.

Greckhamer, T., & Koro-Ljungberg, M. (2004, August 14). Paper presented to American Sociological Association. San Francisco, CA.

Hahn, C. (2008). *Doing qualitative research using your computer: A practical guide.* London: Sage.

Halbwach, M. (1980). *The collective memory.* New York, NY: Harper Colophon Books.

Hammersley, M., & Atkinson, P. (1983). *Ethnography: Principles in practice.* New York, NY: Tavistock.

Hammersley, M., & Atkinson, P. (1995). *Ethnography: Principles in practice.* London: Routledge.

Hardcastle, M.-A., Usher, K., & Holmes, C. (2006). Carspecken's five-stage critical qualitative research method: An application to Nursing Research. *Qualitative Health Research, 16,* 151–161.

Hopkins, C. (2002). "But what about the really ill, poorly people?" (An ethnographic study into what it means to nurses on medical admissions units to have people who have harmed themselves as their patients.) *Journal of Psychiatric and Mental Health Nursing, 9,* 147–154.

Human Relations Area File. eHRAF. Retrieved July 7, 2005, from http://www.yale.edu/hraf/collections.htm

Hurst, I. (2001). Vigilant watching over: Mothers' actions to safeguard their premature babies in the newborn intensive care nursery. *Journal of Perinatal Neonatal Nursing, 15,* 39–57.

Hymes, D. H. (1978). *What is ethnography?* (Sociolinguistic Working Paper 45). Austin, TX: Southwest Educational Development Laboratory.

Jorgensen, D. L. (1989). *Participant observation: A methodology for human studies.* Newbury Park, CA: Sage.

Junker, B. H. (1960). *Field work: An introduction to the social sciences.* Chicago, IL: University of Chicago Press.

Kahn, D. L. (1993). Ways of discussing validity in qualitative nursing research. *Western Journal of Nursing Research, 15*(1), 122–126.

Kaufman, K. S. (1995). Center as haven: Findings of an urban ethnography. *Nursing Research, 44*(4), 231–236.

Keith, J. (1986). Participant observation. In C. L. Fry & J. Keith (Eds.), *New methods for old age research* (pp. 1–20). South Hadley, MA: Bergin & Garvey.

Kleinman, A. (1988). A method for the care of the chronically ill. In A. Kleinman (Ed.), *The illness narratives: Suffering, healing, and the human condition* (pp. 227–251). New York, NY: Basic Books.

Lahman, M. K. (2009). Dreams of my daughter: An ectopic pregnancy. *Qualitative Health Research, 19*, 272–278.

Leininger, M. (1987). Importance and uses of ethnomethods: Ethnography and ethnonursing research. *Recent Advances in Nursing, 17*, 12–36.

Leininger, M. M. (Ed.). (1985). *Qualitative research methods in nursing*. Orlando, FL: Grune & Stratton.

Leiter, K. (1980). *A primer on ethnomethodology*. New York, NY: Oxford University Press.

Liebow, E. (1993). *Tell them who I am: The lives of homeless women*. New York, NY: Penguin Books.

Lincoln, Y., & Guba, E. (1985). *Naturalistic inquiry*. Beverly Hills, CA: Sage.

Lipson, J. G. (1989). The use of self in ethnographic research. In J. M. Morse (Ed.), *Qualitative nursing research* (pp. 61–75). Rockville, MD: Aspen.

Lofland, J. (1976). *Doing social life*. New York, NY: Wiley.

Lofland, J., & Lofland, L. (1984). *Analyzing social settings: A guide to qualitative observation and analysis* (2nd ed.). Belmont, CA: Wadsworth.

Malinowski, B. (1922). *Argonauts of the Western Pacific*. London: Routledge and Kegan Paul.

Malinowski, B. (1948). *Magic, science and religion*. Prospect Heights, IL: Waveland Press.

Mauss, M. (1967). *The gift: Forms and functions of exchange in archaic societies*. New York, NY: W. W. Norton.

Miles, M. B., & Huberman, A. M. (1984). *Qualitative data analysis*. Beverly Hills, CA: Sage.

Mulkay, M. J. (1985). *The word and the world: Explorations in the form of sociological analysis*. London: Allen and Unwin.

Omery, A. (1988). Ethnography. In B. Sarter (Ed.), *Paths to knowledge: Innovative research methods for nursing* (pp. 17–31). New York, NY: National League for Nursing.

Pannowitz, H. K., Glass, N., & Davis, K. (2009). Resisting gender-bias: Insights from Western Australian middle-level women nurses. *Contemporary Nurse, 33*, 103–119.

Patton, M. Q. (1990). *Qualitative evaluation and research methods* (2nd ed.). Newbury Park, CA: Sage.

Pearsall, M. (1965). Participant observation as role and method in behavioral research. *Nursing Research, 14*(1), 37–42.

Pellatt, G. (2003). Ethnography and reflexivity: Emotions and feelings in fieldwork. *Nurse Researcher, 10*(3), 28–37.

Powers, B. A. (2001). Ethnographic analysis of everyday ethics in the care of nursing home residents with dementia. *Nursing Research, 50*, 332–339.

Ragucci, A. T. (1972). The ethnographic approach and nursing research. *Nursing Research, 21*, 485–490.

Reid, B. (1991). Developing and documenting a qualitative methodology. *Journal of Advanced Nursing, 16*, 544–551.

Richardson, L. (1988). The collective story: Postmodernism and the writing of sociology. *Sociological Focus, 21*, 199–208.

Riemann, G. (2005). Ethnographies of practice—Practicing ethnography: Resources for self-reflective social work. *Journal of Social Work Practice, 19*(1), 87–101.

Robertson, M. H., & Boyle, J. S. (1984). Ethnography: Contributions to nursing research. *Journal of Advanced Nursing, 9*, 43–49.

Roper, J. M., & Shapira, J. (2000). *Ethnography in nursing research*. Thousand Oaks, CA: Sage.

Ruwell, M. E. (1985). Introduction. In M. A. Kenworthy, E. M. King, M. E. Ruwell, & T. Van Houten (Eds.), *Preserving field records* (pp. 1-6). Philadelphia, PA: University Museum, University of Pennsylvania.

Sapir, E. (1924). Culture, genuine and spurious. In D. G. Mandelbaum (Ed.), *Selected writings of Edward Sapir in language, culture, and personality* (pp. 308-312). Berkeley, CA: University of California Press.

Shokeid, M. (1988). Anthropologists and their informants: Marginality reconsidered. *European Journal of Sociology, 29*(1), 31-47.

Simmons, M. (2007). Insider ethnography: Tinker, tailor, researcher or spy? *Nurse Researcher, 14*(4), 7-17.

Smyer, T., & Chang, B. L. (1999). A typology of consumers of institutional respite care. *Clinical Nursing Research, 8*(1), 26-50.

Spradley, J. P. (1970). *You owe yourself a drunk: An ethnography of urban nomads.* Boston, MA: Little, Brown.

Spradley, J. P. (1979). *The ethnographic interview.* New York, NY: Holt, Rinehart & Winston.

Spradley, J. P. (1980). *Participant observation.* New York, NY: Holt, Rinehart & Winston.

Stocking, G. W. (1983). *Observers observed.* Madison, WI: University of Wisconsin Press.

Tedlock, B. (2005). The observation of participation and the emergence of public ethnography. In N. K. Denzin & Y. S. Lincoln (Eds.), *The Sage handbook of qualitative research* (3rd ed., pp. 467-481). Thousand Oaks, CA: Sage.

Thorne, S. E. (1991). Methodological orthodoxy in qualitative nursing research: Analysis of the issues. *Qualitative Health Research, 1,* 178-199.

Turner, V. (1967). *The forest of symbols: Aspects of Ndembu ritual.* Ithaca, NY: Cornell University Press.

Turner, W. (1957). *Schism and continuity in an African society.* Manchester: Manchester University Press.

van Manen, M. (1990). *Researching lived experience.* Albany, NY: State University of New York Press.

Varcoe, C. (2001). Abuse obscured: An ethnographic account of emergency nursing in relation to violence against women. *Canadian Journal of Nursing Research, 32*(4), 95-115.

Ward, J. J., & Werner, O. (1984). Difference and dissonance in ethnographic data. *Communication and Cognition, 17,* 219-243.

Weiss, R. S. (1994). *Learning from strangers: The art and method of qualitative interview studies.* New York, NY: The Free Press.

Whittemore, R., Chase, S. K., & Mandle, C. L. (2001). Validity in qualitative research. *Qualitative Health Research, 11,* 522-537.

Wilson, H. S. (1989). *Research in nursing* (2nd ed.). Redwood City, CA: Addison-Wesley Publishing Company Health Sciences.

Wolcott, H. F. (1994). *Transforming qualitative data: Description, analysis, and interpretation.* Thousand Oaks, CA: Sage.

Wolcott, H. F. (1995). *The art of fieldwork.* Walnut Creek, CA: AltaMira Press.

Wolf, Z. R. (1986). *Nursing rituals in an adult acute care hospital: An ethnography.* Ann Arbor, MI: University of Pennsylvania School of Nursing, University Microfilms.

Wolf, Z. R. (2003). Exploring the audit trail for qualitative investigations. *Nurse Educator, 28*(4), 175-178.

11

Exemplar: War Stories: Frontline Reports of the Daily Experiences of Low-Income, Urban, Black Mothers[1]

Roberta Cricco-Lizza

There are broad racial, ethnic, and income disparities in maternal and child health in the United States. These disparities have been well documented, yet many questions remain as to how these differences emerge (Smedley, Stith, & Nelson, 2002). Smedley et al. recommend prospective studies to explore the cultural knowledge and resources used by those affected by disparities. My purpose in this paper is to portray the everyday lives of low-income Black mothers and describe the strategies that they use to survive in an inner-city environment. In this manuscript I focus on the day-to-day life experiences of these women during pregnancy, childbirth, and the first year postpartum. Public health professionals can use this information to gain understanding and insight into factors that influence maternal child health in this population.

Background

In the United States' Healthy People 2010 initiative, public health leaders called for the promotion of healthy pregnancies and healthy infants and the elimination of racial and ethnic disparities in health. According to the latest Healthy People 2010 progress report, racial and ethnic disparities persist as a significant problem, and Black women continue to have the highest maternal death rate and the highest infant mortality rate (United States Department of Health and Human Services, 2007). The maternal mortality rate is 3.7 times higher for Black women than White women (Minino, Heron, Murphy, & Kochanek, 2007).

Black infants have mortality rates that are more than twice those of White babies (Heron et al., 2010).

There is a critical need to understand the factors that contribute to these high mortality rates for Black women and infants. Differences in health behaviors and socioeconomic status, stress, racism, and variations in neuroendocrine, vascular, and immunologic, stress-related processes have been linked to adverse birth outcomes (Giscombe & Lobel, 2005). More research is needed to delineate the nature of stress in Black women (Hogue & Bremner, 2005). It is also important to recognize that there is variation within specific racial and ethnic groups, and efforts should be targeted toward the needs of specific populations within particular social contexts (Duchon, Andrulis, & Reid, 2004; Mullings et al., 2001; Stanton, Lobel, Sears, & DeLuca, 2002). Black women who were born in Africa (David & Collins, 1997) or the Caribbean (Cabral, Fried, Levenson, Amaro, & Zuckerman, 1990) generally have better infant birth weights than Black women born in the United States. This suggests social and contextual dynamics should be looked at more closely for their influence on maternal child health. Hogan, Njoroge, Durant, and Ferre (2001) contend that understanding the social context of women's lives can lead to insight into the factors related to perinatal health issues and can help to identify interventions to reduce disparities. Bhutta (2005) noted contemporary failure to understand sociocultural determinants of health and disease in mothers and children and has called for qualitative studies to fill this gap.

Shambley-Ebron and Boyle (2004) have noted that patriarchal viewpoints have often influenced previous research about Black women. It is important to obtain input from the women who actually experience these health disparities and hear and document their own voices about their lives. There are few qualitative inquiries about the everyday experiences of Black mothers. In most studies the focus is on adolescence and the concerns of this age group as they became mothers (Burton, 1990; Clifford & Brykczynski, 1999; Danziger, 1995; Oxley & Weekes, 1997; Wayland & Rawlins, 1997). Gichia (2000) used an ethnographic approach with low-income, African American, mostly adult women and found that motherhood was a key marking point shaped by familial and cultural practices. Dunlap, Sturzenhofecker, and Johnson (2006) demonstrated that impoverished, African American women were motivated to become mothers because of a desire for lasting, loving relationships. In other qualitative studies with mixed-income Black women, a lack of material and emotional resources, racism, stereotyping, and negativity were identified as stressful parts of motherhood experiences (Mann, Abercrombie, DeJoseph, Norbeck, & Smith, 1999; Sawyer, 1999). Shambley-Ebron and Boyle (2006) conducted an ethnographic study of mixed-income, African American adult mothers and found that these women believed in relying on their own strength to withstand the trials in their lives. Black Caribbean women of varying ages and incomes were interviewed 6–12 months after childbirth about their responses to adversity and psychological distress associated with pregnancy, childbirth, and early motherhood (Edge & Rogers, 2005). These women emphasized the importance of resilience for their well being. Most of the data for these qualitative studies were collected during pregnancy, after childbirth, or retrospectively. The following study was conducted to supply longitudinal, prospective data about this perinatal period.

Method

An ethnographic design incorporates researcher–participant interaction in natural settings over an extended period of time and allows for the collection of contextually detailed descriptions of participants' daily activities (Germain, 2001). My overall goal during this ethnography was to examine the infant feeding beliefs and experiences of urban, low-income Black women within the context of their everyday lives. All of the mothers were enrolled in the Special Supplemental Nutrition Program for Women, Infants, and Children (WIC). The U.S. government–sponsored WIC program provides supplemental foods, infant formula, healthcare referrals, and nutrition education for lower income women and children. Infant feeding beliefs (Cricco-Lizza, 2004), the influence of WIC (Cricco-Lizza, 2005), and influences of nurses and physicians (Cricco-Lizza, 2006) have been discussed elsewhere. In this chapter I focus on the women's descriptions of their everyday lives and the strategies that they used to cope with urban challenges.

Procedures for the Protection of Participants

The Human Subjects Committees gave approval for observations and interviews with written informed consents required for tape-recorded interviews. I paid special attention to potential barriers of distrust during all research procedures. I used trust-generating strategies which included: respectful entry into the field, recognition of issues of power, sensitivity to time and timing, and a relational style (Cricco-Lizza, 2007). The women who were recruited for audiotaped interviews were approached in the WIC waiting room and given verbal and written information about the study. Interviews were conducted privately at times and places selected by the women. Consents were reviewed with participants and the women were encouraged to select their own pseudonyms. These pseudonyms were consistently used to protect their confidentiality.

Setting

The mothers who participated in this study lived in the local neighborhood that was served by a New York metropolitan area WIC clinic. This urban area was a former industrial center which has undergone a considerable economic downturn in the last 30 years. The residents currently have high unemployment rates with related problems of poverty. With an ethnographic approach, I was able to obtain contextually rich descriptions of how these mothers negotiated these challenges on a day-to-day basis. The mothers were followed in the WIC clinic, homes, hospitals, and in community settings.

Participants

There were 130 Black mothers of varying ages and parity who served as general informants. They were observed and informally interviewed on a one-time basis in the WIC waiting room or nutrition classroom. These general informants provided a broad overview of their perceptions of daily life. From this group of 130, I purposefully selected 11 key informants to obtain in-depth information about everyday experiences. I specifically recruited English speaking, adult, pregnant women who were willing to be followed over time. These key informants were all primiparous so that their first experiences as mothers could be acquired prospectively. They were followed from pregnancy to 1 year postpartum, and will be referred to by their pseudonyms. Ten key informants were born in the neighborhoods surrounding the WIC clinic, and one was born in the Caribbean. All 11 grew up in this immediate vicinity. Their average age was 22.9. They completed 10–15 years of education with a mean of 12.5. Ten of the 11 key informants were single.

Data Collection

I used participant observation and interviewing to gather a detailed picture of the women's behaviors and the ways that they talked about their lives.

Participant observation

The level of my involvement varied from observation to active participation in the lives of the participants across the 18 months of data collection. Initially, I sat in the waiting room or nutrition classroom and observed the 130 general informants as they interacted with their babies, relatives, friends, partners, other WIC participants, and staff. I initiated conversations with the general informants and introduced myself as a nurse studying infant feeding. The women talked with me about their daily lives, as well as their pregnancies, birth, motherhood, and infant feeding experiences. I tried to be helpful by opening doors or holding their babies when they filled out forms, but mostly I just listened and observed. I dressed casually in the style of the women who used this multiethnic clinic and tried to be sensitive to my racial/ethnic/economic differences as a White, middle-class woman of Italian–Irish heritage.

The key informants were observed more extensively and in multiple contexts. As I selected and developed rapport with the key informants, observations were extended from the WIC clinic into the community. I met these women in their homes, malls, fast food outlets, and hospitals, and observed them in these varied contexts throughout pregnancy and the first year postpartum. I used these observations as windows into their everyday experiences, and our shared time together contributed to the development of trust. Each observation lasted about 2 hours, and events and conversations were documented immediately after each encounter.

Interviewing

Key informants were formally interviewed once during pregnancy and one or two times during the postpartum. In keeping with the larger aims of the study, each hour-long interview was focused on infant feeding within the context of their daily lives. Not only did the women talk about infant feeding, they also reflected about their childhood, pregnancy, childbirth, motherhood, recovery, and return to work or school. I asked the mothers about their daily activities, and they described the challenges they faced along with the strategies they used to overcome them. These formal interviews were tape recorded, labeled with a pseudonym, and sent to a confidential transcriptionist. I reviewed each transcript alongside the tape for accuracy and clarified any questions during the next contact with the key informant.

With the continued permission of the key informants, the formal interviews were augmented with informal interviews conducted through telephone calls and face-to-face meetings. During this time, there were 147 telephone calls that kept me updated about current events and concerns in the lives of the key informants. All of these informal interviews were typed immediately afterwards.

Data Management, Analysis, and Verification

The 130 general informants were observed and informally interviewed during 63 WIC clinic observations over the course of this investigation. Each of the 11 key informants was also formally or informally interviewed between 11 and 32 times depending on their availability and time of entrance into the study. Field notes, audio-taped transcripts, and analytic memos were entered into NUD*IST. I used this software program to facilitate data management, retrieval, and analysis. The data were reviewed line by line, coded for meaning, reorganized into categories, and analyzed for patterns. I identified a recurrent key informant–generated battlefield metaphor during analysis. The findings were verified through prolonged engagement, triangulation of interview and participation observation methods, and member checking. My continued access to key informants meant that I could prospectively check the meaning of the findings with them throughout the study. My access to the wider pool of general informants in the WIC clinic also allowed me opportunities to observe for evidence of phenomena that were reported by the key informants. In addition, I used peer review groups from the university to critique raw data and interpretation of the findings.

Findings

Many general and key informants had compromised health issues. My observations and informal interviews in the WIC clinic waiting room demonstrated that many general informants had complicated pregnancies. It was common to see tiny babies and apnea monitors in this clinic and to hear mothers talking about neonatal intensive care unit (NICU) experiences. The key informants provided greater detail about these health issues as they were followed over time. Eight of the 11 key informants prospectively reported the development of problems with hypertension, preeclampsia, premature contractions, diabetes, or congenital defects. Three of their babies were transferred to NICUs. General and key informants alike regularly referred to life as a battle as they sought to meet day-to-day needs. In the first section of the findings I address their daily fight for survival. In the second section I detail the warlike strategies the women used to deal with these challenges.

The Mothers Fought for Survival on Multiple Battlefronts

The women described adversity in their lives and talked about daily battles to meet their basic needs. General and key informants reported high levels of stress and struggles related to a lack of material and human resources. As they described their daily lives and activities, I heard repeated concerns over financial problems, housing, education, employment, safety, loss, and racism. While any one of these battles might be formidable, these women had to fight simultaneously on all fronts for daily survival. In their words below, one can hear evidence of race, gender, and class inequities. The women were most verbal about the class issues associated with poverty. Over time they also revealed the scars related to racism. In regard to gender inequities, most of the participants took it as a given that the labor associated with reproduction would be borne by women.

Finances

Constrained financial resources comprised an incessant battle for the women in this study. In the WIC clinic the general and key informants freely talked to each other and the clerks about the unremitting struggle to meet the costs of living. Aja said, "It's so hard out there, money-wise." Almost half of the key informants had to move during the investigation and several had disconnected phones. WIC counselors said that the women often ran out of money by the end of the month. Numerous general and key informants reported, "We don't have any money."

Without financial resources, these women struggled to meet basic needs for food and clothing. For example, one of the pregnant key informants came to the WIC clinic on a winter day wearing a short-sleeve shirt and old, stained pants. She said that she was hungry and had not eaten anything all day. In a similar fashion, many general informants talked about children going without food and told of the fight to make ends meet while they lived from "paycheck to paycheck."

Housing

The informants lived in urban environments where they continually grappled with rundown housing and crime. The general informants said that the residents in the local high-rise housing complexes were afraid to venture beyond their locked doors. Julie, a key informant, provided additional details. She said, "It's a lot of crime up there. It's like a lot of drugs up there." She said that she lived with her mother after childbirth and that the landlord did not supply a refrigerator or stove in the apartment. Julie stated that there were holes in the ceiling which leaked when it rained, and that the landlord refused to make any repairs. Other key informants reported similar tribulations. Karen stated that her landlord charged too much for rent and supplied no heat. She said, "Sometimes we have no choice. We don't have the money. We have to take whatever is there." She described her housing conditions in this way:

> It's a lot of drug addicts around. *A lot!* The whole block is like drug addict city. I grew up on that block . . . It's not a good place where I would want to raise my baby. I'm only living in a room.

My field notes from a home-based interview scheduled with another key informant described my perceptions of her neighborhood:

> Abandoned factories were interspersed with dilapidated, two- and three-story wooden dwellings. The paint was peeling; many of the windows were broken, encased in bars or fencing material or boarded up with plywood. Several empty lots were strewn with tires, garbage bags, and barrels. Occasional plots of dirt in front of the homes were filled with trash bags. Loose refuse was strewn all over the street and sidewalks. There was no sign of any public worker, police officer, or mail carrier in the area.

Education

The general and key informants valued education but identified barriers that were difficult to conquer. Julie said that the local schools were very overcrowded and that there was no individual help available. She stated that she always had a problem reading in school, but teachers "let the kids pass to the next grade cause they wanted them out." Other informants also stated, "They weren't teaching me anything."

Several general and key informants talked about dropping out of school due to the demands of motherhood or the need to care for sick or dependent relatives. Some of the women were too tired to continue school when they became pregnant. Others felt the fatigue more in the postpartum period when they assumed total responsibility for their own and their babies' care. The women also experienced difficulty cobbling together resources for babysitting when they did return to school. For example, Aja, like many of the women in this study, said that she relied on several different sources to watch her baby so she could attend class. She tried to obtain daycare assistance but was 51st on a waiting list.

Job availability
There were limited jobs available on the front lines of this urban environment. Most of the study participants held a series of positions in fast food outlets, car rental agencies, telemarketing firms, department stores, and community health agencies. The women felt compelled to return to work soon after childbirth because of mounting bills. One general informant said that she had to go to work shortly after her cesarean section in order to feed her children. Another woman, suspended from a supermarket because of illness-related absenteeism, immediately went to work on the night shift of a hamburger franchise.

The key informants talked about the dearth of jobs with adequate salaries, security, or benefits. Julie and Helena both said that a car was needed to get to the better jobs in wealthier neighborhoods. Gloria relied on public transportation to get to work and stated that she had to get up at 5 a.m. to get her asthmatic infant ready to leave the house at 6:30 a.m. She said:

> I have to be on the 6:45 a.m. bus and then catch a 7 a.m. bus to the next place. I walk three blocks and drop off the baby at day care. I walk back the three blocks and get another bus to get to work for 8:30 a.m. I am tired but the burnout is worse than anything.

Gloria did not get home until 7 p.m. and said that she needed at least another 3 hours to complete all of the work there. Although she was exhausted, she was still grateful to get a paycheck. Julie was not so fortunate in her job search. She said, "Everybody has dreams . . . [I have] dreams for my child. I want him to be able to say that his mother has a good job." She went for government-sponsored job training but was told that she could only be trained for baby sitting.

Safety
The general and key informants voiced concern for safety in public and at home. Gloria said that in her local area there was "plenty of crime, from robbery to

drug dealing to just all shooting." One little boy in the WIC waiting room said loudly to his mother, "Remember when my daddy hit you and you were crying?" This general informant mother looked embarrassed and did not respond to this question about domestic violence. Personal safety also came up with the key informants. Julie's mother stated that Julie's bouts of premature contractions were caused by beatings from the baby's father. Imani's eye was markedly swollen and discolored in the postpartum period. Ella's blunt affect, reports of emotional numbness, and difficulties with trust and eye contact also suggested emotional trauma but she, like the others, dealt with this on her own.

Missing or dead family members

The women spontaneously talked about the loss of their loved ones. These casualties took many forms but the net result was decreased numbers of human resources in times of need. Only one of the 11 key informants had both parents alive and actively involved in her life. Some of their parents had died young or had been missing for years. Karen, whose father died when she was a young teen, talked about the problems that she and her friends had experienced because of loss. She initially talked about the effects of early loss on her friends but then included herself as well. She said:

> They don't have anyone there for them . . . Because most of their moms and dads, you know, they're separated or their dad is way beyond yonder somewhere in another state, somewhere, and the mom is doing really bad. Most of us don't have a role model or someone to look up to. We have to look up to ourselves.

Seven out of 11 key informants were no longer with the fathers of their babies by the end of the first year postpartum and this served to place the demands of child rearing squarely on the shoulders of the women. For five of these seven key informants, the relationship had floundered when the men were not able to provide needed resources. The boyfriends of the other two key informants were abruptly imprisoned in the early postpartum period.

Many of these women reported multiple losses of parents, family members, and partners. Imani said that her own father had died when she was a young girl and her younger brother had died from "the virus" a few years ago. Imani confided in me that her mother had been very depressed after the death of her son, and she died soon afterwards. She said, "A lot of questions that I have since I got older, I wasn't able to ask her." Imani cried when she spoke about all of these losses. Before the first postpartal year was completed, she was also separated from her husband.

These stories of loss were common amongst the women and strained the ability of the survivors to keep going without the aid of their loved ones. The women felt this loss acutely when they had to contend with the extra demands of childbearing. Most of the women had to resume full activities immediately after returning home from the hospital. Gloria said, "When I arrived home, it was just me alone." Gloria recounted problems caring for herself and her baby and said that she felt very depressed and overwhelmed.

Racism

Living with racial discrimination was a chronic battle for general and key informants. Several informants demonstrated distrust during recruitment. Over time, and as trusting relationships ensued, the key informants talked about discrimination in job searches, racial hostilities in personal relationships, and poor treatment by hospital and store employees. Helena said that potential employers always greeted her faxed resume with enthusiasm. She said that she had problems when she went in for the interview because "my face does not match my resume." She told me that she could tell by the expression on the interviewer's face that the company was not expecting a Black woman and she would usually not be hired. She also noted that she always had to be aware that "if anything turned up missing, I'm afraid I would be blamed." She said of her daily life, "In every nook and cranny, you just can't hide from prejudice." Julie also maintained that she saw discrimination in her life and that it was hard to live with this every day. Julie was particularly angry that a local fast food restaurant served mostly Black people but would not hire them to work there. She said that when she goes into some stores, they don't even acknowledge her. She stated, "They act like they don't hear me."

The Mothers Used Military-Like Strategies to Deal with Life Experiences

The women used various strategies to fight for survival, and these strategies resembled those used in war. They assumed the role of soldiers, developed new tactical maneuvers, trusted in God for justice, shared their resources with their comrades, took short-lived breaks when they were wounded in action, and used escape mechanisms.

Soldiering

Gloria used the specific words, "Be your own soldier" (Cricco-Lizza, 2004) to describe how she negotiated her everyday struggle to survive. She indicated she had been on her own since her mother developed a drug problem when she was 9 years old and said that she had to be a "soldier" to fight her way through adversity in life. Gloria said, "Bad things happen. If I let them bother me, I would never get on with my life." She valued independence, strength, and tenacity, and relied on herself to get things done. Karen had similar life experiences and believed that she had to strive to do things to make a better future for herself and her child. She said:

> I look up to myself . . . It's kind of hard . . . I was very independent [as a child]. When I see that my mom was not going to do it for me, after a while I try to do it for myself. Become good at it, keep doing it myself. Sometimes you don't have any other choice . . . [Children] have to be independent and learn what to do for themselves cause their mom not gonna be there to do it for them. The children don't have any other choice . . . But I wouldn't want my child to grow up the way I did. I want the best for my child . . . I'm gonna go back to school. Sometimes everyone needs somebody to help. And I just don't have that, so I have to do it myself. I think I'm capable of it.

This soldiering strategy was the one most frequently used by the women in this study, evidenced in the words of almost every woman encountered. Helena said, "I can deal with it. I am strong." Karen said, "[I] have never been one to give up. I'm not that type." Julie stated, "I got to survive." Cherise asserted, "I think, like, my sisters and I . . . were all independent because mother worked and we couldn't be babied all day."

The women described life as hard work and a daily battle to be waged. Helena told me that if you were weak, you didn't stand a chance. Ella said that she had to keep going, as she had no time to be tired. Cherise and Helena stated that they learned from their mothers how to deal with adversity. Cherise reported that her mother and aunt worked hard. She said:

> And you know if they did have a problem, they didn't complain. They just worked. They got through it. Well, we had a single-parent household and so I would say if you are a strong person, you're gonna do it. It's not on the basis of you need a husband or you need help, or . . . NO. If you know you can do it, you'll get out there and do it on your own.

I also saw evidence of soldiering amongst the general informants in the waiting room. A middle-aged mother confided to her waiting room friend about all the difficulties that she had with her teenage son. She described her struggle to "straighten him out" and realized that she had to do this on her own. She said:

> I asked God to harden my heart and He said no. I asked Him to close my eyes and He said no. I asked Him to shut my tongue and He said no. And then He told me that I had to walk the path and find my way.

During my data analysis I found that the intensity of "soldiering" also exacted a toll on the women. Anger, anxiety, distrust, and sadness were the most frequent emotions displayed by the women who held this soldiering belief. For example, the middle-aged general informant who said that she had to walk the path and find her way talked as well about walking to the clinic next door for treatment for anxiety attacks. Helena also discussed the cumulative toll of fighting adversity. She said, "And because so much stuff has happened to me, it was just one more thing I had to deal with . . . So I was just devastated."

Trying new tactical maneuvers

Many of the general and key informants demonstrated readiness to learn new behaviors during their transition to motherhood. The women were curious about pregnancy and readily described nutritional facts they learned from WIC nutrition sessions, posters, and videotapes. Half of the key informants initiated breastfeeding even though formula feeding was the norm among their families and friends. Most of these key informants credited education, emotional support, and trusting relationships with WIC staff for their initiation of this behavior. The initial week of breastfeeding was difficult for these women, but I found that they voiced pride in their success and greater satisfaction with motherhood thereafter. Cherise said, "It's like the best feeling. I never realized how happy you really could be." Helena specifically mentioned how breastfeeding decreased stress for her and her baby. The breastfeeding key informants also believed that their babies would be healthier and better prepared to face the daily struggles that they believed were inherent in their future (Cricco-Lizza, 2004).

Trusting in God for final justice

For many of the general and key informants in the study, spiritual beliefs and church services were sources of comfort and hope as they battled adversity. Helena said, "In my religion, Judgment Day will come and the just will be restored . . . The world is full of suffering. Everyone's faith gets tested. My time is now." There were many references to God interspersed in conversations among the general informants in the WIC waiting room. Gloria told me that she looked to God to help her through her struggles. She said:

> It's not easy for me to give up . . . just because it hurts a little. Instead I rather just try to conquer it as much as I can, and if I can't bear it, God will take it away from me.

Several of the key informants referred to their spiritual beliefs during their interviews. Aja's plans for the future included "giving my life to God." Gloria told me that she felt suicidal during her early days postpartum. She said that there "was nothing left than . . . to just pray. . . I guess it was just through prayer that I got through it." Helena said, "Faith keeps us going." She continuously referred to her trust in God throughout her difficult pregnancy and her baby's massive neurological defects. Helena told me, "God watches out for me." She said:

> God has blessed me every step of the way . . . I couldn't do it by myself. God was with me. My mom said I can't be listening to the doctors, that I shouldn't put my faith in imperfect people, that I should have faith in God. So I gave my problems to God.

The general informants also talked about their spiritual beliefs. One mother said that God was a source of solace for her throughout her life. She stated that previous perinatal losses still hurt her "terribly" but that she took comfort in thinking that her babies were with God. Spiritual beliefs buffered injustice and disappointment for the women and their families.

Sharing resources with comrades

The women were generous with their resources and shared them with family, friends, and strangers. Mothers commonly supported each other in the WIC clinic. The general informants would watch each other's babies when they had to use the restroom and offered words of encouragement to other tired or beleaguered mothers. One general informant had a particularly difficult pregnancy and was still feeling poorly postpartum. During her WIC appointment, her neighbor accompanied her and assumed total care of the low-birth-weight infant.

The key informants' words also reflected this same type of generosity. Gloria said, "The best, the highest point of me has always been a person that likes to help other people." Julie also said, "I'm a nice person. I have a good heart." The women's words matched their actions. Helena routinely gathered up clothing her baby had outgrown and distributed it to others in need. Despite her own serious pregnancy problems, she extended herself to other women who suffered pregnancy losses and was generous in spirit, even when confronted with insensitivity. During the heart-wrenching time when her baby was expected to die, Helena was hurt that her cousin told her that "bad things happen because you deserve it." She said that she told him that most people who say that have never had anything bad happen to them. But she told her cousin, "When something bad happens to you and you come looking for sympathy, I will be there for you."

Because so many of their significant others were missing or dead, the study participants sought assistance from a wide net of people. One general informant told me that she relied on a girlfriend to watch her children while she worked the night shift. Another said that she could not afford to get to work without a ride from a friend. Ella lived with several different relatives during the course of the investigation. Most of the women relied on varied female relatives and friends for childcare assistance. These sources of aid were subject to the same difficult living conditions, and help could often not be sustained. Julie, for example, had great trouble finding someone to watch her infant when she went for job training. Her father was "shot to death" when she was three, her boyfriend was incarcerated, her aunt had recently died, and her only sister had lost custody of her own children. She felt compelled to ask her sick mother who lived on the other side of the city. This provided a temporary solution until the mother's car broke down and there was no money to repair it. Stories like this were common and the women often had to scramble to find alternative solutions to meet the everyday demands of their lives.

Catching their breath when wounded in action
General and key informants fought their way through their daily lives until they reached a point where they paused to regroup. The women varied in their threshold of tolerance for daily demands. For some, the diagnosis of pregnancy was a shock and elicited fears about management of additional responsibilities. Several key informants admitted to sleepless nights when they cried over the news. For others, the postpartum period was overwhelming in its demands and Gloria stated, "I felt, I actually felt feelings of suicide." For Helena, the 24-hour demand of caring for a disabled baby sometimes caught up with her and she said, "There have been times I have sat on the floor and cried." Rarely did these women have more than a short-lived surrender to these feelings. Because of the constant demands in their lives, they had to pick themselves back up to fight additional battles.

Escaping
Several general informants in the WIC waiting room were overheard talking about "smoking and drinking and getting high." Some of the key informants talked about friends who liked to drink and Dena said, "A lot of young girls in my age group do a lot of drugs and do a lot of drinking." None of the key informants admitted to using drugs or alcohol while they were pregnant or in the postpartum period, however a few of these women mentioned substance abuse by others. Karen said that most of her old friends were "going from one drug to another. They were looking different; I mean really bad and I'm watching them fall." Only Imani and Karen described a past history of illicit drug use, and they relayed their stories in ways that suggested that they had used drugs to numb pain and escape their daily struggles. During a prenatal interview I asked Imani to tell me what she thought was important for me to know about her. She responded that she was born with a major facial defect and had five operations between birth and age 18. She said that other children did not understand her condition and she had to endure "picking and name calling and stuff like that." I asked her how she responded to that and Imani said, "I didn't take it well." She immediately went on to tell me that she started "experimenting

with drugs." She stated that she went into a drug rehabilitation program and said that she had been "clean" for the past 6 years. Karen talked about similar experimentation. She acknowledged that when she was younger, "I started dangerous things that my friends were doing. You know, I wasn't good. I used to smoke grass, smoke a lot of marijuana." She said that she now smoked cigarettes to deal with all of the stress in her life. She stated:

> It's just all there. It's all on my mind. I don't think it's good for me to be stressing like that, but it's just all there . . . I don't know sometimes everything just pops in my head and I just start thinking and thinking and thinking. It's like I look around for a cigarette and start smoking. I mean it doesn't ease the pain or anything. I don't know.

Discussion

Through the use of an ethnographic approach, I gained a contextually detailed view of the everyday experiences of the mothers in this study. Both general and key informants reported challenges associated with a lack of resources and described how they experienced gender, race, and class inequity on a personal level. Their words reflected their daily battles to survive under hostile conditions. They spontaneously relayed their concerns with finances, housing, education, employment, safety, loss, and racism and problems with one of these issues often magnified the others. The women's reports suggested that significant infrastructural problems constrained the choices available to them and their significant others. The women found it difficult to meet their basic needs in their own neighborhoods despite much effort. Those who sought opportunities in more resource-rich areas perceived that racism thwarted their attempts. Many of the women's everyday activities entailed a battle and the findings indicated that there were unmet mental health needs from chronic stress and unresolved loss. Lack of human resources due to lost family members further increased the burdens imposed by inadequate material resources.

Military leaders have demonstrated the tenuous position of troops that fight without adequate resources. In his classic treatise on military strategies, Sun Tzu delineated how a war cannot be won without sufficient resources (Kaufman, 2001). Public health researchers have also repeatedly shown that those with fewer resources have the highest morbidity and mortality rates (Kasper et al., 2008; LaVeist, 2005; Schulz, Parker, Israel, & Fisher, 2001). These views are supported by the findings from the current investigation. There were many high-risk pregnancies and sick infants among the general and key informants. It was also apparent that major stressors in the lives of these participants began before their pregnancies and were ongoing. Racism was a continuing struggle for the informants. Schulz et al. (2006) have demonstrated that discrimination is associated with poor physical and mental health outcomes for Black women.

In this ethnographic study I have documented the varied strategies the women used to deal with their life experiences. The key informants initiated the *soldiering* metaphor to portray their daily battles for survival. French (1992) and Hooks (1995) have described the struggles of women against racism and sexism and this also supports the soldiering metaphor. Collins (1991) has said that Black women's experiences with hostile and hazardous environments have encouraged the development of independence and self-reliance. The strength of Black women to resist discrimination and to carve out their own paths has also been captured in the fictional characters portrayed in *Sula* (Morrison, 1973), *Beloved* (Morrison, 1987), *Meridian* (Walker, 1976), and *The Color Purple* (Walker, 1982). The women in this study demonstrated the same everyday strength and valor under continued adversity.

One of the ways that these women carved out their own paths was in *trying new tactical maneuvers*. Although community norms favored formula feeding, half of the key informants initiated breastfeeding. Researchers have identified the multiple health benefits of breastfeeding for mothers and babies (American Academy of Pediatrics, 2005) and this process may have particular advantages for stressed populations. Similar to the key informants in this study, breastfeeding mothers have reported less perceived stress (Mezzacappa & Katkin, 2002). A diminished stress response may protect the breastfeeding mother and baby from environmental demands (Groer & Davis, 2002) and this strategy holds promise for ameliorating some of the daily strain.

Many of the women in this study derived hope and comfort from the *trusting in God* coping strategy. With this trust, the women were able to look beyond their daily battles and create visions of a just future. The participants also obtained additional social support from church activities, which is consistent with the findings of others (Holt, Lewellyn, & Rathweg, 2005; van Olphen et al., 2003).

During wartimes, a sense of camaraderie is fostered through the common experiences of enduring the many hardships of the battlefields (Wiener, 2005). *Sharing resources with comrades* was an important strategy that aided both the giver and receiver in this study. Ladner (1971), Stack (1974), and Collins (1991) have described the long tradition of blood mothers and other mothers for sharing mothering responsibilities among Black women. The women in this current study engaged in this tradition but were impeded in their efforts by the loss of so many significant others in their networks. This important finding reflects a serious hindrance for normative coping mechanisms for these women.

The informants used military strategies to resist destructive forces in their lives but they also pinpointed the high personal costs of incessantly fighting the structural barriers to their well being. The women used the *Catching their breath when wounded in action* strategy to take short-lived breaks, but the heavy demands of *soldiering* also exacted feelings of anger, anxiety, distrust, and sadness. Some of the women in this study resorted to *escape* strategies and this is similar to Ehrmin's (2002) findings that alcohol and drugs were used to numb the emotional pain of loss, abandonment, abuse, and racism.

The findings in this study support the weathering conceptual framework developed by Geronimus (2001). She emphasized that Black women undergo premature health deterioration as a result of the cumulative effects of enduring social, political, and economic exclusion. Chronic stress can lead to wear and tear on the major body systems with long term consequences of cardiovascular disease, diabetes, obesity, and premature aging (McEwen, 1998). Black women who persistently use high-end coping may experience the greatest weathering effects on their health (Geronimus, Hicken, Keene, & Bound, 2006). This high-end coping is similar to the *soldiering* reported by the informants in this study.

Conclusion and Implications

The voices of the women in this study clearly resounded with the stories of their battles. In spite of their heroic efforts they cannot win this war without reinforcements of material and human resources. The women's strength reflected in the soldiering strategy should be recognized, but should not be perceived as a replacement for substantive infrastructural change. They need opportunities to use their strength in ways that nurture hope. The women conveyed the need for safe, affordable housing, educational and social support, and job options. Public health interventions must also address gender and class inequity along with racism. The development of these interventions should be built on self-determination by Black women, rather than be imposed from the outside. The women in this study were vocal about their needs and clearly described their normative coping strategies. Their voices should be central to the development of interventions to address the maternal child health disparities experienced by this group.

Everyday experiences might vary in different settings and with different cultural groups. In this study I focused on an urban setting in the United States but women in many varied locales also battle for survival on a daily basis. It is important to listen to their voices so that culturally sensitive interventions can be developed to spare women and children from living under such war-like conditions.

References

American Academy of Pediatrics. (2005). Breastfeeding and the use of human milk. *Pediatrics, 115*, 496–506.

Bhutta, Z. A. (2005). Bridging the equity gap in maternal and child health. *British Medical Journal, 331*, 585–586.

Burton, L. M. (1990). Teenage childbearing as an alternative life-course strategy in multi-generation Black families. *Human Nature, 1*, 123–143.

Cabral, H., Fried, L. E., Levenson, S., Amaro, H., & Zuckerman, B. (1990). Foreign-born and US-born black women: Differences in health behaviors and birth outcomes. *American Journal of Public Health, 80*, 70–73.

Clifford, J., & Brykcznski, K. (1999). Giving voice to childbearing teens: Views on sexuality and the reality of being a young parent. *Journal of School Nursing, 15*, 4–15.

Collins, P. H. (1991). *Black feminist thought: Knowledge, consciousness, and the politics of empowerment.* New York: Routledge.

Cricco-Lizza, R. (2004). Infant feeding beliefs and experiences of Black women enrolled in a New York metropolitan area WIC clinic. *Qualitative Health Research, 14*, 1197–1210.

Cricco-Lizza, R. (2005). The milk of human kindness: Environmental and human interactions in a WIC clinic that influence infant feeding decisions of Black women. *Qualitative Health Research, 15*, 525–538.

Cricco-Lizza, R. (2006). Black non-Hispanic mothers' perceptions about the promotion of infant feeding methods by nurses and physicians. *JOGNN, 35*, 173–180.

Cricco-Lizza, R. (2007). Ethnography and the generation of trust in breastfeeding disparities research. *Applied Nursing Research, 20*, 200–204.

Danziger, S. K. (1995). Family life and teenage pregnancy in the inner-city: Experiences of African-American youth. *Children & Youth Services Review, 17*, 183–202.

David, R. J., & Collins, J. W. (1997). Differing birth weight among infants of US born blacks, African-born blacks, and US born whites. *New England Journal of Medicine, 337*, 1209–1214.

Duchon, L. M., Andrulis, D. P., Reid, H. M. (2004). Measuring progress in meeting healthy people goals for low birth weight and infant mortality among the 100 largest cities and their suburbs. *Journal of Urban Health, 81*, 323–339.

Dunlap, E., Sturzenhofecker, G., & Johnson, B. (2006). The elusive romance of motherhood: Drugs, gender, and reproduction in inner-city distressed households. *Journal of Ethnicity in Substance Abuse, 5*(3), 1–27.

Edge, D., & Rogers, A. (2005). *Dealing with it: Black Caribbean women's response to adversity and psychological distress associated with pregnancy, childbirth, and early motherhood. Social Science & Medicine, 61*, 15–25.

Ehrmin, J. T. (2002). "That feeling of not feeling": Numbing the pain for substance-dependent African American women. *Qualitative Health Research, 12*, 780–791.

French, M. (1992). *The war against women.* New York: Ballantine Books.

Germain, C. (2001). Ethnography: The method. In P. Munhall (Ed.), *Nursing research: A qualitative perspective* (pp. 277–306). Sudbury, MA: Jones & Bartlett.

Geronimus, A. T. (2001). Understanding and eliminating racial inequalities in women's health in the United States: The role of the weathering conceptual framework. *JAMWA, 56*, 133–137.

Geronimus, A. T., Hicken, M., Keene, D., & Bound, J. (2006). "Weathering" and age patterns of allostatic load scores among Blacks and Whites in the United States. *American Journal of Public Health, 96,* 826–833.

Gichia, J. E. (2000). Mothers and others: African-American women's preparation for motherhood. *The American Journal of Maternal Child Nursing, 25,* 86–91.

Giscombe, C. L., & Lobel, M. (2005). Explaining disproportionately high rates of adverse birth outcomes among African Americans: The impact of stress, racism, and related factors in pregnancy. *Psychological Bulletin, 131,* 662–683.

Groer, M. W., & Davis, M. W. (2002). Postpartum stress: Current concepts and the possible protective role of breastfeeding. *JOGNN, 31,* 411–417.

Heron, M., Sutton, P. D., Xu, J., Ventura, S. J., Strobino, D. M., & Guyer, B. (2010). Annual summary of vital statistics—2007. *Pediatrics, 115,* 4–15.

Hogan, V. K., Njoroge, T., Durant, T. M., & Ferre, C. D. (2001). Eliminating disparities in perinatal outcomes—lessons learned. *Maternal and Child Health Journal, 5*(2), 135–140.

Hogue, C. J., & Bremner, J. D. (2005). Stress model of research into preterm delivery among Black women. *American Journal of Obstetrics and Gynecology, 192*(5 Suppl), S47–S55.

Holt, C. L., Lewellyn, L. A., & Rathweg, M. J. (2005). Exploring religion-health mediators among African American parishioners. *Journal of Health Psychology, 10,* 511–527.

Hooks, B. (1995). *Killing rage: Ending racism.* New York: Henry Holt.

Kasper, J. D., Ensminger, M. E., Green, K. M., Fothergill, K. E., Juon, H. S., Robertson, J., et al. (2008). Effects of poverty and family stress over three decades on the functional status of older African American women. *The Journals of Gerontology Series B: Psychological Sciences and Social Sciences, 63*(4), S201–S210.

Kaufman, S. F. (2001). *The art of war: The definitive interpretation of Sun Tzu's classic book of strategy.* North Clarendon, VT: Tuttle.

Ladner, J. A. (1971). *Tomorrow's tomorrow: The Black woman.* Garden City, New York: Doubleday.

LaVeist, T. A. (2005). *Minority populations and health: An introduction to health disparities in the United States.* San Francisco, CA: Jossey-Bass.

Mann, R. J., Abercrombie, P. D., DeJoseph, J., Norbeck, J. S., & Smith, R. T. (1999). The personal experience of pregnancy for African-American women. *Journal of Transcultural Nursing, 10,* 297–305.

McEwen, B. S. (1998). Protective and damaging effects of stress mediators. *New England Journal of Medicine, 338,* 171–179.

Mezzacappa, E. S., & Katkin, E. S. (2002). Breast-feeding is associated with reduced perceived stress and negative mood in mothers. *Health Psychology, 21,* 187–193.

Minino, A. M., Heron, M. P., Murphy, S. L., & Kochanek, K. D. (2007). Deaths: Final data for 2004. *National Vital Statistics Reports, 55*(19), 1–120.

Morrison, T. (1973). *Sula.* New York: Penguin Books.

Morrison, T. (1987). *Beloved.* New York: Penguin Books.

Mullings, L., Wali, A., McLean, D., Mitchell, J., Prince, S., Thomas, D., et al. (2001). Qualitative methodologies and community participation in examining reproductive experiences: The Harlem birth right project. *Maternal and Child Health Journal, 5,* 85–93.

Oxley, G. M., & Weekes, D. P. (1997). Experiences of pregnant African American adolescents: Meanings, perception, appraisal, and coping. *Journal of Family Nursing, 3,* 167–188.

Sawyer, L. M. (1999). Engaged mothering: The transition to motherhood for a group of African American women. *Journal of Transcultural Nursing, 10,* 14–21.

Schulz, A. J., Gravlee, C. C., Williams, D. R., Israel, B. A., Mentz, G., & Rowe, Z. (2006). Discrimination, symptoms of depression, and self-rated health among African American women in Detroit: Results from a longitudinal analysis. *American Journal of Public Health, 96,* 1265–1270.

Schulz, A., Parker, E., Israel, B., & Fisher, T. (2001). Social context, stressors, and disparities in women's health. *JAMWA, 56,* 143–149.

Shambley-Ebron, D. Z., & Boyle, J. S. (2004). New paradigms for transcultural nursing: Frameworks for studying African American women. *Journal of Transcultural Nursing, 15,* 11–17.

Shambley-Ebron, D. Z., & Boyle, J. S. (2006). In our grandmother's footsteps: Perceptions of being strong in African American women with HIV/AIDS. *Advances in Nursing Science, 29,* 195–206.

Smedley, B. D., Stith, A. Y., & Nelson, A. R. (2002). *Unequal treatment: Confronting racial and ethnic disparities in health care. Institute of Medicine Report.* Washington, DC: National Academies Press.

Stack, C. B. (1974). *All our kin: Strategies for survival in a Black community.* New York: Harper & Row.

Stanton, A. L., Lobel, M., Sears, S., & DeLuca, R. S. (2002). Psychosocial aspects of selected issues in women's reproductive health: Current status and future directions. *Journal of Consulting and Clinical Psychology, 70,* 751–770.

United States Department of Health and Human Services/Healthy People 2010. (2007, September, 20). *Progress Review: Maternal, infant, and child health.* Retrieved March 5, 2010 from http://www.healthypeople.gov/data/2010prog/focus16/

van Olphen, J., Schulz, A., Israel, B., Chatters, L., Klem, L., Parker, E., et al. (2003). Religious involvement, social support, and health among African-American women on the east side of Detroit. *Journal of General Internal Medicine, 18,* 549–557.

Walker, A. (1976). *Meridian.* New York: Pocket Books.

Walker, A. (1982). *The color purple.* New York: Pocket Books.

Wayland, J., & Rawlins, R. (1997). African American teen mothers' perceptions of parenting. *Journal of Pediatric Nursing, 12,* 13–20.

Wiener, T. (2005). *Forever a soldier: Unforgettable stories of wartime service; The Library of Congress Veteran's History Project.* Washington, DC: National Geographic Society.

Endnotes

[1]Source: Adapted from Cricco-Lizza, R. (2008) Voices from the battlefield: Reports of the daily experiences of urban, Black mothers. *Health Care of Women International, 29,* 115–134. Reprinted by permission of the publisher. (Taylor & Francis Ltd, http://www.tandf.co.uk/journals)

12

Case Study: The Method

Patricia Hentz

According to Yin (2009), case study methods are well suited when the researcher's aim is to retain the holistic and meaningful characteristics of real-life events. Additionally, the case study method is appropriate when the study of a complex phenomenon is inseparable from the contextual conditions related to phenomena. For example, Goffman's (1961) classic study of mental institutions describes an "underlife" culture that demonstrated the interconnection between the phenomenon of being in a mental institution and the context, the culture of the institution (Yin, 2003; Yin, 2009). As illustrated in Goffman's work, the experience of being institutionalized uniquely affects behavior and the expression of mental illness.

Before delving into the case study method, it is important to note that there are no hard and fast rules or standardization on how to conduct case study research (McKee, 2004). It is a highly flexible research approach that ranges from simple to complex. It can focus on a single individual, a group of individuals, an organization, processes, neighborhoods, institutions, or events. It is a research approach used extensively in social science research, including psychology, sociology, political science, anthropology, history, and economics. Practice disciplines such as nursing, medicine, social work, urban planning, public administration, and education have utilized case study methods based on the rationale that human experiences are often best understood within their social context. An essential point is that the social context is critical to analysis and understanding irrespective of the disciple or research paradigm.

Review of the literature on case study has revealed that this approach is quite varied and includes qualitative and quantitative approaches. Therefore, due to its paradigmatic flexibility, case study research can be difficult to conceptualize (Rosenberg & Yates, 2007). Case studies can be inductive, involving descriptive and exploratory research approaches, and it can be deductive, focusing on hypothesis and theory testing. It could involve a single unit or case or multiple units or cases. Given the scope of case study research this chapter briefly refers to quantitative case studies, however, its primary purpose is to provide an overview of case study from a qualitative perspective. "To understand the nature of case study research, it is useful to conceptualize it as an *approach* to research rather than a methodology in its own right" (Rosenberg & Yates, 2007, p. 448). The structure and function of case study research depend on the qualitative or quantitative research method employed.

The usefulness of case study is explored along with its common features. Key to understanding the case study approach is that the methodological approach stems from the research questions. As stated by Rosenberg and Yates, "the methods used in case study research are pragmatically—rather than paradigmatically—driven" (p. 448). In essence the phenomenon of interest and the research question determine the method and design. To illustrate this, examples will be presented that reflect phenomenological, ethnographic, and grounded theory research methods. Consistent with the literature on case study, emphasis will be on identifying the "object of study within its social context" and the importance of the bond between the object of study and the social context. These are discussed in more depth within the chapter.

Case Study Research: What It Is and What It Is Not _____

The concept *case study* has multiple definitions and has been applied in a variety of ways. Within the social sciences it has been defined very broadly. Case study has been divided into four categories; however, only the fourth category exclusively focuses on case study as a research approach. The first category is the teaching case that does not need to accurately depict a specific individual, event, or process. Its primary aim is to enhance learning. The teaching case is illustrative, and while it often has been derived from case study observations it does not necessarily comply with any specific research methodology. For example, case studies depicting specific psychiatric disorders are grounded in research and are often developed using a combination of evidence-based diagnostic criteria and clinical observation. The second category, case histories, is used for the purposes of record keeping. Here again the primary aim is not research, however, the cases may be useful as data in a research study aimed at examining healthcare delivery. Casework, the third category, is used to describe the management of health care for a patient or population. Similar to case histories, the purpose is not research. The fourth category, case research or case study research, is intended for the purpose of "investigating activities or complex processes that are not easily separated from the social context within which they occur" (Cutler, 2004, p. 367).

Yin (2009) describes key aspects of case study. First, it "investigates a contemporary phenomenon in depth within its real-life context, especially when the boundaries between phenomenon and context are not clearly evident" (p. 18). Second, since the boundary between the phenomenon or "single unit" is quite blurred, the researcher has little or no control over the context within which the phenomenon exists. Thus, the justification for choosing a case study approach is the awareness that it is essential to understand the social context in order to understand a phenomenon. An example of the blurring of the social context and the phenomenon is illustrated in the 2003 film *Monster* (written and directed by Patty Jenkins). The movie depicts the life story of the first female serial killer. Strikingly apparent in this portrayal is that the process of becoming a serial killer is inseparable from the woman's life experiences; a tragic and tortured history of dysfunctional and abusive relationships. The rich contextual detail of her life story provided insights into her becoming a serial killer. In essence the process and eventual outcome are seamlessly interconnected.

Characteristics of Qualitative Case Study Research

Stake (1995) discussed the following characteristics of qualitative case study research that are critical to choosing a case study approach.

- *Holistic.* Focus is on a comprehensive understanding of the phenomenon with rich contextual detail. The sum of the whole is greater than its parts.
- *Empirical.* The researcher maintains a naturalistic orientation for data collection. Understanding the social context requires a firsthand view. Interviewing and participant observation are often strategies of choice because they facilitate an in-depth view of the social context.
- *Interpretive.* The researcher acknowledges the importance of the researcher-subject interaction, personal meanings, and biases. The aim is to uncover the participants' understandings and meanings and to present them with clarity and authenticity. The quality of the findings weighs heavily on the researcher's awareness of his or her personal biases and personal meanings as well as his or her ability to separate personal biases and meanings. In qualitative research, the researcher is the instrument and thus the credibility of the findings relies heavily on the skill of the researcher.
- *Empathic.* Qualitative case study research as a human science maintains the value of and respect for persons.

Case study method is guided by the research question. And, even though case study method has been touted as a flexible approach, the research question provides the guide for creating structure aimed at specific research outcomes. Thus, the data-collection approaches one incorporates must be appropriate in relation to the research question and aims of the study. Considering the fact that case study method draws upon various research methodologies, the researcher embarking on this approach needs to be well grounded in qualitative methodologies and their theoretical underpinnings. In qualitative research, the question is linked to a specific research methodology which in turn directs the data-collection strategies, data analysis, and presentation of the study. For example, a case study that focuses on how an organization has incorporated an innovative healthcare delivery approach may utilize elements of grounded theory research with the research aim of exploring the process of change within the social context. Key members of the organization may be interviewed and observation may be incorporated as a data-collection approach. The theoretical lens for the study might be symbolic interactionalism and the researcher may incorporate theoretical sampling and constant comparison as the approach to data collection and analysis.

Qualitative case studies are often presented as concrete narratives detailing actual experiences. The story, as research narrative, involves a blend of description and analysis aimed at answering the research question. It is important to note that case studies research differs from a traditional sense of story in that it is guided by the research question, follows a specific research process, and its aim is to understand the phenomenon within a social context. The researcher clearly identifies the significance and relevance for the case study along with a detailed explanation on how prior research and/or theories have led to this research topic. Since the qualitative research topic and question form the foundation for the case study, it is recommended that the reader refer back to the specific chapters within this text for more detailed information on developing the research question, the philosophical underpinnings, data collection, data analysis, and writing the findings.

Points of Interest: Intrinsic, Instrumental, and Multiple Case Study

Along with thinking qualitatively, one needs to determine the purpose of the study and what one hopes to understand and ultimately convey. As seen thus far, case study research has been conceptualized in a variety of ways. Stake (2005) has conceptualized an approach for categorizing case studies that involves three points of interest—intrinsic interest, instrumental interest, and multiple case study. The first, intrinsic interest, refers to a case study aimed at understanding a particular case of interest. This could involve an individual or group. The purpose of this type of case is not to generalize to other similar cases, although it may. Its purpose is to thoroughly explore a phenomenon within its social context. An example of an intrinsic interest case study is Liebow's (1969) *Tally's Corner*, a study that focused on a single group of men living in a poor, inter-city neighborhood (Yin, 2003, 2009). The results of this research have offered insights into a subculture that exists in many U.S. cities. As an intrinsic case study it has a specific point of interest, however, what is also evident in this intrinsic case is its ethnographic nature. The second type, instrumental case studies, endorses the aim of providing insight and advancing understanding that could possibly be generalized. Goffman's (1961) classic study of mental institutions provides an in-depth description of the "underlife" culture that exists in mental institutions and has been instrumental in understanding similar institutions. Instrumental case studies extend beyond description and offer insights into what is occurring and why. Many portray a social process and have incorporated aspects of grounded theory research. The third, multiple case study or collective case study (as it is also called), involves the use of several cases to investigate a phenomenon, population, or general condition. The study, *The Family Encounter of Depression* (Angell 1936/1965), depicts the experiences of university students whose families had suffered a loss of income during the Great Depression. While aspects of single cases may be depicted, identifying themes and synthesis are the emphasis. An advantage of multiple case study design is that it often offers greater anonymity and confidentiality. The trade off is that it often loses the individual case perspective.

Five Types of Single Case Study Designs

In addition to understanding a phenomenon of interest, single case study designs offer a range of purposes. Yin (2003, 2009) highlights five kinds of single case designs:

- *Critical case testing a well-formulated theory.* In these case studies:

  > The theory has specified a clear set of propositions as well as the circumstances within which the propositions are believed to be true. To confirm, challenge, or extend the theory, a single case can then be used to determine whether a theory's propositions are correct or whether some alternative set of explanations might be more relevant. (Yin, 2009, p. 47)

  An example of critical case is illustrated in Gilligan's (1982) offering of a feminist perspective on moral developmental theory and moral decision making. Her cases challenged Kohlberg's moral developmental theory that was based solely on a sampling of males. Her case examples clearly identify a decision-making process very different from that of Kohlberg. In contrast to Kohlberg's justice perspective, Gilligan presents an approach to ethical dilemmas that is relational in nature and is based on a care perspective.

- *Extreme or unique cases.* Examples of these cases may be seen in psychiatric practice where a specific disorder is so rare that a single case is worth examining. Another example might involve the description and analysis of a unique organization or community.

- *Representative or typical cases.* These cases represent a common experience or pattern. A case study illustrating the common trajectory for developing anorexia and offering insights into the common risk factors and patterns of the illness would be an example.

- *Revelatory cases.* These involve situations where the researcher explores and analyzes a phenomenon previously inaccessible. An example is the study of body memory by Hentz in the exemplar on case study (see Chapter 13). As discussed in the review of the literature, grieving has been thoroughly examined from its cognitive, emotional, and behavioral aspects, but very little had been explored regarding body memory and its role in the grieving process. Hentz provides a case example of body memory and discusses the need to acknowledge body memory as a critical component in the grieving process.

- *Longitudinal cases.* In longitudinal case studies, a single case is viewed at different points in time. Lauterbach's (2000) research on loss of a newborn examines how women experience the loss over time. In her follow-up phenomenological study, Lauterbach interviews the women from her original study, focusing on the meaning and experience of loss after 5 years.

Single case studies stand on their own which raises areas of concern and requires some words of caution. The first area of concern and caution is researcher bias. Researchers who engage in single case study research need to remain vigilant regarding their biases and pre-understandings. They need to maintain an openness to the data and a research stance referred to by Munhall as "unknowing" (1994). Although unintended, researchers often have difficulty separating what is known from what is to be discovered. Another phrase that illustrates researcher bias and pre-understanding is "believing is seeing." Thus, striving toward a stance of "unknowing" is critical to understanding the meanings and experience of the participant. In qualitative research, what is discovered is often very different than what was anticipated. Thus, it is critical that researchers maintain an openness and expect the unexpected. Second, single case designs require careful and thorough exploration of the case in order to minimize the chance of misrepresentation and premature closure. This involves a thorough database to support the analysis and the findings.

Multiple Case Study Design

In addition to the single case study design there are several case study research designs that involve more than one case. In multiple case study design the unit or phenomenon of study can involve a small or large sample. Several cases may be involved that are representative of a phenomenon. According to McDonnell, Jones, and Read (2000), case studies are chosen because they are viewed as illustrative. This type of study is "essentially an instrumental study extended to several cases" (Anaf, Drummound, & Sheppard, 2007). When several cases are utilized in a multiple case study design the cases need to represent a phenomenon and the researcher needs to take care not to blur the boundaries of the unit or phenomenon. Thus, this requires that the cases be as homogeneous as possible. If the phenomenon is too broad, too loosely defined, and/or the social context is too varied the study resembles an exploratory study more than a case study. The concept of *replication* is key in multiple case study design. Each case is carefully selected with the expectation that there will be similar findings. The rationale for multiple case study or collective case study is to enhance the credibility of the findings and its validity and reliability.

There has been the misconception that case studies are simpler in design than other research methods. In reality, there are several types of complex case study designs that are far from simple. One such design is termed *embedded case study*; a study of cases within a case. An example of an embedded case study would be the study of an organization with the smaller embedded units being case studies of individuals within the organization. Another complex case design, *two tailed,* is used to explore variations of a given phenomenon. An example would be exploring how two individuals who have experienced a similar phenomenon present with very different perspectives of the experience. This approach has some similarity to a constant comparison approach seen in grounded theory research. An example illustrative of a two-tailed qualitative design is the exploration of how two individuals respond differently to a traumatic life event. The one case depicts a story of an individual who responds with resilience while the other case story reveals a process of acute stress leading to post-traumatic stress disorder (PTSD).

Case Study Designs: Descriptive, Exploratory, Explanatory

The research design is the logic that links the data and the research findings to the initial research question. Because case study research focuses on a unit of study or phenomenon rather than any one specific research methodology, it can be used at any level of knowledge development, including exploratory, descriptive, or explanatory. Case study research is also used to describe processes, generate theory, and test theory. Therefore, the data-collection approaches and data analysis strategies need to be tailored to reflect the research aims. Given the divergent nature of case study method, researchers need to familiarize themselves with the data collection and analysis approaches appropriate for the level or type of case study research. Thus, descriptive studies that focus on understanding an individual's experience regarding a specific phenomenon might consider using a phenomenological approach. These case studies will be rich in description of the lived experience. If the purpose is to understand how individuals respond differently given a common situation with a *focus on process*, the researcher may choose a multiple case approach and incorporate a constant comparison approach as seen in grounded theory. An ethnographic case study might be suited when the object of study is an organization or group.

Types of Data for Case Study Research

As expected, the data one collects reflects the research question as well as what one hopes to understand from conducting the research. Yin (2009) presents six common types of research evidence: documents, archival records, interviews, direct observation, participant observation, and physical artifacts. The type of evidence or data depends on the research question and the methodological approach. For example, for a phenomenological case study the primary type of data would be open-ended interviews.

Ethnographic case studies may draw upon several different types of data including: observation, structured interviews, focus interviews, open-ended interviews, and archival records and documents. The use of multiple types of data, termed *triangulation of data*, aids in providing depth to the case study (see **Figure 12–1**).

Developing a Topic of Interest for the Case Study

The first step for case study research is to identify the *object of study* and to define its *boundaries*. This unit or object of study could be an individual, group, or process with its social context clearly defined. The following exemplars illustrate the object of study, the social context, and a specific type of case study.

- *Single case study: "The Jack-Roller."* Shaw (1930) presents comprehensive data on one individual, a juvenile delinquent who is the object of study. The case study is presented as a life history, written from the youth's perspective, with material about him from several other sources. The boundary of this case study is clear—a single juvenile delinquent. The social context of his life is presented in depth.
- *Multiple case study: "Street Corner Society."* Whyte (1943/1955) focuses in detail on two gangs within a specific social context, a street corner. The object of the study is the "street corner gangs." The research is exploratory

in nature using participant observation as the primary data-collection approach. The boundaries of this case study are clear—two specific gangs at one location, a single street corner.

- *Case study with emphasis on social process: "Boys in White."* Becker, Greer, Hughes, and Strauss (1961) focus on the effect of medical school on students. The object of study is the medical students and the social context is medical school. Participant observation was the primary data-collection strategy in this study. There was a longitudinal component: Researchers focused on different points of time in medical school rather than on the study of individuals in medical school (Platt, 1992).

- *Explanatory case study: "Teaching effectiveness."* In the late 1950s and 1960s, a group of educators wanted to understand why the changes they had made in educational approaches did not improve test results (Yin, 2003). Case by case, they explored the complexity of the teaching process in practice, widening the lens from the classroom activity to the organizational,

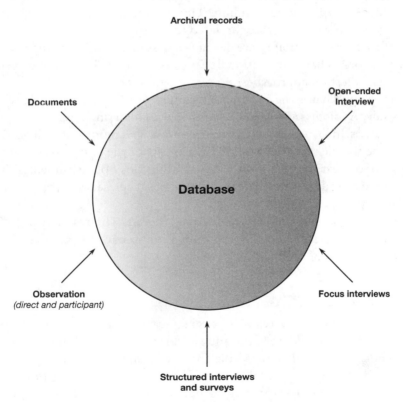

FIGURE 12–1 Convergence of Evidence (Triangulation).
Adapted from Yin (2003). *Case Study Research* (3rd Edition). Thousand Oaks, Ca: Sage.

cultural, economic, and policy contexts in which learning and teaching occur. The object of study involved the educational approaches.

Qualitative Case Study Research: Components of the Research Design

1. The first step is to clearly define the unit or object of study and the social context. Formulation of the research question leads one to the specific qualitative approach or combination of approaches. A key question in this step is to ask if case study is the appropriate approach for the topic? What is the research question? What are the aims and purpose of the research? And, is the social context essential for understanding the phenomenon or object of study?

2. What is already known about the topic? What are the gaps in knowledge? In essence, how will this study add to the body of knowledge or address a gap in understanding? This will include a review of the literature and any relevant theory related to the topic.

3. What data-collection strategies are best suited to address the research question? What is the rationale and justification for selecting specific data-collection approaches?

4. *Sampling.* What is the appropriate sample given the specific type of case study? As discussed earlier, sampling may be for a single case or for multiple cases. In a single case study the questions that need to be addressed are: Is the sample representative and illustrative of the unit of study and the social context? Is the aim of the case study intrinsic or instrumental? Is the aim to provide a critical case, a unique case, a representative case, or a revelatory case?

5. *Data analysis, interpretation, and writing the case.* The research paradigm plays a significant role in determining the approach to data analysis and presentation of findings.

Conclusion

This chapter offers an overview on case study method. Case study method might best be viewed as a versatile and flexible approach well suited to studying phenomenon that is inseparable from its social context. Its application ranges from descriptive to explanatory, from single case designs to multiple case designs. It employs a variety of data-collection and data-analysis approaches based on the aims of the study and the phenomenon of interest. Its strengths include its holistic nature, its in-depth investigation, and its rich description, all of which enhance knowledge.

References

Anaf, S., Drummound, C., & Sheppard, L. A. (2007). Combining case study research and systems theory as a heuristic model. *Qualitative Health Research, 17,* 1309–1315.

Angell, R. C. (1965). *The family encounters the Depression.* Gloucester, MA: Peter Smith. (Original work published 1936.)

Becker, H. S., Greer, B., Hughes, W. C., & Strauss, A. L. (1961). *Boys in white: Student culture in medical school.* Chicago: University of Chicago Press.

Cutler, A. (2004). Methodical failure: The use of case study method by public relations research. *Public Relations Review, 30,* 365–375.

Gilligan, C. (1982). *In a different voice.* Cambridge, MA: Harvard University Press.

Goffman, E. (1961). *Asylums: Essays on the social situation of mental patients and others inmates.* Garden City, NY: Anchor Books.

Jenkins, P. (Director). (2003). *Monster* [Motion picture]. United States: Sony Pictures, Columbia Tristar Films.

Lauterbach, S. S. (2000). In another world: Five years later. In P. L. Munhall (Ed.), *Nursing research: A qualitative perspective* (pp. 185–208). Sudbury, MA: Jones & Bartlett.

Liebow, E. (1967). *Tally's corner.* Boston: Little, Brown.

McDonnell, A., Jones, M. L., & Read, S. (2000). Practical considerations in case study research: The relationship between methodology and process. *Journal of Advanced Nursing, 32*(2), 383–390.

McKee, A. (2004). Getting to know case study research: A brief introduction. *Work Bases Learning in Primary Care, 2,* 6–8.

Munhall, P. L. (1994). *Revisioning phenomenology.* New York: National League for Nursing Press.

Platt, J. (1992). Case of cases . . . of cases. In C. C. Ragin & H. S. Becker (Eds.), *What is a case?* New York: Cambridge University Press.

Rosenberg, J. P., & Yates, P. M. (2007). Schematic representation of case study research designs. *Journal of Advanced Nursing, 24,* 447–452.

Shaw, C. (1930). *The jack-roller.* Chicago: University of Chicago Press.

Stake, R. E. (1995). *The art of case study research.* Thousand Oaks, CA: Sage.

Stake, R. E. (2005). Qualitative case studies. In N. K. Danzin & Y. A. Lincoln (Eds.), *Handbook of qualitative research.* Thousand Oaks, CA: Sage.

Whyte, W. F. (1955). *Street corner society: The social structure of an Italian slum.* Chicago: University of Chicago Press. (Original work published in 1943.)

Yin, R. K. (2003). *Case study research* (3rd ed.). Thousand Oaks, CA: Sage.

Yin, R. K. (2009). *Case study research: Design and methods* (4th ed.). Los Angeles, CA: Sage.

13

Exemplar:
The Body Grieves

Patricia Hentz

This chapter presents an example of an instrumental single case study design using a phenomenological perspective. Instrumental case studies endorse the aim of providing insight and advancing understanding of a phenomenon or single unit. According to Yin (2009) case study methods are well suited when the researcher's aim is to retain the holistic and meaningful characteristics of real-life events. Further, case studies are also desirable when researchers are interested in complex phenomena that are linked to the contextual conditions related to a phenomenon. The following case study is an in-depth view of the experience of loss with specific interest in the experience of body–body memory. This case study narrative provides a rich description of the experience of a 9-year-old girl whose mother died from stomach cancer. The significant finding as illustrated in the case narrative is that the body's experience is relived as it was lived.

Introduction

The grieving process has been well documented, with stages and tasks deemed necessary to facilitate the accommodation of the loss. Within the literature, the concept of uncomplicated grief has been described as a process that transitions from acute grief toward an integration of the loss and a return to the everyday world (see Chapter 7). Evident throughout the literature is that experts differ on the exact timeline for grieving, ranging from several months, to years and even throughout a lifetime. Of interest to this study is that many of the popular theories on grieving have placed particular emphasis on the cognitive, affective, and behavioral domains with little attention to how one's body experiences the loss and the memories it has encoded (Hentz, 2002). Given the lack of attention to body memory related to a significant loss, the aim of this case study has been to bridge this gap by focusing on the involvement of the body in the perceptual experience of loss.

Phenomenological Perspective

From a phenomenological perspective, human behavior is understood as it occurs in the context of relationships to things, people, events, and situations in what Merleau-Ponty (1989) described as embodiment (Oiler-Boyd, 1993). Munhall (2007) discussed how thoughts, feelings, and emotions are deeply embedded in the participant's life world. Thus, understanding the experience of loss as it is linked to the contextual condition requires that one take into account the individual's life worlds which include: spatial, corporeal, temporal, and relational (Munhall, 2007). Spatial life worlds involve exploring the *environment* and its meaning as it relates to the lived experience. Specifically, we understand the experience by taking into consideration the "situated context." Corporeal life worlds or embodiment refer to experiencing the phenomenon as it is lived through one's *body*. Within the context of this study, it is how the body makes sense of the phenomenon as experienced in body memory. Temporal life worlds relate to the element of *time* as well as the perception of time as it relates to the phenomenon. And, relational life worlds are the bonds or connections to self and others in the world. While each of the life worlds has a specific focus, they are interconnected.

Evolution of the Study

As mentioned previously, a research assumption held by this investigator has been that much of the existing theory on the grieving process has not adequately explored the body's experience and, additionally, it has been overshadowed due to the emphasis on the cognitive and affective aspects of grieving:

> This assumption is grounded in a phenomenological perspective and draws from Merleau-Ponty's (1989) description of the body, placing emphasis on the need to move from the views of purely body and purely psychic. The perceiver is not a pure thinker but a body-subject, and there is an unbreakable bond between the human being and the world. (Hentz, 2002, p. 161)

Therefore, understanding the experience of loss and grieving requires that one explore the experiences of mind and body with an awareness of the unbreakable bond that exists between them.

Justification of the Study

The process of grieving refers to the impact of the loss on the individual and the pain and suffering one endures (Cassem, 2000). A strong motivation for pursuing this study stemmed from personal observations of individuals' grieving experiences that did not fit within the expected timeline. Individuals also presented with a physical component related to the loss. This physical component was rarely discussed. It was discovered that many believed that their physical experiences were very unique and that friends and family would not understand or would also think that they were "crazy." As such, this investigation is aimed at uncovering these body experiences in order to understand the body's experience of loss and to bring this phenomenon out of silence.

Review of the Literature

There is an abundance of research and theory devoted to the study of grieving. A common consensus that dominates the literature on grieving is that individuals need to achieve resolution of the loss and experience a degree of acceptance or peace (Cutcliffe, 1998). The process of achieving resolution has been described by Kubler-Ross and Kessler (2005) as five stages that characterize a normal grieving: denial, anger, bargaining, depression, and acceptance. Bowlby (1980) discusses three phases of mourning, beginning with preoccupation with the lost person, followed by focusing on the pain of the experience, then, finally, reorganization characterized by a return to normal functioning. The memories and the pain of the loss may still occur in the final phase but do not interfere with functioning. Symptoms related to grieving have been examined in the field of mental health. Symptoms of grief may include depression and anxiety, anger, suicidal ideation, and even post-traumatic stress disorder (PTSD; Stroebe, Hansson, Schut, & Stroebe, 2008). While grief is an unavoidable and universal experience, for some the experience is much more intense leading to what has been described as unresolved grief, protracted grief, traumatic grief, or complicated grief symptoms similar to PTSD ("Complicated grief (Cover story)," 2006).

The timeline for grieving is quite varied with some experiencing the acute grief phase up to 2 years, and others describing the grieving process continuing throughout a lifetime. According to Rando (1995), although the acute phase may be resolved, subsequent temporary upsurges of grief may occur. Such upsurges include cyclic precipitants such as anniversary reactions, holiday reactions, seasonal reactions, and ritual-prompted reactions (repetitive behaviors).

Theory and research have identified the grieving process. However, grieving as a social construct has not captured the experience of many individuals, especially in the area of body memory. Moving away from these more cognitive models toward a phenomenological lens for understanding grieving shifts how the phenomenon of grieving is viewed. Such an example of understanding the lived experience can be gleaned from the writings of C. S. Lewis (1961):

> To say a patient is getting over it after an operation for appendicitis is one thing: after he's had his leg off is quite another . . . He'll get back his strength and be able to stump about on his wooden leg. He had "got over it." But he will probably have recurrent pain in the stump all his life . . . and he will always be a one-legged man . . . His whole way of life will be changed. (p. 65)

From a phenomenological perspective, "the person with the phantom limb is living his body in the way in which he is accustomed . . . The unity of the human organism can be understood only at this level of preobjective experience" (Oiler, 1986, p. 83). In *Phenomenology of Perception*, Merleau-Ponty (1989) referred to the body as the natural self. One's body holds one's point of view on the world, and one experiences the world concretely through one's body. "The concept of embodiment informs us that consciousness is diffused throughout the body and finds expression through it. We are our bodies" (Oiler, 1986). Work by Merleau-Ponty (1989) has helped shed light on this aspect of grieving and the experience of the body: "[The] haunting of the present by a particular past experience is possible because we all carry our past with us insofar as its structures have become 'sedimented' in our habitual body" (p. 33). Munhall (1992) claimed, "it is through the body that one gains access to the world" (p. 24).

Phenomenology and case studies are well suited to explore the experience of the body following the loss of a loved one. The case study method is desirable in studies such as this one because of its complex and contextual nature. Its application is useful in situations when the researcher's aim is to investigate in-depth, real-life contexts, especially when the boundaries between the phenomenon and context are not clearly evident. As stated by Rosenberg and Yates, " the methods used in case study research are pragmatically—rather than paradigmatically— driven" (2007, p. 448). In essence the research question and the phenomenon of interest determine the research method and design.

Method

This research is a single case study design using a descriptive, phenomenological approach. The participant for this case study was a 21-year-old woman who shared her experience of losing her mother to stomach cancer on Thanksgiving day. The timeline for this story was the year leading up to the death of her mother and the 2 years following the loss. The participant volunteered to be interviewed after she had heard one of my lectures about grieving. I had mentioned that I was about to do a study on grieving with specific interest in how the body experiences grieving.

The type of case study chosen was the instrumental case study approach based on its aim to provide insight and advance understanding of a phenomenon or single unit. The single unit under investigation was the body's experience grieving the loss of a loved one. The social context is the experience of caring for the subject's mother, the relationship between the subject and her mother and the experiences prior to and following her mother's death. The research question under investigation was "How does the body experience grieving after the loss of a loved one?" Qualitative case study research include holistic, empirical, interpretive, and empathic characteristics (Stake, 1995). It should be noted that it was not possible to completely separate the body's experience from this woman's lived experience, however, body experience or body memory can be understood within the context of the life experience.

As stated by van Manen (1990), phenomenology aims at a deeper understanding of the nature or meaning of our everyday experiences. This study incorporated the four concurrent processes described by van Manen. The first process was turning to the nature of the lived experience. This involved developing the research question and the research assumptions and pre-understandings. The participant for the case study was interviewed using open-ended questions exploring the experience leading up to her mother's death and her grieving after her mother's death. The interview focused on concrete examples of the participant's experiences, including occurrences around the time of the loss, her relationship with her mother and other family members, and any specific details she found important to share. There were two in depth interviews lasting 2 hours each. Attention was given to exploring the experience as it was lived rather than interpreted or analyzed.

The second process, the existential investigation, involved exploring the phenomenon with attention to the four life worlds—temporal, spatial, corporeal, and relational (Munhall, 2007). The third process, phenomenological reflection, involved the thematic analysis. The fourth process, phenomenological writing, involved writing a case story that brings to life the body's experience grieving a loss.

Ethical Considerations

The study received approval from the university's institutional research board. The participant was informed of the purpose of the study and how the information would be used. She was informed that she was free to participate and could withdraw at any time. And, I was the only researcher involved in the review and transcription of the audio tapes.

The benefit for the participant was in being able to share an experience with someone who was interested and concerned. The other benefit was in knowing that the story may help others facing similar experiences. Because the actual interview could evoke strong emotions, the participant was informed that if she felt she needed counseling I would be able to give her the names of qualified therapists.

Remembering My Mother: The Body Grieves _____

At the time of the interview Jill was a 21-year-old in her third year of college. The loss of her mother to stomach cancer occurred when she was 9 years old. Jill recounted how the experience was still a vivid memory. Before her mother's death, Jill lived with her mother, grandmother, and younger sister. Her mother had been divorced for 2 years, and both her mother and grandmother worked to make ends meet.

Jill talked in detail about her relationships. Her story follows.

We didn't have much, but we had each other. I was very close to my mom and grandmother and even my 4-year-old sister. I could tell my mother anything, and she would always listen. Somehow she made everything okay. We would cook together and I really did not mind cleaning up, because we all did it together. Then the worst thing imaginable happened, my mother was diagnosed with stomach cancer in January and soon she was unable to work. I spent that year caring for my mother along with my grandmother and my aunt who had taken a year off of work to help. My mother did not do well. She was in a lot of pain and it was hard watching her get thinner and thinner. It was hard on all of us. I remember how scared I was that I would not have my mother with me while I was growing up. My sister did not really understand which was also hard for me.

Things really got worse that November. Each day my mother ate less and less. I found that I also had a hard time eating. I was exhausted. I had a hard time concentrating in school and did not want to be around friends. I just wanted to spend what time I could with my mother. I was losing her. The mother I knew was fading away. She was getting weaker and weaker and even though she tried to listen to me I knew she did not have the energy. I tried to be strong for her, but I was also feeling sick. My stomach was hurting and I had lost my appetite. November was the worst. There was so much suffering. Everyday it was harder and harder to hold on. I felt like I could not breathe and I was scared and anxious. I felt empty. I don't know how else to describe it but emptiness.

My mother died on Thanksgiving and I remember the pain and then just feeling empty.

That next year was very difficult but living with my sister and grandmother made it a little easier. A year later, November, I remember was very weird.

Everything had been going okay. I was going to school and things were going well. I was really happy and had reconnected with friends, and then I just found myself crying. Something was bothering me but I did not know what. I was sad but I did not know why. I felt tired and had low energy and I did not want to do anything with my friends. And then, I lost my appetite, and then by December things did get better and I was feeling better.

The next year went along and things were going well. And again as November approached my stomach was upset and I could not eat. I was now 11 years old and my grandmother took me to the doctor who told us that I was anorexic and therapy was recommended. I went to therapy and we talked about eating and body image but I told the therapist, that I didn't think I was fat and I didn't think I needed to lose weight. My appetite returned after a month. The next year it was the same, and then it hit me that it was not about eating, it was about my mother's death. It was basically the month of November when I lost my appetite and had stomach problems.

I am now 21 years old and Novembers are still hard but it has gotten better over time. I still notice that I get sicker around that time of year. My stomach is upset and I have a hard time eating. I get more colds and I feel tired. My body goes through it first and then my mind knows what is happening. I could not even know what time of year it is and have no concept of time and I would be able to tell it is November every year. It never fails. It is inside of me. Some years when it was too much I basically shut down. All the feelings of anger and the sadness I felt when I was 9 would resurface right around the exact same time. In the last few years I know what it is and I journal and that helps. Each year I feel it and understand it more. It is actually a lot better now. I journal more during November. Each year it gets better and better but there is still always that kind of feeling of floating and not being connected. This year was actually the first year that I was not afraid of that month. I felt like I understood it and I knew I could get through it. I reflect on how I need to move forward.

Body Memory: Relived as Lived

Jill's body experienced the loss as it was lived. Awareness of the body memory had been essential for her to understand her grieving process since the experience had sedimented in her body and continues to be expressed around the anniversary of the loss. As Merleau-Ponty (1989) stated, "[The] haunting of the present by a particular past experience is possible because we all carry our past with us insofar as its structures have become 'sedimented' in our habitual body" (p. 33). The timeline for Jill was around the anniversary of the loss, November. Jill's experience of body memory was not a rational process that she could easily resolve by cognitive strategies or through coping skills training alone. Through awareness of the body's expression of grief, Jill has been able to more fully understand the meaning of the loss and integrate it into her life. For Jill, attempting to suppress or ignore the body was not an option.

Conclusions

In this case study, the researcher has sought to broaden the understanding of the grieving process incorporating body memory as a key element of our consciousness and knowing. Herein lies the potential for new applications for practice. Traditional models of grief counseling with emphasis on cognitive, emotional, and behavioral outcomes need to be revisited. Along with acknowledging the body memory comes the need to develop approaches that give these experiences a voice. There needs to be further exploration of how to help those who are grieving bring voice and meaning to their body memory experiences in order to assist them with finding personal meaning and healing.

Beyond this focus on grieving, the body carries all types of memories. Future studies in the area of body memory offer the potential for a richer understanding and expansion of our view on how to respond to human needs.

References

Bowlby, J. (1980). *Loss: Sadness and depression. Attachment and loss trilogy* (Vol. 3). New York: Basic Books.

Cassem, E. H. (2000). The person confronting death. In A. Nicholi (Ed.) *Harvard guide to psychiatry* (pp. 699–731). Cambridge, MA: Belknap.

Cutcliffe, J. R. (1998). Hope counseling and complicated bereavement reactions. *Journal of Advanced Nursing, 28*(4), 754–761.

Hentz, P. (2002). The body remembers: Grieving and a circle of time. *Qualitative health research, 12*(2), 161–172.

Kubler-Ross, E., & Kessler, D. (2005). *On grief and grieving: Finding the meaning of grief through the five stages of loss.* New York: Scribner.

Lewis, C. S. (1961). *A grief observed.* New York: Harper Collins.

Merleau-Ponty, M. (1989). *Phenomenology of perception* (M. M. Langer, Trans.). Tallahassee, FL: Florida State University Press.

Munhall, P. L. (1992). Holding the Mississippi River in place and other implications for qualitative research. *Nursing Outlook, 10,* 257–262.

Munhall, P. L. (2007). A phenomenological method. In P. L. Munhall (Ed.), *Nursing research: A qualitative perspective* (4th ed., pp. 145–210). Sudbury, MA: Jones & Bartlett.

Oiler, C. J. (1986). Qualitative methods: Phenomenology. In P. Moccia (Ed.), *New approaches to theory development* (pp. 75–103). New York: National League for Nursing Press.

Oiler-Boyd, C. (1993). Phenomenology: The method. In P. Munhall & C. Oiler-Boyd (Eds.), *Nursing research: A qualitative perspective* (pp. 99–132). New York: National League for Nursing Press.

Rondo, T. A. (1995). Grief and mourning accommodating to loss. In H. Wass & R. A. Neimeyer (Eds.), *Dying: Facing the facts* (3rd ed., pp. 211–241). Washington, DC: Taylor & Francis.

Rosenberg, J. P., & Yates, P. M. (2007). Schematic representation of case study research designs. *Journal of Advanced Nursing, 24,* 447–452.

Stake, R. E. (1995). *The art of case study research.* Thousand Oaks, CA: Sage.

Stake, R. E. (2005). Qualitative case studies. In N. K. Danzin & Y. A. Lincoln (Eds.), *Handbook of qualitative research.* Thousand Oaks, CA: Sage.

Stroebe, M., Hansson, R., Schut, H., & Storbe, W. (Eds). (2008). *Handbook of bereavement research and practice.* Washington, D.C.: American Psychological Association.

van Manen, M. (1990). *Research lived experience.* New York: State University of New York Press.

Yin, R. K. (2003). *Case study research* (3rd ed.). Thousand Oaks, CA: Sage.

Yin, R. K. (2009). *Case study research: Design and methods* (4th ed.). Los Angeles, CA: Sage.

14

Historical Research

Karen Saucier Lundy

History does not refer merely, or even principally, to the past. On the contrary, the great force of history comes from the fact that we carry it with us, are unconsciously controlled by it, in many ways, and history is literally present in all that we do.

—James Baldwin

The purpose of any scholarly inquiry in nursing is the production of knowledge that will be of value to the profession. Historical research can advance professional nursing incorporating insights from the past into present practice (Cohen, Manion, & Morrison, 1998). Many of the extraordinary accomplishments of the 20th century and the present are continuations of contributions and innovations from the past (Donahue, 1996). Elements of continuity between past and present also exist. For example, midwives continue to practice in the United States, although in a different role and with a smaller proportion of the childbearing population than in the early colonial period. The 2005 public health crisis resulting from the unprecedented Hurricane Katrina disaster in New Orleans and the Gulf Coast caught most by surprise. By looking at disasters throughout history, such as the sinking of the Titanic in 1912, we can understand more completely how other generations reacted to the unthinkable cataclysmic collision of human progress with nature (Lundy & Janes, 2009).

Health, disease, birth, and death are the most basic of human experiences; their histories are reflections of social conditions and the historical agents of change (Jones & Eren, 2005; Hemphill, 1980). Nursing students are exposed to extensive research on a variety of demographics, such as disease mortality statistics about specific conditions, but rarely are these demographics traced over time. Diseases are covered in terms of present pathological etiologies, but rarely are diseases presented as resulting from political, economic, and social changes (Jones & Eren, 2005). Changes in medical treatment over time from home to hospital and back to the community have all had a significant impact on the everyday lives of Americans and the role of the nurse (Church, 1987). The experiences of health, disease, medicine, and nursing are reflections of social conditions as well as scientific concepts (Libster, 2009). How we conceptualize health and our expectations of who delivers care at what price continues to be a hotly contested political debate at the national level (Reverby, 1987).

Historical research, in an effort to establish *bodies of evidence* from the past allows us to learn something from the past, which will help with the understanding of current and future issues in health care (Streubert & Carpenter, 1999). Scholars can better understand the world and illuminate human nature through historical research, which can "provide us with the potentialities through the course of time and provide hints about the future of humankind" (Dilthey, 1962, p. 12). For example, the history of Alcoholics Anonymous (AA) can be used to explore the rise of the contemporary self-help movement and the changing meaning of substance abuse over time. Our ideas of history reflect our philosophical, political, religious, and moral values and, at the same time, reinforce them. For a more recent historical analysis of U.S. military nursing experience in the Iraqi and Afghan wars, see Scannell-Desch and Doherty's (2010) research.

In addition to creating a body of evidence, historical research can illuminate previous historical accounts. Conflict between what has been written and what was actually experienced in the past can be clarified through historical research (Sweeney, 2005). For example, women's role in society often colored how events about the nurse's role were reported and perceived in the past. As Hallett and Fealy (2009) contend, "Perhaps a clearer understanding of its own history is one of the ways in which the nursing profession can grasp a sense of its own potential for power" p. 2683. Our conceptions govern not only what we select as relevant from the mass of historical facts but also what forces we believe determine the course of events (Dilthey, 1962; Lynaugh, 2009).

When studying a contemporary health issue such as substance abuse or violence, the history of individuals or of the issues themselves provide the critical contextual link of the past to the present (Sweeney, 2005). Backward glances help us "critically evaluate our own convictions," according to Dilthey (1962, p. 14). With the present research focus on evidence-based nursing practice, findings from the past can illuminate potential solutions now. Rapid and unprecedented changes in nursing practice and health care throughout the past century have been paralleled by research development over the past century (Hargreaves,

2008; Reverby, 1987). Earlier research, dating from the middle of the 20th century, focused on what nursing was and what nurses did in practice. One of the earliest writings on the need for historical research in nursing was Newton's (1965) landmark article, "The Case for Historical Research." Prior to Newton's seminal work, there were few published research studies in nursing history.

> *The untrained nurse is as old as the human race; the trained nurse is a recent discovery. The distinction between the two is a sharp commentary on the follies and the prejudices of mankind.*
> —Victor Robinson

Phenomenological research emerged in the last half of the 20th century that explored the nature and meaning of nursing itself. For example, Benner (1984) examined ways in which nurses' experience and education influenced practice. Rafferty (1996) argued that nursing knowledge is a political issue and, as such, the introduction of new ideas and programs into the profession needs to be fully explored in specific historical social context. Using a *historical research design* is of particular relevance to research about contemporary social and cultural issues as it enhances our understanding of the present (Burke, 1991). Any contemporary issue is bound intrinsically with the social and historical milieu of the past (Breisach, 1994; Reverby, 1987; Sweeney, 2005). Lynaugh (2009) remarked that "the history of nursing *is* nursing; nursing historians must help our colleagues and our students to know the history of our profession as it really was and is" (pp. 9–10). Most historical research involves some conceptual idea, theme, or person in history (Butterfield, 1981). For example, the current debate about entry and licensure issues for advanced nursing practice can be more fully understood when examining the role of early leaders, such as Loretta C. Ford. Dr. Ford was the nurse cofounder of the first nurse practitioner program at the University of Colorado, which sparked the development of a new and expanded role for nurses in the United States.

Contemporary nurses stand in a markedly different relationship with society and its powerbrokers than did their forebears in the 19th and 20th centuries (Connolly & Rogers, 2005). However, nurses will always have societal powerbrokers that mediate and intervene on their behalf (Hallett & Fealy, 2009). As Hallett and Fealy (2009) contend:

> Often unable to find their way through the labyrinth of established authority structure . . . nurses frequently were required to work around the margins of authority to set the agenda of their own practice and determine the type of care that they wished to deliver. (p. 2682)

Through historical research, we can better understand how nurses in the present can assume control of their practice, education, and roles in the contemporary healthcare system.

Definition of Terms

Historical research is most often associated with *historiography* as a primary research method. *Historiography* is the synthesis of gathering data in a particular period in history in order to analyze and develop theoretical and holistic conclusions (Austin, 1958). It includes a critical examination of sources, interpretation of data, and analysis that focuses on the narrative, interpretation, and use of valid and reliable evidence that supports the study conclusions. Historiography is considered a meta-level, analytical-historical description of the past. By contrast, a historian studies history or may teach history, while the historiographer writes, analyzes, and interprets history (Austin, 1958; Christy, 1975).

Stages in Historical Research Design

> *Treasure is uncovered by the force of flowing water and is buried by the same currents.*
>
> —Paulo Coelho

Historical researchers are often depicted as "detectives," looking under many different stones for clues, rather than simply describing the appearance and location of the stones (Lundy, 2008). The *first stage* of a historical study is the identification of a researchable phenomenon and includes the reading of relevant literature that reflects the researcher's interest (Austin, 1958; Fox, 1982). Before the researcher begins the formal search process, examining background information on the topic can provide necessary information in developing the focus of the study. The researcher then selects a particular person, phenomena, or era to study in the context of study's focus (Butterfield, 1981). As an example, a nurse historian interested in the contemporary obsession with fitness and appearance among teens and adults might find historical evidence about body image during the Victorian era particularly valuable.

The *second stage* involves developing hypotheses or research questions and identifying a theoretical perspective to guide the data collection process and interpretation of results. A theoretical framework can provide a guide for the historical study, both in data collection and analysis (Lusk, 1997). Although some historians dispute the need for such a framework, many historiographers contend that a theoretical perspective helps the researcher focus and decipher historical events as recorded (Christy, 1975). The historical investigation and analysis concern "knowable truth." The surviving data strongly influence the careful analysis, synthesis, and interpretation of data sources (Lusk, 1997).

The *third stage* involves the data exploration and collection which is usually the most time- and labor-intensive part of the research process, depending on the subject and accessibility of data sources (Lusk, 1997; Austin, 1958). The *fourth* stage includes fact checking, evaluation of the validity and reliability of data and the analysis of evidence from each source. During this stage, the researcher evaluates the data, including the analysis and meaning of missing data, and forms generalizations when possible. At this stage the researcher forms conclusions, answers the research question, or accepts or rejects the hypotheses (Lusk, 1997; Newton, 1965). The *final stage* of historical research involves writing the report that describes findings and their interpretation, and provides detailed supportive evidence in defense of the conclusions (Christy, 1975; Sweeney, 2005).

Data Collection

Historical researchers in their investigation of the past often treat data as "witnesses in a trial." According to Dilthey (1962), history is one of the forms of research "by which the human mind satisfies its curiosity and orients itself in the world" (p. 13). The historical method is more than the simple search for facts about the historical story (Lundy, 2008). A historical investigation includes the meaning of events, which are analyzed based on the availability of surviving data, such as documents, paintings, literature, or secondary resources, which include stories and accounts (Austin, 1958; Breisach, 1994; Hallett, 1998). All the data should be evaluated with a critical eye, using a variety of primary and secondary sources, knowing, as Ginzburg (1992) cautions, that "no archival sources are neutral" (p. 160). Authors of archival material consistently try "to make people believe their version of the truth" (Ginzburg, 1992, p. 160). Dilthey (1962) contends that as historical researchers, "we can never examine our subject first hand in all its complexity. This luxury of present research is forever denied the historian" (p. 14).

Primary sources

Primary sources include first-person accounts of events, in original documents, letters, artwork, literature, music, observational notes, journals, and photographs. Primary sources enable the researcher to get as close as possible to what actually happened during an historical event or time period. Primary sources were either created during the time period being studied or produced at a later date by a participant or eyewitness of the event (as in the case of memoirs), and they reflect the individual viewpoint of a participant or observer. The historical researcher seeks to understand society (i.e., institutions, laws, customs) by tracing the way in which the past has brought about the present (Dilthey, 1962). Primary sources may be in their original format or may have been reproduced later in a different format, including translated, transcribed, or printed documents, books, microfilm collections, videos, and Internet archives, so long as the later version is an authentic and accurate "word-for-word" rendering of the original (Scott, 1990; Haskell, 1998). Handwritten documents, for example, are sometimes published in printed collections by academic presses in an effort to make them easier for researchers to access and to read, such as those that have been translated from the original language. Types of primary sources include, but are not limited to legal documents, such as wills, contracts, or court proceedings; an individual's diary or journal; letters, photographs, music, and art (Howell & Prevenier, 2002). An example of a primary source is the trial transcripts of all the trials of Joan of Arc from the 13th century in France. Written originally in Latin and French, these important first person accounts (albeit legal witnesses) are now available in English translations on the Internet and have been verified by French historical experts. These original sources of data hold the greatest value in the validity and reliability of historical analysis (Lusk, 1997; Sorensen, 1988; Fox, 1982).

Although primary sources are the most critical data for historical research, the use of primary data sources is generally not sufficient proof that the described event actually occurred. A critical analysis of primary resources may reveal that the author, writer, or creator of the primary source reflects the perspective of the writer, observer, or witness, and the accuracy of what truly occurred may be compromised (Foner, 2002). This must be carefully evaluated by the researcher when considering the validity of the original source.

Historical researchers also recognize that original documents are only a trace of what remains of a historical event. They are greatly influenced by the perception, biases, selective survival of the document, and are limited to specific groups of people in society whose accounts have survived, such as the educated and literate (Lusk, 1997; Foner, 2002). People who had little power in a culture—women, lower classes, and minorities, for example—have produced few primary resources. This paucity is primarily the result of illiteracy and the use of oral rather than written historical records, as well as the belief that the work of the powerless was not valuable enough to be preserved. For instance, the recorded trials of accused "witches" during the medieval period in Europe reflect only the version of reality of the officials who conducted the trials and interrogations. There are few first person accounts from the perspective of the women themselves other than forced confessions. The women, who were accused, convicted, and eventually burned at the stake as punishment, were usually illiterate and their stories as primary sources are unavailable to researchers (Lundy, 2008). As George Orwell observed, "History is written by the winners."

Secondary sources
Secondary sources are derived from letters, diaries, and narratives from persons who were not eyewitnesses of the event or did not personally know the person who is the focus of the study. This category of sources is somewhat easier to define, understand, and access. A secondary source is any item that was created after the historical event. Secondary sources also include summaries, personal

interpretations, and views, and include simple descriptions of primary sources that do not reproduce the original "word-for-word" (Denzin & Lincoln, 1998). Types of secondary sources include biographies and accounts written many years after the event, even if written by an eyewitness many years afterward (e.g., a first-person account of a 70 year old who was a child at the time of the event). Critical analysis of these secondary sources follows the same criteria as for primary resources (Scott, 1990; Sorensen, 1988; Christy, 1975). Secondary sources are works that interpret or analyze an historical event or phenomenon; in other words, they are at least one step removed from the event. Additional examples include scholarly or popular books and articles, reference books, biographies, and textbooks. Included in secondary resources are persons who recollect the event, person, or experience even though they were not witness to these experiences (Scott, 1990).

Sampling

Sampling can be quite diverse in nature depending on the availability of existing or surviving documents and other sources. More than in other research designs, the researcher attempts to locate every relevant documentary source related to the phenomena (Fairman, 1987; Lusk, 1997; Sorensen, 1985, 1988).

As previously discussed, the researcher should assume that many documents and other data sources have been lost, destroyed, or deliberately suppressed, thus distorting the true nature of the event or phenomena (Morse, 1995; Foner, 2002). The literate and educated members of societies and cultures (usually males) were in positions of power, such as church and political leaders. They were the primary authors of the vast majority of official primary and secondary sources until the last 2 centuries. Young girls and women often wrote letters or kept diaries, which are considered valuable first-person accounts (Hanson & Donahue, 1996). A well-known example is the diary of Anne Frank, a primary source, written by a young teen girl who experienced the Holocaust by hiding her family in Amsterdam. Anne Frank's diaries gave historians a valuable perspective of the Holocaust and persecution of the Jews in Europe that did not exist in official documents. Artwork created by those in concentration camps of World War II and Third Reich propaganda films are other examples of primary data which add validity and reliability to historical sources. Secondary sources in the example of the German Holocaust include diaries, journals, and interviews with children and relatives of those who died during World War II. Many researchers in all disciplines have examined this horrendous event in our civilizations' history and their collected data sources can provide valuable secondary sources.

> *Historical truth does exist, not in the scientific sense, but as a reasonable approximation of the past.*
>
> —Eric Foner

The selection of data samples is based on the purpose of the research. This may seem obvious, but historical relics are often broad in nature, while only a small portion of the documentary evidence is relevant to the research question. Due to the nature of what humans leave behind, there exist varying degrees of value in historical data (Lundy, 2008). For example, finding documents that include unfamiliar or unrelated information (such as language translation issues and unknown references) can be a distraction from the purpose of the study and is time consuming (Scott, 1990; Haskell, 1998). However, this discovery phase can assist the researcher and further refine the study and/or research question. Essentially, historical research is a "translation of translations."

Locating Data Sources

Diaries, photographs, art, literature, minutes of meetings, eyewitness accounts in newspapers or other official documents, court records, letters, maps, and other relevant sources can often be found in university and specialty collections. Government websites and collections are also excellent beginning points for locating data sources, as are special collections from museums and art galleries (Williamson, Karp, & Dalphin, 2005). Many of these can now be located on the Internet. For example, primary and secondary resources for the Holocaust, including video recordings of Holocaust survivors, can be located on the website of the U.S. Holocaust Memorial Museum: www.ushmm.org,. The largest collection of art in the world, the Louvre Museum in Paris, France now displays art, which can inform historical research, on its website: www.louvre.fr. An excellent website produced by the University of California at Berkeley libraries can assist in evaluating primary sources on the Internet (http://www.lib.berkeley.edu/TeachingLib/Guides/PrimarySourcesOnTheWeb.html). Films from a particular time period can be located easily from the Internet Movie Database (www.imdb.com). Historical research sources often overlooked include a variety of art forms such as paintings, sculpture, poetry, music, and literature. Art can depict the shifts and changes in the social, cultural, and political context of history.

Documentary research using multiple sources and methods of data gathering is defined as *theoretical eclecticism* (Hammersley, 1993). This unique combination of methods to investigate social issues evolved from the Chicago School of Sociology. Specific criteria for inclusion and exclusion of documentary sources should be explicit in the documentation of sources. Justification for documentary inclusion may include the following criteria: authenticity, credibility, representativeness, and meaning (Scott, 1990). *Authenticity* refers to the genuineness of the documents (Hargreaves, 2008). *Credibility* refers to how selective or distorted the contents might be (Platt, 1981). *Representativeness* relates to the relative rank of these documents in the totality of relevant documents that might be available (Hargreaves, 2008). Other documents may be included for comparative purposes, which can speak to the representative status of selected documents for analysis (Brooks, 1969). *Meaning* relates to the ease or difficulty of deriving understanding from the documents. For example, a document source may have been partially destroyed, written in an ancient language, or accompanying images may be illegible (Hargreaves, 2008). Scott (1990) contends that documents seldom tell the whole story; however, the story that is retrieved is interesting in its own right. Hammersley (1993) acknowledges that the reasons why a document was written, the words used, and the intended audience are all significant and should be included in data-collection citations.

Critical thinking and observation should be used in historical research, whether the research involves listening to music or recordings of the era, reading carefully and knowing the language and expressions of the era, taking extensive notes from primary sources that cannot be reproduced, observing art of the era for cultural expression, and examining the artifacts of the era, when possible. Rigor and systematic data collection is critical, including seeking assistance from archivists, historical experts in the subject area, and when possible, visiting physical locations of the historical phenomena (Williamson, Karp, & Dalphin, 2005; Kaestle, 1992). Data should always be labeled and dated, authorship identified, including whether the author was a witness to the events or phenomena and the relation of author to phenomena.

Types of Historical Research

Historical research can take many forms, depending on the purpose of the research as well as the availability and quality of data and resources (and time and finances) available to the researcher. Several types of historical designs are described in this section, but they represent only a select few of the historical research methods that may be used (Gottschalk, 1969).

Oral history is a biographical approach in which the researcher gathers personal recollections of events from a living individual through audio and video recordings (Sorensen, 1985). Oral history can include written works of an individual who has died, but is primarily limited to living individuals. The oral historical method begins with general standardized questions about the person's demographic information, explains the purpose of an oral history, and maintains an informal tone to the entire process (Brooks, 1969). Most researcher questions and comments are unstructured although a general interview schedule may be employed to guide the story when prompting is needed. This method provides the respondent or "storyteller" with a natural and effective environment that allows a reciprocal interchange between the researcher and the respondent. The respondent, as the oral historical interview proceeds, generally moves beyond the initial formality of the standard, focused interview. This allows for nonverbal expression of the listener; such responses can motivate the storyteller to become more involved and energetic. Many oral histories are located in university collections and are available on the Internet. Studs Terkel, an oral historian whose best-selling histories celebrated the common people he called "the noncelebrated," produced oral histories on race relations, older Americans, and World War II veterans. Turkel (1974) advocated moving beyond the famous and powerful in the study of history:

> When the Chinese Wall was built, where did the masons go for lunch? When Caesar conquered Gall, was there not even a cook in the army? And here's the big one, when the Spanish Armada sank, you read that King Phillip wept: Were there no other tears?" (pp. 6–9)

Autobiographical narrative is an account of a person's life that is written or recorded by the respondent. A biographical narrative account of a person's life can be either told to the researcher or found in archives, documents, and other sources.

Life history or *life story* is a biographical writing in the form of an extensive record of a person's life as told to the researchers (Grypma, 2005). The life history of a person involves a living individual. Life stories are used for different reasons, but a predominant theme is "to reach, explore, celebrate, and reveal those who are marginalized and hidden from view" (Maggs, 1985, p. 75).

Case study is a type of historical research that examines individuals, a small group of participants, or a group as a whole. This method sheds light on a phenomenon by studying in-depth a single case example of the phenomenon. The case can be an individual person, an event, a group, or an institution (Lusk, 1997; Hanson & Donahue, 1996). Case studies take a relatively small sample of research subjects as a source of in-depth, qualitative information. An example of a case study is researching the concept of *antisepsis* through historical analysis of 19th-century medical and nursing practice innovators, Nightingale, Semmelweis, and Lister (Larson, 1989).

Reliability and Validity

Establishing authenticity is a challenging and critical aspect of historical research. As has been previously discussed, surviving artifacts of history are often a result of "selection bias"—the survival itself of the documents is significant. *Validity* is related to the external critique of the data. In other words, does the document or artifact represent an authentic representation of what it is intended to be? This can be determined by age of the document, such as the paper, writing style of the author, origin, and consistency with other evidence. Verification by experts is often included in the external validation process (Booth, Colomb, & Williams, 2003; Scott, 1990). Data should include at least two sources of the same type of information (Ashley, 1978). This can be two primary sources, which concur without conflict or disagreement, or one primary source and one independent secondary source, which corroborates the primary source and does not contain any substantial contradictory information. The researcher, even with intense scrutiny of the data sources, must always consider the possibility that primary sources were altered after the original event. Primary sources should always be used when possible, rather than secondary sources (Lusk, 1997; Christy, 1975; Scott, 1990).

Internal criticism of data constitutes the *reliability* of data sources. The researcher attempts to extract meaning from the data and establish the context from which it was derived, the trustworthiness of data sources, such as the author's biases and perceptions of the event, and whether authors are reporting from intimate knowledge or from others' descriptions of the phenomena. The researcher must be vigilant about including both positive and negative criticism of all data sources, including missing accounts and the lack of relevant viewpoints and persons involved in events. Understanding the way in which contemporary words and phrases are used in contrast to past usage and meanings is critical to establishing reliability. *Abortion*, for example, did not always have the social and medical definitions currently ascribed to the term. Reading and analyzing secondary sources can often provide the researcher with clarification of language use and artistic interpretations and alterations of historical events (Lusk, 1997; Christy, 1975; Scott, 1990; Austin, 1958).

Data Analysis

Interpretation of meaning occurs at the analytic stage. Extensive examples should be used, with excerpts from documents and other artifacts. Although most historical research is based on incomplete data, the researcher must extend and derive opinion beyond what is discovered and is known from the data-collection process. A critical description of historical evidence, an evaluation of its historical significance to contemporary society, and creative narratives are provided in the written research report, including the inferences derived, probabilities. The researcher should include all sources in a reference list and footnotes about the sources that reflect the corroboration of facts, as evidence of reliability and validity of the findings. Excerpts from the sources should also be used to enhance the quality of the research (Lusk, 1997; Christy, 1975; Scott, 1990; Sweeney, 2005).

Standards for Evaluating Historical Research

For historical research to be meaningful, standards of professional research should be employed that allow for comparison, replication, and application of results. Streubert and Carpenter (1999) developed specific guidelines for evaluating historical research and include four categories for analysis: *data generation, data treatment, data analysis,* and *interpretation of findings.*

Data Generation

Assessment of data generation includes title appraisal, subject statement, and literature review. An informative title should include the specific population or subject of study without vernacular or culture-bound references. The purpose, subject, or thesis and period in history should be clearly identified (Streubert & Carpenter, 1999). A concise statement of the subject is included in the abstract and defines the topic, justifies the researcher's interest in the subject, and establishes its relevancy to nursing. The literature review establishes the study within a larger framework, substantiates the researcher's knowledge about prior explorations, and inquires into the topic. The literature review should also include the researcher's perspective on how the study adds to prior knowledge and allows the reader to identify divergent viewpoints (Hewitt, 1997).

Data Treatment

Assessment of primary and secondary sources is a critical part of a study's integrity. Historical studies are evaluated by the use of primary and secondary archival sources and this information should be included in the abstract (Streibert & Carpenter, 1999). Primary and secondary sources should be clearly identified by source, location, and conditions of archives in adequate detail for readers to verify and substantiate the study's data sources. The historical researcher works with materials from the past that must be verified as genuine and authentic. As such, historical research must be analyzed through *external criticism* to determine the genuineness of the data and *internal criticism* to determine the truthfulness of the source material. External criticism refers to the historian's accountability to establish that primary sources are genuine and not forgeries or otherwise misrepresented. *Internal criticism* refers to authenticity, which is truthfulness of content. Comparing secondary sources with the primary sources can help establish authenticity and genuineness (Lusk, 1997). Additionally, the research process using a historical design requires corroboration from related research studies and background research of the time period being studied (Hewitt, 1997).

Data Analysis

Study organization involves the identification of a theoretical framework, a research question, and purpose, and should identify bias and potential ethical issues. A theoretical or conceptual framework, if present, provides a structural approach for a historical study and should be evaluated for relevance to the study. The research question should be clearly focused in succinct terms on the nature of the research. Assessing the purpose of the research is closely related to an analysis of the research question. The purpose should clearly state the focus and boundaries of the research in context of the nursing profession. Bias and ethical considerations are critical as with all research. Therefore, the researcher must guard carefully against evaluating the historical findings with a present-day perspective bias. The researcher should state explicitly any personal connection or investment in the study.

Interpretation of Findings

Effectiveness of the narrative and significance to nursing should be described sufficiently. Historical findings must be presented in a clear and interesting narrative manner with connections to the present. This can be done with effective use and selection of quotations from the archival material, as well as with contextual situating of the findings in a holistic framework. Historical research is significant to the nursing profession through the connections of the past to the present from the past (Hewitt, 1997). For example, a recent historical study about the role of nurses in implementing the children's euthanasia program in Nazi Germany can promote an ethical dialogue about the contextual nature of nursing as influenced by the political milieu (Benedict, Shields, & O'Donnell, 2009).

Future Trends in Historical Research

During the past several years, technology has advanced the use of the Internet for correspondence of both primary and secondary sources. As technology has advanced, fewer people keep hard-copy diaries, journals, or handwritten letters. Those who deliver speeches often do not write them verbatim, as was once the case. Oral history is similar to the ancient cultural practice known as storytelling. Storytelling has most often been associated with the oral traditions of the undereducated and less developed cultures and was often expressed as part of a society's entertainment, rather than for leaving historical evidence. Yet, storytelling is an important historical method since stories carry on traditions, community and cultural paradigms, and moral and ethical codes of conduct. Contemporary examples, such as emails, blogs, and instant messaging, create challenges for historians accustomed to depending on handwritten letters and traditional data sources. Historical research will change as most correspondence and eyewitness accounts are recorded on the Internet, challenging the traditional manner in which historical researchers have collected data. This will expand historical research data sources for the researcher through the use of virtual historical research.

The growth of the Internet and other electronic devices used for data storage continue to evolve in the virtual world. A significant body of material of interest to the historical researcher is either created, stored or accessed electronically. For example, Florence Nightingale's extensive journals and letters can now be accessed on the Internet. Prior to this technological availability, nurse historians often had limited access to such primary resources.

Internet data must be evaluated with the same rigor that previous historians have used to ensure credibility of sources. This presents a new challenge in the validation and verification of authentic sources. Rapidly changing technology provides the historical researcher with unlimited access to data while concomitantly challenging scholars with the need to accurately date and reference data sources. Trinkle (1998) cautions the historical researcher to remain vigilant about the ever-present revisionist nature which exists via Internet data sources.

Summary

Historical research is underutilized in nursing. Using historical research design, nurse scholars can expand and illuminate our understanding of the present. It can further promote interdisciplinary collaboration with colleagues in the humanities and social science as we seek to understand more fully the connections and complexity of human experience. Those who engage in historical research understand the need for continuing to study history and, in the process, they will help contemporary nurses better understand not just the past, but the choices we make today. "We are first of all historical beings, and after that, contemplators of history; only because we are the one, do we become the other" (Dilthey, 1962, 1966).

References

Ashley, C. (1978). Foundations for scholarship: Historical research in nursing. *Advances in Nursing Science, 1*, 25–36.

Austin, A. L. (1958). The historical method in nursing. *Nursing Research, 7*(1), 4–10.

Benedict, S., Shields, L., & O'Donnell, A. (2009). Children's "euthanasia" in Nazi Germany. *Journal of Pediatric Nursing, 24*(6), 506–516.

Benner, P. (1984). *From novice to expert: Excellence and power in clinical nursing practice.* Menlo Park, CA: Addison Wesley.

Booth, W. C., Colomb, G. G., & Williams, J. M. (2003). *The craft of research* (2nd ed.). Chicago: University of Chicago Press.

Breisach, E. (1994). *Historiography: Ancient, medieval & modern.* Chicago: University of Chicago Press.

Brooks, P. C. (1969). *Research in archives: The use of unpublished sources.* Chicago: University of Chicago Press.

Burke, P. (Ed.). (1991). *New perspectives on historical writing.* University Park, PA: Pennsylvania State University Press.

Butterfield, H. (1981). *The origins of history.* New York: Basic Books.

Christy, R. E. (1975). The methodology of historical research: A brief introduction. *Nursing Research, 24*(3), 189–192.

Church, O. M. (1987). Historiography in nursing research. *Western Journal of Nursing Research, 9*(2), 275–279.

Cohen, L., Manion, L., & Morrison, K. (1998). *Research methods in education* (5th ed.). London: Routledge Falmer.

Connolly, C., & Rogers, N. (2005). Who is the nurse? Rethinking the history of gender and medicine. *OAH Magazine of History, 19*(5), 45–49.

Denzin, N. K., & Lincoln, Y. S. (1998). *Strategies of qualitative inquiry.* Thousand Oaks, CA: Sage.

Dilthey, W. (1962). *Pattern and meaning in history: Thought on history and society.* New York: Harper and Brothers.

Donahue, M .P. (1996). *Nursing, the finest art: An illustrated history* (2nd ed.). St. Louis, MO: Mosby.

Fairman, J. (1987). Sources and references for research in nursing history. *Nursing Research, 36*(1), 56–59.

Foner, E. (2002). *Who owns history? Rethinking the past in a changing world.* New York: Hill and Wang.

Fox, D. J. (1982). *Fundamentals of research in nursing* (4th ed.). Norwalk: Appleton Century Crofts.

Ginzburg, C. (1992). *Clues, myths, and the historical method* (Trans. J. Tedeschi & A. C. Tedeschi). Baltimore, MD: The Johns Hopkins University Press.

Gottschalk, L. (1969). *Understanding history. A primer of historical method* (2nd ed.). New York: Knopf.

Grypma, S. (2005). Critical issues in the use of biographic methods in nursing history. *Nursing History Review, 13,* 171–187.

Hallett, C. (1998). Historical texts: Factors affecting their interpretation. *Nurse Researcher, 5*(2), 61–71.

Hallett, C., & Fealy, G. M. (2009). Nursing history and the articulation of power. *Journal of Clinical Nursing, 18,* 2681–2693.

Hammersley, M. (1993). *Social research: Philosophy, politics and practice.* London: Sage.

Hanson, K., & Donahue, M. P. (1996). The diary as historical evidence: The case of Sarah Gallop Gregg. *Nursing History Review, 4,* 169–186.

Hargreaves, J. (2008). *The good nurse: Discourse and power in nurse education 1945–1955. Doctoral Dissertation.* Huddlesfield, UK: University of Huddersfield Library.

Haskell, T. (1998). *Objectivity is not neutrality: Explanatory schemes in history.* Baltimore, MD: The Johns Hopkins University Press.

Hemphill, M. M. (1980). *Fevers, floods and famines: A history of Sunflower County Mississippi, 1844–1976.* Indianola, MS: Indianola Press.

Hewitt, L. C. (1997). Historical research in nursing: Standards for research and evaluation. *Journal of the New York State Nurses Association, 28*(3), 16–20.

Howell, M. C., & Prevenier, W. (2002). *From reliable sources: An introduction to historical methods.* Ithaca, NY: Cornell University Press.

Jones, K. W., & Eren, J. (2005). Introduction. *Organization of American History Magazine of History, 19*(5), 4–7.

Kaestle, C. F. (1992). Standards of evidence in historical research: How do we know when we know? *History of Education Quarterly, 32*(2), 360–366.

Larson, E. (1989). Innovations in health care: Antisepsis as a case study. *American Journal of Public Health, 79*(1), 92–99.

Libster, M. (2009). A history of Shaker nurse-herbalists, health reform, and the American Botanical Medical Movement (1830–1860). *Journal of Holistic Nursing, 27*(4), 222–231.

Lundy, K. S. (2008). Historical research. *The SAGE encyclopedia of qualitative research methods,* Vol. 1, 395–399. Los Angeles, CA.

Lundy, K. S. & Janes, S. (2009). *Community health nursing: Caring for the public's health,* 2nd ed. Sudbury, MA: Jones and Bartlett.

Lusk, B. (1997). Historical methodology for nursing research. *Image: Journal of Nursing Scholarship, 29*(4), 355–359.

Lynaugh, J. (2009). "In and out of favour": Scholarship and nursing history. *Windows in Time: A Newsletter from the Center for Nursing Historical Inquiry, 17,* 7–10.

Maggs, C. (1985). *Nursing history: The state of the art.* London: Croom Helm.

Morse, J. M. (1995). *Qualitative health research and critical issues in qualitative research methods.* Thousand Oaks, CA: Sage.

Newton, M. E. (1965). The case for historical research. *Nursing Research, 14*(1), 20–26.

Platt, J. (1981). Evidence and proof in documentary research 1: Some specific problems of documentary research. *Sociological Review, 19*(1), 31–52.

Rafferty, A. M. (1996). Writing, research and reflexivity in nursing history. *Nurse Researcher, 5*(2), 5–15.

Reverby, S. (1987). *Ordered to care: The dilemma of American nursing 1850–1945.* Cambridge, UK: Cambridge University Press.

Scannell-Desch, E., & Doherty, M. E. (2010). Experiences of U.S. military nurse in the Iraq and Afghanistan wars, 2003–2009. *Journal of Nursing Scholarship, 42*(1), 3–12.

Scott, J. (1990). *A matter of record.* Cambridge, UK: Polity Press.

Sorensen, V. J. (1985). *Oral tradition as history.* Madison, WI: University of Wisconsin Press.

Sorensen, E. S. (1988). Historiography: Archives as sources of treasures in historical research. *Western Journal of Nursing Research, 10*(5), 666–670.

Streubert, H. J., & Carpenter, D. R. (1999). *Qualitative research in nursing.* Philadelphia: Lippincott.

Sweeney, J. (2005). Historical research: Examining documentary sources. *Nurse Researcher, 12*(3), 235–246.

Trinkle, D. A. (1998). *Writing, teaching, and researching history in the electronic age.* Armonk, NY: M.E. Sharpe.

Turkel, S. (1974). *Working: People talk about what they do all day and how they feel about what they do.* New York: Pantheon Books.

Williamson, J., Karp, D. A., & Dalphin, J. R. (2005). *The research craft* (3rd ed.). London: Wadsworth Publishing/Thompson Learning.

Resources

Web resources for historical research:

General information on the historical research method with ample web-based resources:
http://history.memphis.edu/history_is.html

General information on the historical research method:
http://www.lawrence.edu/dept/history/HistoryResearchGuides.htm

An excellent web site for evaluating primary sources on the web which is produced by the University of California at Berkeley libraries:
http://www.lib.berkeley.edu/TeachingLib/Guides/PrimarySourcesOnTheWeb.html

Movies from a particular time period can be located easily from this web site:
http://www.imdb.com

Florence Nightingale Museum and Archives at St. Thomas Hospital in London:
http://www.florence-nightingale.co.uk/cms/index.php/florence-introduction

The Louvre Art Museum in Paris, France:
http://www.louvre.fr/llv/musee/alaune.jsp?bmLocale=en

American Association for the History of Nursing is a professional organization open to everyone interested in the history of nursing:
http://www.aahn.org

15

History Exemplar: More Than Good Kind Angels: Exploring the Value of Nursing Service

Marcella M. Rutherford

Adelaide Nutting (1858–1948), in her book *A Sound Economic Basis for Schools of Nursing and Other Addresses*, introduced her work with the statement: "The root of all main problems in nursing will be found, I believe, if carefully studied, to be economic in nature" (1926, p. iv). Later in the book, she touched on one area that has confounded nursing's economic progress and seems prophetic in regard to the phenomena explored in this chapter: "The traditions of the free service of the religious orders which hospitals had long enjoyed strengthened this attitude and made it difficult for them to get a correct point of view on the value of nurses' work" (Nutting, 1926, p. 268). In her writings, Nutting questioned nursing's ability to identify progress and its ability to trace "the lines of development and follow the sequence of events, for such appraisal as we can bring to them" (p. 326). From the historical outset of hospitals in the United States, indeed, nursing services were expected to be free. In 2010 nursing services remain an invisible asset that, although ever present, is ill defined and not quantified for those receiving care (Baer, 2007). It is still difficult to follow the sequence of events that nurses perform so that the value of their services can be accounted for. Rising healthcare costs and limited resources have created the need for data that document nursing's value in order to ensure adequate future investment in the profession. Against the backdrop of nursing history in the 20th-century United States, this chapter presents a case study of one group of the Daughters of Charity who owned and operated a hospital in Jacksonville, Florida, from 1916 through the early 1990s and offers findings that document the evolution of nursing value. This chapter summarizes a historical research project, completed and submitted as dissertational work (Rutherford, 2007).

Method

As stated in Chapter 12, historical research studies events of the past and seeks to accumulate knowledge related to mankind (Christy, 1975; Munhall, 2001). Joan Lynaugh, a nurse historian, stated that history is "memory shaped and formed so as to have meaning; it is the process by which people preserve and interpret the past" (1992, p. 16). Using the historical method, the researcher "deploys the passion to know" (Appleby, Hunt, & Jacob, 1994, p. 271). This passion is grounded in the researcher's "desire to touch the past . . . to anchor oneself in worldliness, to occupy fully one's own historical context by studying its antecedents" (Appleby et al., p. 271). Through the study of lived moments and human experiences, the researcher uncovers the significance of the events, yielding new thoughts, themes, and knowledge useful to today's healthcare practice.

To uncover the themes and knowledge imbedded in a case study, the researcher explores primary and secondary sources seeking the sum total of information to yield a picture of reality that answers the research questions. For this study the archives located at St. Vincent's Medical Center in Jacksonville, Florida, offered invaluable primary source documents, including letters between the Daughters of Charity, Jacksonville and the Visitatrix (Reverend Mother) in Emmitsburg, Maryland; letters written by the Daughters of Charity to those soliciting their help in Jacksonville; documents that contained the announcement of when sisters left and arrived at the hospital; administrative and department meeting minutes; and daily journals maintained by the sister administrators. In addition, the archives yielded administrative reports, financial statements, facility audit reports, articles in newspapers related to the Daughters' activities, hospital newsletters, board meeting minutes, lay advisory committee meeting minutes, administrative presentations, reports compiled by contracted consultants for strategic planning, and governmental reports. Secondary documents included written histories contained in books and journals related to historical accountings on the Daughters of Charity and the city of Jacksonville, marketing documents related to the hospital's services, and documents explaining the U.S. healthcare system policy changes. After the review of archival documents, an interview was conducted with the only remaining hospital administrative Daughter of Charity, Director of Mission Integration Sister DeSales, stationed at St. Vincent Medical Center at the time of the research. This sister had been assigned to the Jacksonville hospital in the 1950s and remained there into the 1960s. She returned to St. Vincent's in the late 1980s and continued to fill an administrative role until the time of this study. She provided additional primary and secondary data for the research.

In this case study, a relatively "typical situation is presented that reflects patterns apparent in many other instances" (Baer, 1989, p. 166). The history of nursing tells a story of women, predominately, seeking to provide better health care for their society. The study explored the support of the Florida community and its willingness to pay for health care and building funds, the sister's belief in the just distribution of resources, their altruistic code of ethics, and their beliefs as members of a religious order known for their strong faith in Christ. In this research, factors were identified that affected the sisters' ability to sustain their professional enterprise. Factors that inhibited the sisters' success primarily included external forces: limited financial resources, competitors seeking to capture paying patients, policy changes affecting payments, society's ability to pay for health services, and the dwindling number of members entering their religious order in the second half of the 20th century. Gender, normally thought of as a limiting factor, was a prerequisite to becoming a Daughter of Charity. As sisters, these nurses and administrators were provided the opportunity to receive education as well as to gain social and economic authority. These sister nurses were able to gain control over their work, often went unchallenged by the medical establishment, and were supported by administrative associates (Wall, 2005). These factors were explored in the research data.

The thesis of the research is that the sisters' unique situation of being nurses and the owners of their own healthcare facility afforded them the special opportunity to demonstrate the valuation of nursing services, in both its tangible and intangible aspects. It argues that economic information is needed to communicate the value of health care and to demonstrate the value of services. This valuation data enhances a profession's ability to acquire money needed to achieve its mission. Valuation as an economic term is used to define worth or value and, as a field or endeavor, involves financial valuing of a company's resources (Copeland, Koller, & Murrin, 2000; Newbold, 1995). The valuation approach, first developed and used in business in the 1960s, was implemented when competition and turbulence within the market made managing value an essential tool (Rutherford, 2008, 2010). Valuation data supports funding and is an important tool in health care, offering providers an ability to influence payers, investors, and decision makers (Rutherford, 2008, 2010).

The purpose of this research was to explore one nursing case history from 1916–1994, examining how the Daughters of Charity in Jacksonville succeeded in demonstrating their value, thereby obtaining the funding and resources needed to care for patients. The social, political, and economic events that took place during this study were examined in order to fully understand the external factors that influenced the findings. The findings uncovered in this historical story provide meaningful and useable information for the nursing profession.

The Story of the Arrival of the Daughters of Charity in Jacksonville

In 1900 Jacksonville's population totaled 28,249 and, according to the 1910 census, the population expanded to 57,699 citizens (Ward, 1985). While the population of the city more than doubled, the number of hospital beds had not kept pace. In 1910 Jacksonville reported only 85 hospital beds available in the city, "not even one bed for every 700 persons" (McGoldrick & Maclay, 1994, p. 37).

On February 2, 1906, the surgeons in Jacksonville opened DeSoto Sanatorium, a 42-bed, for-profit hospital. The physicians opened the facility to provide hospital beds for the community as well as to enrich their practices financially (McGoldrick & Maclay, 1994). In 1906, they also established a nursing school at the sanatorium and used the student nurses to deliver bedside care.

Although the hospital's reputation reported good surgical and medical care, the physicians acknowledged that the facility needed experienced management. Upon honest reflection the physicians realized the facility was poorly managed. By acquiring new managers/owners trained in overseeing the running of the facility, the physicians felt they would be able to focus on what they did best—treating their patients. The Daughters of Charity were the physicians' choice for this role.

One of the earliest documented letters from the community to the sisters was from Father Maher, pastor of the Immaculate Conception Catholic Church, who was enlisted by the surgeons to write a letter to Mother Margaret O'Keefe, Visitatrix and head of the Province of the Daughters of Charity. Father Maher's letter shared that "the DeSoto Sanatorium; under lay supervision it has not turned out satisfactory [sic], and they are anxious now to turn it over to the sisters—to rent, lease or buy on most favorable terms" (December 14, 1910). The physicians at the DeSoto Sanatorium had been educated in other cities and had experienced or heard of the skills of these sisters in hospitals throughout the nation:

> A record has always been made by the sisters for their economical administration, and there is no doubt in my mind that with a good medical staff and under the management of sisters who have devoted years of their lives to this particular work, an institution of this kind in our city would result in untold good for the poor and middle classes, and, at the same time would be so large [sic] patronized by those who are seeking the best care and accommodations during a period of sickness, that it would soon be on a paying basis, or at least, needing very little support on the part of our charitable citizens. (O'Keefe to the Daughters of Charity, Emmitsburg, n.d.)

The Daughters of Charity had displayed their skills as they "dealt with banks, and businessmen with a lawyer's mind, mastered the tendering process for private and state contracts with a mixture of faith and business acumen, dealt with boards of notaries and hostile bishops as a matter of course" (Nelson, 2001, p. 4). The sisters dedicated themselves to an apostolic life, "to seek Christ in every human" (Richardson, 2005, p. 19). The Daughters serve Jesus Christ through their ministries, caring for the poor and marginalized" (St. Vincent's Healthcare, para. 1). No matter how powerful and proficient in their skills they became, any wealth or power they realized was returned in full to the society they served (St. Vincent's Medical Center, 2010).

The Sisters' Competition

By 1916 Jacksonville boasted four other hospitals in addition to the DeSoto Sanatorium. Established in 1870, Duval Hospital became the first hospital to treat patients in Jacksonville. Duval was the first nonmilitary hospital to open in Florida. This facility functioned as a public hospital and asylum, treating both black and white patients. Archival reports described the hospital as being crowded most of the time (Ward, 1995, p. 6). This hundred-bed hospital served charity cases and functioned as a public almshouse—providing marginal care for society's marginal individuals (Reverby, 1993, p. 22).

In 1873, St. Luke's Hospital became the second hospital in Jacksonville. Three women within the Jacksonville community started this private hospital in a two-room facility. In 1916 the facility resided in Springfield, within blocks of the DeSoto Sanatorium. St. Luke's treated primarily paying patients. In 1911 the facility accommodated 35 patient beds but it often ran over capacity and census could be as high as 40–50 patients (Ward, 1995).

The third hospital in Jacksonville opened its doors in 1901. The Boylan House, later named George A. Brewster Hospital, was established by the Women's Society of the Methodist Episcopal Church. These women established the Boylan House in order to provide religious and nursing training primarily to women of color (Ward, 1995). After Brewster sustained damage by fire in 1901, the facility was rebuilt and quickly grew to accommodate 15 beds (Ward, 1995). Brewster provided care to the African American community. The facility in later years changed its name to Methodist Medical Center.

The fourth hospital was started by Dr. Carey Rogers, one of the founding physicians of the DeSoto Sanatorium. In 1911, after Dr. Rogers sold his interests in the DeSoto Sanatorium, he founded Riverside Hospital. Riverside, a three-story brick building soon became "known for its progressive quality health care, and its friendly, caring staff" (Ward, 1995, p. 14).

The Daughters Needed Convincing

In 1910, while St. Luke's campaigned for funds to build its new facility, Desoto Sanatorium surgeons were soliciting the Daughters to come to Jacksonville. After visiting the city, the Daughters of Charity were not convinced that, in light of St. Luke's campaign, the community fit their mission. Dr. C. M. Ottis, a friend of Dr. Gerry Holden, enlisted A. N. O'Keefe, the vice president of the Southern Drug Manufacturer Company, and other community leaders in a letter-writing campaign intended to show the sisters the support they would find in Jacksonville. The numerous letters appeared to be written between 1910, shortly after the first proposal to the Daughters, and 1915.

In 1915, after 5 years of evaluating the competition and the health services available to the community of Jacksonville, in particular to the sick poor, the Visitatrix became convinced of the city's need for the Daughters' services. An important factor that guided the sister's decision was that the number of beds added to the community from 1910–1915 had not improved the health services available to the needy. In this light, the sisters felt the city's needs matched the Daughters' mission. The Daughters of Charity purchased DeSoto in 1916 for $67,000 (Ward, 1995–1996, p. 4).

The Sisters' Letters Tell the Early Story

In 1916, Emmitsburg sent three sisters to Jacksonville and these Daughters routinely documented their experiences and activities back to the Mother Superior. Archival data revealed the dedication of the Reverend Mother of the Daughters of Charity to the education of each of the member sisters, preparing them in the fields of bookkeeping/finance and nursing. Because of this training, the three sisters sent to Jacksonville were well prepared for their assignment. The sisters' letters told of their adjustment to the foreign surroundings. In odd-looking, white-winged habits, they arrived in the city and focused on sharing their knowledge and spiritual intent.

Noted Challenges

Shortly after arriving in Jacksonville, Sister Mary Rose (the first administrator) wrote back to Emmitsburg describing her fellow sister's (Sister Dorothy) experiences, commenting that although the sister was "under a strain all the time, suffers severe headaches with nausea and looks badly; she does try to be generous and has a good spirit" (Sister M. Rose to Mother Margaret, July 16, 1916a).

> We all feel the heat very much, and though it seems to agree with Sr. Andrea, as she seems to be soaking wet all the time, she has gained

about 15 lbs . . . I have had some painting done, five rooms (pts) and the nurses' dining room and a great deal of scrubbing and cleaning; we will not do much this week. I guess you are tired hearing me tell about the dirt, but we will not have the place clean for months yet. (Sister M. Rose to Mother Margaret, July 16, 1916a)

The community in general found the sisters strange looking and had to adjust to these women walking about in their neighborhood. In addition the sisters faced financial difficulties related to the poor performance of the physicians who preceded the sisters at the facility.

The cornette was everywhere an object of curiosity, amusement and even suspicion; the people knew not whether to approach and confide or to withdraw and distrust. . . . In the stores, clerks either ducked behind the counters or fled precipitately to a back room, hoping that a brother clerk would be brave enough and could be grave enough to wait on the new hospital people. Simple cash purchases were alright, but proprietors refused to deliver any supplies—even though absolutely necessary—ordered by Sister Rose on her first extensive shopping tour, because DeSoto [sic] credit was not good. (St. Vincent's Medical Center, p. 4)

It was not long however, before the sisters endeared themselves to the community they would soon call home. The sisters' letters shed light on the financial situation they struggled to manage:

I have no money to pay bills. I had to find $300 for ins. [sic] which came due May 1—and really could not run any longer; the taxes on the cottage and lot are due tomorrow, but I told the party I had no money to pay them $133.04. Shall I renew the ins. which is due on the furniture? It would be a great risk not to carry it. I spoke to Fr. Maher about the rates and he said everyone had to pay them down here. He knew they were high, but there was no way out of it. . . . Oh, how I wish we could have a sister in the O. R.—it is so necessary in a new place in particular, especially as we are trying to get the inside track with the doctors and the doctors themselves are disappointed, I think, that there is not a sister in the surgery. (Sister Mary Rose to Mother Visitatrix, October 24, 1916b)

The original sisters arrived in Jacksonville in the spring, and by the end of summer additional sisters were sent to Jacksonville. In spite of the initial financial obstacles, the sisters continued their work and in 5 months established their credibility with the merchants and patients (McGoldrick & Maclay, 1994).

Developing a School of Nursing

The sisters purchased, along with the DeSoto Sanatorium, a nursing school. Archival documents described these sisters' challenges as they struggled to staff the hospital:

> If I can get some second year girls from some of out [sic] other hospitals, may I take them to finish here? . . . We run between 20 and 25 patients all the time and Sr. Catherine finds it impossible to tend to the 2nd and 3rd floors and see to things as they ought to be seen to and keep after the nurses. Sr. Louise has the operating room, drug room and maternity hall, and as she says herself she does not know a thing about any of these duties. She is under a strain all the time . . . May I be on the lookout for a graduate nurse to look after the maternity and teach some things to the nurses that the Srs. [sic] are not supposed to teach them? If I can get a Catholic for about $40 or $50 per mo., may I engage her? I positively would not offer any more. (Sister M. Rose to Mother Margaret, July 16, 1916a)

Early letters also shed some light on the quality of the nursing students the sisters found when they arrived in Jacksonville. The sisters expressed concerns over the students' training and skills:

> We have two probationers, one very nice Catholic girl the other a non-Catholic who I am afraid is not going to amt. [sic] to much. The probationary [sic] that was here when you and Sr. Bernard were here slipped out one evening early and sent me a note by a dime messenger that she had gone as she was discouraged and has not been heard from since. The very next week another little lassie got married on her afternoon and informed me of it the next day, so nothing surprises me now. The sisters find the girls very unreliable, and incompetent, they don't seem to know how to do the simplest things, are so giddy and loud, extravagant and careless, in fine [sic], very trying. (Sister M. Rose to Mother Margaret, July 16, 1916a)

The sisters quickly upgraded the school's standards. They defined the school's entry criteria and made curriculum changes, setting the new school apart from its predecessor. This school would later be closed in 1973, after graduating 1,279 nurses over its 57-year history, when the costs of running the school were reported on the financial statement as a loss to the facility (McGoldrick & Maclay, 1994, p. 38).

Building a Successful Hospital

On July 19, 1916, on the feast of St. Vincent de Paul, the sanatorium was officially dedicated and renamed St. Vincent's Hospital. Renaming the facility was a priority to the Daughters of Charity. The hospital's new name identified the facility as a Catholic Hospital. In 1919 the Daughters officially renamed the nursing school to St. Vincent's School of Nursing (McGoldrick, & Maclay, 1994). The sisters' works and services soon filled St. Vincent Hospital beds and expansion was needed to meet community needs.

In 1925 the sisters approached the community, aggressively pursuing the funds needed to build their hospital, saying, "if you will donate $200,000, we will build, equip, and operate a modern hospital of two hundred beds" (St. Vincent's Medical Center, n.d., p. 9). Pledges totaling more than $250,000 were collected so quickly that many in the community were unaware of the project. The 200-bed hospital was completed in 1928, costing $1.5 million.

The sisters continued to expand their hospital services, and the facility showed a consistent growth in profits. Even in bleak financial years, such as those noted in the 1930s and 1940s, St. Vincent's experienced growth. St. Vincent's Hospital's *Statement of Properties and Depreciation Year Ended December 31, 1945* demonstrated total fixed assets of $1,104,194.74 (Jarvus, 1945).

By 1951 the hospital was again, like most hospitals across the United States, in need of expansion. The sisters used Hill-Burton funds and planned a $1.6 million construction project, adding a west wing to the Hospital. The original hospital building, built in 1928, consisted of two wings facing the river, with a connecting corridor. This new construction continued the sisters' original design, situating all three wings on the riverfront, allowing each patient's room to have a lovely view overlooking the river (St. Vincent's Medical Center Lay Advisory Board Facts, 1951, p. 6).

From 1945–1990 five major expansion projects were planned and conducted. This healthcare business succeeded because of the funding from the community, making it possible for the sisters to expand the originally purchased 42-bed facility into a 528-bed medical complex. They endured and endeared themselves to the community they served. By 1990, the facility receipts for the year exceeded $141 million (Annual Board of Trustee Meetings, 1990). When looking at how the sisters were able to financially support this growth, a Daughter of Charity, Sister Keehan, offered a statement relevant to this research: "We work very hard to make money because you have to do good *well* . . . . It's not enough to say I'm a sweet little thing and I serve the poor" (Langley, 1998, p. A11).

Themes Identified in the Sisters' Story

The themes uncovered in the primary and secondary data sources told the story of how the sisters successfully built the hospital that would become St. Vincent's Medical Center. The themes identified included: 1) an unwavering commitment to live the mission of the Daughters of Charity; 2) an implicit authority that allowed these sisters to enter into business arrangements not conventionally afforded to laywomen; 3) an emphasis on ensuring that all sisters gained knowledge and mentorship in finance and nursing; 4) an ability to develop a bond, built on trust, between themselves and the community of Jacksonville; and 5) a keen understanding of the role money played in their ability to succeed. In addition the following two themes were not anticipated and were a surprising part of the Daughters of Charity's story: 6) a continued practice of racial separation within the facility, and 7) the limited role of the staff nurse in administration at St. Vincent's Medical Center (Rutherford, 2007, pp. 159–160). These themes reveal the basis of the valuation of the Daughters of Charity's business.

Living the Mission

The "Daughters' spirit of humility, simplicity and charity and their special concern for the advancement of the poor" guided their decisions and acts (Executive Summary of the National Task Force Report, 1986, p. 2). The Daughters of Charity in Jacksonville lived their mission, and this commitment was maintained for more than 80 years. This theme was found throughout the primary and secondary sources contained in the St. Vincent's Hospital archives, documenting the sisters' lifelong commitment to nursing and community care. The Daughters' mission was based on the teaching of St. Vincent de Paul (Dion, 1978). In the early years, without a formal mission statement, the hospital's purpose was found in the corporate bylaws, policies, philosophy, and religious directives made by the sisters. In the late 1980s, a more formal mission and value statement clearly highlighted the sisters' purpose for the patients and community (St. Vincent's Medical Center, 1987).

All of the Daughters of Charity in Jacksonville, from 1916 and throughout the decades that followed into the 1990s, dedicated themselves to the same spirit of purpose. During Sister DeSales's interview, as the only administrator sister still stationed at St. Vincent's Medical Center, she was asked why the Daughters of Charity have remained financially successful over the last 90-plus years? Foremost, she attributed the sisters' success to their dedication to the mission of St. Vincent de Paul. The sisters strived "to see Christ in all people and to assure that no person is forgotten" (Sister DeSales, personal communication, March 16, 2007). Over the decades, all of the Daughters of Charity who took on the role of administrator and sister servant, Sister DeSales stated, had a consistent spirit of purpose. The sister administrators, she pointed out, may have differed on the choice of color for the patient room curtains or on whether to hire physicians and invest in primary care, but they remained unified about the decisions related to the true spirit of their mission. Sister DeSales pointed out that as the numbers of sisters began to dwindle the mission integration program was begun, aimed at infusing the importance of the hospital's mission into the lay administrators.

The primary data found in the financial statements further supported the Daughters' commitment to their mission. Over the years, the expenses related to charity care grew consistently in proportion to the sisters' net profits. In 1993, the Daughters' charity care totaled $7,539,247, while the excess of revenue gains over expenses, after adjusting for nonoperational gains and loss, was $3,563,467 (Johnson, 1994). This comparison of charity expense and net income reflects the sisters' financial commitment to care for the sick and the poor.

Implicit Authority

When the Daughters of Charity in 1916 purchased DeSoto Sanatorium for $67,000, they became solely responsible as the owners and operational administrators of the sanatorium. The Catholic diocese had no connection to or governing voice in the running of the hospital. The money generated by the hospital was controlled by the Daughters of Charity, and was used to support the running of the hospital. In addition, the expenses generated by the facility were the Daughters' financial responsibility.

From the very beginning, the Daughters had to prove their worth and value to the community in order to secure funding support. The community was quickly convinced by the sisters' kindly smiles and nods offered in greeting; their continued commitment during times of community need, their dedication to hard work, their knowledge of health care, and their decision-making ability on issues related to managing the hospital. Through word, action, and deed the sisters demonstrated their continual commitment to the community of Jacksonville and their mission.

These sister nurses proved to be strong-minded business women, knowledgeable in all aspects of running a hospital. The Daughters, upon their arrival, cleaned, painted, cooked, provided medical care to all community members in need, and designed and expanded their facility and services. Hard work, strategic planning, and community partnering provided a recipe for success.

Knowledge of Nursing and Finance

The Visitatrix in Emmitsburg ensured that all of the sisters received training and education prior to appointment to one of the Daughter's hospitals. The Reverend Mothers across the years were dedicated to educating each of the sisters in finance and nursing (Sister DeSales, personal communication, March 16, 2007). Most of the administrators and all of the sisters involved in clinical supervision were graduate nurses (St. Vincent's Medical Center, n.d., p. 7). In the early years the sisters gained their expertise in each specialty area through mentorship. By the 1960s, documents indicated that the sisters were educated in their specialty fields in Catholic universities (Daily Log, September 1, 1960). To gain and maintain their positions of respect and authority, these sisters needed to demonstrate their knowledge and business savvy.

Through the years, the archival data showed the sisters enlisted the help of experts to enhance their knowledge and to obtain the most up-to-date and objective assessment on how the facility could improve operations. The sisters benefited from information shared by other Daughters of Charity facilities, accountants, contracted consultants, and the advice of the lay advisory board. This lay advisory board was established in 1944 and assisted the sisters until 1992 when its name was changed to the System Advisory Board. This board of community leaders was developed by the sisters to not only obtain knowledge related to the community healthcare needs, but its members also provided a bridge that strengthened the relationship between the sisters and the community. These experts and community leader's advice supported and confirmed the sisters' decisions. Recommendations from the consultants were discussed with the lay board. As community leaders, these members championed the sisters' mission. The lay advisors encouraged and enlisted other community leaders to become involved in the mission of the hospital (St. Vincent's Medical Center Lay Advisory Board Facts, 1951). The sisters also knew that the board members could communicate their mission in places the sisters could not gain access.

The Daughters used profits from the hospital to prepare for future patients. They invested in state-of-the art medical advancements, modernized their facility, and provided the latest technology for the citizens of Jacksonville. In the 1970s, the sisters again changed the hospital's name, this time to St. Vincent's Medical Center. In later years, they invested in centers beyond the hospital, targeting resources that offered outpatient diagnostic and primary care. Renovations and expansion of the facility continued throughout all of the study years.

In the 1990s, an era of cost containment in healthcare delivery challenged the Daughters to improve their billing systems and processes. Third-party payer billing rules required computers and software upgrades that were projected to cost $375,000 per year (Moore, 1981). Expenses began climbing faster than revenue and heralded major changes for the facility, as with most facilities across the country. Evidence of the sisters' stewardship practices related to billing and cost efficiencies were noted in the early years and continued throughout their tenure. These ingrained practices helped prepare the facility for the advent of managed care. In 1987 a report conducted by The Hunter Consulting Group to study all the financial viability of all of the hospitals in Jacksonville ranked St. Vincent's financial position as the strongest facility among the competitors reviewed.

Bond Built on Trust

The sisters strived to offer the highest quality of healthcare services to the city of Jacksonville. The sisters' unselfish dedication was at the foundation of the community's trust. In times of need, the community knew the sisters would unquestionably provide the health and spiritual care their community needed. Archival documents displayed the many exemplars from community members recounting the sisters' care, especially noted in the most challenging years, such as the Depression, World War II, the Korean War, and the Vietnam War. During times of dire need the Daughters' knowledge, nature, spirituality, and unselfish commitment shined.

The community's trust was enhanced by the sisters' belief in the worth of the individual. The value of each person was celebrated by the sisters, ensuring each patient was treated with dignity and respect. The sisters' spiritual care offered solace to patients and their families. Spiritual comfort soothed the patient's mind, body, and spirit, in a way not found in secular facilities. Catholicism was an important commitment for each of the sisters, and they included spirituality in care delivery. Patients facing sickness or death, no matter what their personal religious beliefs, benefited from the spirituality they found at St. Vincent's. The sisters respected the patient's own beliefs and provided support to meet these needs. The sisters believed that in critical times of illness the patients found solace and comfort in spirituality.

Sister DeSales spoke of her fear that health care was becoming more secularized. "Seeking God and seeking him in people" creates a relationship between the caregiver and patient and enhances the outcome of the care. At the time of death, patients find comfort in both the medical and spiritual services assisting their journey toward an eternal destiny. The sisters support the beliefs and the god worshipped by each and every patient. It was Sister DeSales' fear that with the increasing movement toward the secularization of health care, the spiritual aspect would be lost (Sister DeSales, personal communication, March 16, 2007).

The Role of Money

The sisters' relationship to money was complex and reflected an intertwining of mission and finance. Archival documents demonstrated how the Daughters of Charity sought money in order to continue their mission. Through the decades, the sisters demonstrated that money was important because it enabled their work to continue. The sisters used the money to make wise investments in order to enhance their ability to care for future patients. Profits allowed the sisters to purchase the technology needed to manage care delivery. The sisters continued to reinvest their income unselfishly back into the hospital to provide quality health services in an atmosphere that fostered respect and compassion.

The Daughters were consistently able to gain the funding needed to not only maintain but also to continually grow their facility. All fundraising campaigns met their targets and exceeded the sisters' campaign goals. This remarkable indication of the community support was noted in its willingness to pay for the Daughter's services and contribute to fund drives. The community communicated its belief in the sisters' worth and value when in 1925 they donated $200,000 within 4 weeks of the Daughters' plea. In 1952 the sisters' fund drive easily collected $700,000 from the community to initiate the planning for hospital expansion. Four additional construction phases occurred between the early 1950s and the early 1990s and the community of Jacksonville continued to willingly fund hospital expansion and renovation.

In 1988, the sisters' companies were restructured into five corporations and a foundation; changes that enhanced their ability to gain greater profits (Sister Celestine, 1984). The community continually invested their paychecks in the sisters' endeavors, because they realized the sisters' work had worth and value to their community. The community "realized that every dollar subscribed would put other dollars to work and the gift will continue to do good to relieve suffering and pain for many years to come" (*Two Hundred Bed Hospital*, 1926, p. 3). The community acknowledged that should they or their family members become sick, the sisters would be there to provide their care.

Sister DeSales commented on the generosity of the community and the St. Vincent's employees. The employees donated money from their paychecks that built an intensive care unit in the 1970s (McGoldrick & Maclay, 1994, p. 39; Sister DeSales, personal interview, March 16, 2007). Sister DeSales shared that this support continues until today, noting in 2000 the employees donated $2 million from their paychecks to build a cardiac diagnostic care unit.

Sister DeSales stated that a focus on money is not where health care should be, and the growth in the players who became wealthy on health care has created an atmosphere of "greed." She commented on the dire effects of the growing distrust between patients and providers. Healthcare delivery has become a very difficult practice environment (Sister DeSales, personal interview, March 16, 2007). The Daughters of Charity's commitment to their mission keeps them focused on what is important in health care, the patient. She offered her insight into the relationship of the Daughters:

> Money is important. Money is very important, but if that's all you're working for then you are missing something, and so is the patient. Without money there would be no mission. The two are intrinsically linked, but the mission comes first. (Sister DeSales, personal interview, March 16, 2007)

Departure from Mission—Racial Separation

The sisters arrived in Jacksonville at a time when "bigotry was rampant" (Curley, 1917). Non-white community members could not seek care from St. Vincent's Hospital until after 1964. The Daughters employed many non-white workers, but these same employees could not avail themselves of the comforting care of their employers. The sisters had Christmas parties for the employees, holding separate gatherings for non-white employees and white employees. These noted practices were in stark opposition to the mission of the Daughters, focusing on serving the sick and the poor, and looking to see Christ in all people.

The context of the times offered some insight into this stark departure from a mission so diligently followed. In 1964 the entire country was struggling with the moral purpose, as African Americans exhibited the courage to seek their rights (Brinkley, 2007). Although modern civil rights legislation was passed by President Johnson in 1964, the struggle for equality began with the emancipation efforts of President Lincoln in 1865, and remains a slow painful pursuit within the community of Jacksonville, as well as other communities across the United States (Brinkley, 2007). The sisters, however, did not challenge the level of racial bigotry within the community. In the early 1960s, Jacksonville was deeply and emotionally segregated, having separate schools, restaurants, churches, drinking fountains, and restrooms. There was a clear separation of whites from non-white members of the community. When the hospital admitted its first black patient in 1964, a PhD friend of a staff physician, the community responded so violently that the patient asked to leave the hospital (Hospital Administrator Daily Log, July 8–10, 1964).

One explanation for this disconnect in the Daughters' actions from their mission might be found in the sisters' wishes to conform to the social norms in a desire to safeguard their patients. To oppose the community's racial norms might have created a strong negative response. Sister DeSales was asked during the March 16, 2007 interview about the inability to provide healthcare services to non-white citizens. Prior to 1964, she described prevailing cultural boundaries and, in those times, crossing these boundaries was not done. Brewster Hospital offered medical care to the non-white citizens of Jacksonville. It is surprising, however, that these strong and courageous sisters failed to take a stand earlier, prior to 1964, in opposition to racial segregation. This type of message would have been in keeping with their mission.

Unanticipated Limited Staff Nurses' Role

The Daughters of Charity are women, nurses, and administrators. These women, as sisters, were granted the opportunity to own and operate a hospital. As nurses, the sister administrators achieved positions as hospital owners that are not offered to many nurses. This environment could have offered a unique opportunity for the sisters to allow lay nurses to participate in management decisions. This did not happen.

Lay nurses were conspicuously absent from administrative meeting minutes. In the early years nursing services was mentioned in the minutes, predominately in relation to the St. Vincent's Hospital School of Nursing, or in connection with needed salary changes. Many entries in the hospital administrator daily log, maintained by the Daughters' administrator from 1951 through 1969, documented the sisters' commitment to the nursing staff (1951–1969). The sisters valued the quality of nursing care provided to the patients and made sure that this employee group was paid well. The sisters also invested in the education of the nurses. Nurses, however, were not part of the hospital's decision-making management team.

Sister DeSales indicated that St. Vincent's followed the standard practices of the healthcare industry of the times. Sister DeSales identified a change in nursing, around the 1970s, whereby nursing departments began to routinely hold nursing meetings. These meetings allowed nursing managers to discuss various aspects of nursing services and implement process-improvement efforts. Nurses were trained in care delivery and nurses had authority at the bedside. Sister DeSales pointed out that when nurses moved outside of their scope, however, they had limited experience in making decisions related to the "big picture." Nurses today are still trying to break down these barriers. Identifying and utilizing nurse leaders from the nursing staff, however, would have offered a valuable perspective and strengthened administrative support for the sisters. At St. Vincent's nurses were not represented at the administrative meetings.

Research Findings

To ensure fiscal health, a hospital system called for "leaders who have vision and judgment—leaders who understand that society is trying to serve many values and who recognize that having more of one thing will often require having less of another" (Fuchs, 1998, p. 215). The sisters knew that competencies in nursing and healthcare finance were required to succeed in health care and to sustain their mission. They recognized the need to make the hard business choices, to set short- and long-range targets, and to anticipate and implement new services created by medical advancements. The sisters demonstrated their vision when they opened a wellness clinic, participated in research seeking the reasons for the high prevalence of lung cancer in the Jacksonville area, implemented the first mobile mammography van in the city, and added the goal of "inventiveness to infinity" to their core values (St. Vincent's Medical Center, 1991, p. 1). The sisters' strongest asset, however, was their simultaneous devotion to three key points—devotion to their mission, the knowledge needed to run their business, and their financial sustainability.

A valuation of the sisters' enterprise, created through an extensive accounting of both its tangible and intangible assets, provides valuable information. Documenting the sisters' assets would require quantifying such cost benefits of the hospital's low ratio of maternal mortality to deliveries, the ratio of neonatal mortality to total live births, the financial savings from reduced infection rates in surgical cases, and a reduction in hospital-acquired pneumonia (*A Picture Visit Through Saint Vincent's Hospital,* n.d., p. 5). Economic analysis also included the cost benefits of reducing the time between illness and returning the patients to their jobs, the worth of increasing the wellness of patients, the study of the cost of one treatment protocol over another, the benefits of early accurate diagnosis, and the outcome of providing supportive care versus the high cost of providing advanced technological interventions to the elderly (Fuchs, 1998). A cost-effective analysis looks at all of the resources that increased the quality of life to the community—aspects of care that not only extended life but also enhanced the quality of life (i.e., the relief of pain and disability) Fuchs, 1998). Measuring economic goods based on the quality adjusted life years may be inadequate however, "because some health care 'does good' by providing sympathy, caring, reassurance, and validation even when it has no effect on health outcomes" (Fuchs, 1998, p. 214). The community members served by the Daughters saw these attributes and recognized value.

Economic valuation includes assessing the threats, as well as the strengths, of a facility. By diligently assessing these factors, St. Vincent's management sustained the value of the hospital. To maintain its value position in the market in the 1990s, for example, St. Vincent's identified threats and then sought ways to minimize each threat. The archival data displayed threats that included staff physicians expanding office services in competition with the hospital; the Mayo Clinic entering into the Jacksonville market; alliances forming between competitive hospitals in Jacksonville; the aging of St. Vincent's physical plant; surrounding communities duplicating market resources; and the prediction of increasing costs that would result in decreased revenues (McManis Associates, Inc., 1990, p. 1). The Daughters identified among their strengths their trusted reputation and consistent dedication to their mission (McManis Associates, Inc., 1990, p. 3). Additional strengths included the financial health of the facility, a dominant position on the west side of Jacksonville for potential program expansions, the ability to leverage existing programs through consolidated services (the for-profit entity added after restructuring), a broad-based primary care delivery system with a good referral base, and a reputation for delivering the highest quality healthcare services (McManis Associates, Inc., 1990).

In an economic analysis of cost-effectiveness, direct and indirect costs, as well as intangible utility, are included in the valuation (Brent, 2003). As health care became more volatile, the sisters needed to explore, document, and seek, at every level, ways to create and communicate value. Although a formal valuation document was not found, the sisters' business value could be noted in a multidimensional blending of their tangible and intangible assets, all focused on their primary commitment to their mission. Thus, a valuation of St. Vincent's Hospital included the value of the sisters' property, investments, cash, equity, business entities, and costs of planned expansion. In addition, the sisters' valuation included the benefits or worth generated from their spirituality, stewardship, trusted position, and knowledge of nursing and healthcare finance. The community throughout several decades recognized the value of the sisters and supported their efforts. The sisters' commitment, knowledge, and hard work were rewarded by the community's willingness to pay for their valued services.

Conclusion

The story of the Jacksonville Daughters of Charity told of the unique relationship these sisters had to the money. Their role as good stewards created a trusting bond with the community of Jacksonville. The sisters' ability to generate money made it possible to build the hospital; their knowledge and hard work, combined with a commitment to a mission, made them successful. But the real basis of their success was trust. In the archival data, the community of Jacksonville spoke of the sister nurses' unselfish dedication to the city and the comforting awareness that the sisters were not interested in making money for the sake of profit. Instead, the Daughters of Charity used all of the profits generated from healthcare services to extend care to a greater number of citizens.

This historical research looked at the story of the Daughters of Charity in Jacksonville, who successfully owned and built a 528-bed Medical Center through steadfast dedication to their mission—to provide care for all people, with a focus on the sick poor. After reviewing the themes identified in this historical case study, one is directed again to Adelaide Nutting (1926) who stated:

> Our golden age, however, is not in the past, it is in the future and the best inheritance we can carry over from the past is the spirit which has brought us through these difficult years, with undiminished courage and unshaken faith in the beliefs and the principles from which we have striven, the spirit which leads one to seek ever for a better way. (p. 338)

Sadly, the sisters are currently disappearing from the landscape of health care. Today the Daughters of Charity need lay administrators to help them maintain the valuation of the business entities they started. Nursing can, however, learn from these sisters. The profession can take the challenge and provide data needed to document the value-driven aspects of its services. The mission of caring for patients is valuable and deserves an adequate investment.

References

Appleby, J., Hunt, L., & Jacob, M. (1994). *Telling the truth about history*. New York: W. W. Norton & Company.

Baer, E. D. (2007). Nursing's ambivalent relationship with money: Introduction. In P. D'Antonio, E. D. Baer, S. D. Ringer, & J. E. Lynaugh (Eds.), *Nurses' work: Issues across time and place* (pp. 81–86), New York: Springer.

Baer, E. D. (1989). Nursing's divided loyalties: An historical case study. *Nursing Research, 38*(3), 166–171.

Brent, R. J. (2003). *Cost benefit analysis and health care evaluations*. North Hampton, MA: Edward Elgar Publishers.

Brinkley, A. (2007). *American history: A survey volume II: Since 1865* (12th ed.). Boston: McGraw-Hill.

Christy, T. E. (1975). A methodology of historical research. *Nursing Research, 24*(3), 189–192.

Copeland, T., Koller, T., & Murrin, J. (2005). *Valuation measuring and managing the value of companies*. New York: John Wiley & Sons.

Curley, M. J. (1917, July 16). [Letter to the Very Dear Mother Margaret] Daughters of Charity History (STVMCA 01-06-01). St. Vincent's Medical Center Archives, Jacksonville, Florida.

Dion, P. E. (1978). *St. Vincent de Paul: His philosophy of health and social services*. Chicago: St. Joseph Hospital.

Executive Summary of the National Task Force Report. (1986, October 30). [Jim Johnson government relations, Daughters of Charity National Health System] (STVMCA 03-18-04). St. Vincent's Medical Center Archives, Jacksonville, Florida.

Fitzpatrick, M. L. (2001). Historical research: The method. In P. L. Munhall (Ed.), *Nursing research: A qualitative perspective* (3rd ed.). Sudbury, MA: Jones & Bartlett.

Fuchs, V. R. (1998). Ethics and economics, antagonists or allies in making health policy? *The Western Journal of Medicine, 168*(3), 213–216.

Hospital Administrator Daily Log (1951–1969). (STVMCA 01-07-01). St. Vincent's Medical Center Archives, Jacksonville, Florida.

The Hunter Consulting Group. (1987). St. Vincent's strategic positioning statement. [Strategic Position Statement (STVMCA 02-03-06). St. Vincent's Medical Center Archives, Jacksonville, Florida.

Jarvus, B. E. (n.d.). *Report of audit year ended December 31, 1945*. [Historic Files] (STVMCA 01-06-01). St. Vincent's Medical Center Archives, Jacksonville, Florida.

Johnson, H. (1994, June 3). *Five-year financial projections*. (STVMCA 02-03-06). St. Vincent's Medical Center Archives, Jacksonville, Florida.

Langley, M. (1998, January 7). Nuns' zeal for profits shapes hospital chain, wins fans but as Daughters of Charity builds $2 billion reserve some, question its goals: No mission no money. *Wall Street Journal*, p. A11.

Lynaugh, J. E. (1992). Historical research, 1989. Unpublished manuscript. In E. D. Baer, American Nursing: 100 years of conflicting ideas and ideals. *Journal of the New York State Nurses Association, 23*(3), 16–21.

Maher, M. (1910, December 14). [Letter to Rev. Mother Superior, Sisters of Charity of St. Vincent de Paul, Emmitsburg] (STVMCA 01-0601). St. Vincent's Medical Center Archives, Jacksonville, Florida.

Mann Wall, B. (2005). *Unlikely entrepreneurs Catholic sisters and the hospital marketplace, 1865–1925.* Columbus, OH: The Ohio University Press.

McGoldrick, T. J., & Maclay, D. M. (1994). History of St. Vincent's Health System: St. Vincent's Medical Center and Riverside Hospital. *Jacksonville Medicine* (August issue), pp. 37–41.

McManis Associates, Inc. (1990, March). *Repositioning for the future executive summary report.* (STVMCA 02-03-07). St. Vincent's Medical Center Archives, Jacksonville, Florida.

Moore, R. (1981, December 4). Finance committee minutes [Finance committee meeting] (STVMCA 02-03-06). St. Vincent's Medical Center Archives, Jacksonville, Florida.

Munhall, P. L. (2001). *Nursing research: A qualitative perspective* (3rd ed.). Sudbury, MA: Jones & Bartlett.

Nelson, S. (2001). *Say little, do much: Nursing, nuns, and hospitals in the Nineteenth Century.* Philadelphia: University of Pennsylvania Press.

Newbold, D. (1995). A brief description of the methods of economic appraisal and the valuation of health states. *Journal of Advanced Nursing, 21*(2), 325–333.

Nutting, M. A. (1926). *A sound economic basis for schools of nursing and other addresses.* New York: G. P. Putnam's Sons.

O'Keefe, A. N. (n.d.). [Letter to the Daughters of Charity, Emmitsburg] Founding Correspondence (STVMC 01-06-01). St. Vincent's Medical Center Archives, Jacksonville, Florida.

Ottis, D. M. (n.d.). [Letter to Reverend Mother Margaret, Visitatrix, Sisters of Charity] Founding Correspondence (STVMCA 01-06-01). St. Vincent's Medical Center Archives, Jacksonville, Florida.

A Picture Visit Through Saint Vincent's Hospital, Jacksonville, Florida (n.d.). [Photostatic Copy of STVMC First 35 Years] (STVMCA 01-07-01). St. Vincent's Medical Center Archives, Jacksonville, Florida.

Reverby, S.M. (2005). Ordered to care: *The dilemma of American nursing, 1850–1945.* Cambridge, United Kingdom: Cambridge University Press.

Richardson, J. (2005). *A history of the Sisters of Charity Hospital, Buffalo, New York, 1848–1900.* New York: The Edwin Mellen Press.

Rutherford, M. (2007). More than good kind angels: The Daughters of Charity's relationship to valuation, mission and money, 1916 to 1994 (Doctoral dissertation, Florida Atlantic University, 2007). *Dissertations Abstracts International* (UMI No. 3287383).

Rutherford, M. (2008). The how, what, and why of valuation and nursing. *Nursing Economics, 26*(6), 347–384.

Rutherford, M. (2010). The valuation of nursing begins with identifying value drivers. *Journal of Nursing Administration, 40*(3), 115–120.

Sister Celestine. (1984, October 12). Review of Legal Records (STVMCA 03-01-04). St. Vincent's Medical Center, Jacksonville, Florida.

Sister DeSales. (2007, March 16). Interviewed by M. Rutherford [Tape recording]. More than good, kind angels: The Daughters of Charity relationship to valuation, mission and money, 1916 to 1994, Florida Atlantic University, Boca Raton, Florida.

Sister M. Rose. (1916a, July 16). [Letter to Mother Margaret, Emmitsburg, Maryland], Founding Correspondence, Administration History (STVMCA 01-06-01). St. Vincent's Medical Center Archives, Jacksonville, Florida.

Sister M. Rose. (1916b, October 24). [Letter to Mother Visitatrix, Emmitsburg, Maryland], Correspondence, Administration History (STVMCA 01.06.01). St. Vincent's Medical Center Archives, Jacksonville, Florida.

St. Vincent's Medical Center, Jacksonville, Florida: St. Vincent's Hospital History 1916–1933. (n.d.). [St. Vincent's Hospital History 1916–1933, p. 1–20] (STVMC 01-07-01). St. Vincent's Medical Center Archives, Jacksonville, Florida.

St. Vincent's Medical Center. (1991). Annual Report. (STVMCA 02-03-06). St. Vincent's Medical Center Archives, Jacksonville, Florida.

St. Vincent's Medical Center. (1987). *Guiding principles and 1989 operating plan.* [1989 Binding Principles and Operating Plan] (STVMCA 03-18-05). St. Vincent's Medical Center Archives, Jacksonville, Florida.

St. Vincent's Medical Center Lay Advisory Board Facts. (1951, May 25). Summary of History of Lay Advisory Board (STVMCA 02-04-09). St. Vincent's Medical Center Archives, Jacksonville, Florida.

St. Vincent's Medical Center. (2010). *The Daughters of Charity.* Retrieved August 14, 2010, from http://www.jaxhealth.com/about-us/mission/daughters-of-charity.aspx

Two hundred bed hospital to be constructed here soon by Saint Vincent's—Two hundred fifty thousand fund raised by citizens to help defray building costs. (1926, March 29). [Historically Relevant Document] (STVMCA 01-07-01). St. Vincent's Medical Center Archives, Jacksonville, Florida.

Ward, J. R. (1995). *In the beginning* (STVMCA 01-601). St. Vincent's Medical Center Archives, Jacksonville, Florida. Unpublished manuscript.

Ward, J. R. (1985). *Old Hickory's town: An illustrated history of Jacksonville.* Jacksonville: Old Hickory's Town, Incorporated Jacksonville, Florida.

Ward, J. R. (1995–1996). *The white-winged Daughters of Charity.* (STVMCA 01-06-091). St. Vincent's Medical Center Archives, Jacksonville. Unpublished manuscript.

16

Narrative Inquiry: The Method

Maureen Duffy

Narrative inquiry is a form of qualitative research that uses a collection of stories as its source of data. These stories are the storied experiences of people's lives as told by themselves about themselves or as told by others about them. In other words, the collected stories may be autobiographical, biographical, or a combination of both. Stories are the primary way that people make sense of their experience and through some form of oral or written conversation reveal and share that experience with others. Riessman (1993) in describing narrative research states that "the purpose is to see how respondents in interviews impose order on the flow of experience to make sense of events and actions in their lives" (p. 2). The meanings that people give to their experience and that shape their lives are collected and organized into story form. Narrative research is a systematic form of inquiry that aims to gather these stories and represent or re-story them to readers and stakeholders (Riessman, 1993, 2007). In this chapter, "story" and "narrative" will be used interchangeably.

However, narrative research does not simply explore the meanings that individuals give to experience or examine the ways in which people tell the tales of their lives. Narrative research is typically more complex than that. Narrative research explores how language reflects the social worlds of people and, in so doing, constitutes their very identities. In other words, narrative inquiry functions at the interface of personal and social identity and of the very social world which is constitutive of such identities. Narratives reveal, sometimes consciously and often unconsciously, the meanings, conventions, dominant beliefs and values of the time and place in which a person lives and develops an identity.

The question of whether narratives collected in research are "true" or not has come up in discussions of narrative research (Phillips, 1997; Polkinghorne, 2007; Schafer, 1992; Spence, 1987). Spence and Schafer, coming from a clinical psychotherapeutic perspective, maintain that factual or verifiable "truth" is much less important than the stories people build up about their experiences, lives, and why they live the way they do. Spence and Schafer maintain that it is the coherence and congruence of a person's life story that determines how the person will live or perform their life story, not whether or not the story reflects actual events that are often impossible to verify anyway. Taking a similar position, Polkinghorne (2007) states, "storied evidence is gathered not to determine if events actually happened but about the meaning experienced by people whether or not the events are accurately described" (p. 479). Phillips, coming from an educational perspective, is more concerned about the "truth" of stories given that educational policy decisions may be made based on good stories that do not necessarily reflect actual events. Educational policy has real effects on children and families that Phillips worries could be based more on the persuasiveness of a good story rather than on the persuasiveness of actual events. The issue of "truth" in narrative research is unresolved and will probably remain so, given that the whole basis of truth involves differing epistemologies and paradigms that are incommensurable. In this chapter, my bias on the question of truth is toward narrative or storied truth rather than empirical truth.

In keeping with the bias towards meaning and storied truth in this chapter, the following questions reflect important underlying issues of narrative standpoint and philosophy. They deal largely with authorial voice, that is, the cultural discourse or worldview that influences the shaping of personhood and creation of personal identity. At any given time and place there are many discourses circulating within a culture, but one or two tend to predominate and more powerfully affect the ways in which people come to understand themselves and perform the identities they take on in their lives. The questions that follow can help to orient the narrative researcher in looking for the large and small stories that come together to form the themes in a person's life and that, together, have shaped the person's identity. A person's identity is laced together by the signatures of multiple interwoven stories.

The following questions can help a narrative researcher think through and plan a research project and gather the back stories of how people have come to see themselves in the way that they do at a particular point in time in their lives:

- Can there be a life without a story?
- Who is the authorial voice of that life/story?
- Is the authorial voice the person who is telling their own story or has the authorial voice been taken over or colonized by another or others who have usurped authorship of someone else's life? (Often, such colonization is "below the radar" of the person telling their life story because they

have internalized and performed versions of their life dictated by the dominant social discourse of their time and place without much awareness of doing so).

- Does the authorial voice change over the course of a lifetime and during critical life transitions?
- In what ways do multiple authorial voices help enrich the creation of a unique story or identity?
- In what ways do multiple authorial voices steal agency and identity from the story of a life?
- Are there many voices authoring the story of a person's life at any given time?
- Who decides and according to what criteria is the dominant version of a person's life told?
- How do people become aware of alternative stories and meanings that might equally or even more satisfactorily describe their lives?
- To what extent is the person aware of the influence of the social world on their constructions of a personal identity?
- How would persons' stories of themselves change if and as they became aware of the connection between their individual life story and the dominant stories about life that circulate in their culture?

From these questions, it should be clear that narrative research is not a passive activity in which the researcher collects frozen memories of life events. Rather, the narrative researcher is a co-participant in the exploration of how a life story came to be understood by someone in the way that it had. Through that very process of mutual exploration, the narrative researcher is often an agent of change, encouraging a person to critically look at how their own life story and identity are so intimately connected to the wider beliefs and values of their families and cultures. Such reflective examination of one's own life and identity, in collaboration with a skilled narrative researcher, frequently results in a changed understanding of one's past, present, and future. In this sense, narrative research can be seen as a radical intrusion into the ecology of a person's life and therefore the narrative researcher must seriously attend to the ethics of narrative research practice.

Questions as Sources of Data and Analysis

The questions presented earlier are exemplars of central questions for the narrative researcher interested in how individual identities reflect dominant social realities and themes. These questions themselves can also be used to analyze the narrative in terms of how it reflects the relationship between individual and social identity. Narrative researchers interested in attending to these kinds of questions are generally situated in the social constructionist paradigm. Within the social constructionist paradigm, researchers are most interested in how meanings are coordinated among participants in local communities and how knowledge generated within local communities can be understood and validated only within them and not outside of them in a larger, more universal way (Schwandt, 1998). Hence, how people come to understand themselves as gendered, sexualized, sociopoliticized, racialized, ethnicized, privileged, or marginalized persons reveals itself through the study of narratives within the social constructionist perspective.

Clearly, narrative research is interested in sensemaking, meaning-making, constructions, and reconstructions of identity and not in an abstracted factual account of "the truth" of a life story. Coherence of a narrative account, congruence between a person's point of view and how they make sense of things, and how well a story is put together are more important and more interesting to the narrative researcher than the positivist illusion of "truth."

Can There Be a Life Without a Story?

Bruner (2004) says "that we seem to have no other way of describing 'lived time' save in the form of a narrative" (p. 692). He takes a decidedly constructionist point of view when he explains the heart of his argument:

> Eventually the culturally shaped cognitive and linguistic processes that guide the self-telling of life narratives achieve the power to structure perceptual experience, to organize memory, to segment and purpose-build the very "events" of a life. In the end we *become* the autobiographical narratives by which we "tell about our lives." (p. 694)

Narrative research, therefore, does not take life stories at face value, but rather explores how the meanings about life stories were built up, amended, deconstructed, and reconstructed again or, in some cases, over and over again.

The case of Terri Schiavo in the spring of 2005 is illustrative of the power of the authorial voice to make critical life and death decisions for another, and, in so doing, to move and shape social dialogue and social meanings. Terri Schiavo had been in what some physicians and her husband called a "persistent vegetative state" for 15 years. They held that her life was basically meaningless because she was for all intents and purposes "dead" and no longer able to process information or in any way to live meaningfully. Her parents and others strenuously disagreed and held that Terri Schiavo was a person in the full sense of the word and that it was possible she was able to process some information and respond to some stimuli, thereby being "alive" and worthy of being kept alive by retaining her feeding tube (Somers, 2005).

The United States and much of the Western world was fascinated by this case and, in the end, maintained a worldwide death watch while also weighing in on the critical issues involved in her case; namely, who had the right to speak for Terri and when, why, and how should a person's life be declared over? Terri's husband and the courts were given the power of authorship over Terri's physical life. In terms of the story of the meaning of Terri's life, her parents, family, friends, and a world of others, as well as her husband and the courts, continue to tell about and author Terri's experiences, values, desires, wishes, and the implications of her life. While she is dead, her story is very much alive and goes on being deconstructed and reconstructed again. As the end time of Terri's life approached, multiple, competing identities of Terri were constructed and circulated by the many authors of her life.

The Structure of Narrative

By necessity, narrative researchers are interested in the structure of a narrative and its structural elements. In a general sense, a narrative is a story that is told according to a timeline or chronology. The story has protagonists or central characters and other characters playing major or minor roles. It has a plotline with critical events that unfold and have consequences and implications for the characters. The story has a theme and tone which provide hints of the meanings generated by the storyteller(s) and characters. The story can often be classified into a genre; for example, a romance or tragedy or tragic-comedy, or story of heroism, among so many other possibilities. And finally, a story includes the act of making sense out of the characters, the actions, and the events that have occurred within the plot. Who tells or narrates the story, of course, is of critical importance. In other words, who has agency in the story must be identified.

Labov (1972) has paid particular attention to the form and structure of narrative and it is not uncommon for some narrative researchers to use a structural analysis of a narrative during the analysis and interpretation phase of the research project. Labov and Waletsky (1967) and Labov (1972) identify the major elements in the structure of a narrative as the following:

- The *abstract* which introduces and summarizes the story.
- The *orientation* which provides details of character, time, place, and events.
- The *complication* which details critical events in the story.
- The *evaluation* which describes the implications and meaning of the actions and events.
- The *result* which gives the outcome (if only a partial one) of the story.
- The *coda* which links the story in the past back to the present of the storyteller's life.

Even though Labov's work can be used to wall off the individual from the broader culture by focusing only on the individual's actions and meanings in the story, a narrative researcher interested in how individual meaning is linked to cultural meaning can also find Labov's structural elements useful by analyzing each element in terms of how it both reveals and contributes to the development of a personal identity that is social rather than private.

In a different vein, Burke (1969) describes the elements of a narrative as consisting of *act, scene, agent, agency,* and *purpose.* In this schema, Burke is interested in what the act was, what the background or context for the act was, who did the act, how the actor did the act, and what the purpose for doing the act was. The focus of Burke's structural elements in narratives is clearly that of the power and meaning of agency and motive.

Steps in the Narrative Research Process

Formulating the Research Question or Focus

The heart and soul of all qualitative research is the development of a research question or focus that lends itself to a qualitative method. In narrative research, common research questions focus on the life story or life history of an individual or a group, as told by individuals. Such narrative research can consist of autobiography, biography, oral history, life history, autoethnography, narrative case studies, and other methods that require collecting the stories of people as the main data sources.

Clinical psychotherapy (Freedman & Combs, 1996; Schafer, 1992; Spence, 1987; White & Epston, 1990) has also demonstrated a strong narrative turn and has focused on helping people to free themselves from constraining life stories and to adopt more satisfying and liberating ones. In the process of focusing on the narrative as a reflection of the manufacture of a person's identity rather than as an essential inborn identity or personality, clinical psychotherapy has made important contributions to narrative research, especially in the area of question construction about the creation and performance of an identity story.

Examples of narrative research questions might include:

- *How did you get the idea that unless you were rail thin you were not acceptable? Where do you think this idea came from and how do you think you got caught up in it? Are there any ideas or notions that are interesting to you yet challenge the idea of needing to be rail thin to be acceptable? And where did these competing ideas come from?* These are clinical research-based narrative questions that seek to explore the development of an identity, in this case a spoiled identity (White & Epston, 1990).

- *What has the experience of being a first-generation Irishwoman in the United States with no extended family been like for you? Who or what did your family fall back on during hard times or during times of crisis?* This is a more sociological-based narrative research question linking the experience of an individual to that of a larger cultural Diaspora.

- *In speaking to members of your extended family and collecting their stories and recollections, as well as reviewing historical and archival material, what have you come to learn about your grandfather who fought in the Irish Revolution during the founding of the Irish Free State? What do you know about his imprisonment in England and his systematic torture by the British by being dragged out in front of a firing squad on multiple occasions without actually being executed?* Responses to these questions would result in a collection of memories or oral histories from people associated with the revolutionary grandfather and would also include use of archival materials to create a biographical story of a captured and tortured founder of the Irish Free State.
- A follow-up identity and relationship-building question with an ancestor the granddaughter never met requiring reflection and imagination might be: *How do you think that your grandfather whom you never knew personally, but knew of in so many important ways through others, would view your contributions to carrying forward the commitments and values to which he was so dedicated? What would he see in how you live your life that would make him swell with pride and delight?*
- *What are the recollections and experiences of survivors of the Holocaust?* Again, this question would generate oral and life histories collected in story form about one of the darkest periods of our time, powerfully connecting personal stories with political events.
- Back to clinical research: *How do you recall your early experiences with your parents or primary caregivers?* This is a question that could be examined narratively for congruence and coherence rather than for historical truth. The focus on coherence and congruence would set the research question apart from traditional psychological or psychoanalytic research questions that seek historical or actual rather than narrative truth (Schafer, 1992; Spence, 1987). The narrative researcher would generally hold that narrative truth is more important than factual or historical truth since such "factual truth" is always situated or contextualized, not least by the plasticity of memory. In fact, the widely used Adult Attachment Inventory (George, Kaplan, & Main, 1996) developed to assess adult attachment styles uses a narrative interview format and analyzes the interview and assesses attachment style based not on the degree of trauma a person experienced as a child, but rather on the coherence, congruence, and completeness of their narrative account about the trauma experience. In other words, in the Adult Attachment Inventory attachment style is assessed based on the degree of a person's ability to tell a coherent, complete story about their early life without significant gaps of time or memory.
- *How do you manage your newly appointed job as Associate Dean when you have just earned your doctoral degree and will be evaluating faculty at full professor rank?*

This question could result in a sociological or symbolic interactionist narrative study inquiring about roles and presentation of self in everyday life similar to the kinds of questions that fascinated Erving Goffman, the classic and utterly original sociologist (1959, 1963, 1974). Goffman (1963) would have been interested in how a person without appropriate credentials manages that fact on the job site and would have viewed such a set of circumstances as stigmatizing, and therefore, as an instance of spoiled identity.

These examples of narrative research questions illustrate some features of formulating a narrative research question to which the narrative researcher should pay attention. No single story will ever capture a life or even a part of a life. Therefore, the narrative researcher must *limit the scope of the research question* and focus on the aspects of the person's life or identity building that are most important or most interesting to the researcher.

The researcher must also clearly identify *who* is the narrator of the story. The narrator could be the *person who experienced the set of events* or it could be a *witness to the experiences*. First person accounts and witness accounts are both powerful forms of storytelling. For example, an aging mother would provide a *witness account* of the story of her daughter's struggle with infertility and the callousness and insensitivity of her daughter's husband to her daughter's experience and emotional torment. The daughter herself would provide a *first-person account* of the experience of infertility and her husband's reactions to her. Witness interviews and stories can also be called collateral interviews and stories.

In biographical and historical narratives, the narrative researcher may collect multiple witness accounts and/or examine the written and oral texts in archival and documentary materials that provide a wealth of witness information. In reflecting on the silence, disguised as love, that prevented her from sharing her own fears with her dying mother, and in wondering how to share her fears about her own cancer experience with her daughter, Kathy Weingarten (2000) invokes the power of witnessing: "We are all always witnesses. People speak, we hear, whether we choose to or not. Events explode in front of us, whether we want to see or not. We can turn on television, see people in moments of extremity, and know their fate before they do" (p. 392).

I would like to suggest that the narrator of a story does not always represent the *authorial voice,* even when that narrator is the person who experienced the events. The authorial voice, especially in examining scripts of identity, is more likely to be the dominant discourse of the culture as represented by key figures in the person's life and by critical cultural signifiers such as the media and advertising. For example, Weingarten (2000) in recounting her mother's impending death, describes the dominant discourse or, we could say, the authorial voice, as the belief that silence and secrecy were the appropriate moral responses to the plight of a middle-aged woman with terminal cancer. It is important therefore for the narrative researcher to examine the source(s) of the authorial voices in a person's life and not to simply represent those voices uncritically as "the" voice of the narrator. Authorial voice does not mean the voice of authority in the strictest sense, but rather the voice of the dominant values, beliefs, and attitudes of the culture that are internalized by the person who is providing an account of experience. For a fuller discussion of dominant discourse and its internalization by persons, see the works of Michel Foucault (1970, 1973, 1976, 1978).

Summary: Key Steps in Formulating the Research Question or Focus

1. Limit the scope of the research question.
2. Identify who is the narrator of the story.
   a. Is the account a first person account?
   b. Is the account a witness account?
   c. Does the account include both first person and witness stories?
3. Understand the discursive or social constructionist distinction (Gergen, 2009; Lock & Strong, 2010) between the narrator and the authorial voice.

Data Collection Procedures

The primary vehicle for data collection in narrative research is the *interview*. The interview could consist of a personal, face-to-face interview with the person or persons who are the participant(s) or subject(s) of the research project and could also include witness or collateral interviews with people who know or knew the subjects of the narrative study. Documentary, historical, and archival material are also important sources of data collection in narrative research. These sources help add to the developing narrative and to confirm or triangulate the accuracy or validity and richness of the information already collected.

Kvale (1996, 2007) provides excellent guidelines that could easily be used as standards for assessing a narrative interview. He emphasizes that the purpose of the interview is to gather information about the life world or everyday experience of the interviewee and that the researcher has the task of seeking and interpreting the meaning of these everyday experiences. Kvale also reminds researchers that global statements from the interviewee are usually not useful and that the researcher has the task of eliciting detailed, specific descriptions of everyday events and their meanings from the interviewee.

The other qualities that Kvale (1996, 2007) outlines as important for the narrative interview are that the researcher have a flexible interview focus, neither too constraining nor too open and unfocused. He also reminds researchers that it is important to develop a willingness to accept ambiguity as a part of the reality of life and therefore to avoid forcing clarity or specificity from an interviewee who is ambivalent or ambiguous about a life situation. Kvale regards the knowledge generated in an interview as an interpersonal act and conversation as the production site of knowledge. Unlike many interview guides and writers, Kvale declares that the process of interviewing may bring about changes in awareness and changes in meaning for the interviewee and that the researcher must be open and sensitive to these possibilities. And finally, the researcher must work to insure that the interview process is a positive one for the interviewee.

The emphasis on the possibility of change and the importance of the interview being a positive experience for the interviewee reminds me of a student's reaction in a class I taught on social and cultural issues in counseling. I had asked the class as one of their assignments to interview someone culturally different from themselves. In reporting her interview experience with a middle-aged Eastern European immigrant woman, the student ended her report by telling the class that at the end of the interview the Eastern European woman commented that she had never realized how interesting a life she had led. I told the student that she could have been paid no finer compliment about her interview skills even as the student expressed doubt about whether a research interview should lead to this kind of change. The memory of the story of the Eastern European woman's powerful positive experience with the student interviewer and her changed and enriched awareness of her own life still delights me many years later. I have no misgivings about the experience of change to which the interview led for this woman.

On the other hand, Parker (2005) warns narrative researchers against believing that their interviewing work is therapeutic for the interviewee and further warns researchers against being too personally intrusive. There is a significant difference between acknowledging that the research interview can function as a catalyst for personal change and holding a position that intensive interviewing is usually therapeutic. The former is a reasonable, theoretically sound constructionist and evidence-based position to hold, the latter is naive and probably dangerous. Parker, however, makes the point: researchers are not therapists and the two roles should not be confused.

Personal and family narratives can be immeasurably enhanced by asking research participants to bring in photographs, drawings, or other special mementos of personal or family life (cf. Banks, 2007). Creswell (2002) notes that such memorabilia can help participants to remember details that they might not have included in their face-to-face interviews. Historical narrative research can be done through the use of such artifacts alone. A both dazzling and heart-wrenching example of historical narrative research using only children's drawings and poems is Volavkova's (1993) book *I Never Saw Another Butterfly: Children's Drawings and Poems from Terezin Concentration Camp, 1942–1944*. This book is a collection of art and poems from some of the 15,000 children under 15 years of age who were imprisoned at Terezin outside of Prague. Fewer than 100 of these children survived. The pictures and poems reflect the juxtaposition of the conditions in the concentration camp and the experiences of the children—hope amidst horror, sunshine amidst darkness and deprivation.

Sources of narrative can be collected from any of the forms of expression that are present in a culture. Music, art, literature, film, advertising, graffiti, dance, theater, letters, web logs, and everyday conversation are examples of readily available forms of cultural expression and narrative that could be studied through narrative research. For example, rap music represents a collection of personal narratives put to beats. Tupac Shakur's 1992 rap song "Brenda's Got a Baby" packs a world of experience, meaning, and story into forty-two short lines. This rap song is an in-your-face storied indictment of how the short life of misery of one illiterate girl affects the whole community. An illiterate girl (Brenda) lives in the ghetto and becomes pregnant as a result of being molested by her cousin. Brenda's family is mainly interested in the welfare check that Brenda's baby will provide. When Brenda has the baby alone because no one acts concerned about her, she throws the baby in the trash, her family kicks her out, and Brenda ends up as a slain prostitute.

Early rap music especially represents a large collection of stories of marginalization, race, race relations, poverty, violence, neglect, death, and rage. Researching rap music for the stories of the meaning of everyday experiences jam-packed into them is an example of doing narrative research without interviewing. Creswell (2002) suggests that the researcher's ultimate retelling or re-storying of a narrative "is based on the assumption that the story told by the participant will be better understood by the listener and the reader if it is resequenced into a logical order" (p. 534). In the case of doing narrative research of rap music, the researcher's retelling of the stories and meanings of rap could function like a Trojan horse—bringing those stories to an audience or a group of stakeholders, usually identifiable by age, class and race, which typically refuses to even hear or listen to the stories of rap.

Summary: Narrative Research Data Collection Procedures

1. Conduct face-to-face interviews with the research participant or subject wherever possible.
2. Do follow-up interviews to add detail, fill in gaps, and check meanings and interpretations.
3. Conduct witness or collateral interviews wherever possible and as appropriate.
4. Ask the interviewee to bring in drawings, poems, pictures, photographs, or other mementos and talk about these, as appropriate.

5. Examine documentary, historical, or archival material, as appropriate for the particular study.
6. Examine forms of expression in the culture; for example, music, art, literature, film, advertising, graffiti, dance, theater, letters, web logs, and everyday conversation, as appropriate for the particular study.
7. Be aware of common interview pitfalls; namely,
   - Paying insufficient attention to the development of an atmosphere of trust and goodwill
   - Not following up with questions about the tone and content of the interviewee's responses when there is little variety in the descriptions
   - Seeking clarity and specificity when the interviewee consistently describes experiences in ambiguous ways instead of accepting the story or a part of it as uncertain or ambivalent
   - Not asking for richer, thicker descriptions and meanings when the interviewee's story seems too pat or glossed or seemingly structured to please the interviewer

The narrative researcher would select the appropriate data-collection procedures from among those listed in this chapter. Of course, not all procedures would be used for every study. The nature of the narrative study, feasibility, time, and budget will determine which procedures are most suitable for a particular study.

Data Analysis Procedures

The narrative researcher has a number of choices to make in determining how to go about analyzing stories and other narrative data that have been collected. A number of options for narrative analysis are outlined and described here.

Structural analysis

One choice the narrative researcher could make is to analyze stories in terms of their structural elements. *Structural analysis* of narratives involves coding the narrative according to its structural elements. If Labov's (Labov, 1972; Labov & Waletsky, 1967) schema is used, then narrative data will be coded by examining the narrative and identifying the *abstract* which introduces and summarizes the story; the *orientation* which provides contextual details of character, time, and place; the *complication* which describes critical events in the story; the *evaluation* which outlines the meaning and implications of the narrative; the *result* which provides the outcome or resolution of the story; and the *coda* which describes how the storyteller brings the events and meanings of the story back into the present. The researcher then fashions a *new story* emphasizing what the key structural elements of the narrative are and how they have come together to form a particular story with a particular meaning pattern.

Burke's (1969) structural analysis could be used in a similar way to analyze a narrative but with the focus on identifying the *act, scene, agent, agency,* and *purpose* of the story. The researcher would then also *retell a new story* but with the emphasis on analyzing the actor's purpose, motives, and intentionality.

There are many other possibilities for examining narratives structurally. These would involve examining the narrative for the literary elements of a story; namely, plot, time, scene or context, characters, events and actions, outcomes and meanings. As in the two other examples of structural analysis above, the researcher would then *retell a new story,* perhaps emphasizing a particular aspect of the original narrative such as character development or the unfolding of events over time or how the plot, characters, and outcomes work together logically or otherwise.

Narrative analysis from a psychological perspective

Narrative analysis from a psychological perspective reflects a movement away from attempting to understand personality, psychopathology, the self, and intentionality through the lens of scientific theories such as psychoanalysis, behaviorism, humanism, and even systems theory. Such theories carry the weight of the scientific worldview that, apart from quantum science, sees human behavior in Newtonian, mechanistic terms. For example, psychoanalysis refers to drives and impulses, ids, egos, and superegos. Behaviorism talks about contingencies of reinforcement and conditioning. Humanism speaks of self-actualization and unhindered free will. Systems theory refers to feedback loops, homeostasis, and interdependence.

Rather, narrative analysis from a psychological perspective moves us toward examining the meanings people attach to their lives and behaviors, how they use language to talk to themselves and to describe themselves to themselves and to others. Narrative psychological analysis attends to the metaphors of self-description and intentionality that are revealed in people's stories and discursive patterns. The researcher interested in psychological narrative analysis will examine narrative for the patterns of metaphors, words, phrases, and speech acts that provide the thread of continuity making up and maintaining the self. This linguistic thread of continuity should be examined for its consistency, coherence and congruence, not for its factual truth (George, Kaplan, & Main, 1996; Schafer, 1992; Spence, 1987). Inconsistencies and discontinuities of self-description, evidenced by significant changes of patterns of metaphors, words, phrases, or speech acts, or incoherent self-description will be marked as reflecting critical narrative turns in the development and maintenance of the linguistic self. As Bruner (2004) points out, it is this linguistic self that becomes the self that is lived out in daily life.

Narrative analysis of identity development

Narrative analysis from a psychological perspective tells the story of a life from the inside to the outside, starting with the individual self as the star and then connecting that already developed individual self to the outside world. Narrative analysis of identity development does just the opposite. It starts with the outside stories of the culture and explores how those outside stories create the inside story of the self. It is a fascinating difference.

The difference emerges in the juxtaposition of the realist view of the self with the postmodern, social constructionist view of the self. The realist view, upon which almost the entire history of psychology is built, regards the self as a separate, self-contained individual entity generally stable over time. The social constructionist view regards the self as relationally constructed, unstable, evolving, and being constructed or manufactured and deconstructed and reconstructed through engagement in multiple roles and relationships over time within the context of a more encompassing, powerful social discourse. It makes sense then that the social constructionist view denies the existence of an essential, real self (Denzin, 2001).

The tool of the narrative researcher interested in identity development is the *reflexive interview*. Reflexivity technically refers to the bending back on oneself. In the reflexive interview, the narrative researcher poses questions to participants that ask them to examine how their ways of thinking, feeling, and being in the world have come to be the way they are. The reflexive interview uses the kinds of questions illustrated earlier in this chapter that relate to authorial voice. These questions invite participants to examine who they are in relation to the larger cultural discourse and to imagine alternative discourses that would result in the production of alternative identities. Narrative research from this perspective assumes the *plasticity of identity* and proceeds to examine how a particular identity has been molded under the direction of what authorial voice(s).

There is no question that narrative research from an identity development perspective has the potential to affect profound changes in people's stories of themselves. The dialogical inquiry that is characteristic of reflexive interviewing focusing on scripts of identity, while respectful, can also be challenging. It can shake a person's self-story to realize through identity development questions that they are living out larger social scripts they may never have thought about before. For example, a wealthy entrepreneur may find it difficult to realize that he is treating money and his family's use of it as if he were still eking out an existence on the side of a hill in the same way that his father was forced to do in his native country. The authorial voice of this man's view of the use of money is located in the larger scripts of poverty and scarcity that long ago ceased to be useful in his own personal and family life, and that, in fact, were now hurtful.

The narrative researcher's role in conducting analysis from the perspective of identity development is to interrogate the scripts of identity that people have come to believe and perform, to identify the interwoven stories and substories that make up a participant's identity, to retell the story of the history of those scripts and stories, and to include in the new story the shifts in identity that have occurred as a result of such inquiry and changed awareness. Clearly, in narrative analysis from the perspective of identity development, the researcher must be aware that every question is potentially an agent of change and therefore ethically charged. In this perspective, every action of the narrative researcher has ethical import. Every question asked or unasked, every story retold or left untold, has ethical significance for both the researcher and participant.

Artistic and aesthetic narrative analysis

Stories are art forms with the language, rhythms, cadences, turns, surprises, and meanings of a narrative bringing a universal form of art—the story—to life. Narrative researchers can be regarded as impresarios encouraging the creation of artistic and aesthetic performances by their research participants through the telling of life stories. As an impresario, the narrative researcher encourages the production and performance of stories by participants and stands in appreciation and awe of the complexity and power of a life story as a form of art. Narrative researchers, in this form of analysis, enter into the emotional and sacred ground of their participants as they tell their life stories and allow themselves to fully emotionally experience and then record their own emotional responses to these stories. Such emotional experiencing by the narrative researcher completes and fulfills the relationship between artist and audience who are in intimate connection with one another. Often, the participants too are surprised by the power of their own artistic performances of their life stories to change the way they think about themselves, others, and their own lives. Thus, the artistic and aesthetic narrative researcher experiences the stories of participants in a holistic and organismic way and retells these stories by including their own emotional reactions and reflections. The appreciation of a life story as a form of art and the retelling of it from the standpoint of this appreciation and with the inclusion of the researcher's own emotional responses is the heart and soul of artistic and aesthetic narrative analysis. The reader also becomes involved in artistic and aesthetic narrative research by becoming emotionally affected and moved by the narrative re-storying.

Summary: Narrative Research Data Analysis

1. Identify the particular method of narrative analysis to be used. For example, structural narrative analysis, psychological narrative analysis, identity development narrative analysis, or artistic and aesthetic narrative analysis.
2. Examine the narrative in terms of the criteria of interest based on the selected method of analysis. For example, elements of literary form and structure; patterns of metaphor and word use, as well as narrative consistency,

coherence and congruence; interrogating the history of persons' scripts and stories of identity and their connection to the larger social discourse; fully emotionally experiencing and appreciating the stories of peoples' lives as art forms and retelling those stories including the researcher's own emotional reactions in them.

3. Retell the story of the narrative from the perspective of the selected method of analysis being mindful to keep the literary elements of narrative present in the new story.

Trustworthiness and Credibility in Narrative Inquiry

Trustworthiness and credibility in narrative research refer to the degree to which the participants have been fully included in the research process and have had the opportunity to reflect upon and comment upon their story as retold by the narrative researcher. Both the researcher and the participant then share the responsibility of the re-storying process. In research that emphasizes collaboration, it seems to me like arrogance to place the entire burden of assuring the faithfulness of an account on the researcher alone. There are many situations in which the participants' only way of being heard and telling their stories is through participating in research and the participants therefore have a strong interest in wanting their stories to reflect the narrative truth of their experiences. The researcher's obligation is to provide meaningful opportunities for the participants to review transcripts and the researcher's retold stories. Any changes, concerns, or objections simply become part of the story of the research and can be included in the narrative, with review again by the participants.

With the increasing trend towards *transparency of procedure* in qualitative research (Chenail, 1995, 2008; Constas, 1992; Flick, 2008), the narrative researcher has an obligation to explicate all procedures followed in the research process. This transparency includes revealing to the reader the following information about the research process: 1) clearly identifying the research question, 2) disclosing where the research data came from, that is, first-person accounts, witness accounts, documentary, archival, historical data and/or samples of a variety of possible cultural forms of expression, 3) identifying and describing the steps in the analysis of the data, and 4) attending to the issues of voice in the re-storying and re-presenting of the narrative by clearly indicating who the narrator is—the researcher, the participant, both in sequential form, both in composite form, or both as interpreted and re-storied by the researcher. A further criterion for assessing the trustworthiness of narrative research that has been the subject of much discussion in my qualitative research classes is whether the *narrative research evokes emotion* in the reader. Indeed, we have discussed at length whether the primary function of narrative research should be to move the reader through the evoking of emotion. If it is not the primary function, I believe it is a critical one.

Summary: Trustworthiness and Credibility in Narrative Inquiry

1. Include the participant fully in the research process.
2. Provide meaningful opportunities for the participants to review transcripts and the researcher's retold story and their comments and reactions to the story of the research.
3. In the interests of transparency, insure that all research procedures and steps are fully described.
4. Consider whether the narrative research story evokes emotion.

Ethics in Narrative Research

The storying of a part of one's life and the sharing of that story with a researcher can lead to a number of different emotional reactions. On the one hand, a person can experience catharsis and relief. On the other hand, a person can become distressed and upset. Or the person can express a strong desire to have their story finally heard and told, even if the telling is anonymously. Knowing that one's story will be told can be validating and powerful. Or the person, through examining their connection to the beliefs and values of their larger social world, can experience rapid and profound change in the understanding of their identity, of whom and how they are in the world. None of these reactions are neutral.

For many, the telling of the story of their life to a researcher is a *dialogical encounter* of the kind that Buber (1958) refers to as "I" and "Thou." The "I" and "Thou" encounter is one of mutuality and reciprocity. In the language of social constructionism, it is one of co-construction. In some forms of narrative research, the co-construction is of the very identity of the person. To some extent, this is moving into territory where angels properly fear to tread. The responsibility of the narrative researcher is clear. The narrative researcher *must be aware of the potential for profound personal change and intense emotional experiencing* that could be generated through the process of narrative interviewing and always approach the participant with sensitivity and respect. Hearing and gathering the stories of peoples' lives also requires that the researcher be fully present to the participants. In addition, the researcher must be comfortable with hearing stories of lives that can reflect the panoply of possible human experiencing. Some researchers are just not comfortable with the kind of intimate knowing of the other that occurs in narrative research and therefore should avoid it. These guidelines fall into the category of ethics that McNamee and Gergen (1998) refer to as *relational responsibility*.

The standard ethical guidelines for any researcher studying human subjects also apply. Consent to participate in the research study should be fully informed, meaning that prospective participants have the opportunity to discuss the study and have any questions they might have fully answered. Prospective participants should have an understanding of the nature and purpose of the study and know that participation is voluntary and that they can discontinue participation at any time without penalty. If Institutional Review Board (IRB) approval is required, the researcher must submit their proposal and obtain approval for the study before beginning. If the researcher is not operating in an institutional context where IRB approval is required, the researcher should still follow the federal guidelines developed for the protection of human subjects in research studies. Issues of identification and confidentiality should be fully discussed and agreed upon prior to the collection of data. Where confidentiality is required, the researcher has an obligation to protect the confidentiality of research participants by using pseudonyms and camouflaging contextual details of the study sufficiently so that readers would not be able to identify the participants. This obligation confers another one on the researcher and that is, the obligation to maintain the integrity of the study by camouflaging identifying information without changing it so much that it no longer reflects the context and experiences of the participants.

Summary: Ethics in Narrative Research

1. Narrative research requires relational responsibility.
2. The researcher must be sensitive, respectful, and fully present to the participant.
3. The researcher must be mindful that personal change and intense emotional experiencing could result from the interview process.
4. The researcher must be comfortable with the intimacy required of narrative research and hearing stories of lives that include the panoply of human experiences.
5. Standard ethical procedures including obtaining fully informed consent, protecting participant confidentiality, and obtaining IRB approval must be followed.
6. The researcher must safeguard the integrity of the study when camouflaging contextual details to protect client confidentiality.

Concluding Comments

Narrative research is about the storied nature of peoples' lives and the nature of how people make sense out of their lives by putting their experiences in story form. Narrative research is not neutral because it sits at the crossroads of individual identity and the culture stories that fashion it. It is not possible to ask people about the stories of their lives without entering into intimate relationship with them. Intimacy changes people. Asking questions and telling stories change people. It is not possible to tell about a life without talking about the people, the place, the time, and the events that were going on during the time of that life and ordering those elements into something that makes sense—a story. Well-told stories of peoples' lives evoke emotion in those who hear or read the stories and then the listeners and readers change too and get hungry for more stories. And in the betwixt and between of art and human science, narrative research provides a way of gathering stories that, in the end, describe all the ways there are of being human and living life. So what it all means is that there are a lot more stories out there just waiting to be told and to be heard.

References

Banks, M. (2007). *Using visual data in qualitative research.* Los Angeles, CA: Sage.

Bruner, J. (2004). Life as narrative. *Social Research, 71,* 691–710.

Buber, M. (1958). *I and thou.* (R. G. Smith, Trans.). New York: Scribner's.

Burke, K. (1969). *A grammar of motives.* Berkeley: University of California Press.

Chenail, R. J. (1995). Presenting qualitative data. *The Qualitative Report, 2*(3). Retrieved July 25, 2010, from http://www.nova.edu/ssss/QR/QR2-3/presenting.html

Chenail, R. J. (2008). Learning to appraise the quality of qualitative research articles: A contextualized learning object for constructing knowledge. *The Weekly Qualitative Report, 1*(9), 49–61. Retrieved July 25, 2010, from http://www.nova.edu/ssss/QR/WQR/appraising.pdf

Constas, M. A. (1992). Qualitative analysis as a public event: The documentation of category development procedures. *American Educational Research Journal, 29,* 253–266.

Creswell, J. W. (2002). *Educational research: Planning, conducting, and evaluating quantitative and qualitative research.* Upper Saddle River, NJ: Merrill Prentice Hall.

Denzin, N. (2001). The reflexive interview and a performative social science. *Qualitative Research, 1,* 23–46.

Flick, U. (2008). *Managing quality in qualitative research.* Thousand Oaks, CA: Sage.

Foucault, M. (1970). *The order of things: An archaeology of the human sciences.* New York: Pantheon.

Foucault, M. (1973). *The birth of the clinic: An archaeology of medical perception.* (A. M. Sheridan-Smith, Trans.). New York: Pantheon.

Foucault, M. (1976). *Mental Illness and Psychology.* (A. Sheridan, Trans.). New York: Harper & Row.

Foucault, M. (1978). *Discipline and punish: The birth of the prison.* (A. Sheridan, Trans.). New York: Pantheon.

Freedman, J., & Combs, G. (1996). *Narrative therapy: The social construction of preferred realities.* New York: Norton.

George, C., Kaplan, N., & Main, M. (1996). *Adult attachment interview.* Unpublished manuscript (3rd ed.), Department of Psychology, University of California, Berkeley.

Gergen, K. J. (2009). *Relational being: Beyond self and community.* New York: Oxford University Press.

Goffman, E. (1959). *The presentation of self in everyday life.* New York: Doubleday Anchor.

Goffman, E. (1963). *Stigma: Notes on the management of spoiled identity.* Englewood Cliffs, NJ: Prentice-Hall.

Goffman, E. (1974). *Frame Analysis: An Essay on the Organization of Experience*. New York: Harper and Row.

Kvale, S. (1996). *InterViews: An introduction to qualitative research interviewing*. Thousand Oaks, CA: Sage.

Kvale, S. (2007). *Doing interviews*. Los Angeles, CA: Sage.

Labov, W. (1972). The transformation of experience in narrative syntax. In W. Labov (Ed.), *Language in the inner city* (pp. 352–396). Philadelphia: University of Pennsylvania Press.

Labov, W., & Waletsky, J. (1967). Narrative analysis: Oral versions of personal experience. In J. Helm (Ed.), *Essays on the verbal and visual arts* (pp. 12–44). Seattle: American Ethnological Society.

Lock, A., & Strong, T. (2010). *Social constructionism: Sources and stirrings in theory and practice*. Cambridge, UK: Cambridge University Press.

McNamee, S., & Gergen, K. J. (Eds.). (1998). *Relational responsibility: Resources for sustainable dialogue*. Thousand Oaks, CA: Sage.

Parker, I. (2005). *Qualitative psychology: Introducing radical research*. Buckingham, UK: Open University Press.

Phillips, D. C. (1997). Telling the truth about stories. *Teaching and Teacher Education, 13*, 101–109.

Polkinghorne, D. E. (2007). Validity issues in narrative research. *Qualitative Inquiry, 13*(4), 471–486.

Riessman, C. K. (1993). *Narrative analysis*. Newbury Park, CA: Sage.

Riessman, C. (2007). *Narrative methods for the human sciences*. Thousand Oaks, CA: Sage.

Schafer, R. (1992). *Retelling a life: Narration and dialogue in psychoanalysis*. New York: Basic Books.

Schwandt, T. A. (1998). Constructivist, interpretivist approaches to human inquiry. In N. K. Denzin & Y. S. Lincoln (Eds.), *The landscape of qualitative research: Theories and issues* (pp. 221–259). Thousand Oaks, CA: Sage.

Somers, A. (2005). *Background: Terri Schiavo's right to live or die. Does Terri's husband have the right to end her life?* Retrieved August 5, 2005, from http://civilliberty.about.com/cs/humaneuthinasia/a/bgTerry.htm

Spence, D. P. (1987). *The Freudian metaphor: Toward paradigm change in psychoanalysis*. New York: Norton.

Volavkova, H. (Ed.). (1993). *I never saw another butterfly: Children's drawings and poems from Terezin concentration camp, 1942–1944* (2nd ed.). New York: Schocken Books.

Weingarten, K. (2000). Witnessing, wonder, and hope. *Family Process, 39*, 389–402.

White, M., & Epston, D. (1990). *Narrative means to therapeutic ends*. New York: Norton.

17

Exemplar: Narrative Analysis: The Effects on Student Learning

Experiencing a Practicum in Marriage and Family Therapy

Paul Gallant

Introduction to Narrative and Narrative Research

This chapter provides an example of narrative research and its focus on the study of the lives of individuals and the stories of their lives as provided by those individuals. More specifically, narrative analysis allows for the systematic study of personal experience and the construction of meaning from the events of one's life (Riesmann, 1993).

A principle of narrative therapy is what has been termed *insider knowledges*, the distinction between objective knowing and the personal knowledge of people who have first-hand experience of a subject (McLeod, 2007). This chapter will bring to light the insider, local knowledge of students who have experienced clinical practice with actual families and live supervision in a marriage and family therapy practicum.

In a pilot for this proposed project, a colleague—a family therapy faculty member of the School of Humanities and Social Sciences at Nova Southeastern University—and I asked students enrolled in internal practicum courses (working with real families while receiving live, in-the-moment supervision) to keep written, ongoing journals of their experiences throughout the 13-week trimester. Our instructions to the students were intentionally vague. The students were instructed to write down anything and everything they believed was a "learning moment" related to their becoming better therapists. Our hypotheses in doing this were 1) it was likely that students who were in training to become therapists were likely learning about working with their clients in methods, times, and places that were not circumscribed within the class syllabus; 2) the things students say they learn in practicum settings may have very little to do with the actual and specific instructions given to them by their supervisor; and 3) the kind of learning students were doing was likely a deeply rich resource from which we could adjust our teaching and supervisory practices. Students' journals would be collected at the end of the trimester, transcribed, and then subjected to a qualitative narrative analysis utilizing a grounded theory methodology. The researchers will be looking for both thematic and unique outcome data.

We hope these data will serve as the basis for better understanding the experiences student therapists find most meaningful when they are being trained in a live supervision setting. Identifying these experiences, and the ways that students perceive them, will allow us to then 1) identify and better understand the learning processes that occur within the context of clinical practica settings, especially as they relate to non-direct instructional interactions between supervisor and student, 2) develop a student-generated narrative that describes the process of learning in a clinical setting from an "emic" or "insider's" point of view, and 3) make adjustments in the way(s) that practicum courses are taught, with an emphasis on promoting those actions and practices that students identify as being most meaningful to their personal learning experiences.

This proposal was submitted to seek to expand this pilot project to include all of the internal practicum courses within the Brief Therapy Institute in the School of Humanities and Social Sciences for a period of 1 year (approximately 24 internal practica). The data generated will: 1) serve as a basis for a comprehensive dissertation research project, seeking to understand those moments that therapists in training find most meaningful to their career development, 2) prove invaluable to the department's curriculum review process, and allow the family therapy faculty to include student voices into the practicum learning outcomes in ways not previously possible, and 3) introduce the process of self-reflection into internal practicum courses as a standard practice.

Why This Research Is Important

A major development throughout all of higher education is the increasing emphasis that all manner of accrediting bodies place on degree programs demonstrating tangible learning outcomes. These requirements are being made of all programs, regardless of whether or not the program is theoretical, technical, or clinical in nature. As a result, faculty teaching individual courses within these degree programs increasingly construct detailed, skill-based rubrics to promote the learning objectives of the course. These rubrics in most cases require students to demonstrate competence(s) and skills along lines preordained by

the faculty or the program. In this way, accrediting bodies can point to the specific skills and abilities that students should possess as a result of their matric-
ulation through a particular curriculum. In theory, this process also allows for
degree granting programs to review and assess their own progress in addressing areas of the curriculum that are lacking, or where student skill sets are
weak. In practice it seems this process has done little to allow actual student input into the development of a course or a curriculum.

Few would argue that the particular skills needed to do family therapy
cannot be outlined in some detail on a checklist of particulars. In fact, the
Commission on Accreditation of Marriage and Family Therapy Education
(COAMFTE) within the past few years has detailed just such a list of skills
and abilities that graduates of all accredited programs must demonstrate.

However, in an interpersonally intensive clinical program like family therapy, where the student is also learning to become a reflective practitioner, this
tangible learning outcomes approach seems to downplay if not actually disregard the importance of personal reflection in becoming an empathic and
competent therapist. It was not long after our program moved to the newly
created program standards described above that some of my colleagues in the
department and I began to recognize a certain gap between our stated training goals and what we thought was most important for our students to learn
before they began their careers.

This perceived gap is supported by a review of the literature addressing
training and supervision. We found a paucity of research aimed at elucidating
how wisdom and experience are accumulated in the training of master's level
marriage and family therapy students. Few studies have successfully investigated measures of professional growth by student therapist interns during
their practicum experience (Paris, Linville, & Rosen, 2006). For the most part
it seems research has focused on the correlation between the development of
clinical skills and positive treatment outcomes.

More than a decade ago Polson and Nida (1998) identified that an area deserving of more attention was exactly which learning experiences are important
to the skill development of therapists in training. Today little has been done
specifically to fill that gap. In 1996 Coward examined the important influences
and events that shaped the personal and professional development of marriage
and family therapists. However, these findings were limited to the study of the
impact of personal characteristics such as motivation, awareness, and resilience
on professional growth; no attention was paid to effects of the learning of experiences of one's training. Wise, Lowery, and Silvergrade (1989) examined the
effects of a supervisor's encouragement on skill development (as well as the
effect of personal therapy on trainees' clinical development) but again their
outcome measurement was client satisfaction. Wolgien and Coady (1997) conducted research that explored therapists' beliefs about the development of

their helping ability. However, rather than examining the effects of their training on their helping ability, this study looked at students' personal life experiences as primary influences on their clinical abilities. Elements such as difficult childhood and adult life experiences and coping with family crises were examined for their effects on participants' ability to be empathic when treating client's difficult situations. Bischoff's (1997) study most closely approximates the interests embodied within this proposal. He looked at how experiences in clinicians' first 3 months of clinical internship affected their personal development. Participants reported on the positive effects that supervisors, peers, and successes had in subsequent clinical interventions. None of these studies, however, entertain the notion that when it comes to acquiring adequate clinical skills, a good deal of student learning may occur outside of the classroom or treatment room setting.

Research Question(s)

In this section state the research question(s) that organize the study. If you want to, you can also describe how you settled on those questions—what your thinking was and whether you changed or modified the questions and what may have prompted those changes.

Since 2004 my primary duties as faculty in two marriage and family therapy programs involved supervising students during their practicum experience of counseling individuals, couples, and families. In both settings the structure has been the same in that six students are assigned to one supervisor for a 6-hour practicum block per week over the course of a semester. Each student is assigned a client. Each client session is observed by the supervisor and the remaining five students. Appropriately, it is called *live* supervision as the students receive immediate feedback, support and instruction by phone-in messages *during* the sessions. Students have the opportunity to look at post-session videos of their work and to discuss their progress with their supervisor and peers in post-session discussions.

Students usually enter the practicum with two anxiety-filled elements. One is the pressure of being observed by others during their first meeting with people who have come to the center requesting help. Adding to this anxiety is the serious nature of the problems they encounter, including relationship tensions between parents and children or between couples, as well as individual problems such as self-doubt, self-abuse, and depression. The second ever-present element is the pressure felt to demonstrate therapy skills that have been taught only previously in the classroom setting. Students struggle with the knowledge of being under the gaze of their peers and the supervisors who grade their performance.

It is in this context that we have developed an interest in knowing how students navigate through this tension-filled initial experience and come out at the end of their practicum at a different place than when they began, in terms of feeling self-confidence and knowing how to conduct therapeutic sessions.

The research questions we pose are:

- What did you learn? (What therapy skills do you know you have demonstrated in your work?)
- How did you learn them? (What were the meaningful moments in the practicum process that enabled this learning?)
- In what ways are you different? (Which was a result of the practicum experience?)

Research Design

As a distinct form of qualitative research, this narrative research design will focus on the development of professional identity in the individual participant's experience of live supervision during their training as marriage and family therapists. Rather than take their stories of their training experience at face value, the narrative research design will explore the meanings given to experience and the changes in these meanings, including the various reconstructions and deconstructions of these meanings over time (Riessman, 2007).

This particular design is strengthened by the following elements: 1) the participants are individuals who are very willing to share their stories; 2) they are invested in their particular clinical training setting; 3) the researcher is interested in the development of a close working relationship with the participants; and, 4) the stories will be processed when the participants are ready to do so and when a chronology of events has been established (Creswell, 2002).

The participants record their experiences at the end of each of the 13 weekly live supervision sessions over the course of a university trimester. Each session consists of a weekly 6-hour block of participating in a therapy session as the primary therapist for an individual, couple, or family; observing therapy sessions conducted by their peers; receiving live feedback from their supervisor either during their actual therapy session or directly after the session; and providing feedback to their peers after observing their sessions. Each participant writes an individual account of their experience for that day, capturing what they have noticed as learning moments, and noting any experience of professional and personal growth. The recordings are limited to the experience during the 6-hour block of supervised clinical experience. These are stories provided by the individual only.

One of the foundations for this narrative research design is found in the theoretical lens of what has come to be known as *narrative therapy* (White, 2007; White & Epston, 1990). More specifically, White's use of the concept of landscape of identity and landscape of identity questions when engaging in what he calls re-authoring conversations strongly supports the design chosen here. The belief is that people act on what they hold precious and important. Thus, an important area of inquiry is into the intentional state understandings of what a person gives value to, including his or her visions, hopes, commitments, and beliefs.

Research Method

Sample

Twelve students in the master's in marriage and family therapy program at Nova Southeastern University were selected for this study. They were chosen because they are entering their first clinical practicum in which they offer counseling to clients at the university's family therapy clinic where they receive live supervision from their practicum instructor. The number of participants more than satisfies the criteria for narrative research sample size (Creswell, 2002).

Data Collection—Use of Interviews

Each participant will be interviewed within the week following the completion of their 13-week practicum experience. The three research questions, cited earlier in this chapter, provide the focus of the interview.

Two prompts will be used to elicit as much information as possible during the interviews. First, the participants will use their written record for reference points. Their journals provide timelines of recorded experiences from the beginning to the end of their practicum experiences. Like a novel, these written records or personal stories establish a sequence of events over time that focus on a particular plot—the three research questions.

A second prompt will be the conversational format of the interviews (Riesmann, 1993) in which the research will ask follow-up questions to obtain more detail of the participant's experience of what happened during the practicum. Questions are asked to fill in the gaps of the story. The intention (Kvale, 1996) is for the questioning process to enable participants to discover new meanings and new relationships among the events of their practicum experiences. The participants themselves start to see new connections in their experiences on the basis of their spontaneous descriptions, free of interpretations by the interviewer.

Data Analysis

The goal of the data analysis in this project is twofold. First we attempt to identify aspects of the participants' written records that describe how they learned the clinical skills they reported learning, and how they developed competence and gained confidence in the process. In searching for these meaningful moments, we assist participants in taking on the posture of a reflective practitioner. The second goal is to write up these meaningful moments from each participant into the form of a coherent, comprehensive story (Polkinghorne, 2004). The concept of time is important to be mindful of here, with a beginning, middle, and end to the process of acquiring skills and the development of professional identity over the course of a trimester.

Narrative analysis of identity development is the method selected for this project. We have a real interest in inquiring about the impact of students' experiences at the clinic on their personal and professional identity development. It is a rich experience to see how external experiences create the inside story of self (Duffy, 2007). The role of a narrative researcher exploring identity development is to conduct interviews, ask good questions, and inquire into the emerging stories of identity the participants have come to believe and carry out in their lives. A critical piece to the process is the retelling of the stories by the researcher to the participants. The questions asked have the potential effect of inviting the participants into a self-reflective posture. The questions serve as a scaffold, helping people to notice changes in their thinking, their self-concept, and their identity. Through the collaboration with the interviewer, participants are enabled to distance themselves from the known and familiar sense of self toward "what is possible to know and achieve" (White, 2007).

Preliminary Finding

The following are four examples of journal entries of students participating in the pilot of the research project described in this chapter. These are samples of the many raw, yet-to-be explored observations of meaningful moments described in their records. Although they were given the same set of questions from which to respond, each participant wrote about their experience in a unique style and in varying detail. To demonstrate the method, in the first three entries, I have inserted a few of the unlimited number of prompt questions that could be asked of each participant to bring forth the rich story development of each student's experience in the practicum. The fourth entry provides an opportunity for the reader to practice inserting your own questions in support of thickening and enriching the written record of that participant. You will notice that in each account of the participant's experience in the practicum, there are abundant opportunities to ask questions that have the potential to engage the person in further meaningful conversation.

As you read the examples that follow, you will most likely observe that the researcher will benefit from being aware that every question offers the possibility of contributing a change to a person's self-concept and therefore calls on the interviewer to maintain a strong ethical posture (Duffy, 2007).

Journal entry 1
Self-reflection: What have I learned?
I've learned that self-doubt is a struggle for me. [May I ask, how did you learn this?] *My perfectionist side of me is hindering my ability to take in this experience as fully as I should be. I need to recognize when self-doubt arises in me, recognize it as self doubt and say to it, "Hey! Buzz off!"*

When/how did I learn this?
I really recognized it from session one but I saw that Dr. G. noticed this struggle of mine early on as well. Now that I know this about myself and see where and how it's holding me back, I can face this head on and actively work to overcome it. [What do you know about yourself that tells you that you can face this head on? Knowing this about yourself, what steps might you take in actively working to overcome it?]

Meaningful moment
I wrote in my first entry that Dr. G. nonchalantly looked at Keri and said, "It seems you've put a lot of pressure on yourself." For some reason that hit me hard and made me realize that I'm the only person putting this pressure on myself. My peers are not. My clients are not. Dr. G. is not. I'm the one who has put this pressure on myself to be a perfect therapist. Thank goodness this turning point happened on day one before any of us had even seen a client. It gave me the tools I needed to view this experience in a way that would make it more beneficial for me. [May I ask, what are these tools that you now have?] *Any time after that I could see self-doubt or perfectionism begin to hold me back in my growth as a family therapist. I could refer back to practicum day one, hour one and it reminded me to be patient with myself.* [Have you continued to notice that you are being patient with yourself? Can you give me an example of this? What was it like for you to notice this about yourself? What does it mean to you to know that you have the ability to remind yourself to be patient?]

Journal entry 2
Skills learned during Dr. G.'s Practicum
1. *Listening*
2. *Showing respect*
3. *Staying in the moment*
4. *Choosing words carefully*
5. *Being at peace*
6. *Curiosity*
7. *Client strengths*
8. *Honoring lives*

1. Listening. *I have become conscious of the need to listen ever so closely or attend to what a client says during a therapy session.* [How did you develop this consciousness? What does it mean for you to know that about yourself, that you developed this consciousness?] *I have also learned to listen to myself*

differently—realizing I am not the expert, but I am there to partner with my client and go for the ride or journey of their thoughts respectfully. [Realizing that you are not the expert, but a partner—is that a big, small, or medium realization, in your opinion?] *I believe I learned to listen better by observing my professor provide feedback to all therapy sessions in practicum. I learned to stop thinking so much and to remain in the client's moments—to really hear what a client expresses.*

2. Demonstrating respect. *I show respect to all, it is my nature, but maybe that has been being polite rather than being truly respectful. Respect is yet another skill I am learning in MFT, respect means being fully enveloped in the moment with the client and not verbalizing or using nonverbal communication signals to express my beliefs. That is not easy at times. I had a client in practicum who told me each session that her husband said ugly things to her. To me it was verbal abuse. Rather than spend time during her therapy session judging her husband or judging her for staying in a marriage whereby someone would say such horrible things to her—I learned the skill of staying in her moments—just staying with her—no words—no nonverbal communication. I stayed still and let her express her world to me. That was demonstrating my respect for her life—even though some things said were not easy for me to listen to.* [You state that some things were not easy for you to listen to—may I ask, what did you have to call on in yourself to be able to listen at these times? What quality or skill of yours do you think you were able to draw upon at those moments?]

3. Staying in the moment. *Initially, I was trying to stay one or two steps ahead of my first client in practicum in order to provide better options or solutions to problems being discussed. I believe I did learn to stay in the client's moment—I learned to enjoy staying in the client's moment. It demonstrates that I am respectful and not working so hard—the client is the expert of their life and their problem(s). I was told by Dr. G. that I will learn this skill by "practice, practice, practice." I believe I also learned this by close observation of all my colleagues and their clients along with such caring feedback from Dr. G. and his doctoral assistant, Ilene.*

4. Choosing words carefully. *I am a New Yorker—fast, quick . . . next. I learned to slow down and reflect upon the power of words. I did not want to appear to stumble as a new therapist—sometimes the correct word does not come to mind immediately with a client—I learned it is OK to stumble finding the right words and the client(s) wants to help me find the right word(s) to reflect upon what they are saying. I developed this skill by looking at recordings of my therapy sessions.*

5. Being at peace. *It is important that clients view me being at peace with whatever they present during therapy. It demonstrates respect for them and their realities. I learned this skill watching Dr. G. in action as a therapist. Dr. G.'s voice is so calming and I learned that using my voice to make a client, or anyone for that matter, feel at ease or at peace is important.* [What does it mean for you to know that you now possess this skill? Who else knows this about you? What might they say about knowing you are a person who has learned to be at peace?]

6. Curiosity. *Engage a client by being curious about what they say and their reality. I demonstrated being curious by posing questions to a client's narrative. It is fun to be curious—again a non-expert's position. Developed this skill by studying various MFT models and watching my professors demonstrate ways to ask curious questions in therapy.*

7. Client strengths. *I have learned to see that whatever a client presents in therapy, I can bring out or take notice of their strengths.* [How did you learn this? Was it easy or hard to develop this skill? In your opinion, is this an important skill for therapists to possess?] *Strengths they demonstrated or used to get through a tough situation. It is very empowering to help a client who is going through a negative situation see their inner strength. I learned this in all my NSU MFT classes and I now look for my inner strength when I am going through a negative situation. That is empowering and helps me to think differently . . . more positively. Neuroplasticity is a new area of study that Dr. G. has introduced me to. Thank you!*

8. Honoring lives. *We normally honor a life after someone has died. Why not honor a life while a person is very much alive? I try my best to honor a client who is brave to come to therapy and expose their lives and their situations . . . even those who are court mandated to be in therapy at BTI. I demonstrate this by being respectful and engaging. I am always looking for good in people.*

Journal entry 3

The first six sessions I participated in were quite embarrassing. Although I always demonstrated respect and care for my clients, I kept trying to fix the client's problems after 5 minutes of conversation, and would move the conversation way ahead of where they might have wanted to go (had they had a chance to do so). I also got carried away in two of the sessions and completely forgot to ask questions. I think the turning point for me was when I reviewed my tape of the worst session I conducted with a couple. I am saying the worst ever, because I will work doubly hard to make sure this conduct will never repeat itself again! In that session, I would not stop talking, giving advice, and acting as the expert of things. I didn't ask questions, I finished the client's sentences, and I even tried to sell them on the clinic's services for their daughter! I actually sat in that video room for a few extra minutes that day and cried. I asked myself if I would be able to change. If so, it would depend mostly on myself, on really listening to Dr. G. and getting feedback from the team. My goal is to be the opposite of what I have always been: opinionated and persuasive. [May I ask, why have you set this goal for yourself? And, what does it say about you that you have set this goal? Does this goal mean that when you asked yourself if you were able to change, that you answered, "Yes!" to that question? What tells you that you have the ability to change? Who else knows about this ability of yours? Of all the people in the world who know you, who would be the least surprised that you have the ability to make these changes? Why would he/she be not surprised?]

The journal has been so helpful in writing down great questions that open space for introspective conversation. I read it every week, so that I remind myself of how I want to be, and how I want my clients to feel in therapy. I really want them to find things out on their own so that these discoveries become more meaningful to them. I want to be able to create such an environment. I know time and practice are fundamental, but I will work on doing my part, by being more like a mirror to them. At least now I know what I need to become and that it is possible for me to get there. [What do you know about yourself that tells you it is possible for you to get there? How did you learn that about yourself? What does it mean for you to hear yourself saying that you know that you have the ability to "get there"?] *I see some progress in how I am going about the therapy, like being less "directive" and listening more to the clients' "here and now" concerns. Last week I finally felt comfortable with having my mind "stay in the present." It felt good to feel that no matter what transpired, the session was about them and due to that, was helpful to them in some way. I still have a long way to go but I am confident that continuing my education under a narrative therapist will augment my progress.*

Journal entry 4
Journal summary and reflection

I really didn't think that I would notice so many changes in my journal. Even though I did not write everything that I was feeling at every moment, I could really see my frustration and lack of confidence in the beginning of practicum start to wither away. I really noticed a change in the later entries, even though I did not directly say "I felt more confident," after reading it I think it was evident. The amount of confidence that I had with my last couple was really a turning point for me and you could tell in my entry about it. Even though it was not without hesitation of, "was I helpful enough?" I still think it was a big change from my first family. In the first few entries I could go back and remember the fear I had in the first few sessions. I think that this fear has changed towards the end of practicum. It changed from being scared that you will not know what to say, or that the clients wouldn't take you seriously to, I hope this client has a good week, and I hope that I am useful and that they come back! But even that fear of, "Is this client going to come back?" changed a little. I had some clients not show, which happened to many of us in our team, but I really felt the need to make sure clients would come back, and initially I was of course blaming myself a little for not making a big enough impact. But as I saw Cody, Kelly, and other team members' clients come back week after week I could see that they were doing pretty much the same things as me in the therapy room, and maybe my clients were not in the right place to commit to therapy at that time. Being around the team and seeing their progress helped me enormously, and for a while I think I was starting to let it hinder me too. Even though I went a few sessions without a client or another team member had a good session, I needed to remember that we all go at our own pace and nobody was judging my progress but me. I think now with getting a new client I'm not as scared of not knowing what to say, I think I have more confidence and have acquired a certain method of finding the question in what the client gives you which really takes the pressure off me. This was something that I liked learning more about in practicum. Learning to be myself in a group full of strangers is something that I need to work on in the clinic and is something not as natural for me in other aspects of my life. I am a shy person by nature and it takes a little bit for me to be myself. But being with new clients every week is really helping me open up, I just know I need some more time and practice to make this a more natural process for me. I think learning how to be yourself along with knowing when to joke and keep the session light hearted and when to be serious takes time, and I think that I have made a big step in the direction I need to go in order to feel more comfortable with myself and how I act in the therapy room. I have really learned that you grow everyday in this profession, and you can notice changes not only in your clients but in yourself with every passing therapy session. I hope to continue gaining more confidence and trust in what I am doing with my clients with the knowledge that clients come to see us because we are there to help, which is comfort and therapy in of itself.

Establishing Trustworthiness

Whose story is it? In the writing of the preliminary narrative analysis, I have become the dominant voice. Member checking involves giving participants their story back by checking for the mini story of the individual participant as well as seeking comments on the larger story from all the students (participants) and adding them to the narrative of the findings. This will provide the opportunity for the story to be enriched through corrections to be made and further comments to be added, so the final product will include all their comments. The narrative product will have all the voices of the participants as well as mine. An ethical posture here is to ensure no one is marginalized (Creswell, 2009).

Implications

As described in this chapter, university settings are competency-driven environments. Course syllabi are now 15–plus pages long, listing the program learning objectives, the program competency objectives, the course learning objectives, and the learning outcomes and core competencies. Following then are the rubrics (with their assignments/grading procedures and point scales) designed to measure the mastery of the competencies.

The examples presented earlier illustrate how, when a person contributes to their professional identity and personal and professional growth, it is more than naming a particular core competency, it is part of a human, personal story, unfolding over time. Participants bring the human dimension through the stories they tell and demonstrate that developing competence is a journey, that the competencies learned are living, moving, growing skills. Simply naming them as core standards prevents the deeper, richer description of the development of these skills as they emerge in meaningful moments over time.

This pilot research project and its narrative analysis methodology are intended to bring forth the rich story development of lessons learned, skills developed, and the meaningful moments from which these emerge.

References

Bischoff, R. (1997). Themes in therapist development during the first three months of clinical experience. *Contemporary Family Therapy, 19,* 563–580.

Coward, R. (1996). Significant events and themes in the development of marriage and family therapists. Unpublished doctoral dissertation, Virginia Polytechnic Institute and State University, Department of Human Development, Blacksburg, VA.

Creswell, J. W. (2002). *Educational research: Planning, conducting, and evaluating quantitative and qualitative research.* Upper Saddle River, NJ: Merrill Prentice Hall.

Creswell, J. W. (2009). *Research design: Qualitative, quantitative, and mixed methods approaches.* Thousand Oaks, CA: Sage.

Duffy, M. (2007). Narrative inquiry: The method. In P. Munhall (Ed.), *Nursing research: A qualitative perspective* (4th ed., pp. 401–421). Sudbury, MA: Jones & Bartlett.

Kvale, S. (1996). *Interviews: An introduction to qualitative research interviewing.* Los Angeles, CA: Sage.

Kvale, S. (2007). *Doing interviews.* Los Angeles, CA: Sage.

McLeod, J. (2007). *Counselling Skill.* London: Open University Press.

Paris, E., Linville, D., & Rosen, K. (2006). Marriage and family therapist interns' experiences and growth. *Journal of Marital and Family Therapy, 32*(1), 45–57.

Polkinghorne, D. (2004). Narrative therapy and postmodernism. In L. Angus & J. McLeod (Eds.), *The handbook of narrative and psychotherapy: Practice, theory and research.* (pp. 53–68). Thousand Oaks, CA: Sage.

Polson, M., & Nida, R. (1998). Program and trainee lifestyle stress: A survey of AAMFT student members. *Journal of Marital and Family Therapy, 24,* 95–112.

Riesmann, C. (1993). *Narrative analysis.* Thousand Oaks, CA: Sage.

Riessman, C. (2007). *Narrative methods for the human sciences.* Thousand Oaks, CA: Sage.

White, M. (2007). *Maps of narrative practice.* New York, NY: W.W. Norton.

White, M., & Epston, D. (1990). *Narrative means to therapeutic ends.* New York, NY: W. W. Norton.

Wise, P., Lowery, S., & Silvergrade, L. (1989). Personal counseling for counselors in training. *Counselor Education and Supervision, 28,* 326–336.

Wolgien, C., & Coady, N. (1997). Good therapists' beliefs about the development of their helping ability: The wounded healer paradigm. *Clinical Supervisor, 15*(2), 19–35.

18

Action Research: The Methodologies

Ronald J. Chenail, Sally St. George, Dan Wulff, and Robin Cooper

Action research has a unique place among the many varieties of research methodologies. It is at once a type of formal academic methodology while also being a social enterprise that is, in various and significant ways, conducted by the people affected by the issues. Action research involves the joining of those who recognize and respond to a need for changes in life or work conditions through a systematic inquiry/praxis (Reason & Bradbury, 2008a).

The democratic or participatory nature of action research (process) is coupled with a focus on action or change (outcome). The focal problem and the associated means utilized to make significant changes are integrated such that change is embedded within the steps/phases of the inquiry. The researchers/inquirers are those people intimately invested in the situation undergoing review and change. Action researchers are not dispassionate outsiders—they are insiders who are intent on reforming aspects of their world (Waterman, Tillen, Dickson, & de Koning, 2001).

The term *action research* has been used by many authors in differing ways. To illustrate this, Reason and Bradbury in *The Sage Handbook of Action Research* (2008b) note a sampling of phrases used in chapter titles: "participatory (action) research," "participatory research," "emancipatory action research," "pragmatic action research," "action science," "co-operative inquiry," "appreciative inquiry," "community action research," "action inquiry," "educational action research," "transpersonal co-operative inquiry," and "collaborative inquiry." While these various terms describe characteristics of action research that have the potential to uniquely shape inquiries, they also inadvertently contribute to the confusion of classifying and labeling within the field of action research (Holter & Schwartz-Barcott, 1993). These terms may represent nuanced differences or may be different terms (reflective of personal preferences) used for the same idea or conceptualization. Thus, action research is not a single methodology but rather a family of research approaches, each in some way distinct from the others.

The family of action research methodologies has found a home in the field of nursing for a number of important reasons. Nursing researchers (e.g., Hart & Anthrop, 1996) see action research as a professionalizing strategy as nursing seeks to achieve the status of a research-based profession, as a vehicle for developing reflective practitioners, and as a means for producing knowledge for practice. They also note that the humanistic qualities of these methodologies appeal to nurses who embrace action research as an emancipatory strategy and as a form of collaborative enquiry rooted in reflective practice. Speaking specifically of community-based participatory research, Shelton (2008) notes this form of action research "seems a natural fit methodologically, for what nurses have been doing and will continue to do" (p. 255). In addition, Robinson (1995) suggests that action research offers nurses the potential to develop transformative shifts in nursing culture. Many nursing researchers point to action research's potential to introduce innovation and facilitate change in practice and to generate and test theories relevant to their world of practice (Titchen & Binnie, 1993; Waterman, Webb, & Williams, 1995). Lastly, Walters and East (2001) suggest that action research approaches are appealing mainly because they allow nurse practitioners and researchers to work *with* and *for* (rather than on) patients.

The variety of professional areas in which nurses have employed the family of action research approaches to generate new knowledge and to produce new change is remarkable. These projects include research 1) defining the evolving nursing profession (e.g., Kelly, Simpson, & Brown, 2002; Walsgrove & Fulbrook, 2005); 2) connecting with communities to produce local change (Parsons & Warner-Robbins, 2002; Shelton, 2008; Walters & East, 2001); 3) producing change in hospitals, clinics, and other practice locations (e.g., Mander, Cheung, Wang, Fu, & Zhu, 2010; Reed, Pearson, Douglas, Swinburne, & Wilding, 2002; The Staff of Mountbatten Ward, Wright, & Baker, 2005); 4) assessing and improving education and training (e.g., Chien, Chan, & Morrissey, 2002; Walker, Bailey, Brasell-Brian, & Gould, 2001); 5) improving practice based upon patients' insights and experiences (e.g., Lauri & Sainio, 1998; Olshansky et al., 2005); and 6) improving practice based upon nurses' and other healthcare providers' feedback (e.g., Coetzee, Britton, & Clow, 2005; Glasson, Chang, & Bidewell, 2008; Ives & Melrose, 2010; Mitchell, Conlon, Armstrong, & Ryan, 2005; Reid-Searl et al., 2009).

In this chapter we discuss *action research (basic)*, *participatory action research*, and *appreciative inquiry*. These three varieties of action research are not the only types, but they are selected for two reasons. First, they possess utility for the advancement of the nursing profession and practices, and their usage reflects a large segment of the extant action research found in contemporary nursing research. Second, they allow us to show how specific methodologies within the family of action research approaches can vary along several key dimensions, specifically the *change/mobilization process, theoretical grounding, leadership, decision-making, specific strategies,* and *beneficiaries.* It is also important to remember that even *within* each of the three approaches to action research discussed in this chapter there exists variation in how researchers concentrate on problems, improvements, or level of involvement as well as how experimental, organizational, professionalizing, and/or empowering a particular study may be (Hart & Bond, 1996).

The Family of Action Research Methodologies

Action research (basic) is used to target and solve an identified dilemma or problem. Stringer (2007) states that action research (AR) "provides the means for people to engage in systematic inquiry and investigation to 'design' an appropriate way of accomplishing a desired goal and to evaluate its effectiveness" (p. 6). In AR, people adversely affected by some circumstance carefully examine the problem, form a picture of the problem, and develop actions designed to remediate or eliminate the problem. This whole process is referred to as action research. Lee (2009) contrasts this outcome-oriented approach with other research methodologies, noting that "action research studies focus on everyday life to bring about improvement and change. This perspective differs with other research traditions which may focus on pure or theoretical research that does not have applicability in the social setting or human context" (p. 32).

To illustrate her point, Lee (2009) describes an action research study designed to evaluate a nurse-led approach to care in a community hospital. The study brought together current and former patients as well as a variety of staff members at the hospital to explore levels of satisfaction and ways to improve the quality of experience for all involved. Lee explains:

> The philosophies of action research were evident during the development and implementation of the research study. For example, workshops were used throughout to explore team members' expectations; to identify and discuss key elements of the study; to explore research methods; to have shared ownership of data collection and analysis; to enhance team members' participation in dissemination of findings in the organization and externally. (pp. 31–32)

Participatory action research (PAR) is generally used to counteract oppressive conditions experienced by a particular segment of society (Schwandt, 2007).

The PAR project is used to challenge the social customs and assumptions that keep those persons marginalized and oppressed. In an example of a PAR project, a group of mentally retarded adults joined with one of their residential caretakers to discuss the ways in which they were treated (Valade, 2004). Their discussions led to a consensus that the public transportation system provided by the city failed to meet their needs in many ways. The primary problem they were encountering was that the reservation system for the vans provided by the city was not dependable and these adults were completely dependent upon this transportation to attend their daily programs, medical appointments, and social outings. They approached this issue with the knowledge that they had little power to exact any change—they faced this issue with full awareness of the power differential and subsequent risk that speaking out might pose. In this study the group invited the transportation company officials for a conversation that resulted in some policy changes. A by-product of this project was that the group's level of confidence in taking a public stance grew through this experience. This, perhaps more than the procedural changes, was the most significant development resulting from this study.

Appreciative inquiry (AI) is generally used to join the members of an organization to make internal changes by focusing on what is already working. More elaborately,

> Appreciative inquiry refers to both a search for knowledge and a theory of intentional collective action which are designed to help evolve the normative vision and will of a group, organization, or society as a whole. It is an inquiry process that affirms our symbolic choice and cultural evolution. (Cooperrider & Srivastva, 2000, pp. 85–86)

For example, one company was experiencing difficulties with numerous incidences of sexual harassment of female employees by some of the male employees. Numerous previous attempts to solve this problem had been unsuccessful. *Appreciative inquiry* was utilized to transform the issue from one of simply reducing or eradicating harassment events to inquiring into examples of good cross-gender relations within the organization and ways to build upon these positive events and interactions. The organization moved its thinking from trying to reduce some unwanted behaviors to re-envisioning what it could become (Cooperrider & Whitney, 2005).

Working Inside and Outside of Traditional Qualitative Parameters

Action research is located within the qualitative research tradition because it is grounded in understanding specific and local phenomena in context, privileging the words/language used by participants, and proceeding thoroughly and systematically. Value is placed on the complexities of factors that contribute to the real-world "messiness" of problems to promote increased understanding of the issues in need of change. The language of participants is privileged over researcher interpretations. Such interpretations are carefully acknowledged and explicitly connected to the words and descriptions offered by the participants. Staying so close to the data (the participants' words and ideas) helps to develop a more textured picture of the experiences and issues from which to generate new understandings and possible action steps (Waterman, Tillen, Dickson, & de Koning, 2001).

The research process is intentional, but at the same time is fluid. While deliberate plans are made, there is receptivity to altering the method to suit the ongoing needs of the project and the participants. For example, in describing their action research study as nurses in a children's hospital, Fletcher and Beringer (2009) explain, "It was important that the method was flexible and reflexive, allowing, when necessary, 'Plan A' to morph into 'Plan B', new information to be used, and the myriad of factors impinging on care to be taken into account" (p. 30). In the best qualitative tradition, action researchers are intent on attending to the current/local situation rather than creating generalizable findings. Finally, action researchers work systematically to conceptualize and understand the situation of interest and consistently to reflect upon the decisions made and the steps taken. The research practice of transparency, that is, explaining researchers' positions and research decisions, builds confidence in those who come to know their work.

Although action research is akin to qualitative methods in general, we have identified some procedures and processes in conducting action research that differ somewhat. One difference is that change is both the outcome and the process. Initiating the inquiry itself is an intervention that begins the change process. The act of studying something that is problematic by the people who experience the problem enhances the chances that people significantly invest in the effort to bring about change. As Glasson, Chang, and Bidewell (2008) put it, "We might consider how much more commitment there would be towards change if it is devised and implemented by those most affected, such as the nurses and patients on the ward" (p. 35). Change is not constrained by a linear process of data collection, analysis, and final report of the study, rather it is begun and continued throughout the steps/phases of the project (and beyond). A second difference is that there is a collectivity of persons involved in the inquiry process who all hold responsibility for the actions taken because they are the stakeholders and have voice in the decisions made about study procedures. At the same time the participants are the intended beneficiaries, because the change that is effected will be to their advantage. A third major difference is that the methodology is more described by the process of change rather than the form of analysis employed (a wide range of analytical procedures, including quantified data and statistics, may be combined and used in action research). The fourth distinction is that action research is research carried out in public— this publicness builds relationships, both internally and externally. The steps or phases in the research context are public knowledge and made known as they occur, therefore knowledge and action are revealed before the project is completed (Hope & Waterman, 2003).

Phases of Action Research

The phases of action research have similarities across the three types we discuss. Action researchers operate from the value base that there is a need for some change or correction to a problem or dilemma (Brown & Tandon, 1983). The process is mobilized by this problem and the search for a solution and/or difference. In addition, the process is cyclical with multiple iterations of the questions and the analysis of the data; as noted earlier, the common "result" is that change is activated by the introduction of the inquiry process itself.

There are also differences among the various action research methodologies. According to Brown and Tandon (1983), the differences are primarily located in the *values and ideologies* of the inquiry and the *political economy* of the inquiry. The values are the "preferences for courses of action and outcomes" (p. 280) and the ideologies are the "sets of beliefs that explain the world, bind together their adherents, and suggest desirable activities and outcomes" (p. 280). The political economy of inquiry refers to questions such as: "What actors have interests in the decision? What authority and resources are relevant to the decision? How will decisions affect actor interests and distributions of authority and resources?" (p. 284).

We, too, think it is useful to illustrate commonalities and uniquenesses among AR, PAR, and AI. To do so we will compare each using the following dimensions of inquiry that we have thematically derived from the literature and from our experiences of editing qualitative research. The dimensions are: change/mobilization, theoretical orientation, leadership, decision-making, methods/strategies, and beneficiaries (see **Table 18–1**).

Action Research (Basic)

Action Research (basic) is initiated with a very practical problem within a context. For example, communication between different staff members in a hospital setting, workload issues, or specification of roles and tasks might be problematic areas that are in need of change in order to maximize efficiency and quality care as well as to improve the work environment for health workers (Holter & Schwartz-Barcott, 1993). Some personnel in this context would agree that these issues are interfering with the work and that a systematic proposal for

TABLE 18-1 Comparisons and Contrast Among AR, PAR, and AI.

Type	Change/ Mobilization Process	Theoretical Grounding	Leadership	Decision-Making	Methods/ Strategies	Beneficiaries
Action Research (Basic)	Using praxis to solve a specific problem without threatening the existing structures of the system or organization	Pragmatism, Consensus Social Theory	An outside usually assists the internal group working on the problem.	Cooperation among the various groups involved	Quantitative and/or qualitative methods of data gathering and analysis	All parties affected by the problem.
Participatory Action Research	To solve a problem of inequality or unfairness by challenging and changing oppressive practices/rules	Conflict Theory, Critical Theory, Marxism	Leadership usually arises from within the oppressed group.	Cooperative and collaborative within the group seeking change, but conflictual with the larger organization or society	Quantitative and/or qualitative methods of data gathering and analysis; education	The group seeking change
Appreciative Inquiry	To create change in an organization by using the momentum already present	Social Constructionism	An external consultant is usually brought in to organize the work groups that represent a microcosm of the organization.	Consultant enlists members of the organization to examine what the organization is doing well	Unconditional positive questioning (Ludema & Fry, 2008); 4-D Cycle: discovery, dream, design, destiny (Ludema & Fry, 2008; Whitney & Trosten-Bloom, 2003)	All parties

change is warranted. In this case an outside research consultant may be invited to help by working closely with each of the affected groups (e.g., floor nurses, administrators, supervisors) to develop actions "that are purposeful and aim at creating desired outcomes" (Greenwood & Levin, 2005, p. 53). The guiding theory would be that of pragmatism (Greenwood & Levin) and consensus social theory (Brown & Tandon, 1983). The consultant would facilitate the data collection and analysis of the data information. The data could be collected through a variety of means such as surveys and interviews and could be analyzed statistically and/or qualitatively. Based on the information gleaned, a solution would be developed that improves the conditions for those groups who were experiencing difficulty. It is important to note that such praxis is not intended to dramatically change the current rules or structure of operation; rather, it seeks to improve the functioning of the current overall system.

Walsgrove and Fulbrook's (2005) project designed to develop the nurse practitioner role in an acute hospital exemplifies the usefulness of action research to improve care at a hospital by bringing affected parties together to increase awareness and to enact new strategies leading to change. At the advent of their English study, Walsgrove and Fulbrook found there was a limited understanding of and minimal support for the development of the nurse practitioner role in a hospital. To address this concern they combined practice development theory with four overlapping action research cycles to collect nurse practitioner practice information from hospital personnel via questionnaires, semi-structured interviews, meetings, discussions, and their own field notes. Their concurrent analysis of this stakeholder-provided information led to a grounded understanding of the nurse practitioner value from a knowledge perspective based upon insiders' input which led to greater support for nurse practitioners within the hospital system. This project illustrates how practice development (i.e., the role of nurse practitioners) and action research can be combined in a systematic process to not only develop and support professional roles of nurses, but also to improve the quality of patient care and the effectiveness of healthcare services.

Participatory Action Research (PAR)

The goal of engaging in PAR, like action research (basic), is practical change. However, there is the additional objective of changing the larger rules and structures that keep the problem in place. Coming from traditions of conflict theory, critical theory, and Marxism, PAR is a "social and education process [in which] the 'subjects' of participatory action research undertake their research as social practice [and] the 'object' of participatory action research is social" (Kemmis & McTaggart, 2005, p. 563). This research paradigm addresses issues of power and responsibility. In their study of older, acutely ill patients in a medical ward, Glasson, Chang, and Bidewell (2008) explain that the nurses participating in the research asked themselves, "Why am I acting this way? Who tells me to do this? Who benefits? Whose interests am I serving: the patient's, doctor's, management's, the relative's or my own?" (p. 35).

In the nursing context, hierarchies that determine work conditions, salaries, or status may pose problems that go beyond the "problem-solution" remedies of AR. The issue may center on basic inequalities, marginalization, or oppression of groups that have become part of the status quo in the organization or profession at large. PAR is used to challenge those basic inequities, even if such efforts would bring conflict with those groups in power. PAR serves the mission of changing the status quo for the benefit of the oppressed group (Kelly, 2005). According to Kemmis and McTaggart (2005):

> At its best, then, participatory action research is a social process of collaborative learning realized by groups of people who join together in changing the practices through which they interact in a shared social world in which, for better or worse, we live with the consequences of one another's actions. (p. 563)

PAR is characterized by the collaboration with which projects are planned and conducted. The whole group decides the best ways to gather information and to make sense of it. The entire process is marked by demystification (as all work is made transparent) as well as reflection in which each research decision and interpretation is subjected to a critical review for increased understanding (Patton, 2002).

When faced with a professional development challenge after problems arose regarding the moving and handling of patients in a British stroke unit, Mitchell, Conlon, Armstrong, and Ryan (2005), instead of relying on traditional top-down training from unit management, used participatory action research to facilitate the nurses themselves to take ownership of their moving and handling practices. They accomplished this goal by providing a context in which nurses could share their insights and real-world experiences in moving and handling patients following stroke, identifying facilitators of safer moving and handling practice, and empowering themselves in collaboration with physiotherapists to direct changes in their practice. Mitchell et al.'s insider participatory action research approach featured data generated from focus group meetings, brainstorming sessions, observational studies, and from written reflective accounts which led nurses to identify equipment, environment, communication, and teamwork strategies that would facilitate their use of rehabilitative moving and handling practices. Besides producing this new knowledge and practice wisdom about moving and handling stroke patients, the participatory action research project helped the participants to feel a greater degree of involvement and value along with improved teamwork.

Appreciative Inquiry (AI)

AI fits into the action research family because of its focus on change. However, while what is problematic is acknowledged, the focus of change begins with what is already going well (no matter how small) toward the desired change. Operating from a social constructionist stance, AI begins with an affirmative topic choice. The objective is to have people talk about those issues that describe the "life-giving" forces and practices that those involved would like to have in place (Cooperrider, Whitney, & Stavros, 2003). For example, in nursing, if communication patterns or interactions among personnel were expressed as problematic areas in the workplace, the AI researcher would begin to focus on incidents, behaviors, conditions, and times that communication patterns and respectful interaction were already occurring, regardless of how infrequent or seemingly insignificant (Keefe & Pesut, 2004). AI researchers proceed through the 4-D Cycle in which members of the organization answer four questions. The first question is "what gives life?" This is called the Discovery phase. Second, the members of the organization are asked to enter the Dream phase by considering the question, "what might be?" This is followed by the question, "how can it be?" which is identified as the Design phase. The process concludes with the Destiny phase in which the question, "what will be?" is posed (Ludema & Fry, 2008; Whitney & Trosten-Bloom, 2003).

In conducting AI a consultant enlists a variety of members of the organization who want change to decide what data to collect and the best ways to collect it (Cooperrider, Whitney, & Stavros, 2003). The inclusion of many participants who are talking with each other about successful events begins the change process (creating greater understanding and possibilities for action) and ensures investment in both the method and information obtained.

Nursing researchers have used AI to address a variety of research interests: community health nursing (Lind & Smith, 2008), nursing culture and work environment (Farrell, Douglas, & Siltanen, 2003; Moody, Horton-Deutsch, & Pesut, 2007; Richer, Ritchie, & Marchionni, 2009), patient care (Havens, Wood, & Leeman, 2006; Moore & Charvat, 2007; Shendell-Falik, Feinson, & Mohr, 2007), RN retention (Challis, 2009), and nursing excellence and best practices (Carter, Cummings, & Cooper, 2007; Carter, Ruhe, Weyer, Litaker, Fry, & Stange, 2007; Stefaniak, 2007). For example, in a Canadian university healthcare center Richer, Ritchie, and Marchionni (2009) used AI to promote the emergence of innovative ideas regarding the reorganization of healthcare services. Their center had been faced with ongoing employee dissatisfaction with work environments, so they used AI in two of their interdisciplinary groups in outpatient cancer care to better understand the emergence and implementation of innovative ideas. AI helped them to identify new ideas about work reorganization related to interdisciplinary networks and collaboration. This lead to the creation of a forum to examine healthcare quality and efficiency issues in the delivery of cancer care. Their study not only helped them to improve their center, but their research also made a contribution to the literature on microsystems change processes of interdisciplinary treatment teams.

Evaluating Action Research

Evaluating action research must include assessing the degree of success in achieving the twin purposes of action research methodologies which are to stimulate change and to involve stakeholders in the process of change. Both are vital so no rank order of the two is possible. Achieving set goals without maintaining the participatory nature diminishes AR's success; maintaining participation but not reaching the goals of the effort is similarly discouraging (Livesey & Challender, 2002).

Another criterion by which to evaluate AR is the occurrence of unexpected positive events or outcomes. These serendipitous events add to the overall value of the AR effort, even though they cannot be fully anticipated. These occurrences are likely due to the fact that action researchers are setting constructive processes into motion and their outcomes cannot be wholly predicted (e.g., Farrell, Douglas, & Siltanen, 2003).

In addition to the importance of achieving outcomes along with developing and maintaining participation, some believe that the participatory nature of AR can stimulate persons to generate efforts for future projects that add to the value/importance of the current AR project. Particularly with PAR, the development of confidence in producing change can transform individuals and groups into activists who may develop new change programs (e.g., Lindsey & McGuinness, 1998).

Action researchers who see their work as primarily affecting change in their local setting may not develop scholarly works from the research, seeing such products as tangential to the committed focus of their work. But making the project known (in some form) is inevitable due to the multiple persons involved in the project itself and the performance of the research in the natural setting, whether it be a school, a hospital, or the community at large.

In addition to presenting "as you go," making clear the process and the results of the project are important. Included in these decisions would be the intended audience and the form of presentation. To an academic audience, written scholarly works or presentations at professional conferences/meetings would be necessary. To lay audiences, brochures or informal discussions/presentations may well suffice. To politicians or other policymakers, information from the project regarding potential impact on certain groups or identifying financial resources required to effect specific changes may be necessary in order for decisions to be made.

The issue of theory generation that is a component of most research efforts is also an issue within the field of action research. Greenwood and Levin (2005) see action research as a "disciplined way of developing valid knowledge and theory while promoting positive social change" (p. 55) while Cooperrider and Srivastva (2000) ask, "Why is there this lack of generative theorizing in action-research?" (p. 76). The role or importance of generating useful knowledge and theory is widely supported, but the degree to which action research lives up to this goal is debated (Badger, 2000).

Challenges

In our effort in this chapter to delineate a set of AR methodologies, we have drawn distinctions and highlighted commonalities. This is done for the purpose of reviewing the large contours of the field of AR. The blending of research and action poses some challenging questions regarding whether or not research/inquiry can or should be so intimately connected with action. What is taught about scientific rigor would have us see such connections with action steps to be a source of contamination while others lament the current lack of usefulness of research that is compartmentalized from implementation (Rolfe, 1996).

Besides concerns regarding its scientific validity, action research presents other significant hurdles. Along these lines Coghlan and Casey (2001) highlight the management challenges for nurses when conducting action research in their own professional settings. For example nurse researchers often need to combine their action research role with their regular organizational roles, and this role duality can create the potential for role ambiguity and conflict. Williamson and Prosser (2002) argue that because action research approaches rely on a close, collaborative working relationship between researcher and participants, this close relationship can also be the source of political and ethical problems for the researchers and participants. They suggest that these close relationships can jeopardize some of the usual ethical guarantees concerning confidentiality and anonymity, informed consent, and protection from harm that might not arise with the use of quantitative or other qualitative methodologies. Coghlan and Casey and Williamson and Prosser underscore the importance for nursing action researchers to be aware of the political conditions of their respective organizations and to be prepared to manage the political and ethical dynamics as they inevitably arise through the course of an action research project.

Despite these challenges practitioners and researchers alike find action research particularly appealing and useful given the synchronicity between the practices/procedures of action research and the practices/procedures of practitioners. One could use the steps or phases of action research to outline the essential components of competent practice or to develop new policies and procedures. Shelton (2008) suggests action research, specifically community-based participatory research, is significant in the field of nursing due to "the opportunities offered through its iterative processes, which allow for reflection and positive exchange, which encourage modifications that strengthen projects, benefit community partners, and create environments of mutual respect and trust" (p. 255).

In our work reviewing and editing action research projects from around the world for many years, we are heartened by the creativity and willingness to experiment with action research, often stretching the parameters of what we have come to understand as "legitimate" or "true" AR. With the growing variety within this family of methodologies, action research continues to present nursing with a vehicle to explore many interesting questions and to suggest new and generative ways of thinking about how to positively impact our worlds.

References

Badger, T. G. (2000). Action research, change and methodological rigour. *Journal of Nursing Management, 8*(4), 201–207.

Brown, L. D., & Tandon, R. (1983). Ideology and political economy in inquiry: Action research and participatory research. *Journal of Applied Behavioral Science, 19*(3), 277–294.

Carter, B., Cummings, J., & Cooper, L. (2007). An exploration of best practice in multi-agency working and the experiences of families of children with complex health needs. What works well and what needs to be done to improve practice for the future? *Journal of Clinical Nursing, 16*(3), 527–539.

Carter, C. A., Ruhe, M. C., Weyer, S., Litaker, D., Fry, R. E., & Stange, K. C. (2007). An appreciative inquiry approach to practice improvement and transformative change in health care settings. *Quality Management in Health Care, 16*(3), 194–204.

Challis, A. (2009). An appreciative inquiry approach to RN retention. *Nursing Management, 40*(7), 9–13.

Chien, W. T., Chan, S. W., & Morrissey, J. (2002). The use of learning contracts in mental health nursing clinical placement: An action research. *International Journal of Nursing Studies, 39*(7), 685–694.

Coetzee, M., Britton, M., & Clow, S. E. (2005). Finding the voice of clinical experience: Participatory action research with registered nurses in developing a child critical care nursing curriculum. *Intensive & Critical Care Nursing, 21*(2), 110–118.

Coghlan, D., & Casey, M. (2001). Action research from the inside: Issues and challenges in doing action research in your own hospital. *Journal of Advanced Nursing, 35*(5), 674–682.

Cooperrider, D. L., & Srivastva, S. (2000). Appreciative inquiry in organizational life. In D. L. Cooperrider, P. F. Sorensen, Jr., D. Whitney, & T. F. Yeager (Eds.), *Appreciative inquiry: Rethinking human organization toward a positive theory of change* (pp. 55–97). Champaign, IL: Stipes.

Cooperrider, D. L., & Whitney, D. (2005). *Appreciative inquiry: A positive revolution in change.* San Francisco: Berrett-Koehler Communications.

Cooperrider, D. L., Whitney, D., & Stavros, J. M. (2003). *Appreciative inquiry handbook: The first in a series of AI workbooks for leaders of change.* Bedford Heights, OH: Lakeshore Communications.

Farrell, M., Douglas, D., & Siltanen, S. (2003). Exploring and developing a college's community of interest: An appreciative inquiry. *Journal of Professional Nursing, 19*(6), 364–371.

Fletcher, M., & Beringer, A. (2009). Introduction to action research. *Pediatric Nursing, 21*(2), 30.

Glasson, J. B., Chang, E. M. L., & Bidewell, J. W. (2008). The value of participatory action research in clinical nursing practice. *International Journal of Nursing Practice, 14*, 34–39.

Greenwood, D. J., & Levin, M. (2005). Reform of the social sciences and of universities through action research. In N. K. Denzin & Y. S. Lincoln (Eds.), *The Sage handbook of qualitative research* (3rd ed., pp. 43–64). Thousand Oaks, CA: Sage.

Hart, E., & Anthrop, C. (1996). Action research as a professionalizing strategy: Issues and dilemmas. *Journal of Advanced Nursing, 23*(3), 454–461.

Hart, E., & Bond, M. (1996). Making sense of action research through the use of a typology. *Journal of Advanced Nursing, 23*(1), 152–159.

Havens, D. S., Wood, S. O., & Leeman, J. (2006). Improving nursing practice and patient care: Building capacity with appreciative inquiry. *JONA: The Journal of Nursing Administration, 36*(10), 463–470.

Holter, I. M., & Schwartz-Barcott, D. (1993). Action research: What is it? How has it been used and how can it be used in nursing? *Journal of Advanced Nursing, 18*(2), 298–304.

Hope, K. W., & Waterman, H. A. (2003). Praiseworthy pragmatism? Validity and action research. *Journal of Advanced Nursing, 44*(2), 120–127.

Ives, M., & Melrose, S. (2010). Immunizing children who fear and resist needles: Is it a problem for nurses? *Nursing Forum, 45*(1), 29–39.

Keefe, M. R., & Pesut, D. (2004). Appreciative inquiry and leadership transitions. *Journal of Professional Nursing, 20*(2), 103–109.

Kelly, D., Simpson, S., & Brown, P. (2002). An action research project to evaluate the clinical practice facilitator role for junior nurses in an acute hospital setting. *Journal of Clinical Nursing, 11*(1), 90–98.

Kelly, P. J. (2005). Practical suggestions for community interventions using participatory action research. *Public Health Nursing, 22*(1), 65–73.

Kemmis, S., & McTaggart, R. (2005). Participatory action research: Communicative action in the public sphere. In N. K. Denzin & Y. S. Lincoln (Eds.), *The Sage handbook of qualitative research* (3rd ed., pp. 559–603). Thousand Oaks, CA: Sage.

Lauri, S., & Sainio, C. (1998). Developing the nursing care of breast cancer patients: An action research approach. *Journal of Clinical Nursing, 7*(5), 424–432.

Lee, N.-J. (2009). Using group reflection in an action research study. *Nurse Researcher, 16*(2), 30–42.

Lind, C., & Smith, D. (2008). Analyzing the state of community health nursing: Advancing from deficit to strengths-based practice using appreciative inquiry. *Advances in Nursing Science, 31*(1), 28–41.

Lindsey, E., & McGuinness, L. (1998). Significant elements of community involvement in participatory action research: Evidence from a community project. *Journal of Advanced Nursing, 28*(5), 1106–1114.

Livesey, H., & Challender, S. (2002). Supporting organizational learning: A comparative approach to evaluation in action research. *Journal of Nursing Management, 10*(3), 167–176.

Ludema, J. D., & Fry, R. E. (2008). The practice of appreciative inquiry. In P. Reason & H. Bradbury (Eds.), *The Sage handbook of action research: Participative inquiry and practice* (2nd ed., pp. 280–296). London: Sage.

Mander, R., Cheung, N. F., Wang, X., Fu, W., & Zhu, J. (2010). Beginning an action research project to investigate the feasibility of a midwife-led normal birthing unit in China. *Journal of Clinical Nursing, 19*(3/4), 517–526.

Mitchell, E. A., Conlon, A.-M., Armstrong, M., & Ryan, A. A. (2005). Towards rehabilitative handling in caring for patients following stroke: A participatory action research project. *Journal of Clinical Nursing, 14*, 3–12.

Moody, R. C., Horton-Deutsch, S., & Pesut, D. J. (2007). Appreciative inquiry for leading in complex systems: Supporting the transformation of academic nursing culture. *Journal of Nursing Education, 46*(7), 319–324.

Moore, S, M., & Charvat, J. (2007). Promoting health behavior change using appreciative inquiry: Moving from deficit models to affirmation models of care. *Family & Community Health, 30*(Supplement 1), S64–S74.

Olshansky, E., Sacco, D., Braxter, B., Dodge, P., Hughes, E., Ondeck, M., Stubbs, M. L., & Upvall, M. J. (2005). Participatory action research to understand and reduce health disparities. *Nursing Outlook, 53*(3), 121–126.

Parsons, M. L., & Warner-Robbins, C. (2002). Formerly incarcerated women create healthy lives through participatory action research. *Holistic Nursing Practice, 16*(2), 40–49.

Patton, M. Q. (2002). *Qualitative research & evaluation methods* (3rd ed.). Thousand Oaks, CA: Sage.

Reason, P., & Bradbury, H. (2008a). Introduction. In P. Reason & H. Bradbury (Eds.), *The Sage handbook of action research: Participative inquiry and practice* (2nd ed., pp. 1–10). London: Sage.

Reason, P., & Bradbury, H. (Eds.). (2008b). *The Sage handbook of action research: Participative inquiry and practice* (2nd ed.). London: Sage.

Reed, J., Pearson, P., Douglas, B., Swinburne, S., & Wilding, H. (2002). Going home from hospital: An appreciative inquiry study. *Health and Social Care and the Community, 10*, 36–45.

Reid-Searl, K., Dwyer, T., Happell, B., Moxham, L., Kahl, J., Morris, J., & Wheatland, N. (2009). Caring for children with complex emotional and psychological disorders: experiences of nurses in a rural paediatric unit. *Journal of Clinical Nursing, 18*(24), 3441–3449.

Richer, M.-C., Ritchie, J., & Marchionni, C. (2009). 'If we can't do more, let's do it differently!': Using appreciative inquiry to promote innovative ideas for better health care work environments. *Journal of Nursing Management, 17*(8), 947–955.

Robinson, A. (1995). Transformative 'cultural shifts' in nursing: Participatory action research and the 'project of possibility'. *Nursing Inquiry, 2*(2), 65–74.

Rolfe, G. (1996). Going to extremes: Action research, grounded practice and the theory-practice gap in nursing. *Journal of Advanced Nursing, 24*(6), 1315–1320.

Schwandt, T. A. (2007). *The Sage dictionary of qualitative inquiry* (3rd ed.). Thousand Oaks, CA: Sage.

Shelton, D. (2008). Establishing the public's trust through community-based participatory research: A case example to improve health care for a rural Hispanic community. *Annual Review of Nursing Research, 26*(1), 237–259.

Shendell-Falik, N., Feinson, M., & Mohr, B. (2007). Enhancing patient safety: Improving the patient handoff process through appreciative inquiry. *JONA: The Journal of Nursing Administration, 37*(2), 95–104.

The Staff of Mountbatten Ward, Wright, M., & Baker, A. (2005). The effects of appreciative inquiry interviews on staff in the U.K. National Health Service. *International Journal of Health Care Quality Assurance, 18*(1), 41–61.

Stefaniak, K. (2007). Discovering nursing excellence through appreciative inquiry. *Nurse Leader, 5*(2), 42–46.

Stringer, E. T. (2007). *Action research* (3rd ed.). Thousand Oaks, CA: Sage.

Titchen, A., & Binnie, A. (1993). Research partnerships: Collaborative action research in nursing. *Journal of Advanced Nursing, 18*(6), 858–865.

Valade, R. (2004). *Participatory action research with adults with mental retardation: "Oh my God. Look out world."* (AAT 3134205). Retrieved August 27, 2005, from ProQuest Dissertations and Theses database.

Walker, J., Bailey, S., Brasell-Brian, R., & Gould, S. (2001). Evaluating a problem based learning course: An action research study. *Contemporary Nurse, 10*(1–2), 30–38.

Walsgrove, H., & Fulbrook, P. (2005). Advancing the clinical perspective: A practice development project to develop the nurse practitioner role in an acute hospital trust. *Journal of Clinical Nursing, 14*(4), 444–455.

Walters, S., & East, L. (2001). The cycle of homelessness in the lives of young mothers: The diagnostic phase of an action research project. *Journal of Clinical Nursing, 10*(2), 171–179.

Waterman, H., Tillen, D., Dickson, R., & de Koning, K. (2001). Action research: A systematic review and guidance for assessment. *Health Technology Assessment, 5*(23). Retrieved July 31, 2010, from http://www.hta.ac.uk/execsumm/summ523.shtml

Waterman, H., Webb, C., & Williams, A. (1995). Parallels and contradictions in the theory and practice of action research and nursing. *Journal of Advanced Nursing, 22*(4), 779–784.

Whitney, D., & Trosten-Bloom, A. (2003). *The power of appreciative inquiry: A practical guide to positive change.* San Francisco: Berrett-Koehler Communications.

Williamson, G. R., & Prosser, S. (2002). Action research: Politics, ethics and participation. *Journal of Advanced Nursing, 40*(5), 587–593.

19

Exemplar: "I've Waited for Something Like This All My Life": PAR and Persons with Intellectual Disabilities

Rita M. Valade

Participatory Action Research (PAR) is a qualitative research method that facilitates the identification and redress of particular problems by persons most affected by these issues. Internationally, it is a powerful method of social change that is slowly becoming recognized as a valid research methodology within the United States. While there may be an initiating or lead investigator (a healthcare provider, academician, or community member struggling with an issue), persons from the community who are affected by the concern are invited to join together to engage in a collective, ongoing rhythm of planning, action, and reflection/assessment over a period of time (Kemmis & McTaggert, 2000; Valade, 2004).

Persons with intellectual disabilities (ID) have often been disregarded or relatively silenced over the ages. Western preoccupation with intelligence as an indicator of personhood is reflected in Descartes', "I think therefore I am", or in the casual way persons in comas are regarded as "vegetables," having lost their humanity because of an inability to communicate and presumably think. As a result, persons who struggle to navigate abstract thinking or communication have tended to become marginalized or held in suspicion. They are considered strange, or "other," not possessing the same qualities of humanity because their intellectual processes may differ or be slower. Professionals are not exempt from this bias. As a result, most research literature available on persons with intellectual disabilities are studies that focus upon what caregivers, family members, or professionals believe are best for this population (Gilson, Bricout, & Baskind, 1998; Trent, 1994). While the studies may be valid, it is important that some studies actually engage the persons themselves who are most affected by intellectual disabilities, namely, persons with ID.

This chapter relates a participatory action research project with adults with intellectual disabilities in Louisville, Kentucky. PAR is an ideal methodology to engage this population, especially in support of one of the disability movement's most prominent maxims: "Nothing about us without us." (Charlton, 1998). It is perhaps the most ethical research approach, because persons who are most affected by a problem become active participants in its research decisions, approaches to resolution, and its solution. Ensuring that the participants are truly in central decision-making positions is essential. What might be the greatest risk is making an uninformed choice. Having many persons involved in the decision-making process helps to limit the potential of making harmful choices about the process and intervention used.

PAR requires extensive involvement on the part of the initiating researcher, because that person also becomes involved in the collective research process (Chenail, St. George, & Wulff, 2007). PAR differs from focus groups, an important part of many research approaches. PAR engages all participants (initiating researcher, coresearchers/community members) over the course of months or years. It is essential for the initiating researcher to acknowledge that those "being studied" have some innate wisdom and self-knowledge. Just as the initiating researcher (e.g., community health nurse or a community member suffering from a health concern related to ground pollution in the neighborhood) has some specific knowledge pertinent to a particular concern, so do the coresearchers or those affected.

The PAR Experience

Most of the literature studied in preparation for this research endeavor offered only limited methodological information and focused more on results. As in all research, in PAR the method helps to shape the results. In this light, the rest of this chapter tells the story of engaging adults with intellectual disabilities in a PAR project through the phases of reflection on experience, planning for action, and action.

Initial Design

Working and living among adults with intellectual disabilities, I have heard some horrifying stories of prejudice, mistreatment, and disrespect by adolescents, educators, bus drivers, and human service and healthcare providers. I decided to engage some portion of this population in a PAR project. The plan included a two-phase PAR research design. Phase One included personal interviews of 25 persons with intellectual disabilities to ascertain what bothered them the most and what they would like to see changed in their lives. Hoping for a consensus of opinion relative to one or two major concerns, I invited 10–12 participants into Phase Two, an ongoing group that would problem-solve and address the issues identified in Phase One. The plan was for the Phase Two participants to decide the frequency and location of their meetings, agendas, and plan for solution. The group discussed and became familiar with the Kemmis and McTaggert (2000) PAR spiral as adapted by Valade (2004; see **Figure 19–1**), integrating planning, action, reflection. As their planning discussions led to

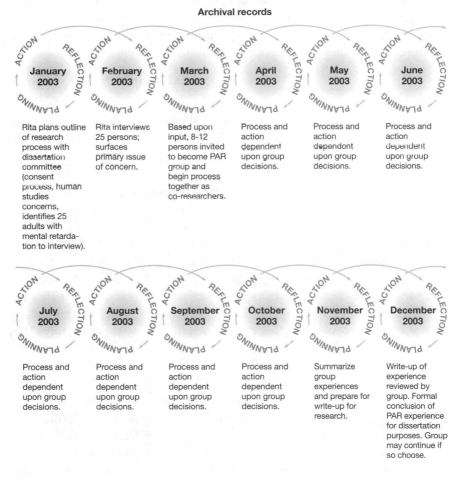

Participatory Action Research with Adults with Mental Retardation

STUDY DESIGN

Archival records

January 2003	February 2003	March 2003	April 2003	May 2003	June 2003
Rita plans outline of research process with dissertation committee (consent process, human studies concerns, identifies 25 adults with mental retardation to interview).	Rita interviews 25 persons; surfaces primary issue of concern.	Based upon input, 8-12 persons invited to become PAR group and begin process together as co-researchers.	Process and action dependent upon group decisions.	Process and action dependent upon group decisions.	Process and action dependent upon group decisions.

July 2003	August 2003	September 2003	October 2003	November 2003	December 2003
Process and action dependent upon group decisions.	Process and action dependent upon group decisions.	Process and action dependent upon group decisions.	Process and action dependent upon group decisions.	Summarize group experiences and prepare for write-up for research.	Write-up of experience reviewed by group. Formal conclusion of PAR experience for dissertation purposes. Group may continue if so choose.

FIGURE 19–1 Participatory Action Research with Adults with Mental Retardation: Study Design.
Source: Valade, 2004, p. 70.

action, they reflected upon what had been done and decided their next steps. My role was to help facilitate the meetings, videotape the gatherings (for peer supervision) to ensure that I would not take control, and take minutes as the basis for the ongoing and final report. I wrote the report and described it to the group to receive feedback to assure veracity. Appropriate informed consent was developed and Institutional Review Board (IRB) clearance was obtained to engage over a period of time with this group of persons with intellectual disabilities in a two-phase research design.

The design as conceived was a thorough and helpful template, but life often takes different directions than planned. This following section describes some of the detours that occurred when individuals populate a plan. After struggling with and subsequently educating the university IRB due to their unfamiliarity with PAR and the vulnerable population that was the focus of the study (including the use of an informed consent form adapted for persons with limited vocabulary) permission was granted.

Phase One

Working with and living among adults with ID in a residential community in Louisville, I was known by many professionals and family members in the area. I was able to bring a certain level of trustworthiness to this study, particularly as I began coordinating interviews. Beginning with individuals I knew personally, I attempted a snowball participant sample approach that did not work. Despite years of immersion in this group of persons, my own discomfort with asking interviewees if they knew of others with ID, I asked them if they had other "friends with disabilities." I was subsequently referred to a few persons with physical disabilities who were not impaired in their cognitive functioning. I learned that it was very important to be aware of my own prejudices and discomforts. In the long run, 25 participants of varying demographic characteristics (sex, living arrangements, age, race, guardianships, marital status, etc.) were engaged in personal interviews for the study. They were identified through referrals from professionals or family friends who knew of appropriate potential participants.

Guardianship status was always in need of clarification. It is often assumed that adults with ID have guardians, but that was not the experience. Only 2 out of the 25 interviewed had guardians. The guardian, potential participant, and I met to explain the overall study and this first phase in particular for which consent was being requested. If the participant wished to participate in Phase Two, then a separate consent meeting with the guardian was scheduled.

Interviews were held at locations of participants' choice. If they preferred to travel to a coffee shop or fast food restaurant, I drove and paid for their snack.

If I was unable to transport them, I brought a small gift of appreciation to their home. I gave each participant a copy of the informed consent, allowing them time to read it and then I explained it in detail. I developed a basic three-point summary: 1) You can talk to me only if you want to—it has to be something you want to do—it is voluntary; 2) You can stop any time and you will not get in trouble; 3) No one will know what you say—what you say will be private between you, me, and maybe my college teacher if it is necessary. All participants signed the form and were provided with a copy. In total, 13 women and 12 men participated; age ranged from 19-52; there were two African American males and 23 European Americans. Seven persons lived in housing sponsored by residential providers, ten lived with their families of origin, and eight lived in other settings. Eighteen were employed. Three respondents walked with assistance, six used wheelchairs exclusively, and 16 walked without assistance. All persons had an intellectual disability based upon their involvement in various programs or schools at some point in their lives. Retrieval of records or individual verification of IQ scores were not required for this study as the programs the individuals had participated in would have already required confirmation of the diagnosis.

In the course of the interviews, some of the participants were able to identify immediately "things that bothered or bugged them" in their lives. Others had more difficulty and were relieved with any prompts I was able to offer. I took special care to listen and report on what the participants said with a clear spirit, withholding my conjectures or projections on what they were trying to say. All of the interviews were completed within 6 weeks.

As the interviews progressed, it became clear that no single concern was surfacing from among interviewees. Persons responded with myriad issues that they wished they could change in their lives. There were very few repetitions among them. Some loose grouping of responses was possible. **Table 19–1** shows their responses. Respondents may have had more than one concern, so the total exceeds 25. One person with ID and physical disabilities summarized her thoughts by saying, "I have the same needs as everyone else; I just have a few more." What became apparent was that the needs these respondents experienced were in fact the same range of needs as persons without any socially defined disability. In my field notes I noted, "Everyone seems to speak out of her or his place and experience. This 'sub-population' has less in common with each other than with the rest of the world" (Valade, 2004, p. 95). It is particularly noteworthy that none of the respondents indicated any desire to change anything about themselves. From my field notes and their responses, no one mentioned any level of dissatisfaction about their body type, physical disability, or mental acuity. As one participant said, "I'm slow but I'm not stupid. I don't like being talked down to, but that's their [the insulter's] issue, not mine. I am fine."

TABLE 19–1   Identified Issues and Frequency Mentioned

Issue	Total Each
More independence; Supported housing; TARC 3 (Louisville's transportation system for persons with disabilities)	6
Loneliness/Desiring more companionship	4
Physical disabilities accommodations; Aging parents not being able to care for participant	3
Better jobs/job coaches; State budget issues; Illness of family member	2
Medical transportation issues for persons who use wheelchairs; Better media coverage of advocacy activities; Vocational training; Society's focus upon being disabled; State waiver for services for persons with mental retardation; War in Iraq; Prettier Environment; Britney Spears CD; Better staffing; Death of a pet.	1

(Valade, 2004, p. 98)

Two Emergent Themes

Although there was no groundswell or consensus of concerns that were clearly articulated by the interviewees, two themes emerged from the data. These themes came from "between the lines" of the conversations, whether just in chatting prior to or after the interview, or waiting in line for a beverage, etc. I was the one who named them, not the participants themselves. I was committed to refraining from interpreting their concerns through my own experience as much as possible. Perhaps they felt there was nothing to be done about these areas, so they did not suggest them as "things that bug them." But I needed to adhere to my boundaries and guidelines for this study, and if the respondents did not name issues in response to the questions posed, I did not include them. Possibly if I were to redo this study, I may have made a different decision. However, it was very important to be clear and not project my years of observation and experience with adults with intellectual disabilities onto their fresh words in these interviews. The two themes that emerged from the "sidebars" of the interview process were the desire to be treated with respect and complaints about the transportation system for persons with disabilities.

Respect

By the third interview, respect began to emerge as a key focus area in the lives of the respondents. Persons who used wheelchairs and had cerebral palsy (CP) in addition to other complications told stories of recent medical appointments. One middle-aged woman who is quite bent over with rigid muscles due to spastic CP spoke about the lengths she went through to get a PAP smear. She had never had one because no medical provider would take the time to help her make special arrangements. She related a story of calling a referred provider to make the office aware that she had spastic CP, used a large wheelchair, and needed a PAP smear. The appointment was made and she was reassured there would be no problem. She arrived at the appointment, only to find that the door to the exam room was not wide enough for her to enter. In addition, she learned that the exam table was not able to be lowered enough for her to get onto it even if she could get in the room. On other occasions, healthcare professionals had scolded her on multiple occasions when she was unable to extend her arm for blood to be drawn. Her spastic CP is so strong that both arms are pulled up tight to her shoulders and she needs someone to literally pull them down and hold them to have access to her veins or inside of her arms. She is tolerant of persons not knowing how to address her needs, but she is exhausted and angry about being ignored, as if she does not know how to instruct them: "Sometimes when people see me in my wheelchair, that's all they see. They act as if I've got no mind whatsoever" (Valade, 2004, p. 103).

Other participants shared numerous stories about being taunted, harassed, physically accosted (as children), and belittled because of their intellectual disabilities. Many of the respondents felt irritation with service providers addressing questions to their attendants and not to them directly. This happens in medical settings, restaurants, grocery stores, and myriad other locations. All participants shared that they knew they didn't always understand questions providers asked, but they hated not being directly addressed.

Transportation

Louisville's transportation system for persons with disabilities (who are unable to drive based upon a disability) is called TARC-3 (Transportation Authority of River City). My awareness of the various stories around TARC-3 began to surface around the edges of interviews by about the seventh individual interview. Complaints about TARC-3 overtly surfaced in five out of the total 25 interviews. But it was only upon further reflection did I begin to realize that almost everyone who used TARC-3 had unpleasant stories about using the service. Some of these complaints focused upon improper tie-downs for persons who used wheelchairs, being on the bus for over the 80-minute maximum TARC-3 rule, rude drivers, and not showing up when scheduled. Most of the time these complaints were interwoven into the fabric of informal chats before or after interviews:

> Ron, a soft-spoken man who uses a wheelchair told about a driver who told him, "You don't tell me how to drive this bus. I'll get you home when I get you home." Another time the driver did not lock his chair properly and Ron jostled and rolled with every movement of the

van. When Ron asked the driver to secure the locks, the driver told him, "You'll be okay until I get you home." Ron was very afraid during that ride. He recounted the feeling of helplessness when being totally dependent upon others to assure his safety. He has learned to be pleasant at all costs, so as to not anger the drivers upon whom he is so dependent. (Valade, 2004, p. 104)

Living and working with persons who rely on TARC-3 daily, even I had become immune to new stories. Complaining about TARC-3 had become part of the cultural norm within my own life. It had become like water to fish, not even noticeable.

Conclusion of Phase One

A variety of issues surfaced during Phase One, but no one or two specific issues were identified overtly by the participants to use as the core concern(s) for Phase Two, the establishment of a group to engage in a PAR experience. For whatever reasons, whether it was out of a sense of helplessness or hopelessness or some other dynamic, the majority of the persons interviewed never mentioned the two themes of respect or transportation as areas that bothered them and that needed change. An important learning moment of this phase was the profound realization that the issues that persons with intellectual disabilities are most worried about and desire change in are the same issues that many persons without cognitive disabilities have. They just may have a few more.

Transition Between Phase One and Phase Two _____

In the early stage of Phase One when describing the entire project to the 25 participants, I explained the different parts of the study in broad terms. All Phase One participants knew of the formation of an ongoing, action-oriented group that would meet over the course of a year. I made notes relative to persons' expressed interests in possible involvement in the group-action phase. These notes helped me to discern who to invite into the second phase of the PAR project. As there was no clear topic articulated around which to form the group, I needed to invite persons into a group that would identify a concern, develop plans, and make decisions about addressing it.

Phase Two _____

It was my hope that our PAR group would have approximately 9–12 members from varying demographics. I was cognizant of the practicality of effective group size (Yalom, 1995), cost (paying for TARC-3 rides, snacks, and space rental for the group), and overall interpersonal relationships among a group larger or smaller than around 12. There were 12 participants from Phase One who had previously indicated interest in the ongoing group. I was grateful that all excitedly agreed to commit to group membership for the next year. I shall never forget Donna's[1] response to my invitation.

A European American woman in mid-life with cerebral palsy, Donna uses a wheelchair and owns her own home. Despite myriad efforts at advertising and following leads, she could not locate a woman to hire to assist her with her care at the hourly rate that her state funding would pay. Ultimately, her 80-year-old mother moved halfway across the state to provide her daughter with in-home care. Donna's mother and family had worked very hard to provide for Donna and to help her be as independent as possible. I sat in Donna's kitchen sharing a pot of coffee as we talked about Phase Two of the study and my hopes for her participation. Bent over from her CP and looking years older than her age, Donna took a deep breath and trained her eyes on mine. She said in her halting speech affected by her CP, "I have been waiting for something like this all my life" (Valade, 2004, p. 110). I was speechless. She proceeded to tell me that she has tried to be a self-advocate but needed the support of other persons. She was glad that the group would need to decide on an issue rather than anyone interpreting for them which issue was important. I felt confirmed in my choice of noting the emergent themes of Phase One, but not building a PAR group around them.

All potential participants were encouraged to think about this year-long commitment. Some checked it out with family members, asking me to call them. Others knew immediately that they wanted to get involved in this project. Regi typified this energy when he said to me, "Don't worry Rita, I'll be there. I want to do this real bad. . . . Do you hear me (with a smile on his face)? REAL BAD. I'm so glad to be in the group" (Valade, 2004, p. 110).

Informed consent for Phase Two was discussed with each individual, including guardians when necessary. All agreed to be videotaped and to have these tapes reviewed by some other "teachers" (my colleagues—a psychologist and a social worker) who would look at them to make sure I wasn't controlling the group. They also agreed to allow another colleague in the meetings who would videotape the meetings. Otherwise, no other persons were allowed (e.g., attendants, family members, etc.). It was important to have only the group control and lead the group. We were offered space at the Louisville Council on Mental Retardation Leadership Institute offices (subsequently renamed the Council on Developmental Disabilities), a totally accessible facility. I told the participants that I had been and would continue keeping a PAR journal, noting events and insights. They would have access to the journal from the beginning of Phase Two should they wish. They would be considered coresearchers in the project. Whatever insight about the group that surfaced I felt belonged to the group.

Throughout the study, it would be very important for all coresearchers to have a sense of empowerment and control in the group. They would decide the timing, length of meetings, focus, and ultimate action steps toward addressing the problems they would identify. Data would emerge through the group interaction, videotapes, and transcripts of the videos. Analysis would occur through group reflection on our collective experience, peer supervision of my group facilitation and participation, and journaling. To the best of my ability, nothing would be written about them without them.

The Group and Our Action

Initially, 13 individuals expressed interest in ongoing participation in the action group. Through struggles with schedule and transportation, nine persons returned faithfully to the Thursday night monthly meetings. It was very important that only the group members were present for the gatherings. True to PAR, the initiating researcher even if not directly affected by the concern as experienced by the majority of the group, is integral to the project. I was a group member. It was a delicate line to walk: My participation was important, but no more important than any participants'. Each member brought talents and experiences to the group. Some of the members' speech was affected by cerebral palsy but eventually group members learned to ask for clarification or grew to understand each other.

Using the transcripts from the videotapes in addition to my journal, I describe some of the dynamics of the PAR group in chronological order. There were a total of nine meetings. The Group One narrative that follows gives a taste of how I reported some of the details of the group process and interaction in addition to processing with my peer supervisors after each group. All group meetings were powerful experiences, but for purposes of this chapter, I have synthesized their insights and movement toward their group action. Being mindful of the PAR spiral of reflection on experience, planning, and action, each group was able to be best summarized by one aspect of the spiral.

Group One: Reflection on Experience

After myriad phone calls and various interactions, a decision was made for the date and time of our first meeting. Persons gathered, clearly feeling awkward during the initial settling in. As introductions began, the group relaxed a bit and the group members began to make connections with each other—some went to the same day program or worked together, one member's father shared a hospital room with another's grandfather, and so on.

About halfway through the introductions, a woman unknown to me entered the room. She introduced herself as Adrian's mother. She had dropped him off and had searched for a parking spot. I was committed to this group being only open to those personally invited. I tried to figure out how to ask her to leave graciously when I realized I could perhaps help everyone out.

I knew where Adrian and his family lived from our Phase One interview. I suggested that I was happy to take Adrian home after our group so that she would not need to stay. She checked with Adrian who thought it was a good idea and she thanked me. She was relieved to be able to return home rather than stay for 90 minutes until we were finished.

After she left, I processed with the group. Donna verbally affirmed my intent of only allowing group members in the gatherings. I received affirmation through the nods in agreement with Donna, and therefore relaxed from my fear of being too exclusive.

The group was then reminded of its focus: It was an opportunity for adults to develop a plan how to best address a problem that they experience firsthand. It was also a research study, "my homework from the University of Louisville." Group rules were established: no guns, safety first, no violence, no making fun of people, be respectful, no nasty tone of voice, and do not call each other "retarded." Issues and concerns surfaced in the midst of brainstorming group rules. Stories abounded. Jackie shared:

> You know, another thing we might want to address is not a rule or anything. . . . But the way the doctors . . . some of the way the doctors don't think you know what you are talking about. . . . Experiences like when you go to the doctor they don't ask you, they ask your parents or they ask your . . . well they ask anybody else.

Sandy continued:

> It just doesn't happen at doctor's offices. It happens everywhere. Just today. I've never been to this dentist's office, the one at Hazelwood [state residential facility for persons with severe mental retardation and physical complications in Louisville] . . . and he came and he asked Tina [caseworker] what was my disability. . . . Instead of asking me, he asked her. And sometimes I get the feeling when people call on the phone they don't like the way I sound on the phone. They feel like they don't want to talk to me because, you know they put that label on me. . . . They said, "I don't want to talk to you. You act too retarded or something like that." (Valade, 2004, p. 124)

As our first meeting drew to a close, the group unanimously and enthusiastically agreed to meet again. A date was established and the participants grumbled about TARC-3 as they left to get on their buses to head home. Despite their complaints, they were interacting and laughing, clearly having been energized by the group experience.

Upon reviewing the videotape during peer supervision, the unconnected responses of some group members after persons with CP spoke indicated the possibility that some group members did not in fact understand each other. I made a note to encourage all to ask for clarification during our next meeting.

We also discussed possible reasons persons without intellectual disabilities make persons with intellectual disabilities invisible through not directly addressing them. Furthermore, we noted that the group members' social skills were highly developed. They spoke one at a time, were patient with each others' speech patterns, stayed on topic, and no one dominated the group. Only two members were silent during the entire meeting. I made a note to encourage their participation in subsequent meetings.

Groups 2 and 3: Reflection on Experience, Group 4: Planning

The progression of the group was rocky with many starts and stumbles. Group dynamics were as profound and convoluted as any group of persons trying to gather, work together, agree on a topic, and plan an action. Politeness and gentility gave way to episodic irritation and limited patience. However, everyone returned to the meetings.

By the end of Group 2, four topics had repeatedly surfaced: advocacy for the use of the term *intellectual disabilities* rather than mental retardation, problems with the medical profession, quality continuing education for adults with intellectual disabilities, and TARC-3 concerns. By the end of Group 3, the members clearly identified TARC-3 as the primary focus of its actions. The group decided it did not want to engage in civil disobedience but would wait until the next meeting to make plans.

Group 4 had struggles on multiple levels. The decision to address concerns with TARC-3 seemed to have organically emerged from among the members by the end of Group 3. But the group engaged in a total change of heart by this fourth meeting. Cindy was unable to attend the meeting because of a TARC-3 issue. She had been at softball practice and scheduled her ride as she had many times before. The bus went to another ball field across the property. Although Cindy jumped and waved and screamed to grab the driver's attention, the bus drove away. Cindy borrowed the coach's cell phone and called TARC-3. She had been given a "No Show" by TARC-3 at the ball field and she would have to wait 2 hours for another ride. Cindy called me as she waited for the next TARC-3 bus, telling me about her anger and frustration. I related the story to the group. The responses were not what I had expected. Overall, there was a growing expression of "blaming the victim," asserting Cindy probably did something wrong in the reservation system.

I was becoming very frustrated, confused, and impatient with the group's change of attitude. As there was a clear withdrawal from the commitment to challenge TARC-3 as the focus of their collective action, I was not sure of the best course of action. Todd's attitude reversal confounded me. A 33-year-old man with a history of being outspoken and strong-willed, he was attempting to recant his history of problems with TARC-3, becoming an advocate for the good drivers and the system as a whole. Finally, as the group progressed,

Todd named the issue that seemed to have stopped the group from pro-
gressing to action.

> Okay. What if we have too many complaints and they've had enough
> and say, "we're going to pull out." What are we going to do then? With
> too many complaints, they'll pull out. You rock the boat too much,
> they gonna pull out. We'll be up the creek.

Others confirmed Todd's observation and fear. Donna reflected, "That's his
fear. You feel like you're at the mercy of TARC-3." Todd continued:

> I feel at the mercy of everybody . . . at Day Spring, at the Mattingly
> Center. It's okay to complain, but you don't want to rock the boat.
> I don't want to get sent back home or not have any way to get out on
> my own. (Valade, 2004, p. 152)

There were multiple dynamic interactions that helped shape the group and
their subsequent action, but Todd's articulation of his fear of losing services
upon which he is dependent was shared by all members. Naming this changed
the tone and attitude of the group. By the end of Group 4, all seemed to be de-
moralized and were fearful of risking. I was unsure who would return to the
group for the next gathering because of the low mood many were in upon departure. Upon further reflection with my peer supervisors, I realized the inner
pressure I felt about the timeline for this endeavor and that we were running
out of time. I also feared that the group members were too vulnerable to engage in an action to better something in their lives. The peer supervisors noted
an interesting pattern: The women expressed less fear of loss than their male
counterparts. Another consideration was that many groups struggle when
there is a shift from ideology/abstract conversation to agreeing upon an action. I needed to be patient and let the group lead.

Group 5: Planning, Group 6: Action

Eight of the nine participants returned to the group. One member was sick
but planned to return next month. I was relieved. Through a lot of hard, honest work, the group decided it would indeed engage in a strategy to address
their concerns and experiences with TARC-3. They decided to invite the executive director of TARC-3 to attend their meeting. They consciously planned
for her to come to their "turf," to provide coffee and cookies as a gesture of
hospitality (versus pop and chips as if it were a party), and to establish an
agenda. Cindy and Regi planned to call the director to invite her.

Acting as a scribe, I wrote down their questions on newsprint and attached
them to the wall.

1. Why are some of the times we request not available?
2. How long can you be on the TARC-3 van?

3. Why do we have to wait 30 minutes and the van only needs to wait 5 minutes for us?
4. Why does my reservation get erased from the computer? If I try to change a round-trip to a one-way trip, sometimes my reservation is lost.
5. Why do the agents act angry when we call to verify that our reservations are still in the computer?
6. Is there any way to verify that I have a reservation?
7. What do the reservation people do when they don't understand me?
8. Signs on the buses say "No eating and no drinking." Why can't we eat or drink but we see drivers eating and drinking?
9. What area does TARC-3 cover?

It was clear that the group had matured in their leadership abilities. They were taking increasing responsibility, asking me to assist in various capacities such as helping with the phone call to Ms. Denison if necessary, writing down the questions on newsprint, and making sure Ms. Denison knew the location of the meeting space. I happily obliged.

Ms. Karen Denison, TARC-3 director, arrived as scheduled during Group 6. The hospitality food was offered and everyone acted, as group member Jackie had advised the month before, "like an adult." The meeting went smoothly. My only role was to introduce myself. The group had developed a plan for introductions. Ms. Denison read through and answered each question posted on the wall. She took each question very seriously and proffered phone numbers and supervisors' names should they encounter similar problems in the future.

Group 7: Reflection, Group 8: Reflection, Group 9: Celebration

The group reconvened a month later and all expressed a sense of empowerment and pride in their work. They reflected upon their work together: "I think we deserve a hand on all we did" (Valade, 2004, p. 172). In reflecting on the tensions they felt along the way, I asked others why they kept coming back. Donna reflected:

> This group helped me to talk about some things that bother me. I wanted to keep coming back because I'm involved in a lot of disabilities things and we were talking about things that interested me. And, there wasn't any staff folks. Not that having staff is bad. A lot of times it is really important and necessary. But it was nice just having us together.

Jackie continued to return "because I made a promise and I do what I have to do to keep my promise." I asked her if it was helpful. Her honest reply was, "sometimes." She continued, "Other times I was too tired to talk about things." (Valade, 2004, p. 174).

It was also in Group 7 that the group members challenged the confidentiality and anonymity of their involvement in the project. In reflecting upon my experience of reading and researching so many articles and books, I told the group that very few actually had folks with intellectual disabilities doing the type of research they did for this project. The group members began to realize on a new level that this project was going to be in a book and that they would not be associated with it because of the agreement they had signed in the beginning. All participants asked that their names and pictures be included in the book. They were proud of their work and wanted credit. This caused my head to spin with thinking about returning to the university IRB committee to explain this unusual turn of events. Receiving the initial permission from them to engage a vulnerable population in a PAR project that was to them an unusual research methodology was difficult enough. But I promised the group I would do my best to meet their request, as they were the coresearchers and deserved all the credit they could get.

By Group 8, I had returned to the university IRB committee and obtained their permission to revoke the participants' anonymity and confidentiality. We brought a camera and tripod to the group session to take pictures of the coresearchers (**Figure 19–2**). I asked all members what information about

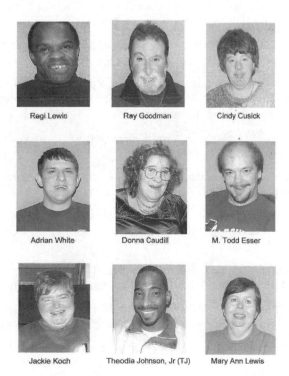

Regi Lewis Ray Goodman Cindy Cusick

Adrian White Donna Caudill M. Todd Esser

Jackie Koch Theodia Johnson, Jr (TJ) Mary Ann Lewis

FIGURE 19–2 Phase Two Group Members.
Source: Valade, 2005.

themselves they wanted included (**Figure 19–3**). During this session, I also offered a detailed overview of my notes and what I had planned to write in the book. They offered little feedback, but expressed gratitude to me for including them in this part of the report.

Energy had waned among the group, and what had been great interest in continuing the group had dissipated by the eighth session. Participants expressed ambivalence about continuing the group but its success was palpable among us all. It was decided that the next (ninth) session should be a party.

For the ninth session, I spliced together highlights of the videos of each of our sessions together. Once we gathered for our party, we set up our tables and chairs to view the DVD of our PAR group. Snacks were served and all sat and watched themselves on the television doing the group work for the past 10 months. All were proud of their work, including me. It was truly a celebration.

---

1. Regi Lewis, 33, works at a local popular restaurant and loves to go out for coffee and to have dinner with his friends.

2. Ray Goodman, 46, works at a local coffee house, rising at 4:30 to get the coffee and muffins ready for his early morning customers.

3. Cindy Cusick is in her late 30's, works at a grocery store and is involved in almost every sport Special Olympics offers and loves working on her computer and cruising the internet.

4. Adrian White, 21, works at a local grocery store and has a passion for music, singing and playing keyboard.

5. Donna Caudill, in her late 40s, proudly owns her own home and is very involved in a variety of recreational and advocacy activities.

6. Michael "Todd" Esser, in his early 30's loves everything to do with the University of Louisville Cardinals, the Minnesota Vikings and his former high school, Manual.

7. Jackie Koch, in her early 50's, lives by herself and is very busy with a variety of local advocacy groups and is proudly pursuing her GED.

8. Theodia Johnson, Jr. (TJ) is in his late 20s, works with Regi and would love to pursue some form of a career as a cartoonist.

9. Mary Ann Lewis, in her 40's, works at a residential center for senior citizens and loves being involved in political advocacy.

FIGURE 19–3   Personal Descriptions.
Source: Valade, 2005.

It was also the end of the group. No one mentioned continuing and all spoke of the group in past tense. They were proud of their work and tired. All expressed gratitude for having been invited into the adventure and gratitude to each other for enduring the tough times. We said goodbye as the TARC-3 buses came to pick them up—a perfect ending.

Conclusion

This PAR experience was powerful and yet did not change the world, but it did alter a slice of it. Selener (1997) notes that PAR has two goals: solving practical problems at the local level and creating a shift in the balance of power in favor of the poor and marginalized. The persons who worked together on this project did just that. They named a practical problem with which they had firsthand experience on a daily basis. In fact it was so much a part of their daily life that they almost did not name it as an issue. As water to a fish, even if the water is a bit dirty, the fish may not actually notice. In both phases of this study, persons who use TARC-3 daily initially did not consider it to be something to challenge or try to improve.

In addition to naming the concern, the group problem-solved to their satisfaction and created a shift in the balance of power with the director of TARC-3 and the supervisors to which the director referred them. The coresearchers overcame their fear of losing services if they challenged the system. They were empowered. They were not invisible. The director spoke directly to them and addressed them as consumers and customers of the service her company provides. As was seen in this study, PAR can change lives.

References

Charlton, J. (1998). *Nothing about us without us: Disability oppression and empowerment.* Berkeley, CA: University of California Press.

Chenail, R., St. George, S., & Wulff, D. (2007). Action research: The methodologies. In P. L. Munhall (Ed.), *Nursing research: A qualitative perspective* (4th ed., pp. 447–462). Sudbury, MA: Jones & Bartlett.

Gilson, S. F., Bricout, J. C., & Baskind, F. R. (1998). Listening to the voices of individuals with disabilities. *Families in Society, 79*(2), 188–196.

Kemmis, S., & McTaggart, R. (2000). Participatory action research. In N. K. Denzin & Y. S. Lincoln (Eds.), *Handbook of qualitative research* (2nd ed., pp. 567–605). Thousand Oaks, CA: Sage.

Selener, D. (1997). *Participatory action research and social change.* Ithaca, NY: Cornell Participatory Action Research Network.

Trent, J. W. (1994). *Inventing the feeble mind: A history of mental retardation in the United States.* Los Angeles: University of California.

Valade, R. (2004). *Participatory action research with adults with intellectual disabilities: "Oh my God! Look out world!"* Saarbrucken, Germany: VDM Verlag Dr. Muller.

Yalom, I. (1995). *Theory and practice of group psychotherapy* (4th ed.). New York: Basic Books.

Endnotes _____

[1] Prior to this point, all names were fictitious as Phase One participants were promised anonymity. Towards the end of our work together, Phase Two participants requested that their names and pictures be used in the study as they were proud of their work. Therefore all names from this point on will be participants' real names.

PART III

Internal and External Considerations in Qualitative Research

The following chapters, which comprise Part III, are designed to address a variety of essential considerations to attain the highest level of research science quality. This section answers questions and concerns frequently expressed not only by students of nursing science, but also by faculty, consultants, and reviewers of qualitative research. Many of these questions may be on your mind as you contemplate doing your own qualitative research studies.

Part III of this edition has updated chapters as well as a new chapter (Chapter 24) about combining more than two qualitative methods in one study. This is exciting as many qualitative researchers have seen for themselves as they do their research that there could be a case study within a phenomenological study or a narrative inquiry method could be combined with an action research part of the study. Combined methods may be part of the original study design, or a study might evolve and call for this design to be expanded to include multiple methods. This chapter is followed by the combination of qualitative research methods with quantitative research methods as one study. I have always believed that if a quantitative study emerges from a qualitative study, that study has much greater potential to reflect the "reality" of the worlds in which participants live than the world and the language of researchers.

The chapters on the ethical consideration, institutional review boards, and evaluation are essential reading for starting a qualitative research study. I particularly want to emphasize ethical considerations. If you find yourself doing a qualitative research study, read more about these considerations in Chapter 20. Our research must meet the highest standards for ethics. Chapter 23, which focuses on evidence-based practice, is critical and challenges the assumption that such practice is dependent on quantitative research and statistical probabilities.

In the last edition there was a chapter on using the Internet, strategies of intraproject sampling, and one on reimagining qualitative research. Once again as I have done throughout this book I emphasize going back to earlier editions for other content. As editions change, choices are made but the choice is always made with the knowledge that the previous editions are available to the reader.

These six chapters do not intend to provide the only answers or interpretations to these questions and concerns, and the reader is encouraged to study the references for additional perspectives. For example, the question of combination of methods, especially qualitative and quantitative, is a subject that once provoked heated discussions. Today this combination is more accepted, however if the reader is to be truly informed about these critiques, additional reading is necessary. Another example is evaluation. There are many systems developed for evaluating qualitative research. Most are a difference in language, but it is a good idea to become familiar with those authors' perceptions as well. One important caution about evaluation is that the criteria that are used for evaluating quantitative research do not apply to qualitative research and if used can be very misleading.

By now if you have been reading carefully, you know I am a stickler for reading more and then some! One book does not provide you with all you need to embark on what I hope for you will be a love of "what" qualitative research represents and what it offers humankind.

20

Ethical Considerations in Qualitative Research[1]

Patricia L. Munhall

As members of the scientific community, nurse researchers have become adept at identifying and applying criteria for evaluating the various aspects of quantitative research. We may have even surpassed our colleagues in other disciplines in the level of rigor we apply when evaluating the design, method, and protection of human subjects of a study. With regard to the protection of human subjects, I like to think that rigor is founded on a profound reverence for human beings and their experiences. As nurse researchers, we have become increasingly sophisticated in our qualitative research endeavors and have begun to identify distinct considerations and criteria for viewing the ethical dimensions of qualitative research.

Naturalistic, direct involvement and participation with people necessitate acknowledging the subjective nature and activity of the researcher as the main "tool" of research. Qualitatively oriented nurse researchers prize this direct involvement yet, contextually, are faced with the canonization of objectivity and the resulting detachment of most prevailing conventions. In contrast, qualitative nurse researchers face the nitty-gritty, the serendipitous, the passions, the complexity of subjectivity and attachment to people and their vicissitudes.

The purpose of this chapter is to provide one of the stepping stones needed to differentiate criteria that are essential and appropriate for ethical considerations for qualitative research methods in nursing. This discussion focuses on selected ethical considerations with the following themes interwoven throughout: ethical means and aims (or ends), collaborators as means, conflict methodology, models of fieldwork, and process consent. Potential for role conflict of the investigator is discussed from the perspective of the therapeutic imperative and the research imperative.

Underlying Assumptions and Dilemmas

In the tradition of qualitative research methods, I would like to state, or bracket, here my own beliefs and values and their implications for ethical considerations when doing qualitative nursing research:

1. The therapeutic imperative of nursing (advocacy) takes precedence over the research imperative (advancing knowledge) if conflict develops.
2. Nursing reflects a deontological ethical system (people are not to be treated as means). However, if individuals consent to be part of our research, they have, in essence, joined the research enterprise. Instead of being called subjects or objects, they are now collaborators (Punch, 1986).
3. Informed consent is a static, past-tense concept. Qualitative research is an ongoing, dynamic, changing process. Because of unforeseeable events and consequences, a past-tense consent is not appropriate. We need to facilitate negotiation and renegotiation to protect our collaborators' human rights. Therefore, a verb-like consent seems necessary, and the concept of *process consenting* reflects the ongoing dynamic nature of qualitative research.

Ethical Aims and Means

Bellah (1981) sets our stage for ethical dialogue with the premise that all inquiry has normative commitments. Arguing that all social inquiry is linked to ethical reflection, he uses the expression "moral sciences" interchangeably with "social sciences." He states: "Social science must consider ends as well as means as objects of rational reflection" (p. 2). Laudan (1977) also focuses on the consequence side of science when he states: "Science is essentially a problem-solving activity" (p. 66). Wilson and Fitzpatrick (1984) state that the purpose of nursing science is "to render reality intelligible as it relates to human health and development" (p. 41). The question to be asked from an ethical perspective is: Toward what goal and for what end? For our purposes here, let us suggest that, for the most part, nurse researchers are very much interested in problem-solving or problem-preventing research and that our motives are to produce an end that is in some way considered "good." In this way, research assumes a normative commitment, something that "ought" to be. The most apparent example of this commitment is that many of our research endeavors focus on facilitating health. The search for a means to produce a desired health outcome requires critical ethical reflection.

Other aims that we have in addition or in conjunction to the attainment of health are assisting people to reach their potential, to self-actualize, and to reach their maximum well-being. Actually, many of these ends are equivalent to or similes of the concept of health.

Acknowledgment that our aims have normative commitments is critical because we then move on to ways (means) of achieving our decided good. In essence, our aims become prescriptive. An example may serve to illustrate this point.

Ethical Aims

One of our normative commitments is to help individuals achieve their maximum potential. In this pursuit, we might perform a qualitative study of a group of "underachievers" who are not attaining full intellectual potential or physical health potential. The ethical questions that arise include whether the ethical aim is to assist the subjects we study or future generations. What do the underachievers we study have to gain from our studying them? Further, is it a given that our mission is to help people reach their maximum potential if unrequested?

Although our society has accepted and promoted some goods, we need to reflect on them. Some may actually be in opposition to others. For example, a steady state or some form of equilibrium may indeed be in opposition to an achievement ethic. In qualitative research, knowledge of our collaborators' aims and normative commitments is an intrinsic component of the research process. We need to reflect on our own and, perhaps more important, their normative commitments.

Ethical Means

In *The Prince* Machiavelli proclaims his aim of a free, independent Italy, free from outside governance, as an end that was readily proclaimed as good. However, his means to that end illustrated moral vacuity. Machiavelli believed that corruption is natural to humankind. However, by generalizing a behavior to all "men," he justifies his means to obtain an end. Human experimentation is based on the ends justifying the means principle. Changing people's behaviors, often an aim in the helping professions, contrasts sharply with understanding different behaviors and accepting and supporting those differences. Perhaps not all people need or want to reach their maximum potential. Some philosophers, such as Immanuel Kant, believe human beings have a moral obligation to reach their maximum potential. The question then becomes: Do nurses have a moral obligation to help others attain a moral obligation? This is an example of an ethical consideration that needs in-depth exploration by nurse researchers.

Aims Versus Means

Ethical consideration in qualitative research (and quantitative as well, though it is not spelled out) entails knowing explicitly and implicitly what our ethical means and aims are. Entering into a collaboration and participating with our collaborators seem precious experiences that call on us to reflect, know, and critically evaluate our ethical means and ends. A negotiated view requires such reflection.

Perhaps the most critical ethical obligation that qualitative nurse-researchers have is to describe the experiences of others as faithfully as possible. This ethical obligation is to describe and report in the most authentic manner possible the experience that unfolds, even if it is contrary to your aims. In our example, perhaps we might find it appears healthier not to strive to reach maximum achievement of your potential! Not having to achieve a numerical level of significance to accomplish your aim may be the highest degree of freedom possible when doing research.

Therapeutic Versus Research Imperative

Ethics is a tangled web of principles where one can usually see the position of the opposition as having some legitimacy. That is why ethical dilemmas are thorny, at best. In the instance of the therapeutic imperative and the research imperative, the ethical systems of deontology and utilitarianism potentially conflict. The nurse who is doing research needs to acknowledge what her therapeutic imperative is. Is it deontological, where the individual is not a means to an end but an end as such? Is it advocacy for human beings? Is it based on justice, beneficence, and respect for patients' rights? The researcher also needs to reflect on the research imperative. Is it utilitarian, where people are used as means to further knowledge? Is the researcher imposing possibly uncomfortable conditions on participants? Is the researcher working under a utilitarian posture where the ends may justify the means? In qualitative research, conflicts that present dilemmas for researchers include the following:

- Means versus possible ends
- Entry versus departure
- Confidence versus disappointment
- Elation versus despondency
- Commitment versus perceived betrayal
- Friendship versus desertion

From a utilitarian perspective, the listed results may seem unavoidable in fieldwork. From the deontological perspective, they are ethically problematic. Role conflict evolves from behavioral expectations in the nurse's therapeutic imperative that may differ from those in the researcher's imperative. Given the potential for harm in fieldwork, consideration must be given to these dilemmas to minimize them or prevent them from occurring. Communication is an essential process, as is a team or joint approach to research. Perhaps even the term *participant observer* could be abandoned, and instead we could simply call all those taking part *participants* or, as already mentioned, *collaborators*. It may be helpful to understand, from a human perspective, that, if there is to be a departure, all who take part are prepared and that the researcher, too, often does feel sad. In essence, there is a real "joining" of feelings and understandings.

Is Being a Collaborator a Means to an End?

Suppose a nurse-anthropologist-researcher asked you to participate in her study titled "Contemporary Women's Hassles: An Exploratory Study," and she asked whether she could visit you in your home at various times when you were available to "sort of" observe and interview you. In addition, she asks, "Would it be all right to visit you in your office?" Rock (1979) states: "No sociologist I know would himself agree to become a subject of observational research" (p. 261).

Well, what is at stake here? When I think of this, very much is at stake, and we need to walk in our collaborators' shoes. Sure, there are hassles for the contemporary woman, but having this researcher come into my home seems not only another hassle, but perhaps a crisis! One needs to be concerned about the usual ethical considerations of fieldwork: privacy, confidentiality, achieving accurate portrayal, and inclusion and exclusion of information. In this instance, however, as in many others, the psychological burden and threat that an outsider might pose need serious consideration. Regardless of all of our efforts to act in the collaborators' best interest, some invasion, as it were, occurs to the person or people involved. The end that we hope to accomplish may be laudable, but we are fooling ourselves, I think, if we are not aware that there is some inconvenience or discomfort in the process of being observed. The unknown consequences of the observation could contribute to a pervasive state of anxiety for the participants, whether consciously or unconsciously. Rather than the casual, "Within 2 to 3 weeks the person seemed comfortable with my presence," or "I was virtually unnoticed after 2 or 3 weeks," we need, as advocates, to attend to other possibilities that occur with observations. We can ask ourselves, "Would we comfortable until the results were in?" Empathizing with and attending to the process of being observed must be ongoing on the researcher's part. We may feel blended into a culture, but that does not mean that the observees are experientially where we are.

As already mentioned, nursing seems to espouse the deontological principle that human beings are to be treated as ends and not means. In contrast with that system is utilitarianism, which argues that the ends justify the means.

From that perspective, one can use another person for the good of others and to advance further knowledge. Technically, the research enterprise turns people into means, and—though one could argue that this occurs far less with qualitative research—the potential still remains. We have come to some peace with this issue through the process of informed consent, where, in effect, the individual joins the research enterprise. Joining the effort affords individuals the opportunities of contributing to society, of being of service, and perhaps of advancing a cause of their own. We may not have thought of informed consent from that perspective, but ethically it helps to resolve the means–end dilemma and makes the term *collaborator* much more accurate.

Informed Consent in Qualitative Research

Fieldwork that is existential and authentic requires the negotiation of trust between the researcher and the participants. Entering into fields in the various roles of participant–observer is a privilege. We are "allowed" into someone else's world with its customs, practices, and events, which we promise to describe faithfully and without bias. While we are negotiating entry into this world, we invite the participants to become part of the research enterprise and validate that agreement with an informed consent. Informed consent has been defined as:

> knowing consent of an individual or the individual's legally authorized representative, so situated as to be able to exercise free power of choice without undue inducement or any element of force, fraud, deceit, duress, or other forms of constraint or coercion. (Annas, Glantz, & Katz, 1977, p. 291)

Typically, informed consents include the title, purpose, and explanation of the research and the procedures to be followed. Risks and benefits are to be spelled out clearly. A statement that the participant has had an opportunity to ask questions about and that the participant is free to withdraw at any time is also included (Field & Morse, 1985). This model of informed consent evolved out of experimental research; some of it is applicable to qualitative research, but to resolve some of the aforementioned dilemmas more is needed.

Process Consent

Because qualitative research is conducted in an ever-changing field, informed consent should be an ongoing process. Over time, consent needs to be renegotiated as unexpected events or consequences arise. For example, I may, in a weak moment, sign a consent form for the previously mentioned researcher to observe me in my home, but without the full realization of what the consequences might be. To be ethical in this situation, the researcher needs to assess the effects of involvement in the field and continually acquire new permissions. Maybe children will react negatively to an outsider in their home, or perhaps the contemporary woman will find that keeping some semblance of cleanliness of her home on a daily basis is just the hassle that will take her over the edge.

Common sense plays a large part in renegotiating informed consent. If our focus should change, we need to ask participants for permission to change the first agreement. This is important from the perspective of sensitivity to our collaborators as well. They may wonder why you "lost" interest in a particular part of the field and chose something that you obviously have found "special." Continually informing and asking permission establishes the needed trust to go further in an ethical manner.

Secrets

Another area that needs ethical consideration in fieldwork is confidentiality of the exchanges between the researcher and the participants. Both informed and process consent should carefully delineate the data to be included in the study. Role conflict can be generated when the participant wants to tell you a secret or an off-the-record remark. The "nurse" listens to this, and in fact, knows that a valuable bond has been established. However, the "nurse researcher" and participants will probably be better off if the researcher gently reminds the participant of the purpose of the study and that all communication is supposed to be part of the study (Field & Morse, 1985). If it is possible, as may be the case in a healthcare facility, the participant can be referred to an appropriate person with any information not relevant to the study. The idea here is to discourage participants from telling secrets unless these secrets can be part of the study. This, of course, needs to be done with the utmost care, because secrets are treasures, but, more important, they imply promises to keep them. Most often these problems can be discussed quite openly with collaborators.

Witnessing unethical or illegal conduct can pose another ethical dilemma. If we are nurses and, as such, the clients' advocates, we cannot place the research imperative above the therapeutic imperative. Some (Estroff & Churchill, 1984) suggest that clear procedures be established prior to the start of the study that spell out the channels the researcher will go through if unethical or illegal practices are witnessed. Researchers are morally obliged from the therapeutic imperative to report such violations. The ethical response of whistle-blowing helps us to understand this particular problem.

Findings and Publication

Anonymity of subjects individually or as a group is often a requisite of qualitative research. However, sometimes individuals and cultures allow themselves to be identified. An understanding about anonymity is part of informed and process consent. What is often not mentioned or planned for is publication and dissemination of findings. With all research, what the researcher intends to do with the findings needs to be explained as part of the consent. A longitudinal view from point of entry to publication needs to be agreed upon with the collaborators. The experience of being observed can be quite different from reading a description of yourself or of your culture or hearing from someone who has such information. To prevent misunderstandings, all taking part need to agree on the various stages and activities of the entire project. What will happen to the descriptions? Will they be presented at a conference? Will they be published? If so, where, and for what purpose? All collaborators need to agree to dissemination of findings, from an ethical perspective of deontology, because they are part of the entire project. Because we may not foresee the consequences of publication, it is wise in this litigious society to protect not only our collaborators but also ourselves.

Conflict Methodology

Conflict methodology in fieldwork is built on the interactionist and ethnomethodological perspective, adding the belief that ordinary social life is characterized by deceit and impression management (Douglas, 1979). Opponents of this method maintain that the researcher is justified in using similar techniques, because it is the explicit purpose of research to expose the powerful and that deception is "legitimate" (Punch, 1986, p. 32).

The argument is based on an end that may in itself be highly moral (recall Machiavelli); yet the means are acknowledged as unethical but, within the conflict methodological view, justified. Ethical arguments are advanced for conflict methodology, but, if civilization hangs onto the Kantian principle, certainly this is a most dangerous practice. The counterargument to justifying deceit is nicely summed up by Warwick (1982):

> Social scientists have not only a right but an obligation to study controversial and politically sensitive subjects . . . but this obligation does not carry with it the right to deceive, exploit or manipulate people. My concern with backlash centers primarily on the alienation of ordinary individuals by research methods which leave them feeling that they have been cheated, deceived, or used. (p. 55)

In nursing research, deception, exploitation, or manipulation of people would be ethically antithetical to all that we philosophically and professionally stand for. Our concept of client advocacy precludes the use of conflict methodology. In addition, we need to be alert to nuances in our research that could cause individuals to feel cheated, deceived, or used. I have often heard collaborators comment that they were supposed to receive a copy of the research report but never did; thus, they feel cheated. In some of our methods and consents, the collaborators actually see the report or description before its finalization to elicit their response and agreement on whether the portrayal is accurate. This may also assist in validation. From an ethical perspective, we need to determine which models of fieldwork seem consistent with our belief system.

Models of Fieldwork

The extent to which invasion into a social setting is ethical is often a matter of common sense. The researcher needs to be aware of what is not being told, as well as what is being said. The extent to which the research is a covert or overt operation also is open to ethical evaluation. Here, again, the ethical aim needs to be clear. There is a fine line between doing anthropological research and an investigation in the journalistic or "FBI" sense. Punch (1986) conceives of three models of fieldwork and relates them to ethical features of trust and deceit:

1. The hypothetical "problemless" project: For instance, a graduate student gains entry into a commune, shares daily life, is accepted, departs to write a description, and allows the culture under study to read and validate what has been written. There is no high trauma, drama, or problems, and, as Punch (1986) points out, this type of study is like the classical ethnography when the investigator could be sure that the Ashanti and Nuer would not be scouring the anthropological journals with their lawyers for negative references to tribal life. Today, I am not sure that we can even say that.
2. The "knotty" project: The institution erects barriers against outsiders and gaining access becomes difficult. An example might be a state mental institution where those associated with certain practices fear publication in the interest of preserving the institution's and their own reputation.
3. The "ripping and running" project: There is deliberate concealment, which, in addition to being ethically indefensible, is illegal. This model depends on an unrevealed person posing as a member of the group. This practice has the connotations of spying and undercover investigating and certainly violates civil liberties.

Many of us doing fieldwork like to believe that, as moral agents, we may come to identify problems and abuses within cultures or institutions. Because of that ethical aim, we may be tempted to justify unethical means, such as bending the truth, to gain entry to obtain an accurate portrayal. Such practices again constitute conflict methodology and have serious consequences for collaborators and researchers in the field. The second and third models of fieldwork hold the potential for moral, social, and political change. However, in the long run, using these two models will have the effect of closed doors in the field because of loss of trust, credibility, and confidence in nurse researchers. The last model of fieldwork violates the very foundation of our nursing practice. Whistle-blowing again is the topic that needs to be addressed and certainly is not limited to practices witnessed by researchers. For instance, in any type of healthcare facility where unethical practices exist, the moral obligation of reporting such practices belongs to all involved. However, as was mentioned earlier, preplanning for such events, should they occur, is one way to ensure that your course of action is known and has been agreed on prior to the commencement of the study.

Summary Remarks

There is much more to be discussed within the topic of ethical consideration of qualitative research. There is much still to be discussed about qualitative research methods in nursing. So these remarks are not concluding but contribute to the dialogue centered on the developed interest in these methods. One facet is clear: One cannot adopt criteria for quantitative research and apply them to qualitative research. The static, past tense of informed consent does not adequately protect human subjects in qualitative studies. For that matter, it may not always do so for quantitative methods.

The most glaring difference, however, springs from the dynamic, process-oriented qualities of qualitative research. Qualitative research could be thought of as a verb, a process, with the ethical components constantly being scrutinized. "Process consenting" might be a way to remind ourselves of the ongoing nature of discussing with our collaborators the means and the aims of our study. In addition, our therapeutic imperative and research imperative need to be made as clear as possible. From an ethical perspective, the therapeutic imperative undergirds the research imperative so that efforts to avoid any difficulties for or disadvantages of the collaborator need our constant vigilance if the research is to proceed ethically. Because we, as nurses, have the ethical theme of deontology threaded throughout our philosophies, I think we are humanistically ahead of many other disciplines in considering the ethics of our research enterprise. Our egos are not split. We are patient–client advocates, and trust, compassion, and empathy encompass all our nursing endeavors, including research.

References

Annas, D. J., Glantz, L. H., & Katz, B. J. (1977). *Informed consent to human experimentation: The subject's dilemma*. Boston: Ballinger.

Bellah, R. (1981). The ethical aims of social inquiry. *Teachers College Record, 83*(1), 1–18.

Douglas, J. D. (1979). Living morality versus bureaucratic fist. In C. B. Klockars & F. W. O'Connor (Eds.), *Deviance and decency*. Beverly Hills, CA: Sage.

Estroff, S. E., & Churchill, L. R. (1984). Comment (Ethical dilemmas). *Anthropology Newsletter,* 25(7).

Field, P., & Morse, J. (1985). *Nursing research: The application of qualitative approaches.* Rockville, MD: Aspen.

Laudan, L. (1977). *Progress and its problems: Towards a theory of scientific growth.* Berkeley: University of California Press.

Punch, M. (1986). *The politics and ethics of fieldwork.* Beverly Hills, CA: Sage.

Rock, P. (1979). *The making of symbolic interactionism.* London: Macmillan.

Warwick, D. P. (1982). Tearsome trade: Means and ends in social research. In M. Bulmer (Ed.), *Social research ethics.* London: Macmillan.

Wilson, L., & Fitzpatrick, J. (1984). Dialectic thinking as a means of understanding systems in development: Relevance to Roger's principles. *Advances in Nursing Service, 6*(2), 41.

Resources

Aamodt, A. (1983). Problems in doing nursing research: Developing criteria for evaluating qualitative research. *Western Journal of Nursing Research, 5,* 398–402.

Amason, J. P. (1990). Cultural critique and cultural presuppositions: Hermeneutics and critical theory. *Philosophy and Social Criticism, 15*(1), 125–150.

Cutliffe, J. R., & Ramcharan, P. (2002). Leveling the playing field? Exploring the merits of the ethics-as-process approach for judging qualitative research proposals. *Qualitative Health Research, 12*(7), 1000–1010.

Denzin, N., & Lincoln, Y. (2005). *The Sage handbook of qualitative research* (3rd ed.). Thousand Oaks, CA: Sage.

Denzin, N. K., & Giardina, M. D. (Eds.). (2007). *Ethical futures in qualitative research: Decolonizing the politics of knowledge.* Walnut Creek, CA.: Left Coast Press.

Ensign, J. (2003). Ethical issues in qualitative health research with homeless youths. *Journal of Advanced Nursing, 43*(1), 43–50.

Erlandson, D. A., Harris, E., Skipper, B. L., & Allen, S. D. (1993). *Doing naturalistic inquiry: A guide to methods.* Newbury Park, CA: Sage.

Ferguson, L., Yonge, O., & Myrick, F. (2004). Students' involvement in faculty research: Ethical and methodological issues. *International Journal of Qualitative Methods, 3*(4), article 5.

Flicker, S., Haans, D., & Skinner, H. (2004). Ethical dilemmas in research on Internet communities. *Qualitative Health Research, 14*(1), 124–134.

Hofman, N. G. (2004). Toward critical research ethics: Transforming ethical conduct in qualitative health care research. *Health Care for Women International, 25*(7), 647–662.

Höglund, A. T., Winblad, U., Arnetz, B., & Arnetz, J. E. (2010). Patient participation during hospitalization for myocardial infarction: Perceptions among patients and personnel. *Scandinavian Journal of Caring Sciences* (epub.).

Kayser-Jones, J. (2003). Continuing to conduct research in nursing homes despite controversial findings: Reflections by a research scientist. *Qualitative Health Research, 13*(1), 114–128.

Lemmens, T., & Singer, P. (1998). Bioethics for clinicians: Conflicts of interest in research, education, and patient care. *Canadian Medical Association Journal, 159*(8), 960–965.

Lincoln, Y., & Guba, E. (1985). *Naturalistic inquiry.* Beverly Hills, CA: Sage.

Morse, J. (2005). Ethical issues in institutional research. *Qualitative Health Research, 15*(4), 435–437.

Orb, A., Eisenhauer, L., & Wynaden, D. (2001). Ethics in qualitative research. *Journal of Nursing Scholarship, 33*(1), 93–96.

Patterson, D., & Brogden, L. (2004). Living spaces for talk within the academy. *International Journal of Qualitative Methods, 3*(3), article 2.

Richards, H. M., & Schwartz, L. J. (2002). Ethics of qualitative research: Are there special issues for health services research? *Family Practice, 19*(2), 135–139.

Sandelowski, M. (1986). The problem of rigor in qualitative research. *Advances in Nursing Research, 8,* 27–37.

Schutz, S. (1994). Exploring the benefits of a subjective approach in qualitative nursing research. *Journal of Advanced Nursing, 20*(3), 412–417.

Shenton, A. K. (2004). Strategies for ensuring trustworthiness in qualitative research projects. *Education for Information, 22*(2), 63–75.

Singh, I. (2010). Cryptic coercion. *Hastings Center Report, 40*(1), 22–23.

Strech, D. (2010). How factual do we want the facts? Criteria for a critical appraisal of empirical research for use in ethics. *Journal of Medical Ethics, 36*(4), 222–225.

Taylor, C., Richardson, A., & Cowley, S. (2010). Restoring embodied control following surgical treatment for colorectal cancer: A longitudinal qualitative study. *International Journal of Nursing Studies* (epub).

Ulrich, C., & Grady, C. (2004). Editorial: Financial incentives and response rates in nursing research. *Nursing Research, 53*(2), 73–74.

Van-Amburg, R. (1997). A Copernican revolution in clinical ethics: Engagement versus disengagement. *American Journal of Occupational Therapy, 51*(3), 186–190.

Van den Hoonarrd, W. C. (Ed.). (2002). *Walking the tightrope: Ethical issues for qualitative researchers.* Toronto: University of Toronto Press.

Watson, J. (1990). Caring knowledge and informed moral passion. *Advances in Nursing Science, 13,* 15–24.

Watson, J. (1995). Postmodernism and knowledge development in nursing. *Nursing Science Quarterly, 8*(2), 60–64.

Watson, L., & Girard, F. (2004). Establishing integrity and avoiding methodological misunderstanding. *Qualitative Health Research, 14*(6), 875–881.

Wilde, V. (1992). Controversial hypothesis on the relationship between researcher and informant in qualitative research. *Journal of Advanced Nursing, 17,* 234–242.

Zeni, J. (Ed.). (2001). *Ethical issues in practitioner research.* New York: Teachers College Press.

Endnotes

[1] This chapter is used with permission. Originally published as P. L. Munhall. (1988). Ethical considerations in qualitative research. *Western Journal of Nursing Research, 10*(2), 150–162.

21

Institutional Review of Qualitative Research Proposals: A Task of No Small Consequence[1]

Patricia L. Munhall

Placing the Task in Context

A colleague of mine sent her research proposal to a large university hospital where the sample for her study was to be derived. She followed the format precisely and was somewhat surprised when she was asked to appear before the institutional review board (IRB) of the hospital. When she arrived, she was astonished to find 26 members of the board present. They discussed the project with her for 2 hours and engaged in what appeared to be an internal struggle over the design and conceptual framework of the study before granting her permission to conduct the study.

My colleague's study was a traditional quantitative research project. Ironically, the study was not to be conducted within the institution itself; rather, the nurse researcher wanted to do a follow-up mailing to all patients who had had hip replacement surgery. My purpose in this chapter is to place the review of qualitative research proposals in a perspective from which this context can be understood.

The foregoing example is given to demonstrate that the institutional review of your proposal, whether qualitative or quantitative, can be a challenging task at best. According to Noble (1985), institutional reviews often pose problems for researchers, regardless of the research method: "A frequent solution . . . is to engage in minimally clinical projects, such as research involving healthy, intelligent, middle-class clients" (p. 293). Using this solution, many researchers have looked for subjects outside institutions, which is one alternative. However, because many nurse researchers are committed to research within institutions, the aim of this chapter is to facilitate the IRB process, specifically with qualitative research proposals.

The Setting

In this chapter, the presentation of qualitative research methods to IRBs in institutional settings is addressed. Similarities of IRB requirements for qualitative and quantitative research designs are discussed. Departures and additions specific to qualitative research methods are analyzed, with emphasis on the educational aspect of research proposals. The idea of process consent also is examined, and the appearance of qualitative researchers before IRBs with research proposals is discussed.

IRBs are the conscience of an institution. They are deeply concerned with human rights and human dignity. The principles of patient autonomy and rights of privacy, confidentiality, anonymity, self-determination, and safety are critical components of the philosophical statements of IRBs.

The most important aspect of any research proposal is the education of our colleagues about qualitative methods and the assurance that we have the same concerns for the dignity and rights of our human subjects. A psychological principle pervades this need for education because most people are generally invested in the status quo, that is, the familiar. Individual members of IRBs are, for the most part, accustomed to the traditional quantitative research design and thus feel a certain amount of confidence when reviewing these proposals. Qualitative research designs within the traditional medical science setting present problems for these IRB members and raise questions simply because the reviewers are unfamiliar with the more unstructured qualitative research methods. This leaves the qualitative nurse researcher with a task of no small consequence.

The Challenges

Qualitative research in institutional settings presents challenges different from those of more traditional research methods. The three main challenges in receiving permission to conduct qualitative research in institutions are as follows:

1. The IRB's possible unfamiliarity with the methods, language, and legitimacy of qualitative research
2. The structural-functionalist perspective that pervades most institutions
3. The conscious or unconscious perception of the similarity of qualitative research methods to investigative-type activities

Although these challenges are interrelated, each one is addressed separately.

Unfamiliarity with Qualitative Research Methods

Most IRBs (and, in fact, many grant review panels) have members who are unfamiliar with the aims and outcomes of qualitative research. At present, many IRBs are developing guidelines and are uncertain about the role that the boards play in their institutions. Their task is complex—so complex that a request for the release of names to do a follow-up mailing to former patients (as previously described) can result in a major meeting of the IRB. The receipt of a proposal with a method called "phenomenology" also may result in an invitation to provide further information. Phenomenological studies aim at understanding a phenomenon by studying the essences of a life experience with thoughtful attention, and they search for what it means to be human in the attempt to discover plausible insight. Many members of IRBs are not familiar with such language in a research proposal. They will ask, "What is phenomenology?" or "What is grounded theory?" Although these questions do not spell disaster for proposed qualitative research projects, they do complicate matters because these important questions are asked from the structural-functional perspective of institutions.

The Structural-Functional Approach of Institutions

The structural-functional perspective is often viewed as the sacrosanct way of organizing a bureaucratic institution. Roles are prescribed, functions are distributed, behavior and outcomes are predictable, and all should go well according to fixed rules and procedures. The values in our healthcare institutions seem removed from or, at best, unrelated to qualitative research aims. For the most part, within our healthcare institutions, pragmatic goals prevail. There should be an action, an intervention, and a concrete observable task with a measurable outcome. Pragmatism in research is narrowly perceived—for example, the idea of testing something to solve some problem. The idea that understanding preceding experience or any lived experience has pragmatic value is not self-evident from the highly structured functional perspective. From this perspective, the search for meaning appears irrelevant. It is this search for meaning that creates confusion in some minds about the difference between qualitative research and investigative journalism.

Similarity of Qualitative Methods to Investigative Journalism

All research methods are essentially investigations, but perhaps they are more threatening to individuals when unstructured interviews and the possibility of a participant observation technique are part of the research design. Quantitative research designs are by nature more specific, the variables are already known, and the researcher searches for relations between variables. On the other hand, discovery, the finding out about something otherwise not fully understood, is often the aim of qualitative research designs.

Within institutions, such studies may be perceived as threatening. Interviewing patients may cause staff to worry about negative information that the patient may give—for example, complaints, reporting incidents, and so forth. If there is to be observation, who does not experience some anxiety about the idea of being observed? Fear, then, is an important feeling to consider, and one that cannot be summarily dismissed: What if you do "discover" some "negative" findings that do not reflect well on the institution or staff?

These challenges must be addressed in any proposal presented to an IRB. The strategies for meeting these challenges include education and translation, the establishment of compatible values, and the generation of trust.

Meeting the Challenges

Education and Translation

Becoming sympathetic to the concerns and psychological dynamics of the members of IRBs is the best place to start. In many cases, qualitative research proposals may not be understood by these people, may be contrary to the way that they think, and may be threatening to them. In addressing these challenges, one should realize that the normal human response to change is resistance. Many qualitative nurse researchers in institutions have reported that "resistance" was the only response to their research proposals and that they have had to change their proposals or move out of the institution. Although this situation is unfortunate, it can be prevented if qualitative nurse researchers educate their colleagues who sit on IRBs about the nature and philosophy of qualitative methods.

Most board members are thoroughly familiar with the methods associated with the Western mindset of objectivity, control, prediction, and so forth. No one needs to explain ex post facto correlation, experimental design, or statistical test, but phenomenology, grounded theory, ethnography, or whatever qualitative research method is going to be used must be explained. Not only must it be explained, but it must be presented in language that can be understood by people familiar with deductive, pragmatic, numerical ideologies. There is a need to explain in concrete terms the primacy of perception, embodiment, and the philosophical concepts. All these ideas should be clearly stated in language that the reader will understand. For example, in submitting a proposal for a qualitative research project that will examine the needs of patients who have had a mastectomy so that appropriate nursing interventions can be developed, language such as "the lived experience" of having a mastectomy, "consciousness," and "essences" may be used but need to be explained. Is this a capitulation, a compromising of our principles? On the contrary, it is the recognition that it can take years to understand these concepts and that, in a proposal, there is a limited amount of time and space for explanation. So, instead of a capitulation, it is actually a pragmatic action for a pragmatic setting. If the institution uses a structural-functionalist approach, it is unrealistic to think that this perspective will not also be reflected in the process of an IRB review.

Compatible Values

In structural-functional bureaucracies, the reality is that the search for meaning, the apprehension of essential relations among essences, the thematic analysis of cultures, the perception of another's world, and the discovery of core variables are at odds with the predominant problem-task orientation. Helping patients find meaning does not rank high among institutional objectives. So this objective must be stated in the proposal in pragmatic terms—such as, "This study will result in improved nursing care," or "This study will act as the basis for developing nursing intervention." The qualitative method must also appear structured, even if the design allows for fluidity and some flexibility. As far as possible, research aims should be compatible with the aims of the institution. The members of the IRB must not think that they are making an exception by accepting a qualitative research proposal because it appears different from their value orientation. It is best, from any point of view, to demonstrate the convergence of values between the institution and the qualitative study by stating how the study's quest for discovery is laying the groundwork for nursing intervention.

Generating Trust

Developing trust and alleviating fear or anxiety or both within the institution are critical to a successful qualitative research proposal, and they are also two of the more awkward challenges. This awkwardness arises from the perplexing situation in which the staff worry about the researcher having access to potentially damaging information or observing poor nursing care. They wonder what the researcher is going to do with possible "negative" findings. The difficulty can be dealt with by pointing out that quantitative researchers in institutions may witness and be part of the same environmental activities as qualitative researchers and that the staff are probably aware of whatever problems exist. Ideally, ethics committees or quality assurance programs address these problems, yet there is always the possibility that qualitative research may uncover some problems, and consequently, the staff may feel threatened.

The first step in dealing with this problem is to include a category for "unexpected findings" in the proposal and to carefully spell out what channels the nurse researcher will use to share such findings. If the members of the IRB understand that the discovery of findings that indicate problems is important so that they can then be solved, members and staff might be more assured. Again, education is important for achieving this perceptual shift.

Traditionally, IRBs are familiar with research that attempts to solve problems. The value of research that may identify problems so that they, too, may be addressed needs to be stressed, and stressed, and stressed. Indeed, it is critical to identify the right problem before testing solutions. Sometimes this is difficult to do, such as when patients complain during interviews about poor nursing care. A good qualitative researcher looks at the larger context (before reporting such a result, ethics demands that the lens of the study must be widened) and finds that there is inadequate staffing. Although the administration may not be happy with that finding, the nurses on the unit will be glad to have such an important need substantiated. At other times, the problem is thornier. Perhaps the poor nursing care is the result of an incompetent nurse. Although the nurse researcher cannot be the only one to know of this, he or she is ethically obligated to report such a finding through the channels that are established prior to starting the project.

Although this is essentially whistle-blowing, with its attendant consequences, sometimes good, sometimes bad, this action embodies the belief that the therapeutic imperative of nursing (advocacy) takes precedence over the research imperative (advancing knowledge) if conflict develops (see Chapter 20). These problems have fewer ramifications for researchers not researching in their home institutions, and, if possible, it may be wise not to conduct research in one's home institution. Additionally, IRBs have members who wish to protect their institutions or their own reputations or both. This difficult problem should be addressed in qualitative research proposals in positive, helpful terms and fully discussed with staff. They, too, need to be fully informed about the research project.

Similarities Between Qualitative and Quantitative Proposals

Many similar areas in qualitative and quantitative proposals are of concern to IRBs. More than likely, the same form will be used for both types of methods, and the researcher will be asked to address the following areas:

1. Objective of study
2. Research methodology
3. Characteristics of group(s)
4. Special groups (e.g., children of compromised adults)
5. Type of content
6. Confidentiality of data
7. Possible risks

Although there may be other variables, ensuring that individual rights and human dignity are protected needs to be demonstrated and documented. Often, IRBs have more elaborate requests than those listed here, and qualitative research proposals are often evaluated on the basis of adherence to traditional scientific method. Scientific legitimacy, then, is being evaluated rather than human subjects' protection. This may not be a problem 10 years from now, but, today, proposals come back from IRBs with questions that indicate reluctance of the IRB to approve the proposal because the board does not understand the method and its concomitant language. As previously suggested, educating members of IRBs about the scientific legitimacy of qualitative studies is an additional task for qualitative nurse researchers. What follows are some distinguishing characteristics of qualitative research that need to be addressed in IRB proposals.

Departure and Additions for Qualitative Research Proposals

A brief overview of the aim and purpose of qualitative research methodology may precede the proposal or, perhaps, be the introductory paragraph, depending on the institution. This overview does not have to be a highly sophisticated discourse about worldviews and paradigms, with quotations from Husserl, Erasmus, or Speigelberg; rather, a simple paragraph explaining how qualitative research methodology seeks to discover new knowledge, uses narrative descriptions in the findings, includes interviews with individual participants, and so forth, is all that is necessary. Stating that these aspects of the methodology can be used to build on one another may be important. Nurse researchers often get into difficulty by discussing intersubjectivity, going "to the things themselves," living the question, and so on. Understandable language is critical.

Objective of the study

As previously discussed, the objective of the study should be ultimately stated in pragmatic language. Often the aim of qualitative research is stated in existential terms. Remember the setting and take the existential purpose one step further by showing how the study might, for example, 1) improve staff performance, and 2) assist the patient in recovery. This approach is appropriate because it is the qualitative research baseline that enables quantitative researchers to develop hypotheses for nursing intervention, staff performance, and assisting patients in their recovery. Stress the importance of the study in pragmatic terms.

Research method

Perhaps the most important part of the proposal, the research method, offers the best opportunity for educating members of IRBs. Introduce the method, the rationale for choosing the method, and the outcome of this method. Take the reader through a step-by-step narrative in language that is familiar. This may mean taking the proposal that was written for nursing colleagues of a similar bent and translating it for persons who may be puzzled by the use of the word phenomenon. For example, instead of saying "lived experience," just say "experience." In fact, someone once asked me, "what other kind of experience is there?" Perhaps replacing the phrase "ontological commitment" with "it is my belief that" also would be helpful. Although it may be human to want to impress one's colleagues with a high level of abstraction, it will probably be counterproductive. In any case, it seems paradoxical when qualitative research is actually very interested in the concrete. No one wants to feel inadequate, and it seems unwise to send out proposals loaded with unfamiliar language. Again, to achieve IRB approval, members must be able to read qualitative research proposals without a dictionary!

So, qualitative researchers need to be clear and emphatic about their research methods. They need to teach about the method and its pragmatic usefulness to nursing sciences in language that will not distract the readers but keep them focused on the substance.

Consequence

There is a debate in the literature about whether informed consent is necessary when observations and discourse take place in the course of a nurse's routine work (Noble, 1985; Oberst, 1985). Interviews have often been exempt from formal informed consent procedures if individual verbal consent is given. However, I fear we will be on a slippery slope if too many of these exceptions to the written consent process are allowed. Common sense must prevail.

Within institutions, qualitative researchers need to anticipate a request for informed consent. If more than one interview or observation is going to take place, the idea of a process consent seems to exemplify a negotiated view of not only the phenomenon but also the study itself (see Chapter 20). All consents need to take into consideration the capacity of the person consenting, full disclosure of the research activity, and the freedom of participants to voluntarily enter and withdraw.

A proposal for process consent is suggested because an informed consent represents a past-tense concept. Qualitative research is often an ongoing, dynamic, changing process. A process consent offers researchers and participants opportunities to actualize a negotiated view and to change arrangements if necessary. A process consent encourages mutual participation and, perhaps, mutual affirmation for the participants and the researcher.

A process consent for qualitative nursing research should be developed with the research participants' input, ideas, and suggestions and should be reviewed at specific times if necessary. This approach is appropriate if the researcher is going to be doing observations or participant observations over a period of time. In addition to the informed consent, a process consent should address some of the processes listed in **Table 21–1**.

It is probably wise to have information about self-disclosed secrets in the process consent. It should be stated that all data obtained will be part of the study. In other words, secrets should be discouraged if they cannot be included in the study. It is best to explain to the participants that some secrets pose a dilemma for researchers who are also concerned about patient well-being. The question of secrets and patients' confidentiality needs to be planned, and

---

TABLE 21–1   Process Consent

Researcher and participants as collaborators come to agree on the following:

- How you will enter the field
- How often, for how long
- How you will prepare to leave
- How you will leave the field
- How you will share the information
- How you will keep the information anonymous and/or confidential
- How you will ensure an accurate portrayal of information
- What you will do if the focus of inquiry changes
- What circumstances might arise that require you to contact the person(s) again
- What you will do with "unanticipated findings"
- What you will do with confidential information revealed to you during conversation(s)
- What will become of information acquired, whether or not presented in written reports
- Where the findings are to go

Comments by participant

_____

_____

Comments by researcher

_____

_____

Dates reviewed and changes made

_____

_____

Signatures

_____

_____

Note: Each study would require a specific process consent, depending on the substance of the study. This process consent is in addition to the usual components of informed consent.

ethical dilemmas need to be considered before the proposal is written (see Chapter 20).

Confidentiality and anonymity

The same guarantee of confidentiality of data and anonymity of participants that quantitative researchers give must be made a general principle of qualitative research. This is a general principle because some institutions allow participant identities to be known, especially if the study is going to reflect positively on them. In addition, some participants enjoy being identified in certain kinds of interviews or studies. However, the general principle is to maintain confidentiality and anonymity.

In qualitative research, can we promise confidentiality when we include precise quotations from the transcripts in our publications? The answer is no, but we can provide anonymity by protecting the identity of the participant. Consequently, individuals and institutions will want assurances that only the researcher(s) will have access to the data and that there will be no identifying evidence, such as names on cassettes, names on computer printouts, and so forth. They will also want information about how and where the data will be stored. In this section of the proposal, it might be helpful to identify the lines of communication that have been established for reporting findings. Information concerning the plans for disseminating the findings (i.e., publication, presentation, and who will receive final reports) should be included and mutually agreed on.

Possible risks

Qualitative research is considered noninvasive, but, in a sense, that is a limited perception of the word. Although it is true that qualitative researchers do not physically alter the participants with interventions, there are invasions of their space and psyches. Although such invasion is often therapeutic, it can pose possible risks if certain precautions are not taken.

It is well substantiated that talking has therapeutic benefits. Patients in institutions, or staff for that matter, often find relief just "getting it out of their system" or "off their chest." Nursing intervention often provides opportunities for patients to ventilate their feelings, and interviews provide such opportunities. Attention is usually viewed as a positive experience, and being important enough to study can be viewed positively. That someone's experience is worth studying can have a validating effect.

Are there risks in qualitative research? One reviewer from an IRB asked about "triggering" an emotional response within an informant. This possibility cannot be lightly dismissed if the experiences under study are highly charged. Because of their training, nurse researchers are usually able to intervene appropriately and make good assessments about how a patient is responding. It may be normal if a patient becomes upset in the course of an interview, and the nurse researcher must be supportive and manage the interview with good clinical judgment. Arrangements also should be made with the patient's primary caretaker to support the patient after leaving the field. Aamodt (1986), still very relevant today, writes:

> In the Human Subject Consent Forms we had said there were no psychological or social risks. Because communication in response to client feelings is an expected nursing intervention, to ignore such a need could be classified as irresponsible. We planned that interviewers would not be the primary caretaker of the child, and when the situation demanded it, the child and parent were referred to the primary caretaker. (p. 167)

An inaccurate portrayal of participants or situations can also cause harm. A statement of how you intend to ensure the accurate description of participants and situations should be included in this section of the proposal. Validation by the participants is respectful and necessary for authentic representation. The harm/benefit question is succinctly placed in context by Morse (1988) when she states:

> Are the risks to the participant any greater than the everyday risk from confiding in a friend? And the "friend" in this context is a registered nurse who is accustomed to handling confidential information, counseling the dying and the distressed, observing and listening. Yet, suddenly, because the information is obtained under the auspices of "research" (rather than practice), the activities of the nurse may be considered by the IRB as potentially harmful. We must learn to trust our colleagues. (p. 214)

Presenting to the IRB

When presenting to an IRB panel, anticipate as many questions as possible. Consider the presentation a wonderful opportunity to discuss your study. However, educating IRB members about your research methods and translating them into clear, concrete, pragmatic terms should also be done in the verbal presentation. Know who the board members are and avoid answering questions in a philosophical or existential style. If there is a member of the clergy on the board, he or she might understand your answer, but the lawyer, the physician, the two laypeople, the banker, and the accountant might not, so keep your discussion clear and precise. Remember, the intentions of the IRB are the same as yours: to protect the patient.

In summary, writing clearly (especially philosophical translation), suggesting compatible values between the institution's goals and the research goals, developing trust, and establishing clear lines of communication are important areas to consider when submitting a qualitative research proposal to an IRB.

Conclusion

What I would like to stress again when writing a proposal for the IRB are the parts of this chapter that suggest keeping the language of your proposal as close as possible to understandable, everyday language. Examples have been provided in this chapter. The language of qualitative research is often philosophical and calls for an understanding, for example, of the philosophical underpinnings of phenomenology. Those concepts need to be translated into everyday language and terms.

The rule here is to simplify, simplify, simplify. This is not the time to sound as knowledgeable as you are, when you know that most members of IRBs do not have knowledge of, or familiarity with, the language of qualitative methods.

IRBs and granting organizations are making a concerted effort to include qualitative researchers on their panels, which is encouraging. Look at who is on your IRB to ascertain who your audience is and then you can adjust your proposal accordingly.

References

Aamodt, A. (1986). Discovering the child's view of alopecia: Doing ethnography. In P. Munhall & C. Oiler (Eds.), *Nursing research: A qualitative perspective* (pp. 163–171). Norwalk, CT: Appleton-Century-Crofts.

Morse, J. (1988). Commentaries on special issues. *Western Journal of Nursing Research, 10*(2), 213–216.

Noble, M. (1985). Written informed consent: Closing the door to clinical research. *Nursing Outlook, 33*(6), 292–293.

Oberst, M. (1985). Another look at informed consent. *Nursing Outlook, 33*(6), 294–295.

Resources

Burns, R. (1989). Standards for qualitative research. *Nursing Science Quarterly, 2,* 44–52.

Byrne, M. (2001). Disseminating and presenting qualitative research findings. *AORN Journal, 74*(5), 731–732.

Denzin, N., & Lincoln, Y. (2005). *The Sage handbook of qualitative research* (3rd ed.). Thousand Oaks, CA: Sage.

Denzin, N. K., & Giardina, M. D. (Eds.). (2007). *Ethical futures in qualitative research: Decolonizing the politics of knowledge.* Walnut Creek, CA: Left Coast Press.

Dixon-Woods, M., Shaw, R. L., Agarwal, S., & Smith, J. A. (2004). The problem of appraising qualitative research. *Quality and Safety in Health Care, 13*(3), 223–225.

Erlandson, D. A., Harris, E., Skipper, B. L., & Allen, S. D. (1993). *Doing naturalistic inquiry: A guide to methods.* Newbury Park, CA: Sage.

Holloway, I., & Wheeler, S. (2009). *Qualitative research in nursing and healthcare* (3rd ed.). Somerset, NJ: Wiley-Blackwell.

Jones, M. L. (2004). Application of systematic review methods to qualitative research: Practical issues. *Journal of Advanced Nursing, 48*(3), 271–278.

Kvale, S. (2008). *Doing interviews.* Thousand Oaks, CA: Sage.

Lincoln, Y., & Guba, E. G. (1985). *Naturalistic inquiry.* Thousand Oaks, CA: Sage.

Lincoln, Y. S., & Tierney, W. G. (2004). Qualitative research and institutional review boards. *Qualitative Inquiry, 10*(2), 219–234.

Miller, S., & Fredericks, M. (2003). The nature of "evidence" in qualitative research. *International Journal of Qualitative Methods, 2*(1), article 4.

Morse, J. M. (2003). A review committee's guide for evaluating qualitative proposals. *Qualitative Health Research, 13*(6), 833–851.

Morse, J. M., & Field, P. A. (2003). *Nursing research: The application of qualitative approaches* (2nd ed.). London: Nelson Thornes.

Munhall, P. (1988). Ethical considerations in qualitative research. *Western Journal of Nursing Research, 10*(2), 150–162.

Munhall, P. (2006). *Nursing research: A qualitative perspective* (4th ed.). Sudbury, MA: Jones & Bartlett.

Powell, A. E. (2001). Reading and assessing qualitative research. *Hospital Medicine, 62*(6), 360–363.

Richards, H. M., & Schwartz, L. J. (2002). Ethics of qualitative research: Are there special issues for health services research? *Family Practice, 19*(2), 135–139.

Sandelowski, M., & Barosso, J. (2002). Reading qualitative studies. *International Journal of Qualitative Methods, 1*(1), article 5.

Thorne, S., Joachim, G., Paterson, B., & Canam, C. (2002). Influence of the research frame on qualitatively derived health science knowledge. *International Journal of Qualitative Methods, 1*(1), article 1.

Endnotes

[1] Reprinted with permission from Sage Publications; *Qualitative Nursing Research: A Contemporary Dialogue,* J. Morse (Ed.), 1989, 1991, pp. 258–271.

22

Evaluation of
Qualitative Research

Marlene C. Mackey

Since publication of the fourth edition of this book (Mackey, 2007), scholars have continued to write about criteria to evaluate qualitative research (Cohen & Crabtree, 2008; Miyata & Kai, 2009; Stige, Malterud, & Midtgarden, 2009). As before, the intent of this chapter is *not* to tell you the best way to evaluate qualitative research. Rather the purpose of this chapter is to present an overview of historical and current thinking about evaluating qualitative research. Unlike quantitative research for which evaluation criteria are relatively clear and generally accepted, there is no one set of criteria that can be used to evaluate a qualitative research report. The literature is replete with recommendations, analyses, debates, concerns, and challenges about standards and evaluation criteria for qualitative research. Engel and Kuzel (1992) argued that standards for judging qualitative research may vary according to the discipline of the creators and users of research findings and that one set of criteria may not be appropriate for all types of qualitative research.

When nurses first started to conduct qualitative research, they frequently studied with sociologists, anthropologists, psychologists, or philosophers who taught them the qualitative methods that were developed in their fields. Little was written on the quality of qualitative research—you knew it when you saw it. However, as nurses used these methods to study nursing problems, they began to write about criteria to evaluate qualitative research or sought criteria from other disciplines.

Early Evaluation Criteria

Aamodt (1983) was one of the first nurses to introduce the need for specific criteria for evaluating qualitative research. She proposed that the criteria should include something about discovery/development of constructs, domains of time and space to bracket a territory for study, the reflex activity of the researcher and the phenomenon of study, detailed descriptions of the context of the study, and the contributions of the substantive or theoretical data to nursing practice, research, or theory. The implication is that a reader of qualitative research should expect information about these components of the research process.

Burns (1989) was one of the first nurse researchers to propose specific criteria to evaluate qualitative research. After describing skills needed to critique qualitative studies and elements of a qualitative research report, Burns listed five steps to critiquing a research report, whether qualitative or quantitative. The reviewer needs to understand the report, compare the elements of the report to an ideal version (or standard), judge the adequacy of the logic within the study, evaluate the usefulness of the study for clinical practice, and compare the findings of the study to previous scientific knowledge. She then described five standards (and threats to the standards) by which the reader could evaluate qualitative studies: 1) descriptive vividness, 2) methodological congruence (rigor in documentation, procedural rigor, ethical rigor, and auditability), 3) analytic preciseness, 4) theoretical connectedness, and 5) heuristic relevance (intuitive recognition, relationship to existing body of knowledge, and applicability). These standards can be found in the latest edition of the Burns and Grove (2009) research textbook and have been useful to many reviewers of qualitative reports.

With the publication of the Lincoln and Guba book (1985), nurses and others quickly embraced the guidelines they proposed for conducting qualitative research. The evaluation criteria that Lincoln and Guba described for the naturalistic (or constructivist) paradigm became extremely popular and continues to be used by qualitative researchers today (Denzin & Lincoln, 2005). Lincoln and Guba used the term *trustworthiness* to refer to a quality research report. Trustworthiness consists of four criteria—*credibility* (truth value, replaces internal validity), *transferability* (applicability, replaces external validity), *dependability* (consistency, replaces reliability), and *confirmability* (neutrality, replaces objectivity). A reader/reviewer looks for the following evidence of credibility—prolonged engagement, persistent observation, triangulation, peer debriefing, negative case analysis, referential adequacy, and member checks. An audit trail of methods and decisions from a reflexive journal provides evidence of confirmability.

Drawing from Lincoln and Guba (1985), Leininger (1994) argued for the need to develop and use criteria that fit a qualitative paradigm and criticized reviewers for using quantitative criteria. She presented six criteria to use to evaluate qualitative studies; however, her citations suggest she developed these criteria specifically for her ethnomethod. Her criteria include *credibility* (truth established through prolonged engagement), *confirmability* (repeated and direct evidence from participants and documents), *meaning-in-context* (data became understandable within holistic context), *recurrent patterning* (instances, sequence of events, experiences, or lifeways), *saturation* (redundancy, no new information), and *transferability* (whether findings can be transferred to another similar context) (pp. 105–106).

Later, nurse researchers questioned the appropriateness of the Lincoln and Guba (1985) criteria for evaluating the validity of a qualitative study. The rigid following of procedures in attempts to ensure the trustworthiness of the study may actually threaten validity (Sandelowski, 1993). Research participants do not have the credentials to validate qualitative research findings (Morse, 1998, 1999a; Sandelowski, 1993). Even qualitative research experts do not have the depth of understanding of another's research to be qualified to validate research findings (Sandelowski, 1998).

"Validity is not an inherent property of a particular method, but pertains to the data, accounts, or conclusions reached by using that method in a particular context for a particular purpose" (Maxwell, 1992, p. 284). Using this realist conception of validity, Maxwell described five types of validity used in qualitative research. *Descriptive validity* refers to an accurate, factual description of everything the researcher saw, heard, felt, or smelled. *Interpretive validity* refers to an accurate presentation of the "meaning" that objects, events, and behaviors had to the people engaged in and with them. Meaning encompasses intention, cognition, affect, belief, evaluation, and other kinds of participants' perspectives. *Theoretical validity* refers to the theory the researcher developed, including the concepts and their relationship. *Generalization* is the extent to which the findings (typically the theory) can apply to other people and other settings. *Evaluative validity*, applying an evaluative framework to the study's findings, is typically not a central concern in qualitative research.

Later Evaluation Criteria

When Janice Morse launched *Qualitative Health Research* in 1991 and later the *International Journal of Qualitative Methods*, nurses and other health-related researchers had a forum for a dialogue about evaluating qualitative research. Scholars could test their thinking and share their concerns and ideas about "what is good qualitative research."

Morse (1991) described the four broad guidelines reviewers use to evaluate manuscripts for possible publication in *Qualitative Health Research*. Reviewers assess the importance or "significance" of the study in terms of the development of new knowledge or theory. The article should excite, impress, or at least interest the reader. A "theoretical evaluation" is done by determining if the results extend beyond description to some level of abstraction and if the theory is logical, clear, complete, and intuitively makes sense. Implications of the theory for use in extending knowledge and for praxis and linkages to the literature are clearly described. Reviewers conduct a "methodological assessment" to determine if an inductive approach was used and if the clearly presented research problem or question was studied using an appropriate research method and data analysis. Selection of the sample is evaluated for appropriateness and adequacy and data collection for saturation. Reviewers also evaluate "adherence to ethical standards" in the conduct and reporting of the study.

As editor of *Qualitative Health Research*, Morse (1999b) has witnessed the disagreement among experienced qualitative researchers in their reviews of manuscripts for the journal. Some reviewers accept descriptive reporting of "raw" data, whereas others believe this to be inadequate. "Qualitative research must, in my view, add something more to the participants' words for it to be considered a research contribution, whether it be synthesis, interpretation, or development of a concept, model, or theory" (p. 163). Other manuscripts may report complex theory but fail to link the theory to data from which it was derived, troubling some reviewers but not others. Reviewers also disagree on the type of results that should be published—common sense vs. innovative, intriguing, and surprising findings. Journal reviewers in the process of reviewing are indirectly shaping criteria that may be used to evaluate qualitative research. Morse (2003), however, cautioned us about the trend to use standards to evaluate qualitative studies that focus on the techniques of doing the study rather than on the findings or the contributions to theory.

Revising/Emerging Evaluation Criteria

Lincoln (1995) suggested additional criteria to evaluate the quality of qualitative research. Lincoln urged a dialogue about the following emerging criteria: positionality or standpoint judgments (all texts are partial, incomplete, and never represent any complete truth), community as arbiter of quality (research serves the community), voice (extent to which alternative voices are heard), critical subjectivity or reflexivity (awareness and understanding of subtle differences in the personal and psychological states of others), reciprocity (intense sharing of observer and others), sacredness (create relationships based on mutual respect, granting of dignity, and appreciation of the human condition), and sharing the perquisites of privilege with those we study (sharing financial and other benefits the researcher gains).

Thorne (1997) described four principles of evaluation (epistemological integrity, representative credibility, analytic logic, and interpretive authority) and five principles of critique (moral defensibility, disciplinary relevance, pragmatic obligation, contextual awareness, and probable truth) in qualitative research. The intent and meaning of these principles are presented elsewhere (Fossey et al., 2002; Popay et al., 1998). The one exception is pragmatic obligation in which the researcher must consider that research findings may be applied in practice and therefore must be presented in such a way as to avoid harm.

Stiles (1999) proposed criteria to evaluate the research method and the validity of data interpretation. The reviewer should examine the research report for clarity and justification of the study questions, selection of participants, and methods of gathering and analyzing data. In evaluating data analysis, the reader considers *engagement with the material* (intense, persistent, prolonged), *iteration* (cycle between interpretation and observation), *grounding* (systematically linking interpretations and observations), and *asking "what," not "why"* (participant interviews). The reader of a research report needs information about the investigator's forestructure (preconceptions, values), the social and cultural context, and the investigator's internal processes (personal experiences, relationship with participants). Stiles suggested validity criteria; i.e., readers, participants, and investigators evaluate the impact of data interpretations on their own preconceptions or bias and determine if the findings are either a fit/an agreement or represent real change or growth in understanding.

Patton (2002) proposed criteria to evaluate a number of approaches to qualitative research including artistic and evocative criteria and critical change criteria. His "social construction and constructivist criteria" most closely addresses the types of research nurses typically conduct: subjectivity acknowledged (discusses and takes into account biases), trustworthiness (Lincoln & Guba, 1985), authenticity, triangulation (capturing and respecting multiple perspectives), reflexivity, praxis, particularity (doing justice to the integrity of unique cases), enhanced and deepened understanding (*Verstehen*), and contributions to dialogue (p. 544).

Drawing heavily on the work of Lincoln (1995), Popay, Rogers, and Williams (1998), and Stiles (1999), Fossey and colleagues (2002) organized and discussed the previously mentioned scholars' work under the steps of the research process. The "research design and questions" should be clearly and explicitly presented in order to meet two essential criteria for quality research: 1) the reader can evaluate the congruence (fit) between the purpose of the study and subsequent sampling, data collection, and analysis, and 2) the reader can determine if something was learned from the participants that goes beyond initial assumptions, understanding, and interpretations (i.e., the views of the participants were authentically presented). *Sampling strategies* (both purposive and theoretical) should be clearly presented in order for the reader to evaluate their appropriateness and adequacy to provide the information needed to meet the study's aims. The reader should have enough information about the data collection methods to evaluate whether the researcher could adequately explore the subjective meaning, actions, and social context of the participants. An adequate report of data analysis includes a description of conceptual processes used to explore the meanings, patterns, or connections among data and how the researcher's own thought, reflection, and intuition were used. Quality research reports reflect transparency (openness and honesty) of data collection, analysis, and presentation.

> Qualitative research findings are presented as textual descriptions that should illuminate the subjective meanings of the phenomena, or social world, being studied, but which should also place the findings in context, so as to represent the real world of those studied and in which their lived experiences are embedded. However, the extent to which anyone is able to represent the experiences and intentional meanings of others depends on interpretations that are necessarily personal, experiential, and political, making qualitative findings at once both descriptive and interpretive. Principle issues related to their trustworthiness are related to the representation of views (authenticity); how the findings are presented (coherence); claims about their typicality; and the contribution of the researcher's perspective to the interpretation (permeability). (Fossey et al., 2002, p. 730)

Morse and colleagues (2002) expressed concern about the rejection of the terms, reliability and validity, by qualitative researchers and an emphasis on strategies for evaluating trustworthiness and utility after the research is completed. They argued that reliability and validity were appropriate concepts as an indicator of rigor in qualitative research. They urged qualitative researchers to reclaim responsibility for reliability and validity by implementing verification strategies while conducting research. "*Verification* is the process of checking, confirming, making sure, and being certain . . . the mechanisms used during the process of research to incrementally contribute to ensuring reliability and validity and, thus, the rigor of the study" (p. 9). These verification strategies are *methodological coherence* (congruence between research question and methods), *appropriate sample* (adequacy evidenced by saturation and replication), *collecting and analyzing data concurrently*, *thinking theoretically* (ideas from data reconfirmed with new data), and *theory development* (as an outcome of the research process).

Drawing on the work of Beach (1993), Eisner (1985), and Shapin (1984), among others, Sandelowski and Barroso (2002) challenged readers of qualitative research to reconceptualize the "research report as a dynamic vehicle that mediates between researcher/writer and reviewer/reader, rather than as a factual account of events after the fact" (p. 3). Instead of using rigid standards and criteria to evaluate these research reports, the reader's task should be to read in order to understand the meaning being communicated.

> Although useful, existing guides for evaluating qualitative studies (variously comprised of checklists and/or narrative summaries of criteria or standards) tend to confuse the research report with the research it represents. They also do not ask the reviewer to differentiate between understanding the nature of a study-as-reported and estimating the value of a study-as-reported, nor do they allow that any one criterion might be more or less relevant for any one study and to any one reviewer. We prefer the word appraisal as opposed to evaluation, as appraisal more explicitly encompasses understanding in addition to estimating value. Any work of art—including the research report—must be understood, or appreciated, for what it is before it can be judged as a good or bad example of its kind. Appreciated here means the exercise of wise judgment and keen insight in recognizing the nature and merits of a work. (Sandelowski & Barroso, 2002, pp. 9–10)

Reviewers/readers of qualitative reports may have difficulty in evaluating the studies if they are unfamiliar with the various "forms" (Sandelowski & Barroso, 2002, p. 12) (i.e., structure or "reconstruction of a research study," p. 10) the report comes in. They need to know what they are looking for and at and where to find it. Reviewers also must be able to distinguish between "reporting adequacy versus procedural or interpretive appropriateness" (p. 12) and "actual versus virtual presence or absence" (p. 13) of information about the study.

Therefore, Sandelowski and Barroso developed a reading guide to assist the reader in the health-related practice disciplines to find information in the report—research problem, research purpose(s)/question(s), literature review, orientation to the target phenomenon, method, sampling, sample, data collection, data management, validity, findings, discussion, ethics, and form. The guide includes a comprehensive definition of each category and asks the reader to determine the presence and the relevance of each of the appraisal parameters. The reading guide is readily available online (see References). The authors invite feedback from readers/reviewers in order to enhance the quality and utility of the guide.

Evaluation Criteria for Phenomenological Research _____

Munhall (1994) proposed *One P, Ten Rs* as evaluation criteria to evaluate phenomenological research for rigor and merit (pp. 189–193). The *Phenomenological Nod* (i.e., nodding in agreement when reading or listening to the study's findings) indicates recognition of the findings and agreement that the researcher has captured, at least partially, the meaning of the experience to the participants. In order to evaluate the *Rigor* of the study, the reviewer can consider additional *Rs*:

- *Resonancy*—The interpretation of the meaning of the experience is familiar, sounds correct, "resonates" of past experiences.
- *Reasonableness*—All activities of the study, including the interpretation of the meaning of the experience sound "reasonable," the researcher presented carefully reasoned rationale for all aspects of the study.
- *Representativeness*—The findings represent the many dimensions of the lived experience; this is evidenced by the multiple data sources examined.
- *Recognizability*—The reader becomes more aware of an experience by recognizing some aspects of that experience, which leads to the next criterion.
- *Raised Consciousness*—The reader focuses on and gains understanding of an experience, a new insight not thought of before.
- *Readability*—Writing should be concrete, readable, interesting, and understandable.
- *Relevance*—Research findings "should bring us close to our humanness, increase our consciousness, enable understanding, give us possible interpretations, offer us possible meaning, and guide us in our lives, personally and professionally" (p. 192).
- *Revelations*—As the reader gains a deeper understanding, "behind or underneath what is revealed to us, we have considered what is being concealed or what wishes to be concealed" (p. 192).
- *Responsibility*—Ethical considerations are evident, including process consent, sensitivity to content of conversations, and authentic representation of meanings.

Munhall (1994) challenged scholars to add to the list of criteria for evaluating phenomenological research. She added to her own list by suggesting *Richness* ("a full embodied, multifaceted, multilayered, thoughtful, sensitive, impassioned description of a human experience" [p. 193]) and *Responsiveness* (people are moved to rethink preconceptions or to act in some way in response to the study) as additional *Rs* for evaluating phenomenology.

Evaluation Criteria for Grounded Theory Research _____

Nurses have conducted grounded theory research for many years. The originators of the method, Glaser and Strauss (1967), proposed criteria to evaluate the quality of grounded theory.

"If a reader becomes sufficiently caught up in the description so that he feels vicariously that he was in the field" (p. 230), the credibility of the grounded theory is judged favorably. The reader also judges credibility by assessing the methods the researcher used to develop the theory. Additionally, before using the grounded theory, the reader evaluates the fit of the theory to the area to which it will be applied. The theory should be easily understandable to a layperson and be general enough to fit a variety of changing situations. The theory's concepts can be controlled by the user to fit ongoing variation and change.

Later, Strauss and Corbin (1998) presented six criteria (questions to ask about the adequacy of the research process) for use in evaluating a grounded theory study, such as questions about sampling, identifying major categories, and verifying categories. They also proposed eight additional criteria (questions about concepts, conceptual linkages, conditions for variation, process, and significance) by which to evaluate the empirical grounding of the research.

More recently, Charmaz (2005) offered the following criteria to evaluate grounded theory studies:

1. Credibility
   - Has the researcher achieved intimate familiarity with the setting or topic?
   - Are the data sufficient to merit the researcher's claims? Consider the range, number, and depth of observations contained in the data.
   - Has the researcher made systematic comparisons between observations and between categories?
   - Do the categories cover a wide range of empirical observations?
   - Are there strong logical links between the gathered data and the researcher's argument and analysis?
   - Has the researcher provided enough evidence for his or her claims to allow the reader to form an independent assessment—and *agree* with the researcher's claims?

2. Originality
   - Are the categories fresh? Do they offer new insights?
   - Does the analysis provide a new conceptual rendering of the data?
   - What is the social and theoretical significance of the work?
   - How does the work challenge, extend, or refine current ideas, concepts, and practices?

3. Resonance
   - Do the categories portray the fullness of the studied experience?
   - Has the researcher revealed liminal and taken-for-granted meanings?
   - Has the researcher drawn links between larger collectivities and individual lives, when the data so indicate?
   - Do the analytic interpretations make sense to members and offer them deeper insights about their lives and worlds?

4. Usefulness
   - Does the analysis offer interpretations that people can use in their everyday worlds?
   - Do the analytic categories speak to generic processes?

- Have these generic processes been examined for hidden social justice implications?
- Can the analysis spark further research in other substantive areas?
- How does the work contribute to making a better society? (p. 528)

EPICURE: An Evaluation Agenda

Because of the diversity of qualitative research traditions, general evaluation checklists or shared evaluation criteria may be inadequate. To address this problem, Stige, Malterud, and Midtgarden (2009) proposed an evaluation agenda that included pluralism but did not require consensus on ontological, epistemological, and methodological issues, however, it did require consensus on what themes should be discussed. They proposed using reflexive dialogue rather than rule-based judgment in evaluating qualitative research. The acronym for their evaluation agenda, EPICURE, refers to engagement, processing, interpretation, (self and social) critique, usefulness, relevance, and ethics.

Application of Qualitative Health Research

Swanson, Durham, and Albright (1997) posed 16 questions that practitioners could ask in evaluating theory, or findings, from a qualitative study for use in practice.

1. What is this study about? What is the "storyline" (theory about why something occurs)?
2. Does the "storyline"/theory fit with my experience in my practice, or do I feel I have to force a fit?
3. Can I understand what the investigator(s) is trying to say? Is there jargon, or is it understandable to me or a layperson?
4. Is the theory general enough to apply to situations I encounter in practice on a daily basis?
5. Does the storyline account for the wide range of behaviors seen in my practice over time?
6. What are the concepts presented in the findings? Are they just named or are they supported by their characteristics (properties) and the range and variation of those characteristics (dimensions)? Are the concepts supported by anecdotal data? Are any of the concepts linked to one another? Do any of the concepts give me an "ah-hah" reaction? Have I seen this or experienced it?
7. Are there conditions that show how the theory varies? Are these sufficiently broad to encompass my practice experience?
8. Can I expand on the theory by thinking of other conditions under which the theory would be applicable?

9. Do the investigators state how the theory can be applied in practice? Can I refute their claim(s) or add to their list of applications?
10. Does the theory (e.g., findings) increase awareness of sociological, psychological, moral, ethical, or organizational aspects of practice?
11. Does the theory suggest accountability for sociological, psychological, moral, ethical, or organizational aspects of practice rather than for technical aspects of practice only?
12. Does the theory suggest application/use including pre- and postinstitutionalization?
13. Does the theory suggest application/use such as "trajectory" or "biography"?
14. Are issues presented from the research that can be raised among the general public?
15. Does the research address empowerment issues for consumers, families, and/or communities?
16. Does the research address the role of the social system (such as the healthcare system or the educational system) in addressing the social problem?

Popay, Rogers, and Williams (1998) argued that qualitative research is needed in health services research to provide "evidence on appropriateness (i.e., the extent to which care can be said to meet the self-perceived needs of the person to whom it is being offered) and evidence of the factors that affect decision making among policy makers, clinicians, and patients (i.e., why people, both lay and professional, behave as they do when they do)" (p. 342). In order to assess the quality of a qualitative research report, they presented a list of questions the evaluator should ask in order to determine the usefulness of the research findings. The questions were:

1. "Does the research, as reported, illuminate the subjective meaning, actions, and context of those being researched?"
2. "Is there evidence of the adaption [sic] and responsiveness of the research design to the circumstances and issues of real-life social settings met during the course of the study?"
3. "Does the sample produce the type of knowledge necessary to understand the structures and processes within which the individuals or situations are located?"
4. "Is the description provided detailed enough to allow the researcher or reader to interpret the meaning and context of what is being researched?"
5. "How are different sources of knowledge about the same issue compared and contrasted?"
6. "Are subjective perceptions and experiences treated as knowledge in their own right?"

7. "How does the research move from a description of the data, through quotation or examples, to an analysis and interpretation of the meaning and significance of it?"
8. "What claims are being made for the generalization of the findings to either other bodies of knowledge or to other populations or groups?" (pp. 345–348)

Popay et al. argued that the primary standard for qualitative research is "lay accounts and the privileging of subjective meaning" (p. 344). The evaluator then looks for evidence of responsiveness to social context and flexibility of design, theoretical or purposeful sampling, adequate description, data quality, theoretical and conceptual adequacy, and potential for assessing typicality.

Metasynthesis for Evidence-Based Practice

"Qualitative health research is the best chance for evidence-based practice to realize its ideal of using the best evidence to create the best practices for individuals" (Sandelowski, 2004, p. 1382). The increasing interest in using qualitative research in practice has resulted in multiple publications about *metasynthesis* of qualitative research findings (Beck, 2009; Finfgeld-Connett, 2010; Paterson et al., 2009; Sandelowski, Trimble, Woodard, & Barroso, 2006; Walsh & Downe, 2005). Sandelowski (2006), however, cautions us to recognize that qualitative metasyntheses are "inescapably interpretations at least 3 times removed from the target experiences under investigation; they are themselves reviewers' representations of researchers' representations" (p. 11) and may not be appropriate bases for effective and safe (physical, ethical, and cultural) practices. Sandelowski (2004) also cautions us that metasynthesis is a highly skilled task and that some reports claiming to be metasyntheses are actually little more than literature reviews and present a threat to the perceived usefulness of qualitative findings.

Margarete Sandelowski is the preeminent expert in qualitative metasynthesis. She and her colleagues have published numerous journal articles and a book (Sandelowski & Barroso, 2007) about synthesizing qualitative research. The book contains chapters on searching for and retrieving qualitative research reports, appraising reports of qualitative studies, classifying the findings, synthesizing findings (metasummary and metasynthesis), optimizing the validity, and presenting syntheses of findings.

Conclusions

The search for criteria or standards with which to evaluate qualitative research continues. The increased emphasis on metasynthesis and the use of qualitative research findings to support evidence-based practice highlights the importance of recognizing quality research. The review of the literature demonstrates that reviewers are concerned with the adequacy and appropriateness of the research methods employed and with the validity and usefulness of the research findings. This literature review presents a number of different frameworks that the reader could use when evaluating qualitative research reports. This chapter is intended to give the reader an overview of these frameworks to help the reader understand the complexity of evaluating qualitative research and to help identify criteria to explore in more depth. The reader is urged to consult the original sources of the material presented in this chapter.

References

Aamodt, A. M. (1983). Problems in doing nursing research: Developing a criteria for evaluating qualitative research. *Western Journal of Nursing Research, 5*, 398–402.

Beach, R. (1993). *A teacher's introduction to reader-response theories.* Urban, IL: National Council of Teachers of English.

Beck, C. T. (2009). Metasynthesis: A goldmine for evidence-based practice. *AORN Journal, 90*, 701–710.

Burns, N. (1989). Standards for qualitative research. *Nursing Science Quarterly, 2*, 44–52.

Burns, N., & Grove, S. K. (2009). *The practice of nursing research: Appraisal, synthesis, and generation of evidence* (6th ed.) St. Louis: Elsevier Saunders.

Charmaz, K. (2005). Grounded theory in the 21st century: Applications for advancing social justice studies. In N. K. Denzin & Y. S. Lincoln (Eds.), *The Sage handbook of qualitative research* (3rd ed., pp. 507–535). Thousand Oaks, CA: Sage.

Cohen, D. J., & Crabtree, B. F. (2008). Evaluative criteria for qualitative research in health care: Controversies and recommendations. *Annals of Family Medicine, 6*, 331–339.

Denzin, N. K., & Lincoln, Y. S. (2005). The discipline and practice of qualitative research. In N. K. Denzin & Y. S. Lincoln (Eds.), *The Sage handbook of qualitative research* (3rd ed., pp. 1–32). Thousand Oaks, CA: Sage.

Eisner, E. (1985). Aesthetic modes of knowing. In E. Eisner (Ed.), *Learning and teaching the ways of knowing: Eighty-fourth yearbook of the National Society for the study of education, Part II* (pp. 23–36). Chicago: National Society for the Study of Education.

Engel, J. D., & Kuzel, J. D. (1992). On the idea of what constitutes good qualitative inquiry. *Qualitative Health Research, 2*, 504–510.

Finfgeld-Connett, D. (2010). Generalizability and transferability of meta-synthesis research findings. *Journal of Advanced Nursing, 66*, 246–254.

Fossey, E., Harvey, C., McDermott, F., & Davidson, L. (2002). Understanding and evaluating qualitative research. *Australian and New Zealand Journal of Psychiatry, 36*, 717–732.

Glaser, B. G., & Strauss, A. L. (1967). *The discovery of grounded theory: Strategies for qualitative research.* Chicago: Aldine.

Leininger, M. (1994). Evaluation criteria and critique of qualitative research studies. In J. Morse (Ed.), *Critical issues in qualitative research methods* (pp. 95–115). Thousand Oaks, CA: Sage.

Lincoln, Y. S. (1995). Emerging criteria for quality in qualitative and interpretative research. *Qualitative Inquiry, 1*, 275–289.

Lincoln, Y. S., & Guba, E. G. (1985). *Naturalistic inquiry.* Beverly Hills, CA: Sage.

Mackey, M. C. (2007). Evaluation of qualitative research. In P. L. Munhall (Ed.), *Nursing research: A qualitative perspective* (4th ed., pp. 555–568). Sudbury, MA: Jones & Bartlett.

Maxwell, J. A. (1992). Understanding and validity in qualitative research. *Harvard Educational Review, 62*, 279–299.

Miyata, H., & Kai, I. (2009). Reconsidering evaluation criteria for scientific adequacy in health care research: An integrative framework of quantitative and qualitative criteria. *International Journal of Qualitative Methods.* Retrieved April 5, 2010, from http://ejournals.library.ualberta.ca/index.php/IJQM/article/view/1822/5203

Morse, J. M. (1991). Evaluating qualitative research. *Qualitative Health Research, 1,* 283–286.

Morse, J. M. (1998). Validity by committee. *Qualitative Health Research, 8,* 443–445.

Morse, J. M. (1999a). Myth #93: Reliability and validity are not relevant to qualitative inquiry. *Qualitative Health Research, 9,* 717–718.

Morse, J. M. (1999b). Silent debates in qualitative inquiry. *Qualitative Health Research, 9,* 163–165.

Morse, J. M. (2003). The significance of standards. *Qualitative Health Research, 13,* 1187–1188.

Morse, J. M., Barrett, M., Mayan, M., Olsen, K., & Spiers, J. (2002). Verification strategies for establishing reliability and validity in qualitative research. *International Journal of Qualitative Methods 1*(2), Article 2. Retrieved August 1, 2010, from http://www.ualberta.ca/~iiqm/backissues/1_2Final/pdf/morseetal.pdf

Munhall, P. L. (1994). *Revisioning phenomenology: Nursing and health science research.* New York: National League for Nursing Press.

Paterson, B. L., Dubouloz, C., Chevrier, J., Ashe, B., King, J., & Moldoveanu, M. (2009). Conducting qualitative metasynthesis research: Insights from a metasynthesis project. *International Journal of Qualitative Methods, 8,* 22–33. Retrieved August 1, 2010, from http://ejournals.library.ualberta.ca/index.php/IJQM/article/view/5100/5587

Patton, M. Q. (2002). *Qualitative research & evaluation methods* (3rd ed.). Thousand Oaks, CA: Sage.

Popay, J., Rogers, A., & Williams, G. (1998). Rationale and standards for the systematic review of qualitative literature in health services research. *Qualitative Health Research, 8,* 341–351.

Sandelowski, M. (1993). Rigor or rigor mortis: The problem of rigor in qualitative research. *Advances in Nursing Science, 16*(2), 1–8.

Sandelowski, M. (1998). The call to experts in qualitative research. *Research in Nursing & Health, 21,* 467–471.

Sandelowski, M. (2004). Using qualitative research. *Qualitative Health Research, 14,* 1366–1386.

Sandelowski, M. (2006). "Meta-Jeopardy": The crisis of representation in qualitative metasynthesis. *Nursing Outlook, 54,* 10–16.

Sandelowski, M., & Barroso, J. (2002). Reading qualitative studies. *International Journal of Qualitative Methods, 1*(1), Article 5. Retrieved August 1, 2010, from http://www.ualberta.ca/~iiqm/backissues/1_1Final/html/sandeleng.html

Sandelowski, M., & Barroso, J. (2007). *Handbook for synthesizing qualitative research.* New York: Springer.

Sandelowski, M., Trimble, F., Woodard, E. K., & Barroso, J. (2006). From synthesis to script: Transforming qualitative research findings for use in practice. *Qualitative Health Research, 16,* 1350–1370.

Shapin, S. (1984). Pump and circumstances: Robert Boyle's literary technology. *Social Studies of Science, 14,* 481–520.

Stige, B., Malterud, K., & Midtgarden, T. (2009). Toward an agenda for evaluation of qualitative research. *Qualitative Health Research, 19,* 1504–1516.

Stiles, W. B. (1999). Evaluating qualitative research. *Evidence-Based Mental Health, 2,* 99–101.

Strauss, A., & Corbin, J. (1998). *Basics of qualitative research: Techniques and procedures for developing grounded theory* (2nd ed.). Thousand Oaks, CA: Sage.

Swanson, J. M., Durham, R. F., & Albright, J. (1997). Clinical utilization/application of qualitative research. In J. M. Morse (Ed.), *Completing a qualitative project: Details and dialogue* (pp. 253–281). Thousand Oaks, CA: Sage.

Thorne, S. (1997). The art (and science) of critiquing qualitative research. In J. M. Morse (Ed.). *Completing a qualitative project: Details and dialogue* (pp. 117–132). Thousand Oaks, CA: Sage.

Walsh, D., & Downe, S. (2005). Meta-synthesis method for qualitative research: A literature review. *Journal of Advanced Nursing, 50,* 204–211.

23

Evidence-Based Nursing and Qualitative Research: A Partnership Imperative for Real-World Practice

Patti Rager Zuzelo

Evidence-based practice (EBP) discussion has reached the "tipping point" (Gladwell, 2002) within and between nursing and medical professional organizations. The "tipping point" refers to the name popularized by Gladwell that describes the contagiousness, big effects, and dramatic changes associated with an epidemic, in this case, an EBP "epidemic," when everything changes all at once.

EBP popularity is astonishing given the fact that nursing research utilization of the 1970s and 1980s called for similar practice changes and, yet, was generally regarded noncommittally by nurses providing direct care. The term *evidence-based nursing* (EBN) has become ubiquitous within professional nursing discussions (Meadows-Oliver, 2009). A quick Google search revealed 3,580,000 results containing "evidence based nursing." This is an astounding number considering that a quick look 4 years ago using a similar search engine revealed 1,253,386 "hits." Journals, conferences, academic centers, books, and practice guidelines offer opportunities to develop EBN expertise.

EBN is a phenomenon that appears to have staying power given its emphasis on best practices and the appealing belief that scientific credibility underlies many or most practice decisions. EBN is particularly attractive given the concurrent emphasis on evidence-based medicine (EBM). It is important for nurses to have a firm grasp of EBN characteristics and processes to appraise its potential benefit to patient outcomes and to make informed decisions as to the application of EBN practice recommendations. It is also important for nurses to have a clear appreciation of EBN and EBM characteristics so as to ensure that the unique contributions of nursing practice are not subsumed within the positivistic worldview of medical science. Qualitative research has a critical role to play in EBN and, yet, it is often overlooked because quantitative approaches receive preferential consideration. This chapter addresses the importance of qualitative research to EBN and explores the barriers, opportunities, and contributions of qualitative research methodologies to EBN.

EBN and Qualitative Research: Fundamental Issues and Concerns

EBN is the integration of solid research evidence, patient preference, and clinician expertise (**Figure 23–1**) (DiCenso, Guyatt, & Ciliska, 2005). In general, nurses are advised to 1) make certain to take practice recommendations from good research only; 2) solicit patient preferences and actions; and 3) evaluate these recommendations, preferences, and actions within the context of clinical expertise and resources. These steps seem simple and clear. In reality, challenges are associated with EBN, including concerns that EBN is research utilization with a new name and disagreement as to what constitutes "good" research and "evidence." Some question not only the constituency of evidence in the health sciences but also "who or what constitutes the truth of evidence? What force or agency is behind this constitution? To what effect?" (Murray, Holmes, & Rail, 2008, p. 277). These questions are important and provide the foundation for this chapter.

Ciliska, Pinelli, DeCenso, and Cullum (2001) note that EBN is a fairly recent term that evolved from the initial concept of EBM. Stetler (2001) asserts that the research utilization movement of the 1970s in nursing was actually the forerunner to EBN and that some EBN models are entrenched in prior research utilization work. DiCenso et al. (2005) describe EBN as "much broader than research utilization" (p. 6) because it incorporates clinical expertise, patient values, and clinical resources.

Although DiCenso et al.'s (2005) definition is widely acknowledged in the published literature, it is also important to note that there is variation in the emphasis on the breadth of this definition. Some authors emphasize "evidence" and the hierarchical value of evidentiary types without much mention of clinician judgment and patient input (Moore et al., 1995). This inconsistency is of concern and may be part of the reason why some nurses find it difficult to understand the difference between EBN and research utilization. When EBN or EBP is described without attending to clinical expertise and patient values, it is similar to basic research utilization and may be more consistent with a medical model of disease-based, positivistic, clinical decision making.

It is interesting to note that the terms EBN and EBP are used interchangeably in the literature with shared ideas from EBM. The variations in terms may be important and should be explored as they contribute to the confusion experienced by nurses as they navigate the literature. For the purpose of this chapter, EBP is used to generically refer to the overarching focus on using evidence to identify best practices and improve patient/client outcomes. EBN refers to EBP activities that are unique to nursing. What constitutes "best" practices and "best evidence" is dependent upon the circumstances at the time. In addition to the

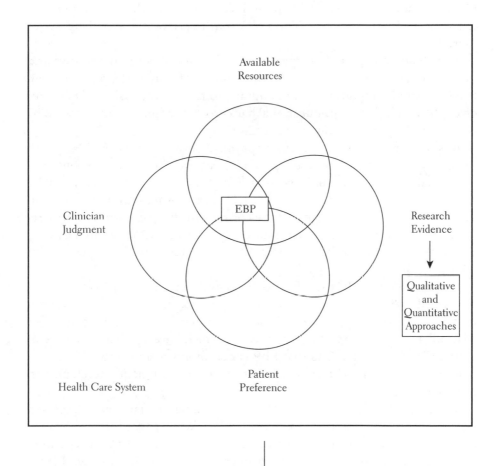

Available
Resources

EBP

Clinician
Judgment

Research
Evidence

Qualitative
and
Quantitative
Approaches

Health Care System

Patient
Preference

Improved Patient/System Outcomes

FIGURE 23–1   EBP and Outcomes Improvement.
Source: Adapted from A. DiCenso and N. Cullum. (1998). Implementation forum. *Evidence Based Nursing, 1*(2), 38–40.

notion of "best" is the lack of conceptual clarity in the literature about variations in terms used to define evidence, research, and knowledge (Rycroft-Malone & Stetler, 2004).

Liberati and Vineis (2004) note that the real failure of medical practice prior to EBM was not that people did not use evidence but that no framework and no set of rules for using evidence in a systematic way existed. The authors identify that acquiring critical appraisal skills is one of the most important tenets of the EBM movement. This point may be relevant to nursing practice as well.

The ability to appraise the quality and relevance of both quantitative and qualitative research studies within the context of real-world practice challenges is vitally important to nursing and difficult to consistently achieve given the widely divergent educational backgrounds of practicing nurses. Why is defining "evidence" so important to nursing?

It is important to have a balanced appraisal of the benefits of EBN. Avoiding the hype of EBN and the resultant tendency to jump on board without careful consideration is critical. What is the "evidence" of EBN (French, 2002)? Nursing, as both a science and an art, needs to actively make certain that qualitative research is as much a part of the considered evidence as quantitative research is. Nurses need to appreciate the complexity of EBP and cannot assume that EBP in its current form is compatible with nursing values and practice (Dale, 2005).

French (2002) conducted a frequency analysis on the key words "evidence-based medicine," "evidence-based practice," "evidence-based nursing," "evidence-based health care," and "evidence-based decision making." Findings revealed a cumulative total of 6,194 papers, most of which have a publication date of 1995 or later. French asserts that EBP is commonly a euphemism for information management, clinical judgment, professional practice development, or managed care.

There is little evidence that EBP has added value to quality assurance and research-based practice. The paradox of EBP is likened to the intense enthusiasm followed by disenchantment that occurred with the Problem Oriented Medical Record, Nursing Process, Primary Nursing, and Reflective Practitioner (French, 2002). French examines the utility of EBP within the context of symbolic interactionism. French provides a selective review of the definitions of EBP and, in agreement with others, points out that these varied definitions have important inconsistencies and reveal two issues: What is the meaning of the word "evidence" (Murray, Holmes, & Rail, 2008), and what is the process of EBP?

There is a wide range of evidentiary sources, including personal reflection, journal articles, policies, guidelines, professional consensus, research, and audit (Dale, 2005; Waters, Rychetnik, Crisp & Barratt, 2009). *Relevance* and *best* are value-laden terms and need to be explored fully within the context of nursing practice—a practice that is inherently different from medical practice. Dale notes that current forms of EBP may be incompatible with nursing because nursing requires a pluralistic approach. Questions drive methods, and some questions are best answered using qualitative methods, particularly those questions that are often of great interest to practicing nurses. Qualitative research varies by type and design with methodologies routed in anthropology, psychology, and sociology with a goal of developing a complete understanding of the reality perceived by the individual and the associated truths (Williamson, 2009). Adding to these concerns is inconsistency within nursing specific to the way that evidence is understood and valued (Waters, Rychetnik, Crisp, & Barratt, 2009).

Some researchers criticize the current EBP paradigm, noting that establishment's endorsement of the Cochrane taxonomy and research database and its promotion of evidence as knowledge is dangerous because it inscribes strict norms and ensures political dominance (Murray, Holmes, & Rail, 2008). The supremacy of the randomized clinical trial (RCT) and systematic review devalues participants' narratives and qualitative research when compared to hard "evidence." Murray et al. decry the EBM movement and assert that EBM "evacuates the social and ethical responsibilities that ought to distinguish health care professions, such as nursing" (p. 275).

Why Use Qualitative Methods for Evidence-Based Practice?

Carper (1978) identifies four patterns of knowing that provide the foundation for nursing. These patterns include empirics, aesthetics, personal knowledge, and ethics. Quantitative research methodologies are applicable to better understanding the science, or empirics, of nursing. The other three patterns are not amenable to "hard" science or positivism. Understanding the whole patient, knowing the patient as a unique individual, engaging with the patient in an authentic relationship, and addressing ethical conflicts relate to qualitative ways of knowing that are vitally important to nursing. Carper's work has been encoded into most approaches to knowledge use within nursing and persists as the hallmark of nursing's relationship to knowledge (Thorne, 2008).

Building on Carper's (1978) knowledge typology, Edwards (2002) notes that aesthetic knowledge relates to expert nursing practice and caring. Aesthetics affirms the artistic nature of nursing by recognizing that the small "tasks" of nursing are truly complicated and important. Empirical knowledge is usually recognized as positivistic and rational but has been broadened to include qualitative methodologies. Personal knowledge is coupled with self-awareness and is connected to experiential knowledge and intuition. Ethical knowledge relates to moral knowledge. Appreciating the various types of knowledge is important because it affirms the duality of nursing research: quantitative and qualitative approaches. Edwards (2002) suggests that in quantitative research people are "reducible and measurable objects independent of historical, cultural and social contexts" (p. 41). Thorne (2008) notes that it is difficult to reconcile nurses' commitment to multiple ways of knowing within the context of the current evidence-based practice agenda and its conventional hierarchy of evidence based on positivism and empirics. Thorne's perspective is consistent with Porter and O'Halloran's (2008) assertion that an overreliance on RCTs can compromise the ability to fathom complex care and may compromise the development of genuine and empathetic nurse-patient interactions.

Qualitative methodologies are often less valued by medical professionals, and hold lower stature in funding requests, and yet, embrace the traditional values of nursing that emphasize personal, connected, holistic caring. Qualitative research questions seek a higher level of intimacy with participants. It is about knowing people and valuing differences. Qualitative research uses the written word to describe feelings and life experiences. This approach shares information in a way that makes patient stories readily accessible to nurses and relevant to their care experiences (Cohen, Kahn, & Steeves, 2002).

Dale (2005) suggests that EBP may potentiate interprofessional conflicts given its particular relevance to medicine with its focus on disease-driven science. Dale notes that the range of research design necessary for generating the evidence base required in medicine is very narrow. Medicine is well suited to quantitative research, and published evidential tiers are very relevant. Quantitative studies require control and measurement. These needs create an artificial experience that can make it difficult for healthcare practitioners to apply research findings to clinical practice. Nursing practice is inherently broader than is medical practice and is built upon the premise that experiences are individual and unique. "Control" and "measurement" may be appropriate concerns in some nursing contexts or situations but certainly not all. As a result, nursing requires a pluralistic, multimethod approach to its knowledge-building endeavors. When nurses apply a positivistic model to nursing practice, qualitative research methodologies become less valuable—despite their relevance and importance to all four patterns of knowing.

Nurses' ways of knowing may include collecting patient stories, learning through experiencing during clinical practice, or generating evidence (Dale, 2005). These knowledge-building activities do not signify that "nursing evidence is less rigorously obtained than that of medicine. It is indicative of the fundamental differences between the two forms of practice and the extent of development of each specific knowledge base" (Dale, p. 51). It is imperative for nurse researchers to generate knowledge in all forms because all forms are relevant to nursing practice and patterns of knowing. The best evidence promotes the most clinically effective practice (Dale, 2005). Interventions specific to dimensions of lived experiences may be more effectively considered via qualitative research methodologies as compared to quantitative research techniques (Rice, 2009). To determine what is "best," nurses must know the patient from a holistic perspective. Qualitative approaches tend to best answer questions that relate to "knowing" patients' preferences, experiences, concerns, and priorities.

The Shortcomings of EBP: Lack of Standardization and a Positivistic Stance

There is no single, agreed-upon process for EBP. The lack of a unifying definition contributes to the confusing array of EBP models that may or may not recognize nursing's unique contributions and perspectives. Nursing discussions tend to recognize a combination of concerns that include research findings, clinician expertise, and patient preference; however, these priorities are not consistently included in EBN and EBM literature. Authors also vary in their delineation of strong to weak research study designs.

Randomized clinical trials (RCTs) are viewed as the evidentiary EBP gold standard by many written accounts. RCTs are quantitative studies that involve randomization with a control group, manipulation of a variable, a double-blind study design, and, ideally, a large sample size. The Moore Hierarchy of Strength of Evidence (Moore et al., 1995) illustrates the importance of quantitative studies by ranking the systematic review of several tightly designed RCTs well above descriptive studies. In fact, this hierarchy groups "descriptive studies" with the opinions of respected authorities and reports of expert committees. It is important to note that this hierarchy is written from an EBM perspective rather than an EBN one. This particular hierarchy is referred to throughout the medical literature (Akobeng, 2005; Chung & Reid, 2001).

Akobeng (2005) asserts that the ability to track down and critically appraise evidence and then to incorporate this evidence into daily practice are key tools of EBM. The discussion centers on evidence and includes such terms as sound and scientific. Akobeng uses a patient or problem, intervention, comparison, outcomes or patient or problem, intervention, outcome(s) format for structuring clinical questions. This structure is only relevant within a positivist paradigm and presents significant challenges when applied to qualitative research (Meadows-Oliver, 2009; Thorne, 2008).

Recommendations for evidence examination include appraising the evidence for validity and its importance and applicability to the patient or patients of interest. Tools are available to appraise randomized controlled trials, systematic reviews, case-control studies, and cohort studies. There is no mention of the need to consider qualitative studies, although it is true that many clinical exemplars in medicine do address topics that are more appropriately investigated using quantitative approaches. This makes sense given the narrow but deep specialization of medicine. It also points out why it is so important for nurses to appraise EBM models and to select the aspects that enhance nursing practice and to disregard or alter the processes that do not enhance practice.

Another example of a positivistic persuasion to EBP is exemplified by Flemming (1998), who offers strategies for asking answerable questions. The examples that are offered suggest that there are three elements to questions: situation, intervention, and outcome. Although this perspective is true in some cases, it provides a narrow view of a researchable question. Questions are not always asked out of a need to "do" or "intervene." At times, important questions address concerns such as "What is it like for people when . . . ?", "What is important to people?", and "What does it mean when people experience, think, believe . . . ?" These questions relate to the art of nursing, the experiential knowing that influences intuition and caring.

An additional concern with the situation, intervention, and outcome model is that it presumes that the situation is well understood and that concepts/ constructs are measurable with one particular interpretation or meaning. For example, grief, pain, anxiety, loss, mourning, love, caring, or knowing hold different meanings and are associated with different possibilities. Flemming addresses strategies for developing questions without first acknowledging that there are questions underlying the questions. This area of research question formulation highlights the unique contributions of a qualitative approach.

The current emphasis on positivistic approaches affects other healthcare disciplines interested in EBP and causes concern. Henderson and Rheault (2004), writing from a physical therapy perspective, note that qualitative research methods are needed if EBP is truly about best evidence. They offer four decision rules for determining the inclusion of qualitative research studies in EBP decisions. These rules pertain to assumptions, qualitative screens, levels of evidence, and grades of recommendation. Several models are offered for appraising the quality of qualitative studies; however, there is no established hierarchy for ranking the evidentiary value of different types of qualitative studies. Given the varied philosophical underpinnings of the major qualitative approaches—phenomenology, ethnography, and grounded theory (Williamson, 2009)—such a hierarchy would not be meaningful.

EBN may differ from EBM in ways that have not been unequivocally addressed. Ciliska et al. (2001) identify five steps of EBN: 1) formulate an answerable question related to a patient problem or situation; 2) search for research evidence to answer the question; 3) appraise the validity, relevance, and applicability of the evidence; 4) make a decision as to whether or not to change practice; and 5) evaluate the decision's outcome. Flemming (1998) offers a slightly different approach to EBN by suggesting that, when making a decision about changing practice, the best available evidence should be used, as well as clinical expertise and the patient's perspective. In addition, Flemming offers that performance should be evaluated using self-reflection, audit, or peer assessment.

Similar to EBN, the steps of EBM are identified as follows: 1) converting information needs into answerable questions; 2) finding the best evidence with which to answer the questions; 3) critically appraising the evidence for its validity and usefulness; 4) applying the results of the appraisal into clinical practice; and 5) evaluating performance (Akobeng, 2005). The major difference between the steps of EBN and EBM appear to be in the meaning of the term evidence. This is a critical difference that cannot be taken lightly. Evidence for nursing needs to be drawn from the entire range of quantitative and qualitative methods. Otherwise, nursing runs the risk of excluding large areas of nursing knowledge from its practice base. In fact, the qualitative area of understanding and knowledge may be exactly why nursing is highly valued and trusted—its continued emphasis on what is human and immeasurable—the qualities that many patients believe is missing from modern health care.

How Does the Evidence Debate Affect Real-World Practice?

One problem area directly related to the rationalism versus empiricism debate is funding priorities. Researchers are pressured to demonstrate measurable effectiveness, an outcome that may be narrowly defined and quantified (Gilgun, 2004). The pressure to demonstrate effectiveness in as short an amount of time as possible is related to the need to keep down costs (Gilgun). In other words, increased effectiveness relates to efficiency, which influences health care costs. The potential for cost savings is an appealing aspect of quantitatively determined outcomes.

In addition to the appeal of potentially impacting healthcare costs, quantitatively designed studies are attractive to funding agencies because of their congruency with established hierarchies of evidence. Most practitioners recognize the difference in status afforded to researchers well versed in the hard sciences as compared to those skilled in qualitative methodologies. Although experienced researchers realize that the research question drives the method, in the real world of competitive funding, nurse researchers may be persuaded to select studies based on the method rather than the value of the particular question to nursing practice. Edwards (2002) concurs and argues that those with power determine what counts as knowledge. Power is equated to financial means, and those questions that are deemed worthy of funding shape nursing practice and affect nursing's definition of itself. Edwards suggests that there should be a much broader perspective of nursing knowledge to include quantitative research findings, qualitative approaches, and other forms using intuitive understanding. Each knowledge form should be regarded equally. Edwards calls for a postmodern view of nursing in which "anything that enhances or informs practice" (p. 44) is justified given nursing's unique practice discipline.

In summary, critical points to consider when examining the idea of evidence in its relationship to nursing practice include 1) the metaparadigm of nursing with its emphasis on holism demands a pluralistic approach to research; 2) nursing's broad discipline requires an evidence-based approach that may differ from medicine or other health professions; 3) defining the nature of evidence is important to EBN; 4) research utilization is connected to EBN, and nursing should credit itself with these early evidence-based endeavors; and 5) once fundamental issues are resolved, there is a need to examine strategies for standardizing EBN practices within the education and practice of nursing, particularly given the various levels of entry into the profession.

The Barriers to Including Qualitative Study Findings in EBN Efforts

The Challenge of Systematically Reviewing Qualitative Studies

Practitioners are increasingly comfortable with accessing systematic reviews to provide practice recommendations. One popular resource for EBP decision-making based upon systematic review is the Cochrane Collaboration. Chung and Reid (2001) identify that the systematic review is a process involving the application of scientific strategies to the assembly, critical appraisal, and synthesis of the studies relevant to a specific clinical question. Cochrane review groups are reluctant to accept studies based on qualitative data and prefer to include papers that are either randomized controlled trials or clinical trials (French, 2002). Ciliska et al. (2001) note that systematic reviews are quantitatively based and tend to have little relevance to qualitative research studies; however, a popular abstraction journal, *Evidence-Based Nursing*, does address both quantitative and qualitative studies. The Joanna Briggs Institute (JBI) is another EBP resource with a broader perspective of the nature of evidence, including the recognition of the need to explore qualitative, textual, economic, and narrative sources (JBI, 2008).

Sandelowski and Barroso (2002) observe that there are challenges associated with "finding the findings in qualitative studies" (p. 213). The researchers analyzed reports (N = 99) of studies that used a qualitative approach to study women with HIV infection. The goal of the project was to design a systematic, practical, comprehensive, and communicable research protocol for conducting qualitative metasyntheses. Qualitative investigators use a variety of reporting formats and tend to use inconsistent and individually determined styles. The lack of standardization makes it difficult to synthesize findings from multiple studies that explore similar questions. The greatest barrier to integrating qualitative study findings is the difficulty of finding them in published works (Barroso et al., 2003; Sandelowski & Barroso, 2002).

Sandelowski and Barroso (2002) also identified challenges with the misrepresentation of data and analysis as findings, misuse of quotes and incidents, inconsistent use across studies with the use of the terms theme and pattern, and theoretical confusion. The researchers challenge qualitative investigators to make certain that findings are clearly evident to readers. Jones (2004) concurs with the urgency of this challenge and notes that identification of qualitative studies relevant to a research question is far more time-consuming than the identification of RCTs for a quantitative systematic review. In addition, Jones notes that the paperwork load is much greater when reviewing qualitative studies, sometimes because abstracts and titles are unclear, compelling the investigator to retrieve whole articles for review.

A set of standardized minimal requirements for qualitative research studies to be published in nursing journals may be one useful strategy for increasing attention to quality and responding to the requirement of usefulness mandated by EBP (Nelson, 2008). Difficulties in clearly identifying research findings as well as the problem with inconsistencies that may diminish the quality of the findings are significant barriers to incorporating qualitative studies into EBN practice guidelines.

Critical appraisal involves reviewing evidence for its validity, reliability, and usefulness. Evidence appraisal is essential to ensure that the best knowledge is being applied. Williamson (2009) notes that the level of evidence should be identified when appraising qualitative research but understanding strategies for assessing the scientific rigor of qualitative studies is challenging, and estimates of rigor for quantitative studies cannot be applied (Rice, 2009).

Suggested strategies for appraising qualitative research vary but often involve structured approaches. The process used to judge the quality of qualitative research is important given that the outcomes of these processes determine what research should be included in systematic reviews (Dixon-Woods et al., 2007). One study compared three approaches to qualitative research appraisal using six qualitative reviewers using three appraisal methods on research papers (N = 12) addressing support for breast-feeding (Dixon-Woods et al.). Results indicated that structured approaches to qualitative research appraisal did not yield higher agreement than when using unprompted evaluation. The researchers concluded by noting that future research should consider how qualitative research appraisals should be included in systematic reviews.

Metasynthesis: Ensuring That the Rich Voice of Qualitative Research Is Heard in EBP

Metasynthesis of qualitative research is comparable to meta-analysis of empirical studies and provides a strategy for integrating findings of multiple qualitative studies on a specific topic (Beck, 2009; Thorne, 2008). Metasynthesis offers a mechanism to help establish qualitative research as a viable source of evidence for EBP (Beck, 2009; Flemming, 2007; Thorne, 2008). Synthesizing qualitative research requires the creation of a systematic logic within which findings from separate studies can be integrated into more robust and generalizable knowledge claims using rigorous, transparent analyses (Thorne, 2008). There are challenges to qualitative metasynthesis including the complex and sophisticated understandings required of those conducting this work. Thorne (2008) observes that until one immerses in the actual work of metasynthesis, it is difficult to appreciate the complexities of the judgments required in "searching, selecting, interpreting, and extracting relevant findings from which to build a new synthetic product" (p. 572). Nonetheless, this work is critically important to EBP given the requisite need for diverse sources of knowledge that fully inform excellent nursing practice.

Misperceptions of Scientific Inadequacies

Russell and Gregory (2003) offer guiding questions to assist with appraising the potential value of qualitative studies (**Table 23–1**). They suggest that whereas quantitative researchers have specific guidelines and strategies for determining sample size adequacy, qualitative researchers have only general principles, primarily based on judgment. Data saturation determines sample size rather than the power analyses associated with quantitative studies. Quantitative researchers unfamiliar with the different yet appropriate sampling plans of qualitative research studies may be skeptical of the smaller sample sizes. In fact, qualitative researchers also identify the need for larger samples without offering explanations as to the rationale for needing a greater number of participants (Cohen et al., 2002). The general critiques related to sample size offered by qualitative researchers when identifying potential limitations to study findings may reinforce the impression that qualitative and quantitative methodologies are best served with large samples.

Terminology Dissonance

Morse, Barrett, Mayan, Olson, and Spiers (2002) identify the challenges associated with establishing reliability and validity in qualitative research. One of these concerns relates to the different terminology used by qualitative researchers when describing processes developed to ensure rigor. The authors

---

TABLE 23–1   Qualitative Research Appraisal Questions

Questions to Help Critically Appraise Qualitative Research

Are the findings valid?
- Is the research question clear and adequately substantiated?
- Is the design appropriate for the research question?
- Was the method of sampling appropriate for the research question and design?
- Were data collected and managed systematically?
- Were the data analyzed appropriately?

What are the findings?
- Is the description of findings thorough?

How can I apply the findings to patient care?
- What meaning and relevance does the study have for my practice?
- Does the study help me understand the context of my practice?
- Does the study enhance my knowledge about my practice?

Source: C. Russell & D. Gregory. (2003). Evaluation of qualitative research studies. *Evidence-Based Nursing,* 6, 36. Reproduced with permission from the BMJ Publishing Group.

---

argue that returning to validity as a process for rigor while using verification techniques enables researchers to be consistent with quantitative scientists while remaining true to the different philosophical perspectives innate to qualitative approaches. The different terms used by qualitative researchers, including trustworthiness and confirmability, exacerbate the perception that qualitative research is "soft" compared to positivistic approaches that emphasize validity and reliability.

Other researchers assert that it is important for researchers to feel confident in the value of using auditability, confirmability, and fittingness as measures of quality (Goding & Edwards, 2002). This dilemma represents more than a debate of semantics. It represents a belief that there is a need to avoid conformity to a positivist, reductionist worldview. This issue requires resolution to facilitate standardization of appraisal guidelines.

The Contributions of Qualitative Approaches to EBN

Studies exploring human behavior, thoughts, emotions, relationships, human experiences, or complex occurrences are best explored using qualitative methods. Quantitative studies emphasize causal relationships. The qualitative approach should be used if it is appropriate to the research question that is being asked. Goding and Edwards (2002) assert that the positivistic approach to EBP suggests that there is one "truth" waiting to be discovered rather than many "truths" to be interpreted. If quantitative research is treated as the best way to approach evidence, how do nurses account for the important, but less tangible aspects of practice such as nursing interactions, interpersonal skills, and intuition?

Thompson, Cullum, McCaughan, Sheldon, and Raynor (2004) suggest that nurses are expected to be active decision makers in health care. This active decision making requires an active command of appraising research evidence. "Evidence-based decision making—like all decision making—involves choosing from a discrete range of options, which may include doing nothing or a wait and see strategy" (p. 68). Nurses deal with differing decision types requiring a variety of research methods and questions. These differing decision types require different questions and different methods. Thompson et al. (2004) offer several examples of decision types. Whereas some, for example, prevention, intervention/effectiveness, or assessment, may be best suited to a quantitative approach, others seem better addressed using an empirical approach. For example, decisions related to communication or experience and meaning relate best to qualitative considerations.

Describing Patient Needs and Experiences: A Phenomenological Exemplar

One example of a qualitative approach to ascertaining patient needs to provide appropriate, targeted nursing care is exemplified by a research study examining the lived experience of having a neobladder (Beitz & Zuzelo, 2003). Neobladder construction is a surgical intervention that has become standard therapy for in situ bladder cancer. Neobladder involves the use of small intestine or small bowel/large bowel combinations to create a low-pressure reservoir that attaches to the person's urinary sphincter following cystectomy (Beitz & Zuzelo, 2003). Many nurses are unfamiliar with this surgical procedure, and, because it is relatively uncommon, patients presented with the opportunity for neobladder construction usually lack basic familiarity with the procedure, unlike more common procedures such as cholecystectomy or coronary artery bypass grafting.

This phenomenological study describes the lived experience and the meanings and essences of the experience of people who chose neobladder construction in response to a diagnosis of bladder cancer. Findings reveal many concerns and worries that should be included in routine neobladder teaching. Participants were very affected by changed sexuality, and this concern was often not manifested until long into the recovery period. Support groups were important to participants and provided them with long-term friendships and companionship as they struggled with the physical changes in voiding and sex while dealing with the potential threat of recurrent cancer.

Beitz and Zuzelo (2003) discovered that the bladder cancer experience profoundly affected the survivors. Thematic analysis uncovered a relationship between time and major themes (**Figure 23–2**). Participants' stories were richly detailed and suggested that areas of patient teaching and counseling required improvement. The study question could have been addressed using a quantitative approach, including survey methodology. However, no published studies explored the neobladder experience from the patient's perspective. Clinicians may have had expertise with the neobladder procedure and familiarity with the typical postoperative trajectory. However, familiarity as an outsider or etic perspective is potentially flawed. Surveys developed from a clinician perspective would have potentially missed the critical importance of support groups; the need for better counseling specific to sexual functioning and sexual loss; the postoperative challenges associated with bladder catheterization and voiding in the day-to-day physical environment in which many people live their lives and work their jobs. This study provided a voice to the many people living with a neobladder. Future questions may be answered using quantitative methods; however, this descriptive study provides important information that would have been missed had a quantitative approach been used. These data may improve the relevance and specificity of future studies concerning neobladder. See **Figure 23–3**.

Oncology Nursing Society (2005)
1. Meta-analysis of multiple controlled clinical trials
2. Individual trials or experiments
3. Integrative reviews of all types of research
4. Nonexperimental multiple studies, including descriptive, correlation, and qualitative research
5. Program evaluation, quality improvement data, or case reports
6. Opinions of experts—standards of practice, practice guidelines

Moore et al. (1995)
I. Strong evidence from at least one systematic review of multiple well-designed randomized controlled trials
II. Strong evidence from at least one properly designed randomized controlled trial of appropriate size
III. Evidence from well-designed trials without randomization, single group pre-post, cohort, time series, or matched case-controlled studies
IV. Evidence from well-designed nonexperimental studies from more than one center or research group
V. Opinions of respected authorities, based on clinical evidence, descriptive studies, or reports of expert committees

FIGURE 23–2   Exemplars of Evidentiary Hierarchies.

Instrument Development and Evaluation: An Exemplar

Qualitative methods are appropriate for instrument evaluation and capture the nuances of instrument use that are not amenable to quantitative discovery. Gilgun (2004) developed the Clinical Assessment Package for Risks and Strengths (CASPARS) for families and children and the 4-D for adolescents who have experienced adversities. Concepts were identified based on Gilgun's long-term qualitative research with adults who had experienced adversities during childhood and adolescence. The qualitative work was necessary for the concept identification important to the instruments' development. Gilgun identified that psychometric testing revealed high instrument reliability. Alpha coefficient, interrater reliabilities, and construct validities were impressive. Gilgun credits the initial qualitative life history research as providing the theoretical underpinnings critical to the integrity and theoretical consistency of the instruments. Qualitative evaluation of the CASPARS reveals that users found the instrument useful and easy to score and interpret. This evaluation, partnered with the quantitative data, reinforced the value of the CASPARS.

Gilgun (2004) also used qualitative evaluation strategies for the 4-D and discovered that the 4-D was not as ideal as the psychometric data suggested. Qualitative evaluation of the 4-D provided the impetus to establishing systems changes that were not revealed as necessary through quantitative evaluation approaches. In addition, practitioner feedback led to modification of instrument scoring. Gilgun concludes by asserting that qualitative research provides information that is at the level of specificity that is required for effective clinical assessment tools.

Theory Development: A Grounded Theory Exemplar

In Chapter 9, Beck adds to the Teetering on the Edge theory of postpartum depression. This grounded theory provides an excellent example of the impact that qualitative research has on theory development. In turn, theories provide a context and framework for subsequent research studies, utilizing qualitative, quantitative, and mixed methodologies, to explore phenomena and conditions of interest to establish evidence that may be used to enhance outcomes and improve nursing practice. Teetering on the edge was the basic social process identified in this study. Findings suggest that practitioners should focus their efforts on assisting women experiencing postpartum depression with interventions targeted to the women's particular stage of the recovery process. The evidence to support these targeted interventions is provided within the context of the grounded theory. This grounded theory assists practitioners in making resource allocation decisions and facilitates the development of individualized plans of care rather than a one-size-fits-all approach to women diagnosed with postpartum depression. A positivistic approach would not have answered the research questions and would not have provided the detail necessary to understanding postpartum depression within and between diverse cultural orientations.

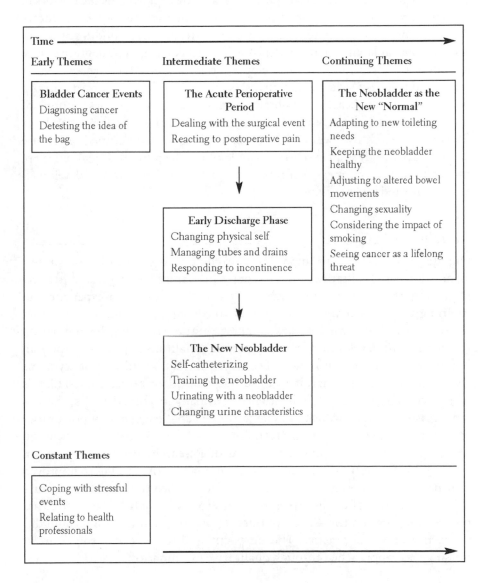

FIGURE 23–3   Major Themes of Living with a Neobladder.
Source: J. Beitz & P. Zuzelo. (2003). The lived experience of having a neobladder. *Western Journal of Nursing Research, 25*(3), 299. Copyright 2003 by Sage Publications, Inc. Reprinted by permission of Sage Publications, Inc.

Developing Definitions to Better Understand Medical Errors in Primary Care: An Exemplar

Kuzel et al. (2003) provide an excellent example of the critical contribution of qualitative research to healthcare practice in a study exploring medical errors in primary care. The authors' proposal was funded by the Agency for Healthcare Research and Quality (AHRQ), thereby demonstrating that funding opportunities are available, although not plentiful, for well-constructed qualitative studies. The study objectives were to develop a patient-targeted typology of medical errors and injuries; understand patients' perceptions of the most common and most injurious medical errors; obtain primary care physician descriptions of medical errors and contrast these with patient descriptions; and provide a basis for other research that will use the study findings to correct medication use systems. This study is an excellent example of the need to use a qualitative approach to develop clear case definitions to gather further data and develop effective, targeted interventions.

Conclusion

Qualitative research is an important contributor to both EBN and professional practice. Qualitative research reports humanize health care. Written research reports put nurses in touch with patient and caregiver experiences in meaningful ways that are rich with detail, in contrast to the reductionist data of quantitatively designed studies. Qualitative studies also lay the foundation for instrument development and evaluation. Qualitative approaches play an important role in the elucidation of concepts and the definitions of key terms that facilitate the meaningfulness of subsequent quantitative studies. EBN is presumed to be important to the science of nursing in a broader sense than its predecessor, research utilization. The combined challenges and opportunities of EBP, outcome indicators, AHRQ (2004) and American Nurses Association (2007) quality indicators, and the Translating Research into Practice program (AHRQ, 2001) emphasize the importance of quantitative studies to improved healthcare systems. As a result, nurses may be inclined to ignore or minimize the contributions of qualitative approaches to research. It is imperative that nurses keep in mind the aspects of nursing practice that are unique and different from medical practice. These aspects tend to be related to the art of nursing, best approached through qualitative examination.

References

Agency for Healthcare Research and Quality. (2001). *Translating research into practice (TRIP)-II.* [Fact sheet. AHRQ Publication No. 01-P017]. Retrieved March 14, 2010, from http://www.ahrq.gov/research/trip2fac.htm

Agency for Healthcare Research and Quality. (2004). *General questions about the AHRQ QI: AHRQ quality indicators.* Retrieved March 14, 2010, from http://www.qualityindicators. ahrq.gov/general_faq.htm

Akobeng, A. (2005). Principles of evidence based medicine. *Archives of Disease in Childhood, 90,* 837–840.

American Nurses Association. (2007). The National Database of Nursing Quality Indicators™ (NDNQI®). Retrieved March 14, 2010, from http://nursingworld.org/ MainMenuCategories/ANAMarketplace/ANAPeriodicals/OJIN/TableofContents/ Volume122007/No3Sept07/NursingQualityIndicators.aspx

Barroso, J., Gollop, C., Sandelowski, M., Meynell, J., Pearce, P., & Collins, L. (2003). The challenges of searching for and retrieving qualitative studies. *Western Journal of Nursing Research, 25*(2), 153–178.

Beck, C. (2009). Metasynthesis: A goldmine for evidence-based practice. *AORN Journal, 90,* 701–710.

Beitz, J., & Zuzelo, P. (2003). The lived experience of having a neobladder . . . including commentary by Artinian BM and Watson LA with author response. *Western Journal of Nursing Research, 25,* 294–321.

Carper, B. (1978). Fundamental patterns of knowing in nursing. *Advances in Nursing Science, 1*(1), 13–23.

Chung, F., & Reid, D. (2001). Evidence-based practice: Assessing the quality of evidence, Part II: Grading the evidence. *Cardiopulmonary Physical Therapy, 12*(4), 117–122.

Ciliska, D., Pinelli, J., DiCenso, A., & Cullum, N. (2001). Resources to enhance evidence-based nursing practice. *AACN Clinical Issues, 12*(4), 520–528.

Cohen, M., Kahn, D., & Steeves, R. (2002). Making use of qualitative research. *Western Journal of Nursing Research, 24*(4), 454–471.

Dale, A. (2005). Evidence-based practice: Compatibility with nursing. *Nursing Standard, 19*(40), 48–53.

DiCenso, A., & Cullum, N. (1998). Implementation forum. *Evidence-Based Nursing, 1*(2), 38–40.

DiCenso, A., Guyatt, G., & Ciliska, D. (2005). *Evidence-based nursing: A guide to clinical practice.* St. Louis, MO: Elsevier Mosby.

Dixon-Woods, M., Sutton, A., Shaw, R., Miller, T., Smith, J., Young, B., Bonas, S., Booth, A., & Jones, D. (2007). Appraising qualitative research for inclusion in systematic reviews: A quantitative and qualitative comparison of three methods. *Journal of Health Services Research & Policy, 12,* 42–47.

Edwards, S. (2002). Nursing knowledge: Defining new boundaries. *Nursing Standard, 17*(2), 40–44.

Flemming, K. (1998). EBN notebook: Asking answerable questions. *Evidence-Based Nursing, 1,* 36–37. Retrieved March 14, 2010, from http://ebn.bmj.com/content/1/2/36.full.pdf

Flemming, K. (2007). Synthesis of qualitative research and evidence-based nursing. *British Journal of Nursing, 16,* 616–620.

French, P. (2002). What is the evidence on evidence-based nursing? An epistemological concern. *Journal of Advanced Nursing, 37*(3), 250–257.

Gilgun, J. (2004). Qualitative methods and the development of clinical assessment tools. *Qualitative Health Research, 14*(7), 1008–1019.

Gladwell, M. (2002). *The tipping point: How little things can make a big difference.* Boston, MA: Back Bay Books.

Goding, L., & Edwards, K. (2002). Evidence-based practice. *Nurse Researcher, 9*(4), 45–57.

Henderson, R., & Rheault, W. (2004). Appraising and incorporating qualitative research in evidence-based practice. *Journal of Physical Therapy Education, 18*(3), 35–40.

Joanna Briggs Institute. (2008). *Joanna Briggs Institute reviewers' manual: 2008 edition.* Retrieved March 14, 2010, from http://www.joannabriggs.edu.au/pdf/JBIReviewManual_CiP11449.pdf

Jones, M. (2004). Application of systematic review methods to qualitative research: Practical issues. *Journal of Advanced Nursing, 48*(3), 271–278.

Kuzel, A., Woolf, S., Engel, J., Gilchrist, V., Frankel, R., LaVeist, T., & Vincent, C. (2003). Making the case for a qualitative study of medical errors in primary care. *Qualitative Health Research, 13*(6), 743–780.

Liberati, A., & Vineis, P. (2004). Introduction to the symposium: What evidence based medicine is and what it is not. *Journal of Medical Ethics, 30,* 120–121.

Meadows-Oliver, M. (2009). Does qualitative research have a place in evidence-based nursing practice? *Journal of Pediatric Health Care, 23,* 352–354.

Moore, A., et al. (Eds.). (1995). Evidence based everything. *Bandolier, 1*(12), 1.

Morse, J., Barrett, M., Mayan, M., Olson, K., & Spiers, J. (2002). Verification strategies for establishing reliability and validity in qualitative research. *International Journal of Qualitative Methods, 1*(2), Article 2. Retrieved March 14, 2010, from http://www.education.wisc.edu/ELPA/academics/syllabi/2006/06Spring/825Borman/Morse%20et%20al%20(2002).pdf

Murray, S., Holmes, D., & Rail, G. (2008). On the constitution and status of 'evidence' in the health sciences. *Journal of Research in Nursing, 13,* 272–280.

Nelson, A. (2008). Addressing the threat of evidence-based practice to qualitative inquiry through increasing attention to quality: A discussion paper. *International Journal of Nursing Studies, 45,* 316–322.

Porter, S., &·O'Halloran, P. (2008). The postmodernist war on evidence-based practice. *International Journal of Nursing Studies, 46,* 740–748.

Rice, M. (2009). The importance of qualitative research to EBP. *Journal of the American Psychiatric Nurses Association, 15,* 200–201.

Russell, C., & Gregory, D. (2003). Evaluation of qualitative research studies. *Evidence-Based Nursing, 6,* 36–40.

Rycroft-Malone, J., & Stetler, C. (2004). Commentary on evidence, research, knowledge: A call for conceptual clarity: Shannon Scott-Findlay & Carolee Pollock. *Worldviews on Evidence-Based Nursing, 1,* 98–101.

Sandelowski, M., & Barroso, J. (2002). Finding the findings in qualitative studies. *Journal of Nursing Scholarship, 34*(3), 213–219.

Stetler, C. (2001). Updating the Stetler Model of Research Utilization to facilitate evidence-based practice. *Nursing Outlook, 49*(6), 272–279.

Thompson, C., Cullum, N., McCaughan, D., Sheldon, T., & Raynor, P. (2004). Nurses, information use, and clinical decision making—the real world potential for evidence-based decisions in nursing. *Evidence-Based Nursing, 7,* 68–72.

Thorne, S. (2008). The role of qualitative research within an evidence-based context: Can metasynthesis be the answer? *International Journal of Nursing Studies, 46,* 569–575.

Waters, D., Rychetnik, L., Crisp, J., & Barratt, A. (2009). Views on evidence from nursing and midwifery opinion leaders. *Nurse Education Today, 29,* 829–834.

Williamson, K. (2009). Evidence-based practice: Critical appraisal of qualitative evidence. *Journal of the American Psychiatric Nurses Association, 15,* 202–207.

24

Simultaneous and Sequential Qualitative Mixed-Method Designs

Janice M. Morse

Mixed methods, defined as one complete method (as the core project) plus a different simultaneous and sequential supplemental strategy, have been well explicated for combining the most difficult designs (Morse & Niehaus, 2009)—that is qualitative and quantitative methods. But as experts in *qualitative* inquiry, we have relatively ignored the issues that occur when we start to describe qualitative simultaneous and sequential designs in which *both* components are qualitative. In this chapter, I argue that qualitative mixed-method designs introduce many of the incompatibility problems of mixed-method design that use qualitative and quantitative components. Various qualitatively driven mixed-method designs are presented. Then, using an armchair walk-through, QUAL–qual designs are contextualized within a hypothetical project of *breaking bad news*, and several examples of QUAL–*qual* mixed-method designs are discussed.

Simultaneous and Sequential Qualitative Mixed-Method Designs

The escalation in the use of mixed-method designs over the past 15 years has resulted in discussions that have centered primarily on the "mixing" of cross-paradigmatic methods—that is, of various combinations of qualitative and quantitative methods—to the extent that it makes us ask the question: When we are referring to mixed-method design, are we referring *only* to combining qualitative and quantitative methods, or can we combine two qualitative or two quantitative methods under the rubric of mixed methods? While some people insist that "mixed methods" refers only to research that uses both qualitative and quantitative methods, other researchers concede that "mixed methods" is a term that may apply to within-paradigm research.

In this chapter, I argue that using a complete method with a supplemental component also from the qualitative paradigm is a legitimate form of mixed-method design.[1] I explore the issues involved with mixing two qualitative methods. When using two qualitative methods, the technical difficulties in mixing textual and numerical data have been removed, but important issues remain in the simultaneous and sequential qualitative mixed-method designs that warrant exploration and discussion.

I begin by presenting issues in mixed-method designs in general, followed by various combinations of qualitative mixed methods as *armchair walk-throughs*. That is, rather than present actual studies that have used qualitative mixed-method designs, I present various qualitative research problems, with proposed solutions that illustrate the use of mixed methods for problems with specific characteristics.

What Is a Mixed-Method Design?

Unfortunately, at this time, there is no real consensus regarding mixed-method design—not even about what it *is*. Leech (2010) notes that some authors define mixed methods as the combined use of qualitative and quantitative methods (e.g., Bryman & Creswell). Other authors would argue that mixed-method design may be applied to the use of two methods within a paradigm (e.g., Morse & Greene). Some consider mixed methods to be the use of two complete research projects within the same study, while others consider this the definition of a *multiple method study* (Morse & Niehaus, 2009); yet others use the terms *mixed methods* and *multiple methods* interchangeably. Here, I define a mixed-method design as follows: *Mixed-method design* consists of a complete method (i.e., the core component), plus one (or more) incomplete method(s) (i.e., the supplementary component[s]) that cannot be published alone, within a single study (Morse & Niehaus, 2009).

In mixed methods, the supplementary component provides explanation or insight *within the context* of the core component, but for some reason the supplementary component cannot be interpreted or utilized alone. Perhaps this is because the supplementary project has an inadequate sample, or lacks saturation, or is simply too narrow to be of interest by itself. The important point is that it is not a complete project in itself and so is not publishable as a separate project.

What Are the Characteristics of a QUAL–qual Mixed-Method Design?

The primary characteristic is that both the core component and the supplementary component have an inductive *theoretical drive*. That means that the project is exploratory-descriptive, with a goal that may range from rich description to theory development. The *core component* (i.e., the complete method) may be classified as a "standard" qualitative method—for instance, as a grounded theory, an ethnography, discourse analysis, phenomenology, a study using some type of observational method, or derived from the use of focus groups or semi-structured interviews, and so forth. On the other hand, the *supplementary component* consists of research strategy(ies) that are used within another qualitative method (rather than a complete method as such), such as a particular style of interviewing or an observational technique. The supplemental component may be *paced* simultaneously (conducted at the same time) or sequentially (after the core component has been completed). The pacing and the type of research strategy used is the one that will best enable the research question to be answered:

1. more fully or *more comprehensively* (with broader scope or increased depth) therefore making the research richer and more useful, *or*
2. to obtain *another perspective*, using a different data type (such as observational data to conduct a core project that uses interviews), *or*
3. to obtain data from a different *level of analysis or abstraction*—for instance the core project may use broadly categorized participant observational data, and the supplementary component may use videotaped data that is microanalyzed, thereby adding detail so that the project better answers the research question; *and*
4. to provide information that may have been inaccessible or unavailable when using one method alone, or to answer a subquestion that cannot be answered within the core component (and therefore moves the research program along).

In addition, designs using a *sequential supplemental qualitative component* (→ *qual*) are used:

1. to answer minor questions that have emerged from the core project, *or*
2. to move the project toward implementation—for instance to develop an assessment guide from a grounded theory core component (Morse, Hutchinson, & Penrod, 1998; Neufeld & Harrison, 2010)

The supplementary component consists of a research strategy from a second qualitative method, usually using separate data, often of a different type. The supplementary component is incomplete as a method—for instance, it may use data that are not saturated—and the supplementary component research continues only until the researcher has the answer(s) that he or she needs for that particular part of the research. The supplementary component continues until the researcher is *certain enough* that his or her analysis regarding that component's subquestion is answered.

Are qualitative mixed methods designed as a class of methods? Or are all qualitative methods mixed methods?

Before going into all of the problems in explicating QUAL $+/\rightarrow$ *qual*>[2] mixed-method design, let us consider if thinking of such designs as mixed-method designs is useful, or are they just normal variations of qualitative studies? Given that qualitative methods are relatively unstructured and good qualitative inquiry is reflexive, two points must be considered:

1. What may be incorporated into a qualitative project as data for a project *not* to be considered as a mixed method? That is, usually qualitative researchers consider anything that is pertinent to the topic to be considered as data, and researchers have the freedom to incorporate that data within the method.

2. As qualitative methods are relatively nonprescriptive procedurally, does this methodological freedom provide the researcher with license to use a variety of strategies within a project, without resorting to the label of "mixed-method design"? That is, generally our methods are not inclusive or exclusive about what strategies must, may, or may not be used within a particular method.

Given these two considerations, it is unclear how qualitative researchers differentiate between a responsive, reflexive qualitative study and a QUAL-*qual* mixed-method study. How, for instance, do we differentiate between an ethnography that uses several data sets and several approaches or differing strategies to each data set and a mixed-method design?

At this time the answer is not always simple, and in part, in the mixed-method continuum, there is certainly a gray area. It is possible that these will differentiate as our understanding about mixed methods increases. Some qualitative methods may be easier than others, such as ethnography, to differentiate. For instance, if we are using conversational analysis (CA), and decide to add an interview or observational supplemental component, the supplemental component adds a new perspective, a different data type, or data that is clearly using a different level of analysis than CA. However, the supplementary component data are incompatible with the CA analysis. Thus, this project would have similar within-paradigmatic incompatibility problems to those that exist with the cross-paradigmatic problems that occur in quantitative and qualitative mixed-methods design, albeit in a slightly different form.

Within-Paradigm Data/Analytic Incompatibilities _____

In qualitative inquiry, little is clear and obvious, and analysis is often a work of compromises and blind attempts at making the best choice. For example, even when designing the most common research question in qualitative health research (i.e., "to study a person's experience. . ."), the various forms of data used consist of compromises that are less than ideal, and some options may result in a loss of quality in the overall study. For instance, if we want to learn about a person's experience, we must make decisions from various alternatives or approaches:

1. *Experiencing it ourselves* (as in autoethnography), transforming the experience into fieldnotes, analysis, and a written article
2. *Recording the experience as it occurs,* using video recordings for observational research or audiotape to record the dialogue
3. *Using interviews to learn about the experience from those who actually experienced it,* as individuals or as a group, using interviews, diaries
4. *Learning about the experience by interviewing others who observed the person(s) experiencing it* (caregivers, relatives, teachers, family members)
5. *Examining records of the experience,* ranging from official records, photographs, diaries, and hospital chart data to historical artifacts
6. *Learning about the experience over time,* as a one-shot event or as a part of a trajectory over time, with antecedents, transitions, stages, phases, and outcomes, interviewing the person as they go through the experience
7. *Examining the observable* behaviors *of those in the setting,* including gross behavioral patterns and/or microanalytical behaviors, including facial expression; the focus may be on the individual, the group, or the interaction among those in the setting
8. *Examining the qualitative descriptions/interpretations of others' research (of other participants),* synthesizing and summarizing the literature
9. *Examining the concepts and theories* that are embedded in the situation, and discussed in the professional literature and in lay discourse
10. *Using fiction, movies, poetry, and insights of others* to explore, for instance, the emotional tone, rather than focusing on the more concrete facts and events

Each of these approaches places us in a different methodological (and analytical) position with a different distance from the most direct datapoint, which, in turn, dilutes and perhaps distorts the actual events and participant experiences. Some of these "locations" give us hard data (or harder data) than others. Some positions provide us with concrete facts and exclude subjective data; others provide us with subjective data, about the *meaning* of the event and emotional data, excluding hard data. Some positions provide us with only indirect perceptions of the experience.

We could use more than one of these approaches, and increase the depth or scope of our analyses. In this case, each data set (or perspective/approach) would then be considered a *component* of the qualitative mixed-method study. They would be a part of one study, and because of the interactions between data sets, may sometimes overlap or they may be separate from the other component. For instance, data from one group may *inform* or facilitate understanding of another group, but because these data are from different sources, are of different types, or are from different levels of abstraction, they *cannot* be mixed, blended, or merged during analysis. Each data set *must* be kept separate, and (unless formally transformed) analyzed separately until the findings from each component can be incorporated into the results narrative. These data used for the supplementary component may verify or add to the core component. When writing up the results (i.e., the results narrative) the investigator moves the findings of each data set into the textual description where the answers to the research question are compiled and addressed as a whole. The researcher then shows how these components contribute to addressing the research question.

Making decisions about the focus of your study—what data types you will have in the original set, and how these data will be presented as they are incorporated at the *point of interface* (i.e., where the two analyses meet) into the *results narrative* to achieve the type of expected results—are important actions of early project conceptualization and proposal preparation (Morse & Niehaus, 2009). Yet, working inductively, qualitative researchers do not know (and cannot anticipate) everything that will happen within the project. But *if* they can envision the possible alternatives, as "if . . . , then . . ." statements within the limits of the type of data they will be using/requiring, the better informed the investigator and the better the study.

We call this preparatory step of envisioning alternatives within a project an *armchair walkthrough* (Morse, 1999; Mayan 2009). An armchair walkthrough enables the researcher to maintain an inductive stance and enables the necessary planning to prepare a proposal. This obviously simplifies the research process—institutional review board (IRB) approval can be obtained for the entire project, funding organized, personnel hired, and timelines estimated.

In QUAL–*qual* mixed-method design, the design is dictated primarily by the method, but also from the objectives or goals of the study, subsequently the study question, from what is known (the literature review), and from the research context (the limitations/advantages of the research participants and setting). Finally, the armchair walkthrough may become a part of the overall audit process for the study, showing the expected course of the study from that which was actually reflexively conducted. Thus, the armchair walkthrough is an important tool for conceiving a project and developing a proposal, including a proposal for a mixed-method study. In the next part of this chapter I illustrate various types of qualitative (QUAL–*qual*) mixed-method design, using armchair walkthroughs.

QUAL+/→ qual Mixed-Method Designs _____

QUAL–*qual* Design Considerations

When planning such studies, methodological considerations are important. *Selecting a method* refers to the best formal method that will enable the research question to be as thoroughly answered as possible. In mixed-method design, this occurs in the core component; in the qualitatively driven mixed-method project, this is one of the major qualitative methods mentioned earlier. The supplemental qualitative component is a research strategy from a different qualitative method, for instance, a particular style of interviewing, such as an unstructured or semi-structured interview. This strategy may be linked to a style of analysis, such as thematic development, constant comparison, or content analysis.

Another design consideration is the mode of sampling and data collection to be used, and these also are directed primarily from the question, but to a lesser extent the context and participants must also be considered. For instance, if the research question pertains only to one group of participants, generally data are collected and pooled within a single data set; if a comparative study is proposed, two or more groups of participants may be identified, data are pooled (and analyzed) by group, and data from each group are compared and contrasted. On the other hand, if a case study design is proposed, data from each participant are collected and analyzed by individual participant. Following this initial analysis, the case study design may be extended, with the common characteristics identified from each participant then compared and contrasted between participants.

Other design characteristics include *level of analysis* (the microanalytic, macroanalytic, conceptual, or theoretical level within which the analysis is conducted); *data type* (the concrete or subjective nature of data to be included in the study); and *data description* (the researcher's operations of inference, interpretation, or objective [hard] description). I refer to *similar participants* as *"groups"* (samples of patients, physicians, or relatives, etc.), and place this terminology into qualitative mixed methods terminology of core and supplemental components, theoretical drive, the pacing of the project, and the point of interface (Morse & Niehaus, 2009).

Types of QUAL–*qual* Designs

In this section, I present various types of simultaneous and sequential qualitatively driven designs, contexts, and examples of methods that may be used, and design considerations. All examples fit the mixed-method criteria that the gap between the core method and the supplemental project is too wide for any "blending" of the data, and the supplemental project is possible but cannot stand alone. Analyses must always be conducted separately. The list is not complete; these examples are used for illustrative purposes only.

Simultaneous QUAL+/→qual mixed-method designs

QUAL + *qual* is most commonly conducted using two data sets and usually two groups of participants. The core method is usually a standard qualitative method, such as phenomenology, grounded theory, or ethnography. Data from the core component are "grouped" for all participants and analyzed by content or thematic analysis according to the method used. That is, these data are not analyzed participant by participant. Rather, data from all participants are pooled as the categories or themes are constructed. The supplementary component consisting of a strategy from another method may be an observational technique or another type of interview, such as focus groups. These data are also "pooled" for all participants. Depending on the questions and the availability of the sample used in the core component, these participants may or may not be the same participants who participated in the core component. However, they are usually from the same population. This is important, because the investigator's approach to these data is different from the approach used in the core component, data are analyzed separately, and the results of each analysis meet in the results point of interface. That is, the results of the core component form the theoretical base of the results narrative and the results from the supplementary component are added to the theoretical base.

Examples of QUAL + qual designs

1. Core component may be conversational analysis (CA) with the supplementary component, focus groups. The conversational analysis provides documentation of dialogue; the focus groups provide group experiential data. Design is QUAL (CA) + *qual* (focus groups).

2. Core component may be a phenomenological study, exploring the meaning of a phenomenon; the supplementary component may be some form of nonparticipant observation. The design for this study pools the data from within the core and the supplementary component. Design is QUAL (phenomenology) + *qual* (nonparticipant observation).

3. A grounded theory is conducted using unstructured interviews of single mothers (employed and not employed outside the home) and their experiences of caring for preschool-age children. Supplementary component consists of semi-structured interview data about the nature of their employment. Design is 2-group comparative design QUAL (grounded theory) + *qual* (semi-structured interviews).

4. Video ethnography of caregivers and patients in an Alzheimer's unit. The QUAL data set are grouped (pooled) data; the supplementary component may have the same videotapes analyzed but at a different level of analysis—for instance QUAL (macroanalysis) + *qual* (microanalysis).

5. Two groups of participants, with data linked between pairs of participants (for instance, physician and patient dyads). The patients may have unstructured phenomenology of the meaning of care, and the physicians, observational data of care provided, observational data of the telling. The design is QUAL (phenomenology) + *qual* (observations).

6. Pooled data linked over a time trajectory (before/after) looking for changes within the groups. The core component may, for instance be an ethnography of a bereavement group; supplemental data may be focus groups 1 year following the bereavement. The design is QUAL (ethnography) + *qual* (focus groups).

Examples of QUAL → qual designs

1. *Building an assessment guide*. The core component may be a grounded theory exploring the process and stages of recovering. Uses this analysis, once the analysis is complete the grounded theory processes (stages and phases) are modified to develop as indicators that may be used in the assessment guide. The design is QUAL (grounded theory) →*qual* (development of indices).

2. *Qualitative evaluation research*. The core component is nonparticipant observations of workers; the subsequent supplemental component is semi-structured interviews *developed from these observations*. The design is QUAL (nonparticipant observation) + *qual* (semistructured interviews)

Summary of Design Types

From these designs, note the following design characteristics:

- When using two independent data sets—different perspectives or different groups of participants—this enables *comparison* of the two data sets (for instance, mothers/fathers; caregivers/patients); those with or without certain significant characteristics (silent diseases versus symptomatic). Such comparison enables the theoretical development of your study to move more quickly.

- If using the same data set, you have a mixed-method design—if you are using different analytic approaches or strategies. The supplementary component elicits additional information or data that may be inaccessible if you are using a single method.

- If your design is using pooled data before and after design, participants are linked by a similar experience. These may actually be different participants in the before and the after groups—but it means that the investigator does not have to wait an extraordinarily long time (even years) for an adequate sample, or for enough time to go by to observe the desired changes.

- Sometimes a question arising from a pooled data set may be answered using "other data" sources (other participants or other types of data). Researchers must evaluate the pros and cons of using alternative data sources in the supplementary components.
- The qualitatively driven designs may be extended to become quite complex "chains" of supplemental components.
- Always diagram your design to prevent confusion.

If conducting research in teams, keep the researchers allocated to separate data sets to prevent cognitive/analytical confusion. This approach has the added advantage of enabling lively analytical/theoretical discussions, making the identification of similarities and differences easier.

Methodological Issues for Qualitative Mixed-Method Designs

Can you use the same data for both the core and the supplemental components? This is an easy question, but the answer is not so straightforward. Whether or not you are able to use the same data for both components depends on the nature of your question, on the requirements for the form of the data, on the adequacy of the data for answering the supplemental question, and so forth. In the previous section, we have an example using the same videotapes for the core and the supplementary components, but data for analysis for each component is prepared differently.

As research is guided by the questions asked, and obviously the question asked of the data set is different for the core and the supplemental questions, different parts of the data set may be used, or the data may be used in different ways—for instance, to develop categories or themes. The ultimate test is asking:

- Will these data provide the information that is needed?
- Are these data good enough to provide that answer?
- Do these data provide the *best* descriptions of the phenomenon that are needed?
- Are these data current and pertinent?

If all of these questions can be answered affirmatively, then use the data set; if not collect new data. Thorne (1994) is a little more conservative and recommends that a few new interviews should always be conducted to ensure that nothing has changed and conditions remain unchanged.

Can you use the same participants in both the core and the supplemental components? The answer to this question depends on what you are trying to find out, what you want to know, and your basic research. If your research design links both the core and the supplemental data set, then the same participants must be used for both components. However, often little is lost if you are forced (perhaps by sequential research design) to use different people for each component, and to aggregate each data set.

QUAL–qual mixed-method design may not always be designed at the proposal stage, and may be implemented to complete a project when unexpected findings leave some important point unanswered. In this case the information needed may be relatively easy to obtain, and considerable delays in the research program eventuate if a separate project must be planned to get that information. It is more efficient to file an IRB approval and to complete the study and then move forward.

Contextualizing Qualitatively Driven Designs

Initially, qualitative inquiry is always context bound. *Context bound* means that the selected research method is dictated by the research question—by what the researcher is *asking* within a particular topic (and often a particular setting). For purposes of these QUAL mixed-method examples, the hypothetical context for the research questions will be studies planned to explore *breaking bad news,* or the information that physicians tell patients about poor prognosis, what patients *hear* when told (and how they learn about their disease and the prognosis), and the context in which the "telling" occurs.

Armchair Walkthrough: Exploring *breaking bad news*

Clinicians have complained that when they are given a prognosis, patients do not hear bad news. Patients say, "I was not told"; clinicians say, "I did tell them!" Such a research design with the goal to determine how "bad news" is given to patients and what they *hear* when given this news demands two sets of paired data.

Project 1: What (and how) do physicians perceive is the best way that they break bad news?
A tremendous amount of research has been conducted from the providers' perspective on the best way to give "bad news" to a patient. Books have been written on techniques of telling; workshops teach techniques. Therefore, if we are to interview providers about *how they tell,* we run the risk of hearing nothing new—but a summary of this in-class learning. But, if we use that information to construct a semi-structured interview schedule, developing questions about patients, for instance, who had various responses to hearing the news, and who was present (supportive) and their response, we would get some interesting data. Semi-structured interview methods are static—that is, all participants are asked the same questions in the same order, and data are analyzed at the same time at the end of the study. Once these data are analyzed, it is highly likely that some interesting new findings will have emerged about the context and breaking bad news.

The focus groups—groups of clinicians—may then be invited to discuss further some part of the findings that had not been on the researchers' "screen" earlier. For instance, the researchers may suggest findings about how clinicians read patient cues—transitory expressions and so forth, when giving back bad news. They may ask the group: What facial and bodily stance cues are observed and how do clinicians make decisions to give the news—do they speak primarily to the patient or her support person, do they remain with or leave the dyad—are decisions that experienced clinicians make almost unconsciously, yet would provide significant supplemental data to this core project. This design would be QUAL (semi-structured interviews) + *qual* (focus group interviews).

Project 2: How do physicians break bad news?

Note that this question differs from Project 1. To solve the dilemma of different physician and patient reports on hearing bad news, we are no longer interested in the perception, but actual behavior.

Data must be collected in two areas:

1. The physician's telling—what the patient is told by the clinician.
2. The patient's hearing. Interview the patient a short time afterwards to determine what the patient has heard. Both data sets are linked (or paired) by patient, as a type of "case study" design with each patient considered a "case." Subsequent analysis may further combine data pairs within the data set (for instance sorting into patients who accurately heard and those who were unable to hear, to identify characteristics of each).

The researcher has a mixed-method project with data from two perspectives. The core component ("what they are told") is a CA project. These data are audio-recorded as each patient is told, and prepared and analyzed according to CA conventions, so that the actual words of the clinician are recorded, along with the pacing and the intonation. However, in order to find out what patients actually *hear*, we must later interview the patients—perhaps get their permission to call them at home later that day, and record a short telephone interview to obtain that information. The supplemental data questions may include, "Would you tell me what happened? What did the doctor say?"

Note the following characteristics in this study:

1. Both data sets are obtained simultaneously—this is a QUAL + qual design.
2. The supplemental data set, that is, the telephone interviews concerning what the patients actually heard, is understandable/interpretable only in the context of the CA data set. The supplementary component is not publishable alone; these data may not be saturated; these are probably truncated targeted interviews seeking particular information, not the "whole story," and must be interpreted within the context of the core component.

3. In this case, the researchers are comparing pairs of data (the CA and the interview data) for each participant in *paired case study*. More often, data for the core and the supplementary projects are kept separate from each other until they are combined at the point of interface (in the write up of the results narrative). Either way, these data are treated more formally than data sets are in ethnographic studies.

4. An additional analysis may be completed near the end of the project. The researcher may wish to categorize the data units (pairs) into group rates as a) excellent comprehension; b) some missing information/misinformation; and c) unable to comprehend. The research might then identify the characteristics of each interaction.

The *point of interface* for this project is within each participant (when comparing the CA data with the interview data).

Project 3: Following a diagnosis of positive breast cancer: What do patients hear when given poor diagnostic bad news?

This time the question places the core component (QUAL) onto what patients hear. In order to answer this question, the investigator must have "evidence" about what the women were *actually* told (the CA becomes the supplemental component) and compare that with the interview data, in which women report *what they heard* the physician tell them. The best design would be to audiotape the interview of the telling, followed by unstructured interviews (perhaps conducted the next day by phone) of the unprompted subjective reports of the interviews.

The core component would be the unstructured interviews, *linked to* the supplemental project—what the women were actually told by the physician, and transcribed for ease of data handling. Thus the analysis would proceed by each pair of data components (what was heard and what was told) compared and described as a unit. The design would be: QUAL (unstructured interviews with women) + *qual* (CA of the physician telling).

Project 4: A more complex and interesting mixed method design would be to increase the number of factors being examined, and thereby increasing the scope of the study. Of course the question would change:

What characteristics enable or inhibit patient comprehension when given poor diagnostic *bad news*?

The question has changed to create a more complex and interesting mixed-method design that increases the number of factors being examined, thereby increasing the scope of the study. The investigator may be interested in whether or not the patient suspected they were about to receive bad news when the patient meets with the doctor; whether or not the physician provides subtle clues about the impending bad news (i.e., foreshadowing [Maynard,

2003]); the patients' response to the bad news and the role of the support person; as well as what they actually heard in the post-interview.

This time we have many data sets:

1. Preinterview with the women about what they expect to be told
2. Audiotaped interviews with the physician, from which we obtain a) transcripts of the physicians giving bad news, b) observational description of the women's response, and c) a description of the support persons' behavior
3. Unstructured telephone post-interviews with the women to elicit what was heard

The core component (QUAL) is the post-interview data; the supplementary components are derived from the other qualitative data sets. Again the data sets are analyzed as linked units and sorted according to various types of responses and comprehension. This design is: QUAL (post interviews) + *qual* (pre-telling interviews) + *qual* (physician's transcript of the telling) + *qual* (women's response) + *qual* (support person's behavior).

Analysis would proceed by sorting the cases into those who had excellent recall and those who had poor recall (and depending on your sample size, possibly other groups between). It would also involve comparing and contrasting each case looking for differences that may be attributed to poor comprehension. Note that the components are placed according to their *contribution to analysis* in the results narrative. The core component is the component that answers the question best, not the one with data that is first collected.

Project 5: Could we do this study using data from the women's post-interviews, with data from all participants pooled into one data set?

Yes, we could—but the design would not be as strong, and the questions could not be answered as definitively. Why? You may be answering the questions in slightly different ways, perhaps answering the questions as "What are the ways (or modes) of hearing bad news?" From these interviews, you would build categories (using content analysis) of similar responses to the news: Perhaps you would have one in which the women were incapable of hearing ("I saw his lips move, but could not comprehend what he was saying"), another in which the women heard some of what was said ("I heard the word 'cancer,' but nothing after that . . ."); some in which the women heard it all, but were incapable at that time of making decisions regarding treatment, and so forth.

Project 6: How do physicians report that they provide bad news? Do physicians "tailor" their message according to the type of message they must give and patient characteristics?

This is yet another approach to the same research problem, this time with the focus on the physicians. The core component may be a semi-structured interview conducted with physicians whose practice requires them to frequently

break bad news. These semi-structured interviews will form the core component pooled and analyzed item by item using content analysis. The information may be important—for instance, the interview could elicit information
about what behavioral cues physicians look for in patients when breaking bad
news and how they decide to pace their message. The supplemental component
may be followed by unstructured nonparticipant observation to observe the
patients' responses. If the project was conducted sequentially, then videotapes
could be used to look for and to confirm those reported cues. This design is
QUAL (semi-structured interview) → *qual* (nonparticipant observation).

Project 7: QUAL + qual, paired data of different levels of analysis

In this study, we decided to explore the spatial orientation (and touch observations) and patterns of touch used in the caregiver interaction when breaking bad news, using participant observations and video microanalytic data.
At this point in the armchair walkthrough, we must decide if we are going
to attempt to rate the efficacy of the telling that appears to accompany the
differing spatial orientation and patterns of touch, for moving the study to
this level of analysis has important implications for increasing the sample
size. You decide that such a study would be very expensive because of the type
of coding and statistical analysis required, and to keep the study as an exploratory QUAL + *qual* of touch observations of touching and microanalysis
of touch.

Data are collected using videotaped consultations during which the prognos-
tic news is given to the patient. Each videotaped interaction is coded two ways:

1. Macroanalytically—coding the proximal location and body action for
   both the caregiver and the patient. Dialogue is transcribed, and the bodily movements are described in concert with the ongoing consultation
   and telling.
2. Microanalytic analysis of touch. To do this analysis, the tape is slowed
   and sometimes separate sequential frames are used to describe the hand
   positions, purpose, type, and duration of touch. If possible, the event preceding the initiation of the touch and following it, and accompanying actions such as eye contact, are included as a part of the touch interaction.

Note that in this study we are using the same data form (i.e., videotapes), but
analyzing them differently—macroanalytically for spatial body position, and
microanalytically for patterns of touch. The two types of data *must* be kept
separate—and analyzed separately. The point of interface is again in the results narrative.

We considered linking these data to patient comprehension earlier, but decided against it. But we may want to consider something like *patient satisfaction,*
or some form of patient rating of the caregiver, extending the mixed-method

design to a quantitative component: QUAL (caregiver interaction) + *qual* (microanalysis of touch) + *qual* (patient comprehension)+ *quan* (patient satisfaction scores).

Conclusions

While some researchers are uncertain if QUAL-*qual* designs *are* mixed methods, in this chapter I argue that they may be a mixed-method design, and deserve attention as such. When qualitative data types, levels of analysis, or participant perspectives are different enough that it is necessary for the two methods to be handled differently and to be kept apart, we have the rationale for using mixed-method design. When one of the components is complete and forms the theoretical base, and the other component supplements the core component, we have a qualitative mixed-method design.

Qualitative mixed-method research has important design considerations, including the planning of the projects, the pacing of the components, and the crafting of the research results and the developing theory. Mixed methods enable qualitative researchers with the designs and principles to handle problems of increasing complexity, and these advances will move qualitative inquiry forward.

References

Leech, N. (2010). Interviews with the early developers of mixed-methods research. In A. Tushakkori & C. Teddlie (Eds.), *Mixed methodology: Combining qualitative and quantitative approaches* (2nd ed.). Thousand Oaks, CA: Sage.

Mayan, M. J. (2009). *Essentials of qualitative inquiry.* Walnut Creek, CA: Left Coast Press.

Maynard, D. (2003). *Bad news, good news: Conversational order in everyday talk and clinical settings.* Chicago: University of Chicago Press.

Morse, J. M. (1994). Emerging from the data: Cognitive processes of analysis in qualitative inquiry. In J. Morse (Ed.), *Critical issues in qualitative research* (pp. 23–43). Menlo Park, CA: Sage.

Morse, J. M. (1999). The armchair walkthrough [Editorial]. *Qualitative Health Research, 9,* 435–436.

Morse, J. M., Hutchinson, S., & Penrod, J. (1998). From theory to practice: The development of assessment guides from qualitatively derived theory. *Qualitative Health Research, 8,* 329–340.

Morse, J. M., & Niehaus, L. (2009). *Mixed methods design: Principles and procedures.* Walnut Creek, CA: Left Coast Press.

Neufeld, A., & Harrison, M. (2010). *Family caregiving: Social support and non-support.* NY: Springer.

Thorne, S. (1994). Secondary analysis in qualitative research. In J. Morse (Ed.), *Critical issues in qualitative research methods* (pp. 263–279). Thousand Oaks, CA: Sage.

Endnotes

[1] If the supplemental method is complete and could be published separately, this would be considered a *multiple method design*.

[2] *Notation:* QUAL indicates a qualitatively driven study, with a qualitative core component; *qual* indicates a qualitative supplemental component; + indicates that two components are conducted simultaneously; → indicates the supplemental component will be conducted sequentially (see Morse & Niehaus, 2009).

25

Combining Qualitative and Quantitative Methods for Mixed-Method Designs

Janice M. Morse and Linda Niehaus

Nurses are interested in the whole person—that is, the psychosocial, the physiological, and the spiritual. Nurses are interested in the individual, the family, and the community; in sick persons, those recovering, and those who are healthy; in elderly persons, adults, children, those newly born, and those as yet unborn. Nurses are interested in the cellular and behavioral; in the environmental and the institutional; in health and illness; in emotions and the unconscious. Given these interests, we need the skills to describe minutely and globally in research designs that allow us to understand mechanisms, associations, and risks. Thus, because of its very broad focus and its encompassing perspectives, nursing research is by its very nature eclectic. Nurse researchers must be versatile and adept at many types of research, both qualitative and quantitative. To grasp nursing phenomena, nursing research often demands that more than one method be used at once and that a mixed- or multimethod research design be used. The purpose of this chapter is to explicate the processes of conducting mixed-method research, both for simultaneous and sequential designs.

Mixed-method research is defined as a research design consisting of one complete method with additional supplementary strategies drawn from a second, different method. It often involves the use of both qualitative and quantitative methods. For instance, a qualitative method with an additional quantitative strategy could be used to allow for measurement of some dimension of the phenomenon under investigation. Alternatively, a quantitative method with an additional qualitative strategy could be employed to allow for description of an aspect or component of the phenomenon that cannot be measured. Qualitative and quantitative research have been described as belonging to different and incompatible paradigms, so how the researcher combines the qualitative and the quantitative components in a single project is essential if rigor is to be maintained.

Terminology and Considerations for Conducting Mixed-Method Research

Before we begin to describe the process of mixed-method design, we review the definitions of all the necessary terms (see **Box 25–1**). The core component of the project is the primary or main study in which the core method is used to address the research question. The supplementary component fits into the core component and consists of strategies added to obtain the necessary supplemental information. The core component is therefore always dominant, complete (i.e.,

Component	A phase of the research, driven by the overall direction of the inquiry, during which one or more methodological strategies are used as research tools to address the research question.
Core component of the project	The primary (main) study in which the primary or core method is used to address the research. This phase of the research is complete or scientifically rigorous and can therefore stand alone.
Method	A cohesive combination of methodological strategies or set of research tools that is inductively or deductively used in conducting qualitative or quantitative inquiry.
Mixed-method design	A plan for a scientifically rigorous research project, driven by the inductive or deductive theoretical drive, and comprised of a qualitative or quantitative core component with qualitative or quantitative supplementary component(s). These supplementary components of the research fit together to enhance description, understanding, or explanation and can be conducted either simultaneously or sequentially with the core component. Mixed-method design can also take place as internal transformation of a single data set.

BOX 25–1   A List of Terms for Types of Mixed-Method Design.

Multi-method design	A plan for a scientifically rigorous research program comprised of a series of related qualitative and/or quantitative research projects over time, driven by the theoretical thrust of the program. The theoretical drive of an individual project may on occasion counter but not change the overall inductive or deductive direction of the entire program.
Strategy	A methodological research tool, drawn from a qualitative or quantitative method, for addressing the research question by either collecting or analyzing data.
Supplementary component of the project	In this phase of the research, one or more supplementary methodological strategies are used to obtain an enhanced description, understanding, or explanation of the phenomenon under investigation. This component of the project can either be conducted at the same time as the core component (simultaneous) or it could follow the core component (sequential). The supplementary component is incomplete in itself or lacks some aspect of scientific rigor, cannot stand alone, and is regarded as complementary to the core component.
Theoretical drive	The direction of the inquiry (Morse, 2003) that guides the use of the appropriate qualitative and/or quantitative methodological core. The nature of the research question determines the theoretical drive of a project.
Theoretical thrust	The overall inductive or deductive direction of a research program. The theoretical drive of an individual project may on occasion counter but not change the theoretical thrust of the research program.

Revised from Morse, J.M., Wolfe, R.R., & Niehaus, L. (2005). Principles and procedures for maintaining validity for mixed-method design. In L. Curry, R. Shield, & T. Wetle (Eds.), Qualitative methods in research and public health: Aging and other special populations. Washington, DC: GSA and APHA.

BOX 25–1   A List of Terms for Types of Mixed-Method Design *(continued)*.

scientifically rigorous), and can stand (and even be published) alone, whereas the supplemental component is conducted only until the researcher is certain the additional supplemental findings are adequate to provide the necessary information. We therefore refer to the methodological research tool used to obtain supplementary information as a strategy rather than a method. Nomenclature for different types of mixed-method designs is presented in **Box 25–2**. Uppercase letters are used to denote the core component of the project, and the supplemental component is indicated with lowercase letters.

QUAL + quan: Qualitative core component of the project (inductive theoretical drive) with a simultaneous quantitative supplementary component.

QUAL → quan: Qualitative core component of the project (inductive theoretical drive) with a sequential quantitative supplementary component.

QUAL + qual: Qualitative core component of the project (inductive theoretical drive) with a simultaneous qualitative supplementary component.

QUAL → qual: Qualitative core component of the project (inductive theoretical drive) with a sequential qualitative supplementary component.

QUAN + qual: Quantitative core component of the project (deductive theoretical drive) with a simultaneous qualitative supplementary component.

QUAN → qual: Quantitative core component of the project (deductive theoretical drive) with a sequential qualitative supplementary component.

QUAN + quan: Quantitative core component of the project (deductive theoretical drive) with a simultaneous quantitative supplementary component.

QUAN → quan: Quantitative core component of the project (deductive theoretical drive) with a sequential quantitative supplementary component.

QUAN ↓ qual: Researchers using experimental design with qualitative data as documentation to describe differences between groups.

QUAL ↓ qual: A quantitative descriptive design using numerical data in the process of description.

BOX 25–2   Nomenclature for Types of Mixed-Method Design.

Recognize the Role of the Theoretical Drive

Research projects are conducted either inductively (usually using a qualitative method) or deductively (usually using a quantitative method). In mixed-method design, the overall inductive or deductive direction of the inquiry is referred to as the theoretical drive, and this encompasses both the core and the supplementary components with the data or findings of the supplemental component contributing to the findings of the core component (Morse, 2003; Morse & Niehaus, 2009; Morse, Wolfe, & Niehaus, 2005). Further, the theoretical drive of the core component overrides the drive of supplemental components (see **Figure 25–1**). For example, if the project is QUAL-*quan*, the theoretical drive is inductive and qualitative, regardless of whether the minor component is deductive and quantitatively driven. If a research program involves a series of interrelated mixed-method projects over time (as in multimethod design), the overall theoretical thrust of the program is maintained, irrespective of the theoretical drive of individual projects (Morse, Wolfe, & Niehaus, 2005). The nature of the programmatic research question determines the overall inductive or deductive direction (thrust) of the research program (see Figure 25–1). Note that a multimethod research program may also include projects using different single methods.

Other aspects that must be attended to when conducting mixed-method design are sampling issues and the pacing of the project.

Sampling Issues

When the mixed-method design involves qualitative and quantitative components, sampling becomes difficult. In a QUAN-*qual* study, the quantitative sample (which is too large and randomly selected) is unsuitable for use with the qualitative component, and in a QUAL-*quan* study, the qualitative sample (which is too small and purposefully selected) violates the needs of the quantitative component. In the next section, we discuss specific ways to overcome these limitations and processes of conducting mixed-method research.

The Pacing of the Project

If the supplementary component is conducted at the same time as the core component, we describe it as simultaneous mixed-method design, and it is indicated with a plus (+) sign; if the supplementary component follows the core component, perhaps because the results are interesting and additional information is required, the mixed-method design is sequential and is indicated with an arrow (→) symbol.

Consider an example for a mixed-method project. Suppose we are conducting a qualitatively driven study in the relatives' waiting room to explore relatives' experiences of waiting for news of the condition of an injured person in the emergency room. The theoretical drive of this study would be inductive, and the core (main) method used may be grounded theory. But, if in the course of conducting the study we noticed that the relatives were anxious, we may decide to measure their anxiety using a quantitative standardized anxiety

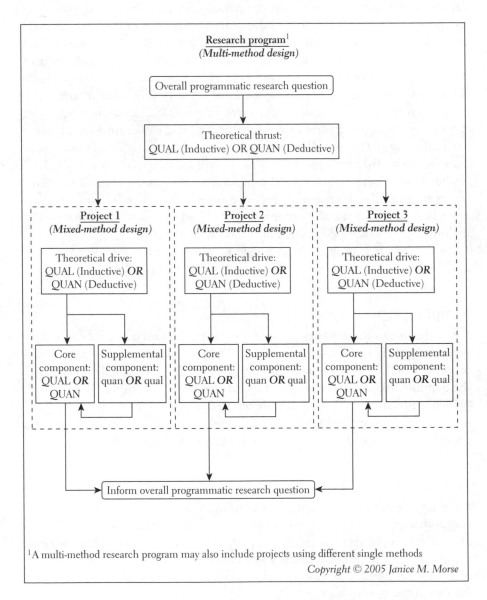

FIGURE 25–1   Mixed-Method Design Versus Multi-Method Design.

scale. In this example, the core component would be qualitative (QUAL) using grounded theory, and the supplemental component would be quantitative (*quan*) using the anxiety scale. Given that the supplementary component is conducted at the same time as the core component, we would describe the design as a QUAL+*quan* study.

Conversely, we could decide to conduct the same project using a theoretical framework stating that waiting for news of an injured relative was anxiety-producing, and this anxiety could be reduced if relatives could receive social support by waiting together. This would be a quantitatively driven study, using a battery of tests such as an anxiety scale and a social support measure. But during the pilot study we observe that the use of television is another variable that eases anxiety, and so we decide to document the nature and use of television by those who are waiting and watching. However, because we cannot find or develop a more suitable instrument to rate this variable, we decide to describe this aspect of the phenomenon qualitatively. This second project has a deductive theoretical drive, is quantitatively driven (QUAN), and has a qualitative supplementary component (*qual*). We would describe the design as QUAN+*qual*. To be even more complex, we may decide then to transpose these qualitative data to form a quantitative variable(s), and our design would be QUAN+*qual→quan*.

Processes of Conducting Mixed-Method Research

The inductive or deductive theoretical drive of a project is determined by the nature of the researcher's question, and the nature of the question in turn determines the selection of the research method and, subsequently, the research design and procedures. **Figure 25–2** shows the process of conducting a mixed-method research design. Important to note is that, although the theoretical drive and the pacing of the procedures (for sequential or simultaneous designs) alter the design of the project, the actual procedures can be represented on the same chart. There are two basic pathways: the core component is described in the left pathway, and the supplementary component in the right pathway.

The Core Component

With both sequential and simultaneous designs, the core component (the left pathway in Figure 25–2) is conducted according to standard procedures for the methods selected until the data have been collected. The core component must always be conducted according to the principles of the selected method, will meet qualitative standards for reliability, validity, and rigor, and may be publishable without the supplementary component. Of most importance, the researcher must remember that the supplementary findings are not methodologically complete and cannot be published alone. Their role is to contribute "missing pieces" to the results of the core component, which are stronger and more comprehensive with the contribution than without it.

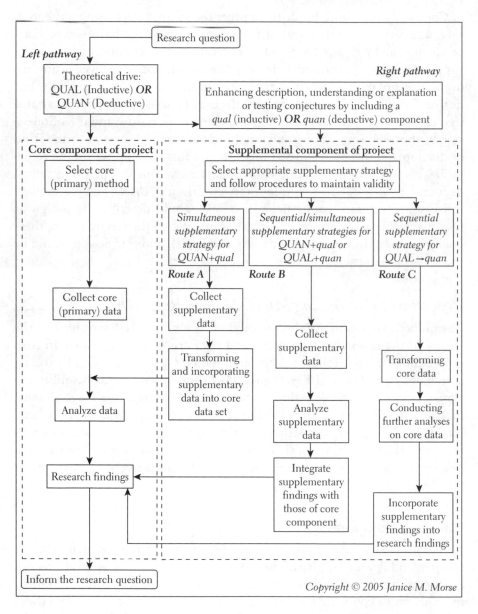

FIGURE 25–2 An Overview of the Process of Mixed-Method Design.

The Supplementary Component

Maintaining validity of the supplementary component (the right pathway in Figure 25-2) is the most difficult task. If the supplementary component is conducted simultaneously and supplementary data have been collected, these data are analyzed with the core data; if the supplementary data are collected sequentially, they are integrated into the findings after the core analysis is completed; if the supplemental analysis is conducted on the primary data following the core analysis, the results contribute to the overall research findings (see Figure 25-2). Also, the researcher must attend to issues in sampling and the type of data used because these problems are exacerbated when the supplementary component is from the opposite paradigm (quantitative with a qualitative study or vice versa).

In this chapter, we describe and illustrate only two qualitatively driven and two quantitatively driven mixed-method research designs because these four designs have the greatest potential for error and threats to validity.

QUAL–*quan*: Qualitatively Driven Mixed-Method Designs

In both types of QUAL–*quan* designs, the theoretical drive of the project is inductive and qualitative. The primary role of the supplemental component (*quan*) is to enhance description of aspects of the phenomenon being studied or to test conjectures by using quantification (see Figure 25-2). This can be done by quantifying qualitative characteristics of the sample that appear to be important during analysis (a supplementary data transformation analysis strategy) or by collecting quantitative data about characteristics of the sample participants (a supplementary data collection strategy). The supplementary strategy is drawn from quantitative methods either during the core component of the project so that qualitative and quantitative methods are carried out simultaneously (QUAL+*quan*) or following the core component so that qualitative and quantitative methods are carried out sequentially (QUAL→*quan*). These types of mixed-method designs are illustrated here:

- QUAL+*quan* (Figure 25-2, Route B): When the core project is qualitative, and the supplementary strategy is quantitative, the qualitative sample (purposefully selected and small) does not meet the quantitative criteria of size (large) and randomization. For a simultaneous design, if the quantitative data are used to enhance description (as in measuring how anxious the relatives were in the earlier example), the quantitative instrument used must have external norms. The scores obtained for the participants in the small qualitative sample may then be interpreted with the normative populations, because the researcher can draw conclusions about how anxious the sample is, and add this to the description. These scores for the qualitative participants are not averaged and presented as group scores unless the sample size meets the minimum requirement of $n = 30$, the minimum number required to estimate a mean score (Pett, 1997).

- QUAL→*quan* (Figure 25-2, Route C): Quantitative data may be used to enhance a qualitative study by transposing the qualitative data collected in the core component and conducting further analyses on the primary data. For this technique, first the nature of the qualitative interviews used must be examined because data transformation can be conducted only if all of the participants have been asked the same questions (as in semistructured, open-ended interviews) or if the answers can be inferred from the interviews (for instance, the same five or six guiding questions have been used for all interviews). Data cannot be transformed if the researcher has used interviews that have evolved as the study has progressed, as is often used in ethnography (Spradley, 1979). Procedures for quantifying qualitative data are well described elsewhere (Bernard, 2000). Briefly, the researchers must develop categories within the qualitative data, code responses numerically, develop definitions for the codes, establish interrater reliability, code the transcripts, analyze the resulting numerical data, and incorporate the supplementary findings into the qualitative results to enhance conclusions and implications. For instance, in our example of the anxiety of relatives waiting, we may observe that those who appear to meditate have less need for the support provided by relatives. In the interviews with these relatives, those who are spiritual have spoken of their use of meditation. This information may be coded and the nonparametric statistical analysis could be conducted to determine whether there are significant associations between relevant variables. Note that this data analysis strategy is sequential because the transformation of the qualitative data cannot be performed until the qualitative analysis is completed, and these results inform the research findings rather than build the findings per se.

QUAN–*qual*: Quantitatively Driven Mixed-Method Designs

In QUAN–*qual* mixed-method designs, the overall direction of the inquiry is deductive and quantitative. The primary role of the supplemental component (*qual*) in these designs is to enhance description, understanding, or explanation about the phenomenon that the core method cannot access (see Figure 25-2). This can be done either by collecting qualitative data using open-ended questions within an otherwise structured instrument (QUAN+*qual*) or by collecting and analyzing qualitative data separately to explain puzzling findings (QUAN→*qual*). These mixed-method designs are discussed in this section with specific attention to issues associated with simultaneous or sequential designs. A decision flowchart for the selection of a sample for a qualitative supplementary component while conducting a quantitatively driven core component is shown in **Figure 25–3**. The decisions for simultaneously driven research are on the left, and those for sequential are on the right pathway.

- QUAN+qual (Figure 25-2, Route A): Simultaneously deductively driven components of a project provide a problem for the qualitative supplemental component: the quantitative sample is too large and randomly selected for the supplementary qualitative component. If the study involves a quantitative questionnaire with several open-ended questions at

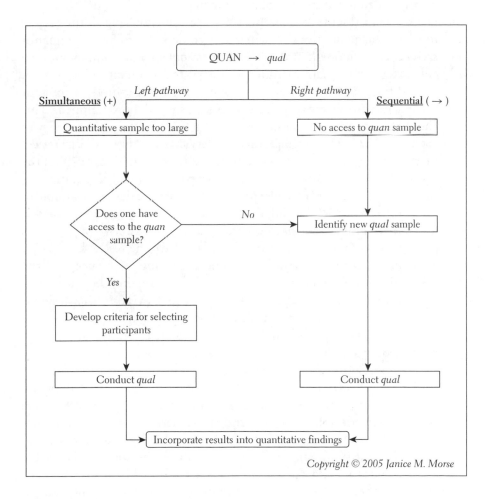

FIGURE 25–3 QUAN–qual Mixed-Method Designs.

the end, although these open-ended questions may be analyzed qualitatively, it is a stronger design to transpose the qualitative data to quantitative data and incorporate these data into the quantitative analysis (for instructions, see Bernard, 2000). An example of this design is a quantitatively driven survey that had 10% of the items written as semistructured open-ended questions used to obtain evidence regarding the incidence and severity of untoward effects on participants of unstructured interviews. The sample size of 500 respondents was not extraordinarily large for the management of the textual data, the transposition of these qualitative data to enable their incorporation into the statistical analysis was not prohibitive, and the inductive qualitative component greatly added to the validity of the overall project.

- QUAN→*qual* (Figure 25–2, Route B): The greater challenge is the project in which the qualitative supplementary component follows the quantitative core component. If the role of the supplemental component is to collect additional data to add description to the quantitative component, if the researcher has access to the quantitative sample, criteria for the purposeful selection of participants should be developed. This should be according to the criteria of a "good informant": the ability to articulate, have knowledge about the interview topic, be willing to reflect on the topic, and have the time to participate (see Spradley, 1979). If the researcher has access to the quantitative participants (for instance, research assistants who are collecting the quantitative data may be able to make referrals), the principles of qualitative sampling should be followed. If the researcher has no access to the quantitative participants (for instance, they cannot be traced or recalled), the researcher has no alternative but to draw another sample, according to the needs of the qualitative supplementary component. Participants may be selected by scores achieved on the quantitative component. Obviously, this design is only slightly weaker than is a multiple-method design in which the sample is that of a complete study and the results are rigorous enough to be published separately. An example of this mixed-method design is a quantitative survey of a neighborhood that reveals no correlation between working mothers of toddlers and the use of daycare facilities. Follow-up qualitative interviews reveal that many of the fathers in these areas were students with flexible schedules, and the fathers organized their schedules to assume care of their children during the day and elected to do their studies in the hours their wives were able to be home. This flexible arrangement for child care had not been anticipated by the researchers, and the subsequent qualitative component was necessary to provide explanation for the unexpected findings.

Discussion

Mixed-method design may allow for more complete understanding than can be obtained by a single method used alone. However, combining a core method with a supplementary strategy, in particular qualitative and quantitative strategies, requires expert understanding of the principles of both qualitative and quantitative methods and knowledge of sampling strategies and data transformation to maintain validity.

Is conducting a mixed-method design rather than a multiple-method design cutting corners? Should not all designs that explore complex phenomena use multiple methods in which all components employ complete methods as in multiple-method design? The answer is that there is a role for mixed-method design and for the completion of the project more expeditiously than for the conduct of a multiple-methods design. In fact, ethnography may be considered a qualitatively driven mixed-method design that has become so institutionalized and eclectic that its very flexibility has become institutionalized as a complete method.

Mixed-method design, if conducted rigorously, is a stronger design than a design in which a single method is used alone because the supplemental component enhances validity of the project per se (see, for example, Locke, Silverman, & Spirduso, 1998, p. 117). Further, with mixed-method design all components are published as a whole, although Morgan (2004) notes that on occasions the supplemental component may be criticized by reviewers as being weak or unscientific, and often can be the cause for the rejection of the article. However, the strongest design—multiple-method design—is often weakened at the point of publication if the researcher is tempted to publish each method separately.

References

Bernard, H. R. (2000). *Social research methods: Qualitative and quantitative approaches.* Thousand Oaks, CA: Sage.

Locke, L. F., Silverman, S. J., & Spirduso, W. W. (1998). *Reading and understanding research.* Thousand Oaks, CA: Sage.

Morgan, D. (2004, September). *Mixed-method design.* Keynote address at the 5th Qualitative Research Conference in Health and Social Care, Bournemouth University, England.

Morse, J. M. (2003). Principles of mixed methods and multi-method research design. In A. Tashakkori & C. Teddlie (Eds.), *Handbook of mixed methods in social and behavioral research* (pp. 189–208). Thousand Oaks, CA: Sage.

Morse, J. M., & Niehaus, L. (2009). *Principles and procedures of mixed-method design.* Walnut Creek, CA: Left Coast Press.

Morse, J. M., Wolfe, R. R., & Niehaus, L. (2005). Principles and procedures for maintaining validity for mixed-method design. In L. Curry, R. Shield, & T. Wetle (Eds.), *Qualitative methods in research and public health: Aging and other special populations.* Washington, DC: GSA and APHA.

Pett, M. A. (1997). *Nonparametric statistics for health care research: Statistics for small samples and unusual distributions.* Thousand Oaks, CA: Sage.

Spradley, J. P. (1979). *The ethnographic interview.* New York: Holt, Rinehart & Winston.

Endnotes

We acknowledge the contributions of Ruth Wolfe and Seanne Wilkins in preliminary work for this chapter. Reprinted and extensively revised from Morse, J. M., Niehaus, L., & Wolfe, R. R. (2005). The utilization of mixed-method design in nursing research. *International Nursing Review (Japanese), 28*(2), 61–66. Copyright (c) 2005 Janice M. Morse. Further details on mixed-methods design may be found in Morse, J. M. & Niehaus, L. (2009). *Principles and procedures of mixed-method design.* Walnut Creek, CA: Left Coast Press.

[1] If the supplemental method is complete and could be published separately, this would be considered a *multiple method design.*

[1] *Notation:* QUAL indicates a qualitatively driven study, with a qualitative core component; *qual* indicates a qualitative supplemental component; + indicates that two components are conducted simultaneously; → indicates the supplemental component will be conducted sequentially (see Morse & Niehaus, 2009).

Epilogue: In Coming to an Open Closing

Patricia L. Munhall

It is my hope that in reading this volume or parts of it you have come to understand how critical qualitative research is to nursing practice and healthcare delivery. Among my goals in this book are to highlight the fundamental role of understanding, to provide a different path to understanding, and to demonstrate the depths of understanding that qualitative research can help us attain. Our philosophies of nursing seem to be concerned with the uniqueness of each human being and that *being* takes place in an individual situated context. We profess in our philosophies a respect for autonomy and self-determination of people, which is to say we honor people's perceptions of the world and their decisions, whatever they may be.

If their perception puts them in harm's way, we are in a role to reflect back to them a different way of viewing the world, but we do not discount their perceptions or make assumptions that individuals should see the world the same way we do. In this book we discussed the importance of recognizing multiple realities and the influence of this recognition as uncovered by qualitative research.

Perceptions originate from an individual's situated context and their life worlds' contingencies that inform for us a perspective of holism. Other beliefs we find in nursing philosophies give voice to humanism, open systems, multiple realities, and the overarching embrace of these beliefs with caring, compassion, and empathy.

Our philosophies of nursing are highly ideal in nature, and often we find the everyday realities impinging on our implementing those beliefs. We want to live them, but the world is often "too much with us," with severely limited human and material resources. In the fourth edition of this book I wrote in the epilogue about our very broken healthcare system, and where healthcare disparities and shortages make our philosophies sometimes look like "pie in the sky."

In this edition I am more hopeful because of the historical passage of healthcare reform by our government in 2010—the intent of which is to relieve the many healthcare disparities and reform (a task of no small consequence) the entire healthcare system. Many challenges are ahead. However, we must strive to actualize those aims and goals to the extent that we are able. One way to accomplish this is through the pursuit of qualitative research.

One reason healthcare reform was passed was because of the characteristics of qualitative research. Many qualitative studies in nursing demand a new morality of equality for health care. While it is unclear how large their role was, the methods of qualitative research did indeed influence the outcome. The power of giving people voice to tell their stories relative to their experience within the healthcare system influenced this historical passage—the case studies; the narratives from families, individuals, and communities; the studies of different economic groups and cultures; and the meanings of the many experiences people came forth to talk about in front of Congress all played a part in this change. Those in charge could not help but be moved when they truly understood how denying health care to people deeply hurt and incapacitated them and destroyed lives and families.

There were statistical reports and quantitative reports but nothing could move some very incalcitrant members of Congress. However, stories of blindness, paralysis, mothers who lost their children, children who lost their mothers or fathers helped to make all the voices heard. Healthcare disparities could no longer be tolerated. This is the power of "giving voice to people," the critical component underpinning all qualitative research.

This journey of learning about qualitative research methods, if you started with this text, is just the first part. Perhaps a qualitative researcher is about to be born and this volume will represent your gestation.

I wish you a very successful birthing process. If this turns out to be your research "home" because of the way you are in the world, I think you and the recipients of your research will indeed be fortunate. You will turn to them and their lives, their individual being in the world and in different situated contexts, giving them authentic voice. You, as a nurse researcher, will have the opportunity to feel and learn things that are inaccessible by other methods. You will gain insights and discover knowledge that comes from listening to another and often hearing interpretations you would never have thought of from your own context. How could you? We really are different!

To paraphrase what was said in this book, qualitative research has the power to liberate us from presuppositions, preconceptions, assumptions, and biases and allows us to see what is real, not what was constructed by others with little or no evidence. This is critical to freeing people and/or emancipating groups from stereotypes that often prevent their acceptance and opportunities to develop.

For us to truly understand the other we must come to know who we are, what we believe, our subjective world. In encounters with others, we enter another world, another subjective space, and we interact in an intersubjective space. Qualitative researchers celebrate subjectivity as the way to knowing: the subjectivity of the other speaks to us, and then we come in contact with that world and we can empathize from a place of understanding.

I once heard that what people want most is to be understood. Think—isn't that what you want? It is a normal human desire. Often I think it is wondrous to watch qualitative researchers when they are not doing research, per se. They are instead *being* qualitative. I watch them either as faculty or practitioners, and I see that they often interact and listen differently to people from the way their colleagues who come from the positivistic paradigm do. They carry over their research practices to their professional and also their personal worlds.

Not everyone who reads this volume will become a qualitative researcher. That certainly would be a remarkable feat, and I am not sure we would want to convert all to qualitative research; however, I would like to see more realization through funding as to the potential of qualitative research. But that is not the main point I want to make here.

You may or may not become a qualitative nurse researcher, but even if you do not, I do hope that you will take some of the understandings that you may have gleaned from this *perspective into your practice*. The foundations through concepts or beliefs of qualitative research when applied to practice, not just research, offer one of the best perspectives in our hope to have our practice characterized by our concern with the individual, the individual's unique circumstances in the world, and our real desire to want to understand from the individual's subjective perspective.

For example, you do not have to do qualitative research to practice unknowing as was discussed in Chapter 5. Nor do you have to be a qualitative researcher to take into account a person's situated context as the most potent influence on the way that person is in this world. Neither do you have to do qualitative research to reach into the subjective world of the other.

However, if you have indeed found an affinity and appreciation for what qualitative research offers to us as human beings and want to pursue this kind of research, I do welcome you to this most meaningful world of research. With its intense focus on meaning, understanding, and interpretation of experience, it is my hope that this book will be a good foundation for you. You will be entering a world that is very intertwined, in that your professional understandings will become much more philosophical, and it will also become more apparent that the separation between the professional and the personal is quite arbitrary.

This method of research embraces subjectivity and, as such, embraces feelings and emotions. I am not sure you can do this kind of research and not sometimes want to cry or laugh with your participants. That is why it does take a special kind of individual to do good qualitative research. Entering into others' experiences is an altruistic act if done for an altruistic reason, and a qualitative researcher must be sincere, authentic, and caring. Participants can tell!

In this open-closing (there is really no closure), I want to remind you that we are always in experience, our patients are always in experience, and so it is incumbent upon us to understand and appreciate their life-worlds as well as our own with all the variations and complexities therein. We enter into another's experience, and thus we are privileged and also indebted—indebted to produce the best quality research, with the most meaning and the most direction for improving practice in all its many domains.

To me it is this complicatedness, sometimes called the messiness of our human lives, the interconnectedness of phenomena, and the appreciation of intersubjectivity that gives qualitative research the authenticity and existential humanness that has the potential to enrich our lives. The knowledge and insight gleaned are essential to compassion, care, liberation, and finding meaning in our everyday experience. The findings provide authentic groundings to develop theory, to critique practice, to understand why different ways of doing something might be more beneficial, to develop new practices based on understanding the meaning of a phenomenon to individuals, and to shed ourselves as "the knower" who can figure out what is best for people from our own perspectives. Qualitative researchers acknowledge that the experts of experience are those that are in or have been in the experience. To think otherwise is quite presumptuous.

To those of you who say, "Yes, this is what I want to do, this is me, I have found a home," I wish you success in your research endeavors. For those of you who will continue along the positivistic avenue, I also wish you success in your research endeavors. What I do hope is that all of you will have found something in this volume that has touched your heart, soul, and mind and that encourages you to reach out in a more authentic way to others, to listen differently, to care more about subjectivity, to shed the knowing of the professional, and to once again come in touch with why you became a nurse in the first place: to help people in a caring, compassionate, and empathic way.

Index